# Outcomes in Speech-Language Pathology

**Second Edition**

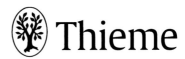

# Outcomes in Speech-Language Pathology

**Second Edition**

**Lee Ann C. Golper, PhD**
Professor
Director, MS-SLP Program
Director, Speech-Language Pathology Clinical Division
Director of Quality and Risk Management
Department of Hearing and Speech Sciences
Vanderbilt University
Nashville, Tennessee

**Carol M. Frattali, PhD‡**
Formerly, Adjunct Professor, University of Maryland
Research Professor, George Washington University
Research Coordinator, Speech-Language Pathology Section
M.G. Magnuson Clinical Center
National Institutes of Health
Bethesda, Maryland

Thieme
New York • Stuttgart

Thieme Medical Publishers, Inc.
333 Seventh Ave.
New York, NY 10001

Acquisitions Editor: Emily Ekle
Editorial Assitant: Elizabeth D'Ambrosio
Senior Vice President, Editorial and Electronic Product Development: Cornelia Schulze
Production Editor: Barbara A. Chernow
International Production Director: Andreas Schabert
Vice President, Finance and Accounts: Sarah Vanderbilt
President: Brian D. Scanlan
Compositor: Carol Pierson, Chernow Editorial Services, Inc.
Cover Illustration: Photo used with permission. Vanderbilt Bill Wilkerson Center, Department of Hearing and
Speech Sciences. Graph used with permission, Professional Research Consultants (PRC), Inc. 11326 P. Street,
Omaha, NE 68137-2316
Printer: Sheridan Books, Inc.

Library of Congress Cataloging-in-Publication Data

Outcomes in speech-language pathology / [edited by] Lee Ann C. Golper, Carol M. Frattali. — 2nd ed.
    p.   cm.
  Originally published: Measuring outcomes in speech-language pathology / edited by Carol M. Frattali.
  Includes index.
  ISBN 978-1-60406-642-5
  1. Speech therapy—Evaluation. 2. Outcome assessment (Medical care) I. Golper, Lee Ann C., 1948–
II. Frattali, Carol. III. Measuring outcomes in speech-language pathology.
  RC423.M39 2013
  616.85′506—dc23                                                                                 2012019883

**Important note:** Medical knowledge is ever-changing. As new research and clinical experience broaden our
knowledge, changes in treatment and drug therapy may be required. The authors and editors of the material
herein have consulted sources believed to be reliable in their efforts to provide information that is complete
and in accord with the standards accepted at the time of publication. However, in view of the possibility of
human error by the authors, editors, or publisher of the work herein or changes in medical knowledge, neither
the authors, editors, nor publisher, nor any other party who has been involved in the preparation of this work,
warrants that the information contained herein is in every respect accurate or complete, and they are not
responsible for any errors or omissions or for the results obtained from use of such information. Readers are
encouraged to confirm the information contained herein with other sources. For example, readers are advised
to check the product information sheet included in the package of each drug they plan to administer to be
certain that the information contained in this publication is accurate and that changes have not been made in
the recommended dose or in the contraindications for administration. This recommendation is of particular
importance in connection with new or infrequently used drugs.

Some of the product names, patents, and registered designs referred to in this book are in fact registered
trademarks or proprietary names even though specific reference to this fact is not always made in the text.
Therefore, the appearance of a name without designation as proprietary is not to be construed as a
representation by the publisher that it is in the public domain.

Printed in the United States

5  4  3  2  1

ISBN 978-1-60406-642-5
eISBN 978-1-60406-643-2

# Contents

Preface............................................................. vii

Acknowledgments..................................................... ix

Contributors ....................................................... xi

In Memory .......................................................... xv

**Section I.   History and Contemporary Issues**

1. Outcomes Measurement: Definitions, Dimensions, and Perspectives........3
   *Carol M. Frattali*

2. Outcomes Measurement: Converging Issues, Trends, and Influences ...... 25
   *Lee Ann C. Golper*

3. WHO's International Classification of Functioning, Disability, and
   Health: A Framework for Clinical and Research Outcomes................ 58
   *Travis T. Threats*

4. Outcomes Measurement in Federal Programs and Public Policy .......... 73
   *Kathleen Romanow and Janet E. Brown*

**Section II.   Clinical Services**

5. Outcomes Measurement in Health Care................................. 91
   *Margaret A. Rogers and Robert C. Mullen*

6. Outcomes Matter in School Service Delivery ......................... 116
   *Jean Blosser*

7. Outcomes in Long-Term Care Settings ............................... 141
   *William P. Goulding*

**Section III.  Organizational Performance**

8.  Outcomes in Health Care: Achieving Transparency Through
    Accreditation . . . . . . . . . . . . . . . . . . . . . . . . . . . . . . . . . . . . . . . . . . . . . . . . 153
    *Paul R. Rao*

9.  Cost-Effectiveness Analysis in Speech-Language Pathology Outcomes . . . . 183
    *Richard M. Merson and Michael I. Rolnick*

10. Defining Quality Through Patient Safety and Satisfaction Outcomes . . . . . . 202
    *Nancy B. Swigert*

11. Outcome Assessment for Improving Organizational Efficiencies . . . . . . . . . 223
    *Tamala S. Bradham*

**Section IV.  Research**

12. Treatment Research . . . . . . . . . . . . . . . . . . . . . . . . . . . . . . . . . . . . . . . . . . . 245
    *Lesley B. Olswang and Barbara A. Bain*

13. Evidence-Based Practice: Applying Research Outcomes to Inform
    Clinical Practice . . . . . . . . . . . . . . . . . . . . . . . . . . . . . . . . . . . . . . . . . . . . . . . 265
    *Kathryn M. Yorkston and Carolyn R. Baylor*

14. Applying Single-Subject Experimental Research to Inform Clinical
    Practice . . . . . . . . . . . . . . . . . . . . . . . . . . . . . . . . . . . . . . . . . . . . . . . . . . . . . . 279
    *Kevin P. Kearns and Michael R. de Riesthal*

15. Meta-Analysis in Outcomes Research . . . . . . . . . . . . . . . . . . . . . . . . . . . . . . 298
    *Katerina Ntourou and Mark W. Lipsey*

**Section V.  Graduate Education**

16. Outcomes Measurement in Graduate Clinical Education and
    Supervision . . . . . . . . . . . . . . . . . . . . . . . . . . . . . . . . . . . . . . . . . . . . . . . . . . 315
    *Sue T. Hale and Lennette J. Ivy*

17. Outcomes in Higher Education . . . . . . . . . . . . . . . . . . . . . . . . . . . . . . . . . . . 338
    *Michael L. Kimbarow, Celia R. Hooper, and Alex F. Johnson*

**Index** . . . . . . . . . . . . . . . . . . . . . . . . . . . . . . . . . . . . . . . . . . . . . . . . . . . . . . . . . . . **359**

# Preface

An outcome is a natural result; a consequence; or, generally, a comparison of a measurement made at one point in time to that made at another point in time (Wertz & Irwin, 2001). An observation about a result does not necessarily explain why the result occurred or if the result can be confidently and logically linked to some event or manipulation that preceded it. Any conclusion drawn about the meaning of an outcome, therefore, requires carefully specifying and defining the factors that may have contributed to the outcome. Consequently, unless specific conditions are met, an outcome does not index intervention efficacy, effectiveness, efficiency, or cost-effectiveness, nor does it necessarily index the impact, meaningfulness, or value of the result to the stakeholders.

Claims about outcomes require qualifiers and are subject to the question "So what?" In the preface of the first edition of this text, Frattali referred to the advice that Dr. Robert T. Wertz had passed along to her from the late Dr. Wendell Johnson (Frattali, 1998), namely that outcome measurement requires us to consider the following questions: *What do you mean? How do you know?* And, *what difference does it make?* In this edition we continue to seek answers to these questions. Here authors contribute commentary and points of view to continue the dialogue and provide operational definitions of outcome measurement (What do we mean?); methodologies to gather data and evidence to support claims (How do we know?); and reflections on ways to translate evidence into a context that is meaningful to stakeholders (What difference does it make?).

This text revisits or expands upon several of the topics related to outcome measurement in speech-language pathology that were initially raised by Frattali in the first edition. To set the stage for the topics examined in this edition, Section I references historical and contemporary issues, anchored by a reprint of Frattali's Chapter 1 from the first edition. The definitions, dimensions, and perspectives provided in this chapter create the central orientation and historical context for this second edition. Chapter 2 reflects upon that history in the context of contemporary developments and convergences in outcome measurement that have evolved since the publication of the first edition. Operational definitions are introduced and refined in Chapter 3, with a review of the current version of the prominent model applied to rehabilitation intervention outcomes measurement and research today: the World Health Organization's International Classification of Functioning, Disability, and Health (WHO ICF). Chapter 4 further contributes to the definitional backdrop with a comprehensive overview of the current federal programs and public policies that are widely influencing outcome measurement in health care and education settings today.

In Section II the focus narrows to setting-specific considerations and methodologies in clinical services, beginning in Chapter 5 with a review of the state of outcome measurement in speech-language pathology within health care settings, followed in Chapter 6 by a discussion of specific concerns for practice in the schools. Chapter 7 discusses current issues and measurement practices that are specific to the long-term care setting.

Section III examines methods for evaluating organizational performance, beginning in Chapter 8 with a review of current issues and mandated data collection that are key features in accreditation processes. Chapter 9 examines the contribution of financial performance data to management and decision support in speech-language pathology programs. This focus on finances is then balanced in Chapter 10 against measurement of quality and patient safety. Chapter 11 discusses methods for performance improvement measurement to achieve organizational efficiencies.

Section IV focuses on research and the use of outcomes to inform clinical practice, beginning in Chapter 12 with a general review of the state of treatment research in speech-language pathology today. Chapter 13 considers the methods and obstacles encountered in the application of evidence-based practice. Chapter 14 then provides a response to some of the questions raised in Chapters 12 and 13 by considering the utility of single-subject research approaches to inform clinical practice decisions. Chapter 15 concludes the section with a tutorial and overview of meta-analysis in intervention outcomes research, with examples from intervention research in communication disorders.

Section V provides the final frame for the discussions on outcome measurement with a focus on graduate education, beginning in Chapter 16 with the role of outcome data in clinical education and supervision, and ending in Chapter 17 with a broad look at national trends in higher education and specifically in communication sciences and disorders programs.

The selection of these chapter topics, the contributing authors, and the organizational design of this text was guided by an overarching objective: to provide both stand-alone and complementary treatment of related topics across chapters. For that reason, while retaining the unique focus of each chapter, there is purposeful augmentation and redundancy across the topics between chapters.

There are two areas that are not addressed in this edition that had been addressed in the first edition: outcomes from an international perspective, and outcome measurements within special populations (fluency, child language, dysphagia, voice, neurogenic communication disorders, etc.). These deletions were made not only because of space limitations but also based on feedback from reviewers who noted that the first edition had a fairly limited international perspective, and that the section on outcomes with special populations did not cover every disorder or population of concern to speech-language pathology. So rather than attempt to expand these areas further, they were deleted.

Finally, appreciating that outcome measurement today is both a "hot topic" and a "moving target," authors were asked to end their chapters with their main conclusions and predictions for future directions, that is, where are we now, how did we get here, and where are we going? In every case, the authors' predictions for the future are positive but cautionary. It is hoped that the perspectives, information, and advice presented in this text will contribute to a positive future for our profession. Time will reveal the outcome.

# References

Frattali, C.M. (Ed.) (1998). *Measuring outcomes in speech-language pathology.* New York, NY: Thieme.

Wertz, R.T. & Irwin, W.H. (2001). Darley and the efficacy of language rehabilitation in aphasia. *Aphasiology, 15,* 231–247.

# Acknowledgments

This text is a co-edited effort. Dr. Carol Frattali's vision and handiwork have been carried forward into this second edition and are evident from the team of contributors assembled to the scope of topics included. Many of Dr. Frattali's original contributors participated as contributors or reviewers for this revision. These reviewers made recommendations for topic deletions, expansions, and additions, and suggested contributors or new topics for this edition. I am indebted to the thoughtful advice and suggestions received from several of the original contributors: Richard Merson, Michael Rolnick, Jean Blosser, Paul Rao, Diane Eger, Katherine Verdolini-Abbot, David Beukleman, Kathryn Yorkston, Connie Tompkins, and Edward Conture. Many of the original contributors to the first edition are among the list of contributors to this second edition. Paul Rao, Jean Blosser, Lesley Olswang, Alex Johnson, Kathryn Yorkston, Michael Rolnick, and Richard Merson have either revised their original chapters or are now authors or coauthors of a new topic in this edition. These authors are now joined by an outstanding group of new contributors: Travis Threats, Kate Romanow, Janet Brown, Margaret Rogers, Rob Mullen, Bill Goulding, Nancy Swigert, Tamala Bradham, Carolyn Baylor, Barbara Bain, Kevin Kearns, Michael de Riesthal, Katerina Ntourou, Mark Lipsey, Michael Kimbarow, Alex Johnson, Celia Hooper, Sue Hale, and Lennette Ivy. I am sincerely indebted to each of the contributors to this second edition for the gift of their precious time to this project and for sharing their expertise and commentary on a topic so timely and crucial to the future of our profession.

I also want to express my gratitude to Emily Ekle, acquisitions editor, and Elizabeth D'Ambrosio, editorial assistant, I was so fortunate to have worked with both of them throughout the development and completion of this text. And a special "thank you" to Barbara Chernow, our production editor, who helped to shepherd the final product to completion and graciously facilitated all of the last-minute figure changes and text edits.

In her acknowledgments in the first edition, Dr. Frattali thanked her colleagues Audrey Holland, Robert T. Wertz, and Martha Taylor-Sarno for their insights and personal philosophies, which were so influential to her, noting these individuals had "crystallized" her thinking on this topic. I, too, feel a personal debt of gratitude to these same, mutual colleagues and friends, and I add Carol Frattali, Bob Marshall, Kathy Yorkston, and Ed Conture to this short list of role models who have been so central to my career and professional development. My sincere, personal thanks to each of you for the guidance and support you have given me, for the examples you have set, and for your enduring friendship.

# Contributors

**Barbara A. Bain, PhD**
Professor Emerita
Idaho State University
Pocatello, Idaho

**Carolyn R. Baylor, PhD**
Acting Assistant Professor
Department of Rehabilitation Medicine
University of Washington
Seattle, Washington

**Jean Blosser, EdD**
Vice President
Therapy Programs and Quality
Progressus Therapy
Baltimore, Maryland

**Tamala S. Bradham, PhD**
Assistant Professor
Associate Director of Quality and Risk
    Management
Department of Hearing and Speech Sciences
Vanderbilt University
Nashville, Tennessee

**Janet E. Brown, MA, CCC-SLP**
Director, Health Care Services in
    Speech-Language Pathology
American Speech-Language-Hearing
    Association
Rockville, Maryland

**Michael R. de Riesthal, PhD**
Assistant Professor
Director, Pi Beta Phi Rehabilitation
    Institute
Department of Hearing and Speech
    Sciences
Vanderbilt University
Nashville, Tennessee

**Carol M. Frattali, PhD[‡]**
Formerly, Adjunct Professor, University of
    Maryland
Research Professor, George Washington
    University and
Research Coordinator, Speech-Language
    Pathology Section
M.G. Magnuson Clinical Center
National Institutes of Health
Bethesda, Maryland

**Lee Ann C. Golper, PhD**
Professor
Director, MS-SLP Program
Director, Speech-Language Pathology
    Clinical Division
Director of Quality and Risk Management
Department of Hearing and Speech
    Sciences
Vanderbilt University
Nashville, Tennessee

**William P. Goulding**
National Director
Outcomes and Reimbursement
Aegis Therapies
Greendale, Wisconsin

**Sue T. Hale, MCD**
Assistant Professor
Director of Clinical Education
Department of Hearing and Speech
  Sciences
Vanderbilt University
Nashville, Tennessee

**Celia R. Hooper, PhD**
Professor and Dean
University of North Carolina at Greensboro
School of Health & Human Sciences
Greensboro, North Carolina

**Lennette J. Ivy, PhD**
Associate Professor and Chair
Department of Communication Sciences
  and Disorders
The University of Mississippi
University, Mississippi

**Alex F. Johnson, PhD**
Provost and President for Academic
  Affairs
MGH Institute of Health Professions
Boston, Massachusetts

**Kevin P. Kearns, PhD**
Interim Provost and Vice President for
  Academic Affairs
State University of New York at Fredonia
Fredonia, New York

**Michael L. Kimbarow, PhD**
Associate Professor and Chair
San Jose State University
Department of Communication Disorders
  and Sciences
San Jose, California

**Mark W. Lipsey, PhD**
Research Professor
Director, Peabody Research Institute
Vanderbilt University
Nashville, Tennessee

**Richard M. Merson, PhD**
Coordinator of Clinical Research
Speech-Language Pathology Department
Beaumont Health System
Associate Professor
Oakland University William Beaumont
  Medical School
Royal Oak, Michigan

**Robert C. Mullen, MPH**
Director, National Center for Evidence-Based
  Practice in Communication Disorders
American Speech-Language-Hearing
  Association
Rockville, Maryland

**Katerina Ntourou, PhD**
Speech-Language Pathologist
Department of Hearing and Speech
  Sciences
Vanderbilt University
Nashville, Tennessee

**Lesley B. Olswang, PhD**
Professor
University of Washington
Department of Speech and Hearing
  Sciences
Seattle, Washington

**Paul R. Rao, PhD**
Vice President, Inpatient Operations &
  Compliance
National Rehabilitation Hospital
Washington, DC

**Margaret A. Rogers, PhD**
Chief Staff Officer for Science and
  Research
American Speech-Language-Hearing
  Association
Rockville, Maryland

**Michael I. Rolnick, PhD**
Director
Speech and Language Pathology
Beaumont Health System
Royal Oak, Michigan

**Kathleen Romanow, JD**
Regence BlueShield
Seattle, Washington

**Nancy B. Swigert, MA**
Director
Speech-Language Pathology and Respiratory
  Care
Central Baptist Hospital
Lexington, Kentucky

**Travis T. Threats, PhD**
Professor and Chair
Department of Communication Sciences &
  Disorders
Saint Louis University
St. Louis, Missouri

**Kathryn M. Yorkston, PhD**
Professor
Head, Speech-Language Pathology Division
Department of Rehabilitation Medicine
University of Washington
Seattle, Washington

# In Memory

Carol M. Frattali's professional career contributions and life example established a high ideal for all who were privileged to have known her. The memory of her grace, wit, and intellect remain with us. I hope this second edition, on a topic she felt so passionate about, continues her legacy.

*—Lee Ann C. Golper*

[Photograph provided by Dr. Michael Kusmick and used with permission]

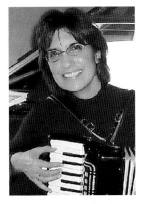

**Carol M. Frattali, PhD**
1954—2004

# I

# History and Contemporary Issues

# 1

# Outcomes Measurement: Definitions, Dimensions, and Perspectives

*Carol M. Frattali*

## ♦ Chapter Focus

This chapter, which is reproduced from the first edition of this text, provides the historical background and definitions for the topics and themes that are referenced, revisited, or introduced in this second edition, and provides a unifying framework for the book's content. It should be noted that some of the governmental and accreditation agency names and health-related quality-of-care models cited here have been revised since the 1998 publication of this chapter. These revisions are described elsewhere in this text. Minor formatting changes were made in this chapter to be consistent with the second edition. References to chapter numbers and chapter authors that were found in the first edition have been deleted and replaced with the current chapter numbers and authors, where appropriate.

## ♦ Introduction

We know surprisingly little about what works in clinical care. Many treatments and technologies in common use have never been evaluated. Many others that have been evaluated remain of uncertain benefit to large patient populations. Why, in this age of technology and information, haven't we learned more about the outcomes of our interventions?

Ellwood (1988) believes that moving even a substantial fraction of the service delivery system in a common direction of data collection is difficult. He describes hard held practitioner notions of patient care (more care; less paperwork) and the begrudging attitude to adopt outcomes technology only to preempt the threat of losing professional control. Iezzoni (1994) says "the devil is in the details" (p. 3). She suggests that meaningful measurement of patients' outcomes requires vigilant application of two basic methodologies: a measure of the outcome itself (few good outcome measures exist), and a way to adjust for patient's risks for various outcomes (often outside experimental control). Deming (1982) blames managers unwilling to break habits of decision making based on hunches instead of data. He labels this prevailing style of management "tyranny," and calls for a transformation routed toward profound knowledge.

We enter an era rich with pioneering deacons and seminal tomes crossing the disciplines of health care, education, economics, engineering, business, and management in a field increasingly known as outcomes measurement, and, if we are to apply outcomes measurement to improving interventions and decision making, outcomes management. Yet, despite advances in computer technology, measures, and methods, knowledge about the effects of clinical interventions has not accrued at the speed the problem demands.

Paul Ellwood (1988) believes it is timing. He quotes Sir Francis Darwin: "In science the credit goes to the [one] who convinces the world, not to the [one] to whom the idea first occurs." He cites ambitious efforts to install integrated management information systems that capture outcomes, help practitioners in making decisions, and feed the results back to decision makers. Yet, most efforts have lost momentum, and have been successful only in capturing the imaginations of the media and the health care professions. None have yet to convince the world.

Nevertheless, strands of optimism are laced in current thinking on outcomes measurement. The time is right for widespread application—an opinion based largely on improvements in our ability to manage information with computers and the demonstration (e.g., by Medicare's diagnosis-related groups [DRGs]) of the effect an expanded database can have on integrating service and financial information. Ellwood affirms, "We have the opportunity to proceed immediately" (p. 6).

The purposes of this chapter are to give you a sense of history about outcomes measurement, offer definitions and classification schemes that can serve to organize your thoughts, and provide an overview of the various methods in use. The chapter constructs a framework intended to unify the book's content.

## ♦ Historical Perspective

Popular opinion holds outcomes measurement as a contemporary concept in service delivery. Outcomes measurement, in fact, actually emerged in the mid-nineteenth century. The leading pioneer of the time was Florence Nightingale (in Iezzoni, 1994). Her motivation was the finding that hospital patients died at higher rates than their cohorts treated elsewhere. Even more troublesome were the comparisons of mortality rates across the principal hospitals of England in 1861. The in-hospital mortality rate in London hospitals was close to 91%, compared with a mortality rate of close to 16% in naval and military hospitals. Nightingale explained the discrepancy, in part, by variations in patient risks (such as age and "state of the cases at admissions"). Her more important findings, however, were her observations that facilities with better outcomes also had better sanitation, less crowding of patients in wards, and a location distant from sewage disposal. In response, Nightingale proposed changes in ward configurations, sanitation, and hospital location that led to reductions in hospital mortality rates. This example became the earliest known account of outcomes measurement (collecting, analyzing, and reporting outcomes data) and management (making changes based on data to improve outcomes).

Ernest A. Codman, a prominent Boston surgeon of the late nineteenth century, also holds a space in history as a proponent of monitoring outcomes of care (Berwick, 1989; Iezzoni, 1994). His contribution was his effort to link specific interventions with their effects on patients. Called the "end-results idea," Codman described it as "merely the common-sense notion that every hospital should follow *every* patient it treats, long enough to determine whether or not the treatment has been successful, and then to inquire 'if not, why not' with a view to preventing similar failures in the future" (Codman, 1934, p. xii).

Unfortunately, Codman's idea led to his fall from grace among his medical colleagues at The Massachusetts General Hospital, who viewed his practices of tracking patients as extreme. Codman reacted:

"So I am called eccentric for saying in public: that Hospitals, if they wish to be sure of improvement,

1.  Must find out what their results are.

2.  Must analyze their results, to find their strong and weak points.

3.  Must compare their results with those of other hospitals. . . .

Such opinions will not be eccentric a few years hence" (Codman, 1917, p. 137). Codman eventually left The Massachusetts General Hospital and opened his own hospital in Boston's Beacon Hill, where he completely installed his end-results tracking system. He categorized, as a result of scanning volumes of data for each patient, types of causes of treatment errors or failures, including (Codman, 1917):

- Errors due to lack of technical knowledge or skill

- Errors possibly due to a lack of judgment

- Errors due to lack of care or equipment

- Errors due to incorrect diagnosis

- Cases in which the nature and extent of the disease was the main cause of failure

- Cases who refused to accept treatment

Thus, Codman linked specific outcomes to specific interventions. He later resigned from The Massachusetts General Hospital, protesting its practice of promotion by seniority (a practice considered antithetical to his end-results idea), and was forced, with few referrals, to close his hospital and live a professional life of discontent.

Where Nightingale succeeded, Codman failed. Today, however, both are recognized for their contributions, which form the conceptual foundation of outcomes measurement and management. The lesson learned here is that it is not enough to know simply about end results, but to know *why* these events occurred (Iezzoni, 1994). Thus, the link of patient characteristics and specific interventions with specific outcomes is crucial to knowledge.

## Modern-Day Leaders in the Outcomes Movement

Two current-day leaders in outcomes measurement, whose contributions largely founded the field of quality improvement, are Avedis Donabedian (1980) and the late W. Edwards Deming (1982). Donabedian, a physician and professor of public health at University of Michigan, spread his knowledge across three volumes exploring approaches to quality assessment and monitoring. He is best known for establishing a unifying framework of quality of care, and coining the terms *structure*, *process*, and *outcome* approaches to its assessment. He defines these terms:

**Structure:** The relatively stable characteristics of the providers of care, of the tools and resources they have at their disposal, and of the physical and organizational settings in which they work. Thus, the concept of structure includes the human, physical, and financial resources needed to provide care (p. 81).

**Process:** The set of activities that go on between and within practitioners and patients. These include technical management (e.g., diagnostic and treatment methods), and interpersonal aspects of care (e.g., the psychosocial interactions between practitioner and patient) (pp. 79–80).

**Outcome:** A change in a patient's current and future health status that can be attributed to antecedent health care. Change includes improvement of social and psychological function in addition to the more usual emphasis on the physical and physiological aspects of performance. By still another extension I shall add patient attitudes (including satisfaction), health-related knowledge acquired by the patient, and health-related behavioral change. All of these can be seen either as components of current health or as contributions to future health (pp. 82–83).

Donabedian's teachings were introduced during a time of intense debate over which approach to quality assessment—process or outcome—was superior. Like his predecessors, he found, through conceptual and empirical study, that process and outcome are inextricably linked:

> Process and outcome are fundamentally linked in a single, symmetrical structure that makes of one almost a mirror image of the other, no matter how many attributes are used to test the relationship. Thus, the emphasis shifts to a more thorough understanding of the linkages between process and outcome, and away from the rather misguided argument over which of the two is the superior approach to assessment. (p. xi)

Donabedian's (1980) triad of structure-process-outcome mirrors the notion of systems thinking by recognizing the fundamental relationship among all three elements.

During the same time period, a similar movement was underway, but in the manufacturing industry. The attention of large corporations in the United States, such as Ford and General Electric, was being diverted to the work of W. Edwards Deming (1982). Deming was an internationally renowned statistician and consultant, based in Washington, D.C., whose work led Japanese industry into new principles of management and revolutionized the quality of their products and service. He called for nothing short of a transformation of the American style of management, one that neglects to plan for the future and foresee problems through use of a systematic process of data collection and analysis to increase knowledge. Deming states, "Anyone in management requires, for transformation, some rudimentary knowledge about science—in particular, something about the nature of variation and about operational definitions" (p. xi).

His work spilled into the industries of education and health care, although the impatience of managers, oriented toward quick fix and pressured by economic constraints, quelled the movement. A wise Deming predicted: "Long-term commitment to new learning and new philosophy is required of any management that seeks transformation. The timid and the fainthearted, and people that expect quick results, are doomed to disappointment" (p. x).

Among Deming's principles for transformation is the fifth of his 14 points for management: Improve constantly and forever the system of production and service. Through a use of statistical tools and knowledge of systems and process variation, he proposes the cycle of Plan (study a work process to decide what change might improve it), Do (make the change), Study (observe the effects or outcomes), Act (standardize the change if it resulted in improvement; if not, decide what other changes might result in improvement and begin the cycle again) to improve continually the quality of products and services. Deming also emphasizes consumer research as the hallmark of innovation. Thus, quality is aimed at the needs of the consumer, present and future. His vigilant focus on systematic and scientifically based process improvement invariably leads to better outcomes at a lower cost, which he believes should be the aim of any service provider who works for the common good of an industry as a whole.

In the field of medicine, the work of John Wennberg is also noteworthy from an historical perspective. John Wennberg, a professor at Dartmouth Medical School, conducted a landmark study of unacceptable variation in performing hysterectomies in the state of Maine (Wennberg & Gittelsohn, 1973). In one county, 70% of women had had hysterectomies by the age of 70; in a nearby county the figure was only 20%. The measured variation passed all tests of statistical analysis to adjust for possible explanatory factors, including age, diagnosis, socioeconomic status, and severity level. If Wennberg is right, states Berwick, Godfrey, and Roessner (1990), "then the health care dollar is not only inflating, it is being spent largely in some colossal game of dice" (p. 8). The study confirmed suspicions of "for-profit" medicine and dissolved consumer trust in the quality of care.

It is perhaps this study that has spurred payers, managed care systems, accreditation bodies, and government agencies to approach any provider with skepticism and scrutinize the care rendered in the service delivery system. Thus, the 1970s marked the end of the practitioner's "our word is our honor," and the beginning of the payer's "prove it."

## Advances in Outcomes Measurement

Another study is credited with accelerating the outcomes movement, at least from a position of public protection. This time it was the release of mortality data by the U.S. Department of Health and Human Services' Health Care Financing Administration (HCFA) (Brinkley, 1986). Its only value is found in a lesson learned about the consequences of looking at outcomes alone.

In the mid-1980s, HCFA was compelled to publicly release death rates of Medicare beneficiaries by reporters' demands under the federal Freedom of Information Act. Based on governmental predictions, 142 hospitals had significantly higher death rates, while 127 had significantly lower rates. One facility had a death rate of 86.7% compared with a predicted 22.5%. The hospital administrators, infuriated by the data and media interpretations regarding quality of care that followed, argued rightfully that HCFA failed to standardize adequately for severity of illness. What the public did not know was that many of the hospitals with high mortality rates were tertiary care centers treating more medically complex patients, and the facility with the most aberrant death rate was a hospice caring for terminally ill patients.

The release of HCFA data spurred the development of other systems that incorporate severity adjustments to level the playing field and allow fair comparisons of "apples to apples." At the same time, systems were becoming more sophisticated with advances in computer technology. Several severity measurement systems were introduced in the health care field. Examples include APACHE (Acute Physiology, Age, and Chronic Health Evaluation; Knaus, Zimmerman, Wagner, Draper, & Lawrence, 1981); CSI (Computerized Severity Index; Horn et al, 1991); MedisGroups (Brewster et al, 1985; Iezzoni & Moskowitz, 1988); and DRGs (diagnosis-related groups) (Fetter, Shin, Freeman, Averill, & Thompson, 1980; Vladeck, 1984). While severity is defined differently by each system, all defined "severity" by linking it to a specific outcome or clinical state. For example, APACHE linked severity to in-hospital mortality; CSI to treatment difficulty based on diagnosis and disease-specific signs and symptoms; MedisGroups to clinical instability as indicated by in-hospital death; and DRGs to total hospital charges or length of stay. Severity is rated by factors such as diagnosis, separate ratings of severity for all diagnoses, and categories of major surgery. While medically based in their designs, these outcomes measurement systems influenced activities in other areas of the service delivery system.

### *Advances in the Field of Rehabilitation*

Outcomes measurement in the multidisciplinary field of rehabilitation is particularly interesting to us as rehabilitation providers. Of perhaps greatest significance was the introduction of the Functional Independence Measure (FIM) (State University of New York at Buffalo Research Foundation, 1993) as an outcome instrument designed to quantitatively measure the burden of care and written in a language understandable to the payer. This minimum data set, which measures communication among other rehabilitation variables, rates functional abilities on a 7-point scale of independence. Due to its ease and efficiency of use, as well as its appeal to payers, the FIM has become an industry standard worldwide. Another database, the Uniform Data System for Medical Rehabilitation (UDSMR), which incorporates the FIM and has catalogued the functional outcomes of hundreds of thousands of patients, has become potentially powerful in its capacity to establish a payment system for rehabilitation. Yet, the database suffers from its neglect in linking specific processes to specific outcomes. Thus, the claims of treatment effectiveness remain largely unfounded. Nevertheless, outcomes measurement studies using the FIM are proceeding to create function-related groups (FRGs) to determine resource use and, thus, set reimbursement rates for rehabilitation (Stineman et al, 1994; Wilkerson, Batavia, & DeJong, 1992).

In the meantime, other rehabilitation outcome measures and automated systems were being designed or refined as outcomes measurement and management became a primary means for survival in a cost-constrained system. These measures or systems include the Level of Rehabilitation Scale III (LORS III; Parkside Associates, Inc., 1986), Patient Evaluation and Conference System (PECS; Harvey & Jellinek, 1979, 1981), and Rehabilitation Institute of Chicago Functional Assessment Scale '95 (RICFAS;

Cichowski, 1995). Some have been designed to overcome some of the weaknesses of the FIM, particularly the problem of low sensitivity in capturing functionally important change. Yet, many continue to lack sufficient reliability and validity that allow sound interpretations of derived data.

### Advances in Speech-Language Pathology

Fueled by flaws in current research activities, accreditation agency outcomes initiatives (e.g., the Joint Commission on Accreditation of Healthcare Organizations' [JCAHO] Agenda for Change and the Commission on Accreditation of Rehabilitation Facilities' [CARF] outcomes management focus in its standards for medical rehabilitation), managed care and regulatory agency demands for data, and consumer choice, professionals began looking to their membership organizations for needed leadership and direction. In response, the American Speech-Language-Hearing Association (ASHA), in 1993, established the Task Force on Treatment Outcomes and Cost Effectiveness (American Speech-Language-Hearing Association, 1995). It was established to generate an outcomes database to assist in meeting current public demands. Among its many initiatives, the task force packaged cost data for use in negotiating managed care contracts, supported the development and dissemination of 10 technical reports summarizing the efficacy of treatment in key clinical areas, and designed a data collection system to aggregate outcomes data in the areas of cost, consumer satisfaction, and functional status. It continues its work in validating new outcome measures, focusing more recently on pediatric measures and measures that can be used by school systems. Concurrently, ASHA completed a 3-year grant project to develop the ASHA Functional Assessment of Communication Skills for Adults (ASHA FACS; Frattali, Thompson, Holland, Wohl, & Ferketic, 1995), and reorganized its research structure (i.e., elevated the Research Division to a Scientific Affairs and Research Department) for, among other important activities, the pursuit of multisite clinical trials research.

Predating ASHA's aggressive outcomes initiative, however, was a landmark conference sponsored by the American Speech-Language-Hearing Foundation, titled Treatment Efficacy Research in Communication Disorders (Olswang, Thompson, Warren, & Minghetti, 1990). This conference injected new life into our field in the area of efficacy research, and, by extension, outcomes measurement. Leija McReynolds, assigned to present an historical perspective of treatment research, admitted

> . . . there is not much history to report. Applied research in the behavioral sciences only began in earnest in the 1960s, and even later than that in speech, language, and hearing. Treatment efficacy research has an even shorter history than applied research in general. . . . So, the history is sparse and short. Very little treatment research has been conducted. (p. 5)

But, McReynolds (1990), in the same stream of thought, continued:

> "There is a new breeze blowing." Certainly it is a gentle breeze, not a strong wind, but it is a kinder wind than it was just a few years ago, and I believe our profession is gradually becoming aware of the need for evaluating our treatment in a controlled manner. (p. 5)

McReynolds (1990) was right. Today, we are hearing about new outcome measures, such as the Voice Handicap Index (Jacobson, Johnson, & Grywalski, 1995), the National Outcomes Measurement System (NOMS) (American Speech-Language-Hearing Association, 1995), and the ASHA FACS (Frattali et al, 1995). New automated outcomes management systems, such as the OUTCOME (Evaluation Systems International, Inc., 1994), Beaumont Outcome Software System (BOSS) (Merson, Rolnick, & Weiner, 1995), and the Functional Outcome and Utilization System (FOCUS) (Focus Rehab, Inc., 1995) recently were made commercially available. Refereed journals devoted to scientifically based clinical practice (e.g., *The American Journal of Speech-Language Pathology: A Journal of Clinical Practice*) were created, thus inviting the conduct and publication of efficacy and outcomes research. National and international efforts in outcomes measurement are mounting, as evidenced by the number of scientific meetings and workshops addressing the topic, and creation of related professional organizations (e.g., The Treatment Efficacy Research Group in Communication Disorders), and study sections (e.g., Quality Improvement Study Section of ASHA Special Interest Division 11: Administration and Supervision), whose missions include the advancement of clinical research or databased quality of care.

But a caveat is offered with recent advances in outcomes measurement. The problem easily could shift from one of "too little evidence" to another of "too much weak evidence." We soon could suffer from division of purpose in outcomes measurement in general, and flawed methods of data collection, analysis, and interpretation in specific. These pitfalls are all too possible in the current environment that is operating with differing, and sometimes conflicting, terminology and conceptual frameworks from which to create new knowledge. Further, various measurement methodologies are being applied, some correctly, some incorrectly, with less than vigilant efforts at acknowledging study limitations and making valid interpretations. Consequently, we must devote considerable attention at the outset to how we are defining our terms and applying our methodologies so that the data collected and interpretations made are both useful and meaningful.

## ♦ Terminology

I have chosen the term *outcomes measurement* as the topic of this book, but not without considering the terms *outcomes research, efficacy research,* and *outcomes management.*

Often used either loosely or interchangeably, these terms and their offshoots (e.g., *treatment efficacy, treatment effectiveness, treatment efficiency, program evaluation, quality improvement*) cause many professionals to stumble in discussions on the topic. I use the term *outcomes measurement* as a broad term that encompasses both outcomes research and efficacy research. Outcomes management, however, overlaps the boundaries of measurement because it involves taking next steps of using outcomes data to improve or make decisions about care. Although outcomes management is addressed throughout this book, measurement is the central theme.

I also use the term *outcomes measurement* with no intention of minimizing *process measurement.* Outcomes measurement, as described by its proponents, is meaningful only if linked to facility, client, and clinician characteristics (to allow comparison of "apples to apples"), and the various processes of care (to allow us to make relational statements about the effects of specific interventions).

### What Is an Outcome?

Given the above qualifications, an *outcome* is simply a result of an intervention. I intentionally use the plural term, *outcomes,* because it is a multidimensional concept defined only in terms of the agent. Agents can be clinicians, teachers, employers, administrators, payers, and the clients/families themselves—all consumers of care. Thus, outcomes can be

- *clinically derived* (e.g., ability to sustain phonation, accuracy in naming, type and frequency of disfluencies in a speech sample, integrity of the swallowing mechanism);

- *functional* (e.g., ability to communicate basic needs, telephone use);

- *administrative* (e.g., client referral patterns, productivity levels in direct client care, rates of missed sessions);

- *financial* (e.g., cost-effective care, rate of rehospitalizations, average lengths of stay;

- *social* (e.g., employability, ability to learn, community reentry); and

- *client-defined* (e.g., satisfaction with services; quality of life).

Donabedian (1985) offers a definition of *outcome* in the context of health care:

> Outcomes are those changes, either favorable or adverse, in the actual or potential health status of persons, groups, or communities that can be attributed to prior or concurrent care. What is included in the category of "outcomes" depends, therefore, on how narrowly or broadly one defines "health" and the corresponding responsibilities of . . . practitioners or the health care system as a whole. (p. 256)

If we use this example in other contexts, we can easily replace the term *health* with terms such as *learning ability* (from the standpoint of education), *costs* (from the standpoint of the payer), and *quality of life* and *satisfaction* (from the standpoint of clients or their families). We quickly understand that we as clinicians are not striving for one outcome only, but for a range of outcomes, as defined by the interests or needs of any given stakeholder, and at any given point in time during or after the provision of care. While a clinician might show initial interest in short-term outcomes (e.g., articulation accuracy from session to session), a client might be more interested, even at the start, in long-term outcomes (e.g., returning to work as a result of improved communication skills required by the job).

If we extend beyond the clinical model, outcomes measurement also can be applied to other contexts, including the professional preparation level in university programs. Methods can allow, for example, investigation of educational outcomes and related outcomes such as student satisfaction with curricula, employers' appraisal of graduates' on-the-job performance, and clinical competency. Management of these outcomes would have strong implications for revising or improving academic programs.

## When Do Outcomes Occur?

The temporal order of outcomes gives rise to three terms, coined by Rosen and Proctor (1981): intermediate, instrumental, and ultimate outcomes. *Intermediate outcomes* let us know, from session to session, whether treatment is benefiting the client. These outcomes allow exploration of the treatment process. Thus, they are of prime interest to investigate all who use them as barometers of adjustment in treatment plans. Studies that investigate outcomes are designed to answer questions such as, What makes a good session? How important is this to the overall goal of treatment (or the ultimate outcome)? Olswang (1990) gives the example of a clinician questioning whether practicing sounds in isolation, syllables, words, and/or phrases is necessary to achieve sound production in conversation.

*Instrumental outcomes* are outcomes that activate the learning process. These are outcomes that, when reached, trigger the ultimate outcome. Once an instrumental outcome is reached, treatment is no longer necessary, for the individual will continue to improve on his or her own. The focus is on how long to treat—a question of particular interest to payers. Citing phonology treatment again, Olswang (1990) recommends that the clinician question at what level of correct production of the target sound is sufficient to trigger correct production in conversation.

*Ultimate outcomes* are those that demonstrate the social or ecological validity of our interventions, such as functional communication, employability, ability to learn, social integration, and so on. Research designed to study ultimate outcomes explores questions about the meaningfulness of treatment. What does it mean to attain functional communication, and how much direct treatment is necessary? Ultimate outcomes are of prime interest to payers and regulators as well as clients and their families: How will this treatment make me a more effective communicator? How will it enhance my ability to learn in school? To get a job?

## How Are Outcomes Defined?

Once outcomes are identified, they must be defined operationally if they are to be measured. For example, if we are measuring functional communication, what do we mean by functional? Do we mean common everyday skills (e.g., telephone interactions, responding in an emergency) that allow one to convey basic needs or interests? Or do we mean more individually defined or higher level skills (e.g., writing business letters, completing forms, reading and comprehending a book) that allow one to return to work, school, or community activities? What do we mean by communication? Do we mean understanding and speaking only, or do we include nonverbal skills? With a partner? In a group? Do we include speech intelligibility? Do we include reading and writing? Very quickly, the business of outcomes measurement becomes weighted in definition.

Deming (1982) devotes an entire chapter of his book, *Out of the Crisis*, to operational definitions: "An operational definition puts communicable meaning into a concept" (p. 276).

Deming continues:

> Adjectives like good, reliable, uniform, round, tired, safe, unsafe . . . have no communicable meaning until they are expressed in operational terms of sampling, test, and criterion. . . . We have seen in many places how important it is that buyer and seller understand each other. They must both use the same kind of centimetre. . . . This requirement has meaning only if instruments are in statistical control. Without operational definitions, a specification is meaningless. (p. 277)

Indeed, if we are to be consistent in our measurement of physical, physiological, or behavioral changes, we must operationally define "changes" by way of measurement instruments. Further, these instruments must be reliable and valid (i.e., in statistical control) if the data derived are to be meaningful. In addition, current demands add to the requirement of sound psychometric properties. Given current payer demands, our instruments should also be quantitative and comprehensible. That is, they should be interpretable in numeric terms (e.g., by means of scores) to objectively and efficiently document or measure change, and the test results must be interpretable by the lay person (often the person who is making decisions about payment or continuation of services).

## Classification Schemes

Useful frameworks in which to define outcomes are found if you consider outcomes along a continuum of the consequences of disease, disorder, injury, or active pathology. Both medical and social models are advanced by the health care community. No one model has yet to be universally accepted; thus, the lack of a uniformly accepted conceptual framework presents one obstacle to development and application of outcome measures, as well as outcomes measurement methods and interpretations. Three frameworks are described.

## World Health Organization Classifications

The most well-known conceptual framework, the *International Classification of Impairments, Disabilities, and Handicaps (ICIDH)* comes from the World Health Organization (WHO; 1980). The ICIDH acknowledges a chain of principal events that occur in the development of illnesses:

1. Something abnormal happens (a pathology occurs).

2. Someone becomes aware of such an occurrence (thus, heralding recognition of impairment).

3. The individual's performance or behavior may be altered and common activities may be restricted (giving rise to a disability).

4. The individual is placed at a disadvantage relative to others, thus socializing the experience (creating a handicap).

The pathology, according to the WHO, is an intrinsic situation which becomes exteriorized by an impairment. The impairment becomes objectified (i.e., the process through which a functional limitation expresses itself as a reality in everyday life) by disability and, in turn, socialized by handicap. The WHO defines the consequential phenomena as follows:

*Impairment.* Any loss or abnormality of psychological, physiological, or anatomical structure or function. It represents deviation from a norm.

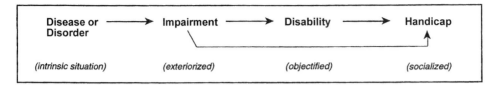

**Fig. 1.1**   The World Health Organization's Consequences of Disease or Disorder. (From World Health Organization. (1980). *International classification of impairments, disabilities, and handicaps.* Geneva: Author. Reprinted by permission.)

*Disability.* Any restriction or lack of ability (resulting from an impairment) to perform an activity in a manner or within a range considered normal for a human being. A disability is the functional consequence of an impairment manifested in integrated activities represented by tasks and skills.

*Handicap.* A disadvantage resulting from an impairment or disability that limits or prevents the fulfillment of a role that is normal (depending on age, sex, and social and cultural factors) for that individual. A handicap is the social consequence of an impairment or disability, defined by the attitudes and responses of others. Thus, the state of handicapped is relative to other people.

As **Fig. 1.1** illustrates, impairment, disability, and handicap can be linked. Although suggesting a simple linear progression along the full sequence, the situation can become more complex. Handicap may result from impairment without the mediation of a disability. For example, an individual who uses an augmentative communication device may not have difficulty with everyday communication (a disability), but may, in fact be socially stigmatized, which leads to social isolation (handicap). Also, one can be impaired without being disabled, and disabled without being handicapped—for example, the individual with a lisp who experiences no problems with communication, or the augmentative communication user whose social and work environments make the necessary accommodations to prevent handicap. If we are to apply the framework to the field of speech-language pathology, we can use the example of the person with cerebral vascular disease who sustains a stroke (disease and disorder). The resultant impairment is aphasia, which leads to a communication disability manifested in the performance of daily life activities such as communicating with family and friends, using the telephone, making grocery lists, and reading the newspaper. The disability leads to social isolation, interruption of community activities (e.g., bridge club, holiday celebrations), and loss of a job as an office assistant.

The WHO framework portrays a problem-solving sequence in the context of clinical intervention. Intervention at the level of one element has the potential to modify or prevent succeeding elements. As Batavia (1992) explains, "with appropriate rehabilitative interventions, an impairment does not necessarily result in a disability. Similarly, with appropriate social and environmental interventions, a disability does not necessarily result in a handicap" (p. 3).

Because each stage along the WHO continuum can be classified as an outcome, three classes of outcome measures are identified. Impairment instruments include our traditional diagnostic and instrumental measures, designed for differential diagnosis and identification of specific phonological, voice, fluency, language, cognitive, and swallowing deficits. Disability measures include the functional status instruments that measure communication in everyday contexts, and also include swallowing measures that assess, for example, independence during meals and adequate nutrition. Handicap measures include health-related quality-of-life measures or handicap inventories, usually designed as self-administered questionnaires that capture social, environmental, and economic disadvantages from the perspective of the client or family.

The WHO framework, while useful universally, has suffered from its simplicity (e.g., excluding certain scenarios of the consequences of disease) and terminology (e.g., use of the term *handicap*). It also has been criticized for its alignment with a medical rather than social model, and its internal inconsistencies and lack of clarity of the terms *disability* and *handicap*. In recent years the term *handicap* has fallen into disuse in the United States primarily because individuals with disabilities consider the term to have socially imposed negative connotations. Numerous proposals have suggested revisions to the WHO, and an ICIDH-2 model is currently in beta testing (Placek, personal communication, 1996). In the meantime, however, other classification schemes, aimed at solving some of the problems of the WHO typology, have been described (see Chapter 3, by Threats, for a discussion of the revised version of the WHO ICF).

*Nagi Classifications*

Saad Nagi (1965) constructed a framework of four distinct but interrelated concepts: active pathology, impairment, functional limitation, and disability. His model is a close variant of the Institute of Medicine Model of Disability and Disability Prevention (Pope & Tarlov, 1991) as well as the Disablement Model of the National Institutes of Health, National Center for Medical Rehabilitation Research (National Institutes of Health, 1993). Nagi's concepts are described as follows:

*Active pathology.* Interruption or interference with normal processes and efforts of the organism to regain the normal state. It refers to cell and tissue changes. Indicators include signs and symptoms and are found in attributes of the individual.

*Impairment.* Anatomical, physiological, mental, or emotional abnormalities or loss. Indicators, again, include signs and symptoms and are found in attributes of the individual.

*Functional limitation.* Limitation in performance at the level of the whole organism or person. Indicators include limitations in various activities such as walking, reasoning, and communicating. Indicators are found in attributes of the individual.

*Disability.* Limitation in performance of socially defined roles and tasks within a sociocultural and physical environment. Indicators include limitations in performance of such roles and tasks as related to family, work, community, school, and recreation. Indicators are found in these relations on the one hand, and in the conditions in the sociocultural and physical environment on the other.

When compared with the ICIDH, many would say that Nagi's "functional limitation" is synonymous with the WHO's "disability"; likewise, Nagi's "disability" is synonymous with the WHO's "handicap." Both frameworks recognize that whether or not a person performs a socially expected activity depends not simply on the characteristics of the person, but also on the larger context of social and physical environments.

According to the Nagi framework, all pathology is associated with impairment, but not all impairments lead to functional limitations. Similarly, all functional limitation and disability are associated with impairment, but not all functional limitations lead to disability. Disability can also exist in the absence of functional limitation (e.g., disfigurement). **Figure 1.2** illustrates the conceptual relationship among the categories in Nagi's framework.

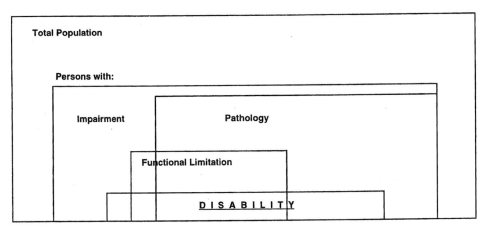

**Fig. 1.2**   Nagi framework. (From Institute of Medicine. (1991). *Disability in America.* Washington, DC: National Academies Press. Reprinted by permission.)

*Wilson and Cleary's Conceptual Model of Patient Outcomes*

Wilson and Cleary (1995) recognize that as therapeutic efforts focus more on improving patient function and well-being, the need to understand these relationships will increase. They also recognize the problem that has hampered progress in this area—the lack of conceptual models that specify how different types of outcome measures interrelate. They believe that such a conceptualization involves the integration of medical and social paradigms of health: the former held by clinicians and basic science researchers; the latter by social scientists.

In the clinical paradigm, the focus is on etiological agents, pathological processes, and biological, physiological, and clinical outcomes. The principal goal is to understand causation to guide diagnosis and treatment. Controlled experiments are its principal methodology. In contrast, the social science paradigm (i.e., the "quality-of-life model"), focuses on dimensions of functioning and overall well-being. Experimental research designs are rarely possible because the focus is on the way numerous social structures influence individuals.

Wilson and Cleary (1995) conclude that none of the current conceptual models include the full range of variables that are typically included in health-related quality of-life assessments. Furthermore, they attest that most models do not specify the links between biological and other types of measures, nor have they been tested empirically. Thus, Wilson and Cleary propose a conceptual model, a taxonomy of patient outcomes, that categorizes measures of patient outcome according to the underlying health concepts they represent. They also propose different specific causal relationships between different health concepts, thereby integrating medical and social models of health (**Fig. 1.3**).

According to the model, measures of health can be thought of as existing on a continuum of increasing biological, social, and psychological complexity. At one end of the continuum are biological measures; at the other end are more complex and integrated measures such as functioning and

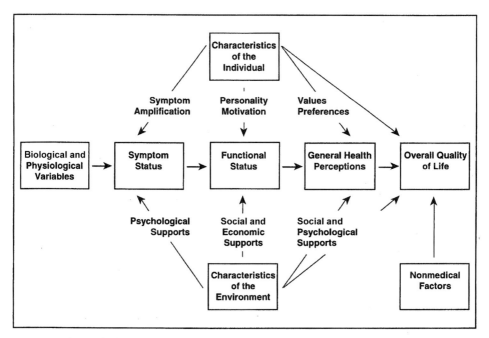

**Fig. 1.3** Wilson and Cleary's conceptual model of patient outcomes. (From Wilson, I. B., & Cleary, P. D. (1995). Linking clinical variables with quality of life: A conceptual model of patient outcomes. *Journal of the American Medical Association, 273*(1), 59–65. Reprinted by permission. Copyright © (1995) American Medical Association. All rights reserved.)

general health perceptions. Dominant causal associations with each level are specified. The five levels in the model are described:

*Biological and physiological variables.* These include the function of cells, organs, and organ systems. Measures include those of physiological function (e.g., pulmonary function, reflexes), and physical examination findings.

*Symptom status.* Assessment focuses not on specific cells and organs, but on the organism as a whole. These include physical, psychological, or emotional symptoms (e.g., weakness, confusion, speech difficulty, fear, worry). Thus, a symptom is a patient's perception of an abnormal physical, emotional, or cognitive state.

*Functional status.* Measures of function assess the ability of the individual to perform particular defined tasks. Four domains of function include physical function, social function, role function, and psychological function. Functional status can vary depending on personality and motivation (e.g., a determination to be self-sufficient), as well as social and economic supports (e.g., supportive family, access to care). Thus, two individuals with similar conditions may function very differently.

*General health perceptions.* These represent an integration of previous health concepts, discussed above, as well as others such as mental health. Thus, they are, by definition, a subjective rating. Variations in health perceptions are associated with individual and preferences, as well as social and psychological supports.

*Overall quality of life.* This concept involves subjective measures of a patient's well-being. These general measures often assess how happy and/or satisfied respondents are with life as a whole. They represent a synthesis of a wide range of experiences and feelings that people have. Overall quality of life, too, is associated with individual values and preferences, and social and psychological supports.

The Wilson and Cleary model (1995) perhaps does the best job of integrating a social model of health with a medical model. As you move from left to right in the model, you move outward from the cell to the individual to the interaction of the individual as a member of society. The concepts at each level are increasingly integrated and increasingly difficult to define and measure. At each level, there are a growing number of inputs that cannot be controlled by clinicians or the health care system as it is traditionally defined.

## How Are Outcomes Measured?

Outcomes measurement involves a range of measures (from physical to physiological to behavioral to self-perceived, and including financial and administrative measures) and methodologies (from experimental, to quasi-experimental, to nonexperimental). These latter classifications have attempted to give order to the multiplicity of methods that can be applied, and the conclusions that can be drawn about the outcomes of clinical interventions. An appropriate precursor to describing these classifications is a discussion of the distinction between outcomes research and efficacy research, which has led to differing views about treatment efficacy and treatment effectiveness.

### Outcomes Research versus Efficacy Research

The terms *outcomes research* and *efficacy research* are found under the umbrella of outcomes measurement. Typically, research carries a definition of scientific or scholarly investigation that implies explicit protocols and well-controlled conditions aimed at proving causation. Not all research, however, is aimed at questions of causation. Thus, important differences have evolved between outcomes research and efficacy research.

Benninger, Gardner, Jacobson, and Grywalski (1997) draw a distinction between efficacy research and outcomes research. Treatment efficacy is the ability of an applied treatment to produce a predicted result. Treatment efficacy is what drives controlled clinical studies. Conceptually, it is distinct from outcomes research that measures the effectiveness of a specific treatment as it is applied to a typical circumstance. Outcomes studies seldom incorporate experimental research designs because their focus is on the influence of the applied treatment over numerous facets of the patient's life that typically cannot be experimentally controlled. Benninger and his colleagues conclude: "In simple terms, outcomes research attempts to demonstrate treatment effectiveness by relating clinical and more objective measures of treatment results to the subjective experiences and responses of patients who have had those treatments" (p. 789).

### Efficacy versus Effectiveness

As noted above, a distinction is made between studies of treatment *efficacy* and *effectiveness*. The U.S. Department of Health and Human Services' Agency for Health Care Policy and Research (AHCPR, 1994), borrowing from the original definitions of the Congressional Office of Technology Assessment (1978), also distinguishes the concepts of efficacy and effectiveness in terms of the different research methodologies applied (**Table 1.1**). *Treatment efficacy* involves the extent to which an intervention can be shown to be beneficial under optimal (or ideal) conditions; treatment effectiveness involves the extent to which services are shown to be beneficial under typical (or real-world) conditions. In this sense, treatment effectiveness involves the extent to which optimal benefits are actually achieved.

Palmer (1990) suggests that the distinction between efficacy and effectiveness was in medical treatment research because of awareness of the loss of control when moving from animal to human experiments. As summarized by AHCPR (1994), efficacy research is reserved exclusively for well-controlled clinical studies; it is only efficacy research that can prove cause-effect. The real-world limitations of "effectiveness" research prevent complete control of conditions and reduce confidence in conclusions about causality. Consequently, studies of effectiveness (i.e., outcomes research) are suited for making statements about trends, associations, and estimates. The efficacy-effectiveness distinction is captured in Sackett's dichotomy of randomized controlled clinical trials into *explanatory* and *management trials* (Sackett & Gent, 1979). Explanatory trials measure efficacy by ensuring ideal conditions in subject selection, strict adherence to an experimental protocol, and only counting outcomes predicted by theory to relate to the treatment process. In contrast, in management trials that measure effectiveness, all comers are accepted as subjects, treatment is given according to usual practice, and all outcomes occurring after randomization are counted. Lipsey (1990), however, argues that it becomes essential to deal with the reality of conditions that cannot be controlled. Therefore, clinical trials increasingly include quasi-experimental features, are conducted in multiple phases, and are accompanied by side studies (in Palmer, 1990).

So far in the discussion, there is agreement that efficacy research is designed to *prove*; outcomes research can only *identify trends, describe,* or *make associations or estimates.* But, if we are to extend

**Table 1.1**   Outcomes Measurement Classifications

| Classification | Description | Examples |
|---|---|---|
| Experimental or class I | Random assignment to intervention and control groups/phases | Randomized controlled clinical trials<br>Time series research (single-subject designs) |
| Quasi-experimental or class II | Nonrandom assignment to intervention and control groups/phases | Case-control studies<br>Cohort studies<br>Program evaluations<br>Quality improvement studies |
| Nonexperimental or class III | No clear comparison groups, or nonrandomized historical controls | Case studies or reports registries and databases<br>Group judgments or expert opinion |

*Source:* Adapted from Fineburg, H. V. (1990, May). The quest for causality in health services research. In L. Sechrest, E. Perrin, & J. Bunker (Eds.), Conference proceedings: Strengthening causal interpretation of nonexperimental data (pp. 215–220). Rockville, MD: Agency for Health Care Policy and Research, U.S. Department of Health and Human Services; and Report of the Therapeutics and Technology Assessment Subcommittee of the American Academy of Neurology. (1994, Mar). Assessment: melodic intonation therapy. *Neurology,* 44(3 Pt 1), 566–568.

the difference to the research concepts of efficacy and effectiveness, there is a parting of the ways. Proponents of efficacy research, as conceptualized by Kendall and Norton-Ford (1982), regard efficacy research as research that can prove treatment *effectiveness*, as well as other characteristics of efficacy, such as treatment *efficiency* and treatment *effects*. Thus, the concept of efficacy versus effectiveness research, in terms of differences in experimental control, becomes illogical. The terms that characterize treatment efficacy are described by Kendall and Norton-Ford as follows:

- *Treatment effectiveness:* Whether treatment does or does not work

- *Treatment efficiency:* Whether one treatment works better than another/whether all components are necessary in a treatment

- *Treatment effects:* Which aspects of treatment differentially influence which behaviors (see Chapter 12 by Olswang and Bain for further discussion)

Treatment efficacy *is* effectiveness; it, too, is efficiency and effects if we ascribe to the nomenclature of Kendall and Norton-Ford (1982). Treatment effectiveness does not, then, suggest research method (both outcomes research and efficacy research can investigate treatment effectiveness, only at differing degrees of experimental control and levels of confidence in interpretations of causality). It does characterize the aspect of treatment efficacy being investigated (i.e., whether or not the specified treatment works).

The term *treatment efficiency* finds yet a different spin on Kendall and Norton-Ford's (1982) definition, if viewed from the vantage of economics. According to the Joint Commission on Accreditation of Hospitals (JCAHO, 1994), treatment efficiency is the proportion of total cost (money, resources, time) that can be related to actual benefits received. Thus, efficiency refers to cost-effectiveness. Studies of this type link costs to clinical outcomes, and are sought by many payers who want to know what kind of value they are getting for the money spent.

### Classifications of Outcomes Measurement Methods

Outcomes measurement methodologies usually involve primary analysis of data (i.e., data from those sources that produce original knowledge about an intervention) and can be classified as *experimental, quasi-experimental,* or *nonexperimental.* Fineburg (1990), who views methodologies from the vantage of group designs, offers definitions:

*Experimental:* Studies that involve random or fully specifiable assignment to intervention and control groups. Randomized controlled clinical trials are included in this category.

*Quasi-experimental:* Studies that involve nonrandom (and not fully specified) assignment to intervention and control groups. Examples include program evaluation and quality improvement studies.

*Nonexperimental:* Studies that involve no clear comparison groups. Case studies and data registries are examples (see Chapter 14, by Kearns and de Riesthal).

Outcomes studies have also been classified, according to the quality of evidence yielded by various measurement methods, as *class I, class II,* and *class III evidence* (Report of the Therapeutics and Technology Assessment Subcommittee of the American Academy of Neurology, 1994). Holland, Fromm, DeRuyter, and Stein (1996) summarize these categories in a brief synopsis of the efficacy of the treatment of aphasia as follows:

*Class I:* Evidence provided by one or more well-designed randomized controlled clinical trials.

*Class II:* Evidence provided by one or more well-designed randomized clinical studies such as case-control, cohort studies, and so forth.

*Class III:* Evidence provided by expert opinion, nonrandomized historical controls, or one or more case reports.

Efficacy research, as described above, could be regarded as experimental or class I; outcomes research as quasi- or nonexperimental, or class II or class III. **Table 1.1** organizes various research methods used by clinical researchers, clinicians, or managers into these classifications. These design methodologies, however, cannot be so neatly catalogued. While we can differentiate efficacy and outcomes research methods, "they more accurately exist on a continuum where at some point in the middle, they overlap" (Olswang, personal communication). Even at the "low end" of outcomes research, certain methods (e.g., case studies), if well controlled, can constitute efficacy research. In addition, criticism has been directed toward study implications in terms of the quality of the methods categorized. Holland et al (1996) identify a weakness of the American Academy of Neurology (AAN) classifications in that they are based solely on the design of a study and do not guarantee the quality of the study itself. For example, they cite a study by Lincoln et al (1984), classified as a class I study, which seriously questions quality of evidence. First, its lack of treatment effects "was likely attributable to the facts that the 'treated' patients received less than 2 hours of treatment per week, given over a very short period of time, and the subjects were heterogeneous and included individuals with dementia and brain tumor" (p. 5). In contrast, a study by Poeck, Huber, and Willmes (1989), classified as a class II study, "incorporated an ingenious method of partialing out the effects of spontaneous recovery in both treated and untreated groups, thereby solving a particularly troublesome issue in relation to the effects of treatment" (p. 5). The same weakness can be extended to experimental, quasi-experimental, and nonexperimental studies because they, too, are classified by study design.

## Experimental (or Class I) Methods

Traditional thinking (Fineburg, 1990) in the medical field reserves randomized controlled trials as the only accepted method of experimental research—a position by clinical researchers who employ small-group or single-subject designs. Holland and colleagues (1996) remind us that large studies may not provide us with much information concerning the results of treatment for excluded subjects with comorbidities or unusual forms of disorders. So, too, they may not provide information on how the treatment works, the duration or intensity of treatment that might affect the efficacy of treatment, or the specific nature and quality of treatment that may or may not be effective with certain patients. These important efficacy questions may be answered more appropriately and economically by small-group or single-subject experimental studies.

According to Olswang (1990), efficacy research involves the use of *group (large or small)* or *single-subject experimental methods.* Group designs allow for the study of subject populations, thus permitting the generalization of results. They typically involve a treatment group and no-treatment or other-treatment control group. Behaviors between the groups are compared to note any differences. These designs, however, often suffer from problems associated with subject homogeneity, thereby threatening the validity of experimental findings.

Single-subject designs solve the problems associated with subject homogeneity in that a subject serves as his or her own control, or heterogeneity among subjects is systematically investigated. These designs methodologically rely on tight experimental control and replication within and across subjects to allow for enhanced generalizability of results. Thus, this type of efficacy research, unlike between-group designs, can reveal the nature of the interaction between the independent variable (treatment) and subject characteristics. The ways in which a subject or different subjects respond to different amounts and types of treatments become a rich source of information about the intervention process.

## Quasi-Experimental (or Class II) Methods

Most investigators would agree that any inferences made about causal relationships are impaired when the premises of the true experiment are breached (Sechrest & Hannah, 1990). But there are several reasons why experimental data are not always available, and why it may not be possible to produce them. Some experiments may not be ethical (e.g., an experiment that withholds treatment for a control group); some experiments are administratively and logistically impossible; some may be too expensive; some may require too much time to complete; some experiments may fail (e.g., due to loss of subjects); and some experiments may lack the ability to control all variables to draw conclusions. A quasi-experiment is one in which the researcher falls short of meeting all the parameters of the experimental research design, but with much of the study methodology in place.

The methodological and ethical dilemmas that underlie randomized clinical trials research have given rise to the slow but steady acceptance of less rigorous or quasi-experimental methods of outcomes measurement) including methods in the realms of program evaluation and quality improvement.

**Program Evaluation and Quality Improvement Methods**   *Program evaluation* methods were designed primarily to determine whether a program is meeting its goals. Both clinical and administrative goals are monitored. Program evaluation is defined in the Commission on Accreditation of Rehabilitation Facilities' Standards Manual for Medical Rehabilitation (CARF, 1997) as a system that enables the organization to identify the outcomes of its programs, the satisfaction of persons served, and follow-up on outcomes achieved by persons served.

As implied by CARF's definition, program evaluation activities must be outcome-oriented. Patton (1982) describes program evaluation as the systematic collection of information about the characteristics (structure), activities (process), and outcomes of programs and services that help administrators reduce uncertainty in the decisions they make regarding those same programs and services that they administer. Thus, program evaluation is a planned process of gathering and analyzing data to help reduce the risk of decisions.

*Quality improvement* methods were designed to determine primarily whether actual services comply with pre-established gold standards (e.g., accepted practice parameters).

In this sense, the methods constitute comparison testing. However, with recognition that methods also can be designed to acquire new knowledge, quality improvement activities can result in establishing or refining gold standards. Quality assessment and improvement are defined broadly by the Joint Commission on Accreditation of Healthcare Organizations (JCAHO, 1997) in its standards for improving organization performance:

PI.1. The hospital has a planned, systematic, hospital wide approach to process design and performance measurement, assessment, and improvement.

PI.3.1. The hospital collects data on important processes and outcomes related to patient care and organization functions.

PI.5. The hospital systematically improves its performance (pp. 134–136).

The methods typically involve a systematic process, as described above, of Plan–Do–Study–Act. With the introduction of systems thinking in quality improvement activities, all structural inputs and processes (including clinical, organizational, support, and administrative) share equal importance in influencing positive outcomes. As managers acquire advanced computer technologies and statistical knowledge, both program evaluation and quality improvement methods are becoming more sophisticated from theoretical and scientific standpoints.

**Other Methods**   Other quasi-experimental methods include case-control studies and cohort studies, catalogued in the field of epidemiology (i.e., the study of the nature, cause, control, and determinants of the frequency and distribution of disease, disability, and death in human populations) (Timmreck, 1994). Both studies are considered observational because no one attempts to intervene or to alter the course of the disease.

*Case-control studies* are retrospective studies because they are conducted after the onset of an outbreak and "look backward" to the possible causes of the outbreak. "Case-control" refers to the way in which the study group is put together. These studies begin assessment of the persons or groups with a disease, condition, or disorder (cases) and identify a separate control group that has not been affected (controls). The possible causes of the disease, condition, or disorder constitute the outcome under study (Riegelman & Hirsch, 1989).

*Cohort studies* are prospective studies because they are conducted before the onset outbreak and "look forward" to assess morbidity and mortality. "Cohort" means a group of persons who share a common characteristic, especially age. Cohort studies begin with a study group that possesses the characteristic(s) under study and a control group that is free of this characteristic. Both groups are followed forward in time to determine whether they will develop a particular condition. The occurrence of the condition is the outcome under study (Riegelman & Hirsch, 1989).

### Nonexperimental (or Class III) Methods

*Case reports*, use of databases or registries, group judgments, and expert opinion are among the nonexperimental methods. These methods, while subjective and fraught with a lack of experimental controls, are useful in that they can be conducted by clinicians and managers for large groups of clients, and lend support to quasi- and experimental studies of treatment efficacy or outcome. These methods can also help to prompt and shape causal hypotheses.

### Synthetic Analysis

In contrast to outcomes measurement methods that involve primary analysis of data, methods that involve synthetic analysis (i.e., studies that refer to available knowledge, which involve synthesis of information to gain new insights) should be mentioned. Some of these methods include meta-analysis, cost-benefit or cost-effectiveness analyses, and technology assessment.

*Meta-analysis* is a method for reviewing and summarizing clusters of prior studies, irrespective of their differences. The results of studies are statistically combined, thus producing a single estimate of an intervention or an effect from studies that use different scales to measure the effectiveness of an intervention (Eddy, 1990; Smith & Glass, 1977).

*Cost-benefit* or *cost-effectiveness analyses* are conducted to determine how outcomes compare with their costs. They also are conducted for comparative purposes in determining which provider can achieve the same outcomes at a lower cost. Thus, costs and outcomes are linked in data analysis, often via use of automated management information systems or existing data banks available from large payers, such as Medicare, Medicaid, and Blue Cross/Blue Shield. A cost-benefit analysis determines the economic efficiency of a program expressed as the relationship between dollars spent and dollars saved. A cost-effectiveness analysis explores the effectiveness of a program in achieving targeted intervention outcomes in relation to the program costs (e.g., dollars spent per points on a functional outcome measure) (Rossi & Freeman, 1982).

*Technology assessment* denotes any process of examining and reporting properties of a technology used in clinical care, such as safety, efficacy, feasibility, and indications for use, cost, and cost-effectiveness, as well as social, economic, and ethical consequences. Assessment ideally includes evaluation of immediate results of the technology as well as its long-term consequences. A comprehensive assessment of a technology may also include an appraisal of problems of personnel training and licensure, new capital expenditures for equipment and buildings, and possible consequences for the health insurance industry and social security system. Currently, the predominant assessment methods are literature reviews and consultation with experts.

Technology assessments historically have been conducted on a reactive, ad hoc basis (e.g., in reaction to inquiries by third-party payers) rather than by systematic review and priority setting. Consequently, rigorous clinical evaluation of technologies (e.g., clinical trials research) largely has been confined to the final regulatory step of premarket approval (Institute of Medicine, Committee for Evaluation of Medical Technologies, 1985).

## Multiple-Attacks Approach

Perhaps the most effective approach to outcomes measurement is one of multiple attacks. By this I mean the measurement of outcomes from multiple but independent sources using various methods. Mosteller (1990) believes a multiple attacks approach is more influential in shaping public policy than outcomes data from one study or a collection of studies using the same method. Considering the spectrum of methods, the concept of multiple attacks has appeal for both the researcher and the clinician.

As explained in an earlier publication (Frattali, 1996), we have looked historically to our scientists to conduct the needed experimental research to amass outcomes data and prove that what we do makes a difference. Given the various outcomes measurement methods either advanced or in use today, such a view is myopic. Outcomes research methodologies, because of their less stringent design characteristics, are amenable for use in real-world settings with large patient populations. While causal interpretations must be qualified by study design limitations, findings can lend support to experimental evidence of efficacy. Outcomes research methodologies, in fact, may be a bridge to the longstanding schism between clinicians (who argue that research is seldom clinically relevant) and researchers (who argue that clinicians seldom apply research findings to clinical practice).

### How Are Outcomes Managed?

Once we measure outcomes, we must manage them if they are to have any purpose at all. The management of outcomes gives rise to the development of new standards of practice and management tools such as critical paths (i.e., treatment regimes, supported ideally by patient outcomes research, that include only those vital elements that have been proved to affect patient outcomes) to increase both treatment- and cost-effectiveness. Thus, we can move from assumption-driven to data-driven clinical methods. Ellwood (1988) concisely defines the field of outcomes management in the context of health care:

"Outcomes Management is a technology of patient experience designed to help patients, payers, providers make rational [health care]-related choices based on better insight into the impact of these choices on the patient's life. Outcomes Management consists of:

- Common patient-understood language of health outcomes;

- A national database containing clinical, financial, and health outcome information and analysis that estimates as best we can the relationship between [health care] interventions and health outcomes, as well as the relationship between health outcomes and money;

- An opportunity for each decision maker to have access to those analyses that are relevant to the choices they must make" (p. 4).

The best outcomes data can exist without anyone knowing and, thus, without any influence on clinical practice. In order for us to manage outcomes, outcomes data must be translated into practice guidelines and protocols, which in turn should be distributed widely in efforts to change practitioners' ways of doing things and, thus, reach desired outcomes in a more predictable manner.

## ◆ Conclusion

There is no need for euphemism on what is driving the need for outcomes data. We all know it is cost pressures. But it was costly, under a retrospective payment system, to support practitioners who were paid for any service they wished to provide with no accountability for the end result. It is equally worrisome to wonder if practitioners in a prepaid system might withhold needed care because they stand to gain financially from doing so (Berwick et al, 1990). Outcomes data, then, become the link to knowledge about the appropriateness and quality of care.

Many practitioners believe that in a cost-driven system, money saved, not outcomes gained, is the object. This view is short-sighted. As quality of care suffers, consumers (e.g., clients, families, managed care systems, regulators) will not remain passive, particularly if given a choice of providers. In the long-term, practitioners who can prove both cost-effectiveness and quality of care will gain a strategic advantage in what has become a competitive game of service delivery.

We have a task before us—to cumulate outcomes data, not only to prove that what we do works, but to continually upgrade what we do. Thus, we have a second task—to apply new knowledge to new practice patterns. Fineburg (1990) speaks about the connections of causality, convincingness, and change. He explains that one measure of success in research is the extent to which the knowledge produced by researchers leads to action. In the design of studies, analysis of data, and presentation of findings, we should never lose sight of the purposes of the investigation and what audiences we want to convince. For whom is the investigation being conducted? What are their needs, beliefs, interests, and incentives? It is naive not to recognize that surprising or unwelcome results will be met with much more skepticism and scrutiny than will results that confirm preconceptions or satisfy political agendas. But, if we are to do our jobs, we must engage controversial and political topics.

Holland (cited in Goldberg, 1993) believes we must be masters of our fate—for our professional integrity and for the sake of our clients. To do that, "we must take what we know from efficacy studies, see that the results are translated into practice guidelines, and make sure that those guidelines are widely disseminated and followed" (p. 45). Every individual has the right to expect the best of what exists in clinical practice.

Outcomes measurement begins with inquiry. Clinical questions are subjected to systematic study. The findings lead to yet other questions that are explored, answered, and generate more questions. Clinical inquiry and its subsequent study form the foundation of any clinical discipline. We must ask the questions, and seek to answer them intelligently using various methodologies under the rubric of outcomes measurement.

# References

Agency for Health Care Policy and Research. (1994). *Distinguishing between efficacy and effectiveness.* Rockville, MD: Author

American Speech-Language-Hearing Association. (1995). *ASHA Task Force on Treatment Outcomes and Cost Effectiveness: Project overview and status.* Rockville, MD: Author

Batavia, A. I. (1992, Jul-Sep). Assessing the function of functional assessment: a consumer perspective. *Disability and Rehabilitation, 14,* 156–160

Benninger, M. S., Gardner, G. M., Jacobson, B. H., & Grywalski, C. (1997). New dimensions in measuring voice treatment outcomes. In R. T. Sataloff (Ed.), *Professional voice: The science and art of clinical care* (2nd ed., pp. 789–794). San Diego, CA: Singular Publishing Group

Berwick, D. M. (1989). E.A. Codman and the rhetoric of battle: A commentary. *The Milbank Quarterly, 67,* 262–267

Berwick, D. M., Godfrey, A. B., & Roessner, J. (1990). *Curing health care: A report on the National Demonstration Project on Quality Improvement in Health Care.* San Francisco: Jossey-Bass

Brewster, A. C., Karlin, B. G., Hyde, L. A., Jacobs, C. M., Bradbury, R. C., & Chae, Y. M. (1985, Winter). MEDISGRPS: a clinically based approach to classifying hospital patients at admission. *Inquiry, 22,* 377–387

Brinkley, J. (1986). U.S. releasing lists of hospitals with abnormal mortality rates. *New York Times,* 12 March: 1

Cichowski, K. (1995). *Rehabilitation Institute of Chicago Functional Assessment Scale-Revised.* Chicago: Rehabilitation Institute of Chicago

Codman, E. A. (1917). *A study in hospital efficiency as demonstrated by the case report of the first five years of a private hospital.* Boston: Thomas Todd Company

Codman, E. A. (1934). *The shoulder: Rupture of the supraspinatus tendon and other lesions in or about the subacromial bursa.* Boston: Thomas Todd Company

Commission on Accreditation of Rehabilitation Facilities (CARF). (1997). *Standards manual and interpretive guidelines for medical rehabilitation.* Tucson, AZ: Author

Deming, W. E. (1982). *Out of the crisis.* Cambridge: Massachusetts Institute of Technology, Center for Advanced Engineering Study

Donabedian, A. (1980). *Explorations in quality assessment and monitoring. Volume 1: The definition of quality and approaches to its assessment.* Ann Arbor, MI: Health Administration Press

Donabedian, A. (1985). *The methods and findings of quality assessment and monitoring: An Illustrated analysis. Volume 3.* Ann Arbor, MI: Health Administration Press

Eddy, D. M. (1990). The role of meta-analysis. In L. Sechrest, E. Perrin, & J. Bunker (Eds.), *Conference proceedings: Strengthening causal interpretation of nonexperimental data* (pp. 173–176). Rockville, MD: U.S. Department of Health and Human Services, Public Health Service, Agency for Health Care Policy and Research

Ellwood, P. M. (1988, Jun). Shattuck lecture—outcomes management. A technology of patient experience. *The New England Journal of Medicine, 318,* 1549–1556

Evaluation Systems International, Inc. (1994). *OUTCOME TM.* Denver, CO: Author

Fetter, R. B., Shin, Y., Freeman, J. L., Averill, R. F., & Thompson, J. D. (1980, Feb). Case mix definition by diagnosis-related groups. *Medical Care, 18*(2, Suppl), iii, 1–53

Fineburg, H. V. (1990). The quest for causality in health services research. In L. Sechrest, E. Perrin, & J. Bunker (Eds.), *Conference proceedings: Strengthening causal interpretation of nonexperimental data* (pp. 215–220). Rockville, MD: U.S. Department of Health and Human Services, Public Health Service, Agency for Health Care Policy and Research

Focus Rehab, Inc. (1995). *The Functional Outcome and Utilization System* (F.O.C.U.S.). Nashville, TN: Author

Frattali, C. M. (1996). Childhood language perspectives: Clinical outcome perspectives. In M.D. Smith & J.S. Damico (Eds.), *Childhood language disorders.* (pp. 3–16). New York: Thieme Medical Publishers

Frattali, C. M., Thompson, C. K., Holland, A. L., Wohl, C. B., & Ferketic, M. M. (1995). *The American Speech-Language-Hearing Association functional assessment of communication skills for (ASHA FACS).* Rockville, MD: ASHA

Goldberg, B. (1993, Jan). Translating data into practice. *ASHA, 35,* 45–47

Harvey, R. G., & Jellinek, H. M. (1979). *Patient evaluation and conference system: PECS.* Wheaton, IL: Marianjoy Rehabilitation Center

Harvey, R. F., & Jellinek, H. M. (1981, Sep). Functional performance assessment: a program approach. *Archives of Physical Medicine and Rehabilitation, 62,* 456–460

Holland, A. L., Fromm, D. S., DeRuyter, E., & Stein, M. (1996). Efficacy of treatment for aphasia: A brief synopsis. *Journal of Speech and Hearing Research, 39,* S27–S36

Horn, S.D., Sharkey, P.D., Buckle, J.M., Backofen, J.E., Averill, R.E, & Horn, R.A. (1991). The relationship between severity of illness and hospital length of stay and mortality. *Medical Care, 29*(4), 305-317.

Iezzoni, L. I. (Ed.) (1994). *Risk adjustment for measuring health care outcomes. Ann* Arbor, MI: Health Administration Press

Iezzoni, L. I., & Moskowitz, M. A. (1988, Dec). A clinical assessment of MedisGroups. *Journal of the American Medical Association, 260,* 3159–3163

Institute of Medicine, Committee for Evaluation of Medical Technologies. (1985). *Assessing medical technologies.* Washington, DC: National Academy Press

Jacobson, B. H., Johnson, A., & Grywalski, C. (1995). *The Voice Handicap Index.* Detroit, MI: Henry Ford Hospital, Division of Speech-Language Sciences & Disorders, Department of Neurology

Joint Commission on Accreditation of Healthcare Organizations (JCAHO). (1997). *Hospital accreditation standards.* Oakbrook Terrace, IL: Author

Joint Commission on Accreditation of Hospitals (JCAH). (1994). *Accreditation manual.* Oakbrook Terrace, IL: Author

Kendall, P., & Norton-Ford, J. (1982). Therapy outcome research methods. In P. Kendall & J. Butcher (Eds.), *Handbook of research methods in clinical psychology* (pp. 429–460). New York: John Wiley and Sons

Knaus, W. A., Zimmerman, J. E., Wagner, D. P., Draper, E. A., & Lawrence, D. E. (1981, Aug). APACHE—acute physiology and chronic health evaluation: a physiologically based classification system. *Critical Care Medicine, 9,* 591–597

Lincoln, N. B., McGuirk, E., Mulley, G. P., Lendrem, W., Jones, A. C., & Mitchell, J. R. (1984, Jun). Effectiveness of speech therapy for aphasic stroke patients. A randomised controlled trial. *Lancet, 1,* 1197–1200

Lipsey, M. W. (1990). Theory as method: Small theories of treatments. In L. Sechrest, E. Perrin, & J. Bunker (Eds.), *Conference proceedings: Strengthening causal interpretation of nonexperimental data* (pp. 33–52). Rockville, MD: U.S. Department of Health and Human Services, Public Health Service, Agency for Health Care Policy and Research

McReynolds, L. (1990). Historical perspective of treatment efficacy research. In L. B. Olswang, C. K. Thompson, S. E. Warren, & N. J. Minghetti (Eds.), *Treatment efficacy research in communication disorders* (pp. 5–14). Rockville, MD: American Speech-Language-Hearing Foundation

Merson, R. M., Rolnick, M. L., & Weiner, R. (1995). *The Beaumont Outcome Software System (BOSS).* West Bloomfield, MI: Parrot Software

Mosteller, E. (1990), Improving research methodology: An overview. In L. Sechrest, E. Perrin, & J. Bunker (Eds.), *Conference proceedings: Strengthening causal interpretation of nonexperimental data* (pp. 221–230). Rockville, MD: U.S.

Department of Health and Human Services, Public Health Service, Agency for Health Care Policy and Research

Nagi, S. Z. (1965). Some conceptual issues in disability and rehabilitation. In M. B. Sussman (Ed.), *Sociology and rehabilitation* (pp. 100–113). Washington, DC: American Sociological Association

National Institutes of Health. (1993 March). *Research plan for the National Center for Medical Rehabilitation Research.* NIH Pub. No. 93–35091. Bethesda, MD: U.S. Department of Health and Human Services

Office of Technology Assessment. (1978). *Assessing the efficacy and safety of medical technologies.* (OTA Publication No. OTA-H-75). Washington, DC: Author

Olswang, L. B. (1990). Treatment efficacy: The breadth of research. In L. E. Olswang, C. K. Thompson, S. P. Warren, & N. J. Minghetti (Eds.), *Treatment efficacy research in communication disorders* (pp. 99–103). Rockville, MD: American Speech-language-Hearing Foundation

Olswang, L. B., Thompson, C. K., Warren, S. F., & Minghetti, N. (Eds.). (1990). *Treatment efficacy research in communication disorders.* Rockville, MD: American Speech-language-Hearing Foundation

Palmer, R. H. (1990). Small theories of programs. In L. Sechrest, E. Perrin, & J. Bunker (Eds.), *Conference proceedings: Strengthening causal interpretation of nonexperimental data* (pp. 57–60). Rockville, MD: U.S. Department of Health and Human Services, Public Health Service, Agency for Health Care Policy and Research

Parkside Associates, Inc. (1986). *Level of Rehabilitation Scale III.* Park Ridge, IL: Author (Now available from Formations in Health Care, Chicago)

Patton, M. Q. (1982). *Practical evaluation.* Beverly Hills, CA: Sage Publications

Poeck, K., Huber, W., & Willmes, K. (1989, Aug). Outcome of intensive language treatment in aphasia. *The Journal of Speech and Hearing Disorders, 54,* 471–479

Pope, A. M., & Tarlov, A. L. (Eds.). (1991). *Disability in America: Toward a national agenda for prevention.* Washington, DC: National Academy Press

Report of the Therapeutics and Technology Assessment Subcommittee of the American Academy of Neurology. (1994, Mar). Assessment: melodic intonation therapy. *Neurology, 44*(3 Pt 1), 566–568

Riegelman, R. K., & Hirsch, R. E.(1989). *Studying a study and testing a test.* Boston: Little, Brown and Company

Rosen, A., & Proctor, E. K. (1981, Jun). Distinctions between treatment outcomes and their implications for treatment evaluation. *Journal of Consulting and Clinical Psychology, 49,* 418–425

Rossi, P. H., & Freeman, H. E. (1982). *Evaluation: A systematic approach* (2nd ed.). Beverly Hills: Sage Publications

Sackett, D. L., & Gent, M. (1979, Dec). Controversy in counting and attributing events in clinical trials. *The New England Journal of Medicine, 301,* 1410–1412

Sechrest, L., & Hannah, M.(1990). The critical importance of nonexperimental data. In L. Sechrest, E. Perrin, & J. Bunker (Eds.), *Conference proceedings: Strengthening causal interpretation of nonexperimental data* (pp. 1–8). Rockville, MD: U.S. Department of Health and Human Services, Public Health Service, Agency for Health Care Policy and Research

Smith, M. L., & Glass, G. V. (1977, Sep). Meta-analysis of psychotherapy outcome studies. *The American Psychologist, 32,* 752–760

State University of New York at Buffalo Research Foundation. (1993). *Guide for use of the Uniform Data Set for Medical Rehabilitation: Functional Independence Measure.* Buffalo: Author

Stineman, M. G., Escarce, J. J., Goin, J. E., Hamilton, B. B., Granger, C. V., & Williams, S. V. (1994, Apr). A case-mix classification system for medical rehabilitation. *Medical Care, 32,* 366–379

Timmreck, T. C. (1994). *An introduction to epidemiology.* Boston: Jones and Bartlett Publishers

Vladeck, B. C. (1984, Apr). Medicare hospital payment by diagnosis-related groups. *Annals of Internal Medicine, 100,* 576–591

Wennberg, J., & Gittelsohn, A. (1973, Dec). Small area variations in health care delivery. *Science, 182,* 1102–1108

Wilkerson, D. L., Batavia, A. L., & DeJong, G. (1992). Use of functional status measures for payoff medical rehabilitation services. *Archives of Physical Medicine and Rehabilitation, 73,* 111–120

Wilson, I. B., & Cleary, P. D. (1995). Linking clinical variables with health-related quality of life: A conceptual model of patient outcomes. *Journal of the American Medical Association, 273,* 59–65

World Health Organization(1980). *International classification of impairments, disabilities, and handicaps.* Geneva: Author

# 2

# Outcomes Measurement: Converging Issues, Trends, and Influences

*Lee Ann C. Golper*

## ♦ Chapter Focus

This chapter reflects upon several of the evolutions in outcomes measurement that have transpired since the publication of the first edition of this text, 14 years ago. This author examines broad contemporary issues including "tail spinning" economic pressures, political and social changes, technological advances, and changing expectations for efficiencies and accountability within health care and education. These issues are raised to create a backdrop for more focused treatment of their impact and influence in speech-language pathology in other chapters and to demonstrate how global events are converging to promote outcome measurement as a fundamental concern in all speech-language pathology clinical service settings and graduate education.

## ♦ Introduction

In the preceding chapter, reprinted from the first edition of this text, Frattali made several observations about the future of outcome research, and predicted that outcome data will

- become the link to knowledge about the appropriateness and quality of care;
- help practitioners gain a strategic advantage in service delivery;
- enable consumers to expect the best practices in clinical services; and
- ensure the advancement of clinical disciplines.

This chapter considers these forecasts in light of several contemporary developments that have pushed outcome research and outcomes measurement toward greater and greater prominence across all of the settings in which speech-language pathology clinicians and educators work. The past decade in particular has brought a steep march toward greater demand for efficient, cost-effective, and accountable services in health care and education at a time when electronic data storage capacity is measured on an *exabyte* scale (Stewart, 2011). The ability to crunch bigger numbers faster has resulted in easier and more varied ways to capture, share, and apply outcome data for greater transparency and an increased reliance on data for decision making in all industries.

Regardless of the type of professional work we perform or the setting where we perform it, outcome data are now the "scorecards" against which the value and utility of our work are measured. The increasing demand for meaningful, cost-effective outcomes from policy makers and stakeholders is both a common *threat* and a common *thread* reaching into all corners of the profession. But, when understood and embraced, outcome measures should improve the quality and appropriateness of services, strengthen the position of practitioners, promote best practices, and ensure the continued advancement of the profession (Frattali, 1998a).

## ♦ The Elephant in the Room

No discussion about the current emphasis on outcome measurement within health care and education in the United States could proceed without acknowledging the elephant in the room—the worldwide economic crisis. Although jobs that are allied with health care and education have been relatively spared compared with other industries, the ultimate effect of corrective actions with federal budgetary cutbacks is pervasive. The present and predicted future economic stresses are at the heart of all of the pencil-sharpening actions and mandates from the federal government that are discussed in Chapter 4 and elsewhere, aimed at budget reconciliations and spending course corrections

To illustrate this trend, **Fig. 2.1** provides a graph from the Congressional Budget Office (CBO) that combines historical data and projected revenue and expenditures as a percent of the gross domestic product (U.S. Federal Budget, n.d.; CBO, 2011, n.d.). The trends shown across the revenue versus expenditure lines amply demonstrate the point that cost-containment and accountability are going to

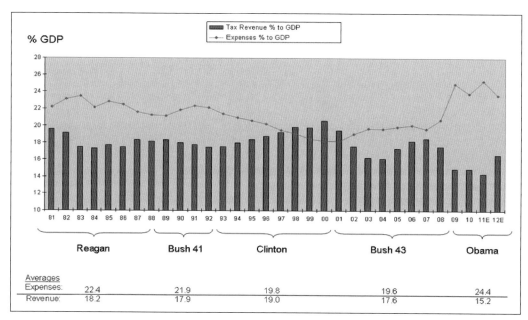

**Fig. 2.1** Tax revenue and expenses as a percent of the gross domestic product (GDP) 1981–2012. (From http://en.wikipedia.org/wiki/United_States_federal_budget. Original data sources: Congressional Budget Office, Office of Management and Budget: historical tables [http://www.whitehouse.gov/omb/budget/Historicals/] and Congressional Budget, 2011 [http://www.cbo.gov/ftpdocs/120xx/doc12039/HistoricalTables%5B1%5D.pdf].)

be permanent fixtures in publicly funded programs. At this writing, there are strident debates within the U.S. Congress over measures to balance the federal budget that are predicted to result in funding cuts in programs in the Department of Health and Human Services and the Department of Education. The new rules for Individuals with Disabilities Education Act (IDEA) Part C, published in September, 2011, include major changes related to eligibility criteria, and currently there are five bills sitting in Congress proposing changes in "No Child Left Behind."

Economic stress is a primary "converging factor" heightening the importance of outcome measurement in education and health care. The many references to initiatives, mandates, measurement tools, and incentives for efficiencies that are peppered throughout this text would not have developed at such a rapid pace or have been so far-reaching were it not for acute fiscal concerns. These factors have elevated the discussion and scrutiny of *cost* as a factor in the public's assessment of the relative *value* of education and health care services. The terms *value, value analysis, value-based purchasing,* and *value-added service* appear in several chapters in this text, all essentially referencing the outcome equation: *quality/cost = value.*

# ♦ Enhancing Quality Through Research

When clinical practices are informed by the best available evidence, the value of these services is enhanced. In the estimation of worth, scientific evidence adds weight to the "quality" side of the *quality/cost = value* equation. A quotation from John Eisenberg, the administrator for the Agency for Health Care Policy and Research (AHPR) within the Centers for Medicare and Medicaid Services (CMS) in 1997, is frequently used to define quality: "At its most basic level, quality is doing the right thing, at the right time, in the right way, for the right person" (Eisenberg, 1997, p. 1). If quality means doing the right things, then the definition of quality should be derived from unbiased evidence, not economic, social, or political influences. The application of scientific methods to the definition of what the *right* procedures (in clinical service or graduate education) are and how to best apply them and with whom, is the essence of *evidence-based practice* (EBP). The persistent question is: How do we rationally and realistically integrate scientifically proven interventions (EBP) into the unpredictable, individualized, end-user world of clinical practice (Justice, 2008; Kamhi, 2011)? Responses to that question are evident in the growing emphasis on "bench-to-bedside" research, or *translational research* (Zerhouni, 2003); a call for more of $N = 1$, case-based studies, and single-subject experimentation (Kamhi, 2011; Tsapas & Matthews, 2008); a growing acknowledgment of the role of empirically based evidence generated from clinical practices, also called practice-based evidence (PBE) (Westfall, Mold, & Fagnan; 2007); and comparative effectiveness research (Fenstermacher, 2010).

## Treatment Outcomes Research

Treatment efficacy research, ranging from large-scale, randomized-controlled trials (RCTs) to carefully controlled, single-subject experimental designs (SSEDs), seeks to compare therapies, to compare treatment to no treatment, to determine who is likely to benefit or not benefit from a given intervention, and to identify optimal procedures (timing, dosage, sequence) in interventions.

*Translational* research in medicine typically involves questions that are tested in the research laboratory, followed by clinical trials, and then, if the treatment effects remain promising, introduced into point-of-service clinical practice (effectiveness research). *Effectiveness* research essentially tests to see if procedures demonstrated as efficacious in the research laboratory are indeed effective in real-life clinical practice, where the pristine controls of the laboratory are not practical. Effectiveness research helps to establish the degrees of allowable variations outside of ideal conditions. *Systematic reviews* (SRs) of research literature are measures taken to scrutinize the research methods of a group of studies addressing a related question that meet predetermined criteria, to identify potential bias or methodological flaws, and elucidate the conclusions that can confidently be made from the collective findings. Well-executed systematic reviews are the backbone of EBP. *Practice guidelines* and *standards of care* ideally are based on the *best available*, or least biased, evidence. The processes of executing, analyzing, and making recommendations based on treatment outcomes research provide the guideposts for clinicians so they can consistently do the right things, in the right way, at the right time, and with the right person.

## ◆ Outcome Data

References to *outcome data* are evident throughout this text from several perspectives: to define quality, cost, and value of results; to address federal mandates and public policies; to ensure compliance with accreditation processes; to evaluate interventions with individuals; to inform and improve clinical services; to evaluate organizational performance; and to determine if teaching methods are effective. The demand for good data comes from all corners of our professional globe, and the significance of the potential impact of data has never been more acute. Quoting an observation made by a medical department chair recently,

> I remain absolutely steadfast in thinking that good data presented coherently, persuasively, and persistently will have an impact. But today it's not just laboratory-based research or even population-based science, it's also economics, law, sociology, examination of medical care delivery systems, issues of human behavior, and how people respond in seeking medical care. (Schaffner, 2011)

Outcome data can come from quantitative, objective measures, such as biometric assessments (vital signs, laboratory findings), behavioral measures (test scores, behavioral observations), instrumental measures (endoscopies, acoustic analysis), or measures of a nonobservable trait (satisfaction, perceived level of handicap). The scales used to measure outcomes can range from within-person change measures to large compendia of data sets across vast populations. Computer technology has engendered the latter with the phenomenal growth in electronic data storage and sharing capacity. The capacity to gather and manage big data, coupled with the application of *metadata* technologies, is providing another of the factors converging on outcome measurement today.

### Big Data

Readers born after the time when personal and general purpose computing had become second-nature and electronic communication devices a standard appendage, let's say sometime after the mid-1980s, may find it difficult to appreciate the mind-boggling expansion in information captures and availability that has taken place in recent years. The growth in computerized information *storage capacity* is documented in a study by Hilbert and López (2011), who found the per capita capacity of the world's general-purpose computers doubled every 18 months over the two decades studied, from 1986 through 2007. The authors note, "The majority of our technological memory has been in digital format since the early 2000s (94% in 2007)" (p. 60). This data storage trend is illustrated in **Fig. 2.2**. The increased capacity for information storage has created millions of virtual warehouses of vast amounts of structured and unstructured "mega" data, with data storage worldwide having reached an *exabyte* scale (one billion gigabytes) proportion (Stewart, 2011), illustrated graphically in **Fig. 2.3**. The ever-expanding volume of information generated within individual organizations and the demand for information by business, health care, government, researchers, and various auditing and oversight groups is keeping individuals with expertise in information technology in high demand. Information technology (IT) teams are continuously challenged to design new ways to capture, store, and retrieve massive amounts of structured data (e.g., spread sheets) and unstructured

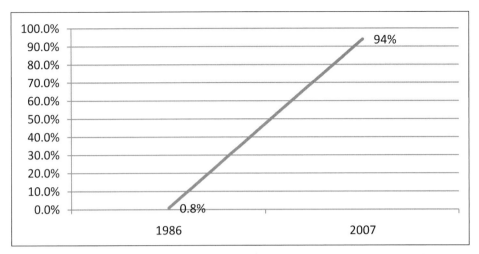

**Fig. 2.2**   Trajectory of technological memory in digital format. [Data from Hilbert, M., & López, P. (2011, Apr). The world's technological capacity to store, communicate, and compute information. *Science, 332*(6025), 60–65.]

data (e.g., verbatim interviews, word documents, PDFs, audio and video files, security data from video canvassing) efficiently. IT is also challenged to manage the security of the data to protect their use for the intended and appropriate purposes. To appreciate that immensity of that challenge and the security risks to electronic data, a must-read for every computer user is *Worm: The First Digital World War*, by Mark Bowden (2011).

## Metadata

*Metadata* is the cornerstone of information technology, particularly in bioinformatics. It provides the indexing and search methods necessary to sort and use vast amounts of information. The term *meta-data* first appeared in an English-language dictionary in 1983 and has been defined as data that

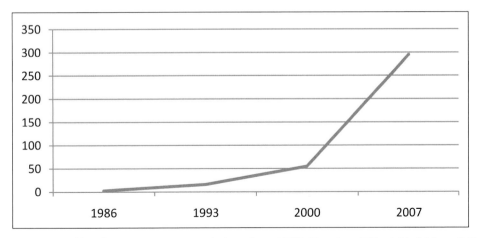

**Fig. 2.3**   World's information storage capacity in exabytes ($10^{18}$). [Data from Hilbert, M., & López, P. (2011, Apr). The world's technological capacity to store, communicate, and compute information. *Science, 332*(6025), 60–65.]

provide information about other data (Mish, 1983); or "data, information and knowledge on data, information and knowledge" (Execution Make It Happen, n.d.). In bioinformatics, metadata refers to data that describe other data in the databases applied to medical science and health-related questions (Fenstermacher, 2010). Although computerization has allowed for extraordinary advances in metadata capacity, storage, management, and applications, metadata should not be thought of as strictly an electronic, computer-age phenomenon. Some of us can recall using our university or community libraries' physical card file, with its 3-by-5 file cards listing the title of the book, author, year of publication, publisher, subject, the location of the book within the library stacks, and handwritten entries on the back of the card listing who checked out the book, when it was checked out, and when it was returned. This information is metadata—information about information. When authors check a reference to verify the provenance of a quotation or citation in the research literature, by searching either the paper copy or electronically accessed articles, they are performing operations on metadata. Appreciating that metadata do not necessarily require a computer, electronic computers are mighty handy when faced with large, master data files requiring abstracting critical data sets that need to be organized efficiently, accessed quickly, and, more importantly, shared across users. Computers provide an efficient means to sort and abstract information of interest from large data sets to identify relationships, draw inferences (knowledge), and create documents (worksheets, tables, reports) that can then be automatically represented in multiple languages and formats (dash boards, scorecards, graphs) and shared by geographically remote users.

Creating metadata simply means storing an underlying backbone of descriptive and definitional information about a piece of data in a way that will allow for capturing particular *information elements* or the *content collection* that is contained in the data files. Metadata make it possible to design compatible networked files, so content can be exported or new content can be imported. Information elements for a file's content can then be defined to keep track of who created it and when it was created, as well as the *semantic knowledge*—the descriptive characteristics of the information contained in the file and the associated data sets that are in the database. An example of metadata operations is found in the designs of electronic classroom support platforms commonly used in universities, such as *Blackboard* (Blackboard Inc., n.d.; http://www.blackboard.com), which has metadata features. These electronic classroom platforms enable instructors to create metadata fields for data file sharing within and between courses, and track predefined functions. Instructors can create metadata content pages that specify fields such as the title of the file, the source, the date of creation, the contributors, the authors and roles of the authors, any technical information related to the format of the file, the intended use of the content, and so forth. Files can then be saved to the content collection and shared with others.

## Predictive Modeling

*Predictive modeling* refers to constructs and statistical regression analysis methods to make certain predictions based on patterns within the data that are collected. The use of predictive modeling statistics originated in the field of archeology in the 1950s (Geisser, 1993). Predictive modeling is now used extensively in business, where the methods are referred to as *data mining,* to predict customer behavior and manage customer relationships. When you make a purchase online or conduct a Google search, you are both accessing information from databases and entering data about yourself (your email or IP address, search patterns, interests, reading preferences, spending patterns, and so forth). Those data are then used to make predictions about the likelihood of your engaging in certain future actions. When Netflix "suggests" a movie for you based on your movie rental patterns, say, "other movies starring George Clooney," those recommendations come from predictive modeling.

Various filtering methods and predictive modeling are part of the heuristic tools used to screen out spam messages, based on key words within the sender address, URL, subject line, type style, content of the message, and so forth. In health care, biostatisticians use predictive modeling to calculate the probability of an individual's developing a particular medical condition based on key words and values (data) in the patient's history and the patient's familial history of the incidence of that condition. Predictive modeling has been a centerpiece of *disease management risk stratification* for many years (Cousins, Shickle, & Bander, 2002), but the application of predictive modeling to health care decision making is a fairly recent development linked to cost containment, quality management, and implementation of standards of care and best practices. *Disease-specific predictive models* are increasingly being applied to inform the decisions about the suitability of particular care settings and clinical interventions in high-risk populations such as elders with multiple chronic health conditions (Rogers & Joyner, n.d.; Sylvia et al, 2006). One needs to be cautious when applying statistical tools such as predictive modeling to health care data. Statisticians warn us that no matter how well-designed the IT models are, erroneous conclusions may be drawn and wrong decisions made if the contributing data are biased, conflicting, or incomplete (Axelrod & Vogel, 2003).

## Data-Driven Risk Management

As is discussed later in this text, two consensus reports published by the Institute of Medicine's (IOM) Committee on Quality of Health Care in America—*To Err Is Human: Building a Safer Health System* (IOM, 1999) and *Crossing the Quality Chasm: A New Health System for the 21st Century* (IOM, 2001)—have been particularly influential in shaping the course and magnitude of outcome measurement in health care organizations. These companion reports spotlighted epidemiological data demonstrating the devastating effects of medical errors, resulting in tens of thousands of deaths annually (IOM, 1999), and defined six broad targets for improving care delivery (IOM, 2001). Care should be *safe, effective, patient-centered, timely, efficient,* and *equitable*. These publications are often credited with shifting the emphasis in health care error reporting from merely observing and reporting the occurrence of errors, toward *identifying the sources* and *preventing the problems* by strategically redesigning the processes of care.

Following the publication of those IOM reports, data-driven processes in *organizational behavioral management* (OBM) have proliferated to engender continuous monitoring of large-scale performance outcome data and "small samples of events" to provide timely data to organizations and providers (IOM, 2001). It is important to note that small scale audits and a single devastating incident within an organization can be just as powerful as a large-scale trend analysis when identifying potential problems.

Initiatives from policy makers have resulted in mandated reporting and analyses that examine the evidence of the prevention of medication errors, the quality of care in specific settings (rural communities and in mental and substance abuse programs), the implementation of performance measurements in health care facilities, and individual provider performance, for example Medicare's Pay-for-Performance (P4P) program. The Agency for Healthcare Research and Quality (AHRQ) has Patient Safety Indicators (PSIs) to ensure medical error prevention programs are in place in acute care facilities, by looking at factors such as delays in diagnosis and treatment, postoperative complications (postoperative hemorrhage, physiological and metabolic derangement, respiratory failure, pulmonary embolism or deep vein thrombosis, sepsis, wound dehiscence), decubitus ulcers, transfusion reactions, complications of anesthesia, and other risk management problems (AHRQ, n.d.; Miller, Elixhauser, Zhan, & Meyer, 2001). Organizational performance data across these specific risk areas must be gathered and reported.

As stated earlier, the megadata revolution, coupled with the demand for outcome data, has increased the reliance on information technology for monitoring and reporting purposes, and for clinical documentation. Under the Administration Simplification Compliance Act, CMS recently implemented mandatory electronic filing for Part A and B billing and cost reporting. This mandate not only facilitates more efficient filing and processing of claims, but also allows CMS to scrutinize billing patterns, Current Procedural Terminology (CPT) code usage patterns, and costs for delivery of services across providers, facilities, and regions. Electronic documentation and claims submission have also enhanced the oversight of fraudulent submissions. For example, claims are electronically "edited" before submission to ensure duplicated procedures are not being billed and only allowable combinations of procedure codes (CPTs) are being billed for a given patient on a given date. Automated claims are now screened to ensure the claims for services provided or medical equipment distributed matches the data in the medical history.

The reporting of ongoing, timely, and transparent "consequence data" to payers and consumers is mandatory and aimed at reducing errors, improving delivery processes, and achieving cost-efficiencies. Thus, financial data, administrative data, and patient care data collection (including reporting, sharing, auditing, and feedback methods) are now an integral part of health care service delivery and another *converging issue* for the profession.

The opportunities to provide central repositories for clinical data have also primed the pump for research into prevention, diagnosis, and treatment. For example, the Federal Interagency Traumatic Brain Injury Research (FITBIR) database, funded at $10 million by the National Institutes of Health–National Institute of Neurologic Disorders and Stroke (NIH-NINDS), will be built over the next four years and designed to store large volumes of structured (values, scores) and unstructured (functional MRI images) data related to traumatic brain injury (TBI). This mega-database will enable comparisons of results across TBI intervention studies. The database is also expected to aid in enhancing diagnostic markers and predictive markers, provide a better understanding of mechanisms and factors in TBI recovery, and improve evidence-based practice guidelines for patient recovery from the incident of injury through rehabilitation (Merrill, 2011; NIH, 2011).

## Health Care Data

### Personalized Care

One of the most significant transformational examples of metadata in the advancement of health care science in the past decade is the *Human Genome Project* (NIH, 2008), which would not have been achievable without a metadata backbone (Fenstermacher, 2010). The immensity of that project demonstrated how metadata management methodologies and bioinformatics can collaborate to accelerate the analysis of large amounts of structured and unstructured information. The Human Genome Project laid the groundwork for "personalized" medicine (Fenstermacher, 2010), whereby medical therapies are tailored to an individual's genetic characteristics. In addition to considering genetic factors, personalized medicine also considers the individual's physical, environmental, and social factors as those variables strongly influence intervention choices and alternatives. The movement toward personalized health care is a key feature of the Obama administration's health policies (Dalton, Sullivan, Yeatman, & Fenstermacher, 2010). During her Congressional confirmation hearing, Secretary of Health and Human Services Kathleen Sibelius articulated that policy: "Personalized medicine represents a key strategy of health care reform. The potential application of this new knowledge, especially when supported through the use of health information technology in the patient care setting, presents the opportunity for transformational change" (Sibelius, 2009).

### Electronic Health Records

Electronic health records (EHRs), with their computerized physician order entry (CPOE) features, reduce the incidence of medical errors, morbidity, and mortality, and thus EHRs translate into billions of dollars in savings per year nationwide (Leapfrog Group, 2008). Some EHR systems contain software enhancements for clinical decision support, such as embedding links to generic alternatives for drug orders and to evidence-based research articles, standards of care, or practice guidelines. When certain key words (diagnostic conditions, procedures) are entered in the record, or when certain parameters, such as pharmaceutical dosing orders that are outside normal values or drugs that are known to have an adverse interaction, are ordered, embedded-associated links are automatically activated to query the user before the order entry can be completed. EHRs can allow researchers and quality auditors to explore deviations from standard medical protocols (HHS, 2009; Kahol, Vankipuram, Patel, & Smith, 2011) and prevent diagnostic errors (Croskerry & Nimmo, 2011). EHRs that provide a patient with Internet access to e-health or e-patient features (whereby patients can access laboratory results or communicate directly with providers in a HIPAA-compliant format) encourage better compliance with health care regimens and engagement in care (Evers, 2006; Evers, Cummins, Prochaska, & Prochaska, 2005). In a study of adults living with disability and chronic disease, Fox (2007) found patients with disabilities were less likely than other patients to go on line, but once they were encouraged to do so, they become avid health consumers. Fox found that providing e-patient systems allowing patients with disabilities to access their own medical records resulted in better compliance, more engagement with diet and fitness regiments, greater interactions with physicians, and an increased ability to cope with their condition (Fox, 2007).

**Preventing Errors**   Elimination of medication errors has been a prime objective in health care safety regulations for decades. As stated above, one of the safety features of EHRs is the capacity to detect when doctors are going to make a serious error in medication prescribing (Coleman et al, 2011). That feature alone is a sufficient explanation for CMS's current financial incentives for the adoption of EHRs. The EHR is touted as a way to provide better communication generally across the care team, and specifically during between shift "handoffs" between providers, as well as reduce mistakes when entering and reading drug orders.

It is now generally agreed that serious errors made during care team handoffs could be reduced and errors from drug interactions and dosing errors resulting in morbidity and mortality could be largely prevented by embedding safety precautions (alerting queries) in the EHRs. Proponents of the use of information technology and the EHR to improve communication and reduce medical errors, Bernstein, MacCourt, Jacob, and Mehta (2010) state, "The overwhelmingly most common source of handoff-related error was a failure to transmit information" (p. 2629). These authors suggest, "The ideal handoff system, therefore, would support a multimedia approach such that pictures, trend graphs, radiographs, and the like can be shared efficiently" (p. 2630). Thus, to improve patient safety through better communication among the care team members, the implementation of EHRs has become one of CMS's central objectives for physicians and health care organizations in the U.S. today and into the next decade.

**Centers for Medicare and Medicaid Services' Electronic Health Record Initiatives**   Since 2011, the CMS has provided substantial incentives to eligible physician providers and critical access hospitals (CAHs) to implement electronic medical/health records. Even though only approximately 20% of doctors and 10% hospitals are currently using electronic health records (Pear, 2010), starting in 2015 hospitals and doctors will be subject to penalties by CMS if they are not using EHRs. The last year that an eligible hospital can transition to electronic records is 2016.

**Meaningful Use and Clinical Quality Measures**   There are several infrastructure and process criteria that have been established by CMS for the EHRs in order for facilities to comply with the new requirements and be eligible for the substantial bonus incentives. For example, certain data parameters must be included in the electronic record (demographic information, height, weight, medications, and smoking history). To receive the EHR incentives after 2015, eligible providers and hospitals and CAHs must also demonstrate they have met CMS's standards for *meaningful use* of the electronic record. Included in the expectations for meaningful use are *clinical quality measures* (CQMs), which means there must be a "mechanism used for assessing the degree to which a provider competently and safely delivers clinical services that are appropriate for the patient in an optimal time" (CMS, 2011a,b). CMS's CQMs include "process measures," defined as "scientifically acceptable measures" that increase the probability of achieving a certain outcome, and "outcome measures," which index the result of the performance, or nonperformance, of a function or process. The CMS criteria and definitions for meaningful use are described on their Web site as follows:

"The American Recovery and Reinvestment Act of 2009 specifies three main components of Meaningful Use:

1. The use of a certified EHR in a meaningful manner, such as e-prescribing.

2. The use of certified EHR technology for electronic exchange of health information to improve quality of health care.

3. The use of certified EHR technology to submit clinical quality and other measures.

Simply put, 'meaningful use' means providers need to show they're using certified EHR technology in ways that can be measured significantly in quality and in quantity" (CMS, 2011b, p. 1).

**Accessing Electronic Health Record Data**   Electronic health records necessarily contain person-specific information. Creating usable and flexible electronic health record data for clinical outcomes and research purposes is not the primary purpose of the electronic medical record; thus, either "consenting" the participants before providing an intervention that is a part of a research protocol or de-identifying the personal information in the record according to institutional review board (IRB) policies is required. Once captured into a research database, the data entries become nodes, variables, and values that can be defined hierarchically and expressed either as a set of patient-specific data elements or de-identified (Kirklin & Vicinanza, 1999). EHRs contain an individual's data from a single visit or several procedures across an extended episode of care, and are a treasure trove of potentially trackable personal identifying information, or *protected health information* (PHI), such as the individual's name, age, medical record number, address, zip code, diagnoses, procedures, laboratory values, and so forth. Consequently, for research purposes, traceable information must be *de-identified*, so it can then be sorted, profiled, patterned, compared, and referenced within that database for queries and reports that are anonymous and not relatable back to a specific person. It may be advantageous for patient-specific research data to be *re-identified* when opportunities for clinical trials come up and offered to candidates likely to benefit. The best way to build a research database with de-identified information from clinical records is via an auxiliary metadata capture system, of the sort provided by REDCap, discussed later in this chapter.

**Data Privacy**   Access to an individual's EHR is strictly monitored in accordance with the privacy protections contained in the Health Insurance Portability and Accountability Act (HIPAA). The language and implementation of the HIPAA statute was initially intended to ensure that legal protections are in place governing the transfer of electronic health information between payers and other entities to prevent prejudicial disclosures. These regulations were designed to ensure that the confidentiality of an individual's electronic health data would be protected, so that the individual would not be at any disadvantage when data are shared between entities. For that reason, one of the reporting features of all EHR data management is an electronic audit trail on every key entry into the medical record. Electronic "fingerprints" are traceable back to every device and individual who accessed the file, along with when the record was accessed, the sections that were viewed, and so on. Access to EHRs is restricted to only those individuals who have a "need to know" purpose.

With appropriate precautions, or use of a secure data capture system such as REDCap, the electronic medical record can be a rich source of data for comparative effectiveness research and best practices studies. For example, Fisher and Burton (2010) describe a methodology developed for ICU patients with heart failure, in which data abstracting measurements were embedded within the facility's existing documentation system to automatically restructure from the piecemeal clinical data a coherent measurement of heart failure severity to then predict the likelihood of the individual's requiring an ICU admission. They found they could reduce the volume of clinical data needed to refine and define intervention strategies without sacrificing information. In that example, data abstracting and analysis methodologies applied to the medical records of certain patients were used to develop local "best practices" by reducing errors, making laboratory results more meaningful to the user, selecting the most likely candidates for ICU admissions, and improving outcomes.

Data from EHRs can also be used for purposes of monitoring organizational performance improvement, to improve quality and patient safety, and enhance efficiency and cost-effectiveness. EHRs are mined to ensure compliance with national quality standards and to conduct audit reports (e.g., the incidence of surgery-related pneumonias, rapid readmissions, and dosing errors).

**Electronic Health Record Data Captures for Speech-Language Pathology Outcomes**   As with other areas of clinical service delivery, electronic medical record documentation of speech-language pathology services can be formatted to allow for a variety of storage and retrieval purposes, depending on the EHR's built-in documentation and reporting features. Some electronic records are little more

| CLINICIAN | | | | | |
|---|---|---|---|---|---|
| | **VISIT DATE** | **CLIENT** | **REC #** | **UNIT/AUDIT** | **TYPE OF NOTE** |
| Smith, Robyn | | | | | |
| | 9/30/2011 | | | | |
| | ☐ Interrupted | N. Jones | 005511550 | HS/S-L 12:37pm | Ped SLP Progress Note |
| | ☐ Interrupted | K. Wright | 005750071 | HS/S-L 11:57 pm | Ped SLP Feeding Asses |
| | ☐ Interrupted | N. Frum | 007878211 | HS/S-L 1:44 pm | Ped SLP Feeding Note |
| Ashmore, Penelope | | | | | |
| | 10/05/2011 | | | | |
| | ☐ Interrupted | L. Shuster | 009823204 | HS/S-L 2:34 pm | Ped Goldman-Fristoe Test of Articulation-2 Sounds in Words Subtest |
| | ☐ Interrupted | J. McCarthy | 006744325 | HS/S-L 3:02 pm | Ped SLP Preschool Language Scale-Fifth Ed |

*Electronic Health Record: MediServe Rehabilitation Therapy Documentation

**Fig. 2.4**   Example of a documentation audit report for interrupted or incomplete charting.

than the electronic equivalent of paper files, and hospitals and outpatient clinic providers are only beginning to ramp up to use of electronic records, to align with CMS initiatives. For many of us, data capture for speech-language pathology outcomes reporting is an aspiration, not the current reality. However, there are several commercially available software packages specifically designed for rehabilitation therapy provider documentation and reporting purposes, for example *Chartlinks* (2010), *UnichartsTM* (n.d.), *Source Therapy NetTM* (n.d.), and *MediServe* (n.d.). These software packages may require site licenses and on-site IT support. Most systems are designed to be integrated into a medical facility's existing electronic documentation, billing, and appointment systems (e.g., Cerner, EPIC, MediPac, McKesson, Eclipsys, Siemens), or may serve independently as the electronic medical record system in small outpatient clinical operations. In addition to meeting CMS's mandated billing and documentation needs, most rehabilitation documentation and reporting systems have features to ensure that CMS compliance rules for rehabilitation are followed, such as the "8-minute rule" for certain therapy procedures and national Correct Coding Initiatives (CCI) edits. These automated systems can ensure that (1) documentation requirements are met, (2) authorizations and referrals are processed appropriately, and (3) certifications and recertifications are filed in a timely manner. The report shown in **Fig. 2.4** provides an illustration (with fictitious data inserted) of an automated EHR compliance audit of missing or incomplete records performed on speech-language pathology clinical documentation.

For purposes of targeting cost-effectiveness, most EHR enhancements can perform automatic and more efficient charge captures (which eliminate the need for paper "encounter forms," and data-entry personnel, and reduce errors in billing data). These systems track productivity data and missed appointment data, and provide business growth indicators. Some commercially available programs have a data abstracting and reporting feature enabling speech-language pathology departments or units to set up the specific report fields of interest to them. Some systems require additional reporting software enhancements, such as *Crystal*, that can be integrated into the rehabilitation documentation software to create and configure the reports (e.g., productivity, management, financial, and clinical outcome reports).

Ideally, a clinical program serving communication-impaired clients should have features that allow users to abstract testing and clinical performance data and any functional status ratings that have been entered into the record during routine procedure documentation, so that those data can be abstracted into outcome reports for cost and results comparisons. To be able to use electronic documentation for those purposes requires selecting the right product configuration and having knowledgeable clinical staff who can work with the IT team during the initial development of the documentation templates and reporting system. The clinical staff and IT team need to establish ahead of time exactly what questions will be asked from the data. Again, ideally, clinical programs should be able to use data from electronic documentation for their local reporting needs and to have in hand the financial decision-support information that Merson and Rolnick call for in Chapter 9.

# ♦ Demand for Evidence of Effectiveness and Best Practices

### Evidence-Based Practice

Except to point out a few observations about trends over the past decade in this chapter, we will leave the topic of evidence-based practice (EBP) and outcomes research for more elaborated treatment in other chapters in this text. Suffice it to say that the demand for EBP and practice guidelines described by Frattali (1998b) in the first edition of this text continues. The profession of speech-language pathology, supported by its professional associations, has demonstrated a good track record of strong commitment to the principles of EBP in graduate education and in clinical service delivery. Nearly 15 years ago the Academy of Neurologic Communication Disorders and Sciences (ANCDS) became one of the earliest professional groups in speech-language pathology to recognize the importance and the future of systematic reviews (SRs) for evaluating the quality of the evidence in neurogenic communication disorders and prepare practice guidelines for speech-language pathology practitioners. Writing committees within ANCDS initiated a series of SRs leading toward the development of practice guidelines for the management of neurogenic communication disorders (Golper, 2001), resulting today in over three dozen peer-reviewed articles on the SR process, meta-analysis, and practice guidelines for the management of neurological communication disorders associated with traumatic brain injury in children and adults, dementia, acquired apraxia of speech in children and adults, aphasia, and various modalities for the treatment of the dysarthrias and related disorders (ANCDS, n.d.; http://ancds.org). With the establishment of the National Center on Evidence-Based Practice in Communication Disorders (ASHA N-CEP, n.d.) in 2005, the talents and resources of the American Speech-Language-Hearing Association have been directed toward focused initiatives in EBP, including developing systematic reviews and an outcomes research repository, dissemination of intervention research evidence to members and consumers, and member education about evidence-based practices (Rao, 2011). The ASHA/N-CEP Web site provides a compendium of SRs that have been published in speech-language pathology and recently has conducted internal SRs of treatment evidence for specific conditions and questions, with additional reports forthcoming (see Chapter 5). **Figure 2.5** illustrates this growth in systematic reviews of speech, language, cognition, and dysphagia research, as documented by the number of studies listed on the N-CEP Web site between 1998 and 2008.

Systematic review of intervention outcome research is an essential component of EBP. Over the past decade, as experience with EBP, or evidence-based medicine (EBM), has evolved and gained popularity and prominence in medicine and rehabilitation decision making, questions have been raised about how to best conduct these reviews and how to integrate EBP into routine clinical practice. The methods for conducting SRs have been critiqued, and recommendations for improving those reviews have been made (for example, see Elamin et al, 2009; Marshall et al, 2011; O'Mathúna, 2010; Schlosser, 2007). The relative weighting of RCTs as the "gold standard" reference for evidence is less a matter of concern to critics than the dogma that RCTs are the *only* evidence worth considering when defining best practices. In a recent report in the journal of the Royal College of Speech Therapists in the United Kingdom, Marshall and her colleagues (2011) review and comment on the state of SRs specifically in speech and language intervention research. They recommend that alternative reviewing systems and criteria be considered when the criteria for systematic reviews are not met: "Systematic reviewing should not be seen as a single method; there are as many ways to con-

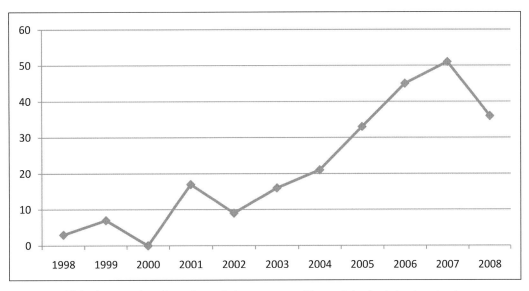

**Fig. 2.5**  Published systematic reviews of speech, language, cognition, and dysphagia treatment outcome research in speech-language pathology. [Data from American Speech-Language-Hearing Association National Center on Evidence-Based Practice (ASHA N-CEP). (n.d.). Compendium of evidence-based practice guidelines and systematic reviews 1998–2008. http://www.asha.org/members/ebp/compendium/.]

duct systematic reviews as there are questions. There is a need to engage in developments in reviewing approaches in order to develop appropriate methodologies for SLT" (Marshall et al, 2011).

Marshall et al (2011) reference several resources for evidence reviews that are specific to speech-language pathology/speech-language therapy, including *Evidence-Based Practice Brief,* a quarterly Web-based site maintained by Pearson publishers (http://www.speechandlauguage.com/ebp/); *Speech Bite^(TM),* an open-access Web site maintained by the University of Sydney and *Speech Pathology Australia* (http://www.speechbite.com); and the journal edited by Schlosser and Sigafoos, *Evidence-Based Communication Assessment and Intervention* (EBCAI).

## Evolving Notions About Evidence-Based Practice

Haynes, Devereaux, and Guyatt (2002a,b) recommend revising the original and often reproduced EBP model from that of Sackett, Richardson, Rosenberg, and Haynes (1996) and Sackett, Rosenberg, Gray, Haynes, and Richardson (2000) to that shown in **Fig. 2.6**. This revised version takes into greater account the patient's/client's *clinical state* and *circumstances* (e.g., the distance from home to the clinic) and places *clinician expertise* in the middle of the decision triad, with the argument that "evidence does not make decisions, people do." That conceptual restructuring of the evidence triangle into these overlapping Venn diagrams maintains consistency with basic tenets of EBP, such as using the best available evidence to guide decisions, but acknowledges the validity of weighing other factors, such as patient choices and clinician expertise, during decision making. This balance is stressed by Dollaghan (2007) in her discussion of the E[3]BP model (Kamhi, 2011).

In his thoughtful commentary on the conundrum of balancing research evidence with patient preferences and the clinician's experience, from an E[3]BP perspective, Kamhi (2011) considers the differences and diversions between scientific methods and clinical methods. The objectives, the built-in mechanisms for critique and corrections, and, most important, the consequences of mistakes are ways in which research and clinical methods are fundamentally different. Kamhi notes clinical practice does not apply experimental controls; does not have mechanisms for objective, independent evaluation and verification; and is not constrained by theory. Clinical practice lacks these

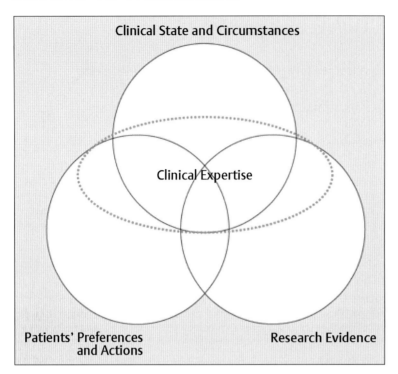

**Fig. 2.6**   An updated model for evidence-based decisions. [Reproduced from Haynes, R. B., Devereaux, P. J., & Guyatt, G. H. (2002b). Physicians' and patients' choices in evidence-based medicine: evidence does not make decisions, people do. *British Medical Journal, 324,* 1350 [Editorial]. Reprinted with permission from BMJ Publishing Group Ltd.]

basic tenets of scientific inquiry. Thus, unlike scientists, clinicians have "the option of being theoretically agnostic because clinical outcomes are almost always more important than theoretical coherence" (p. 61). He notes the inherent risk with using clinical practice/experience as "evidence" is that clinical evidence will be used to *prove* what one already believes, a contradiction of the core principle of EBP. In EBP, evidence is valued or ranked based on the potential degrees of bias in the findings. If one appreciates the potential for clinical practice data to be biased, then practice data are a questionable form of evidence at best. But Kamhi (referencing Tonelli) admits there is, "still some question as to how much weight clinicians should assign to high-quality empirical evidence versus practice-based, experiential evidence" (Kamhi, 2011, p. 61), and he suggests the relative weighting of any one of the three sources of EBP depends on the particular person being treated. Ultimately, an intervention decision is personalized; consequently, Tonelli (2006), Kamhi (2011), and others (Tsapas & Matthews, 2008) propose a *case-based approach* as a way to integrate the dogma of high-quality empirical evidence (such as RCTs) into evidence-based clinical practice: "When high-quality evidence is available and the patient resembles the average patient in the clinical research, EBP is the model of choice. When high-quality evidence is not available or the case is atypical, a case-based approach may be preferable" (Kamhi, 2011, p. 63).

In a similar argument, Tsapas and Matthews (2009) note the paucity of strong evidence from RCTs in the majority of interventions across health care, which means treatment guidelines often rest on the weaker forms of evidence: consensus opinion and clinical knowledge. They suggest:

> When faced with increased therapeutic uncertainty, a safer alternative for making individualized therapeutic decisions would be $N = 1$ trials, which help formalize therapeutic decision-making, transferring to single-patient decisions the safeguards of RCTs. Therapies are tested sequentially and final medica-

tion is decided on a shared basis. This incorporates objective data, patient values, and preferences, and patient-important outcomes. (Tsapas & Matthews, 2008, p. 925)

## *N* = 1 Models: Single-Subject Experimental Designs and Case-Based Reports

Because evidence must ultimately come down to the individual, Tsapas and Matthews (2008) call for more *N* = 1 intervention trials, of the sort found in single-subject experimental designs (SSEDs). SSED intervention trials are *N* = 1 *experiments* as compared with *nonexperimental* case reports containing descriptive and observational data. Typically, case reports in health care–related journals do not include the experimental controls that are characteristic of single-subject research. In speech-language pathology intervention, treatment studies that are buttressed by the application of SSEDs to the intervention design can make a significant contribution to the clinical literature. Case reports and single-subject research contribute to the pre-efficacy phases of research, as with phase I and II research questions (Beeson & Robey, 2006). *N* = 1 studies are valuable in the post-efficacy research phase, where treatment intervention is tested in real-life conditions (i.e., the effectiveness research phase), and well-designed single-subject experimental methods can index efficacy.

### *Effect Size in Single-Subject Research*

As Kearns and de Riesthal discuss in Chapter 14, SSEDs apply rigorous procedural controls and experimental methods, with individual subjects serving as their own controls. The iconic graphic data plots one associates with these various experimental designs can be scrutinized visually to verify the treatment effects, but in recent years single-subject researchers are compelled to include calculations of the *effect size,* the degree of variation from the null state, within the report of results (Beeson & Robey, 2006). Effect-size calculators for SSED data are available through several sources online, and are described in the methods of SSED articles (for example, Campbell, 2004). Single-subject performance data also can be subjected to precision *estimation models* of the change values (levels), slope, and trends to examine for bias (Solanas, Leiva, & Salafranca, 2010; Solanas, Manolov, & Onghena, 2010). As Beeson and Robey (2006) point out and Kearns and de Riesthal amplify more fully in Chapter 14, *single-subject research* (SSR) is both popular and often the most appropriate research method to use with communication disorders intervention research. There is a preference for SSR over group designs in early intervention research with infants and toddlers (Wolery & Dunlap, 2001), and SSR is the predominant experimental design in the treatment literature with certain conditions, such as aphasia. In a compendium of over 600 articles related to aphasia treatment contained in the ANCDS aphasia treatment Web site (http://www.u.arizona.edu/~pelagie/ancde/index.html), 288 articles were group designs and 332 were single-subject designs (Beeson & Robey, 2006). Although *N* = 1 SSR studies obviously are not randomized-controlled between group experimental trials, and for that reason systematic reviewers usually rank SSR results lower then group studies in evidence scaling, Beeson and Robey (2006) argue that since effect size calculations and their standard deviation units are quantifiable, SSR studies are amenable to meta-analysis, which is higher ranked evidence (level I or II) in most SR systems. Ntourou and Lipsey discuss the topic of meta-analysis involving SSR in Chapter 15.

## Practice-Based Evidence

The debate over the practical utility of infusing what Kamhi (2011) called the "certainty" of scientific research (EBP) findings into the "uncertain" world of clinical practice has resulted in a predictable recommendation: *practice-based evidence* (PBE). PBE in its various forms is viewed as a "promising" bridge between science and practice (Kamhi, 2011). PBE refers to outcome data that "can range from unsystematic observational evidence obtained by practitioners about the effectiveness of their treatments to systematic research that evaluates in depth, comprehensive information about patient characteristics, process of care, and outcomes" (Kamhi, 2011, p. 62).

Practice-based evidence is increasingly viewed as a way to bring laboratory evidence into clinical practice. Westfall et al (2007) observed, "What is efficacious in randomized clinical trials is not always effective in the real world of day-to-day practice. . . . Practice-based research provides the laboratory that will help generate new knowledge and bridge the chasm between recommended care to improved care" (p. 403; cited in Horn & Gassaway, 2007). Systematically comparing a series of different treatments for a particular condition within an individual (such as testing a series of drug therapies to treat an individual patient's hypertension) is a form of PBE. When systematic, experimental methods are applied to a between-group or between-treatments comparison, these comparisons may be referred to as *comparative effectiveness research* (CER).

### Comparative Effectiveness Research

Comparative effectiveness research applies *systematic* research methods to compare different interventions and strategies to prevent, diagnose, treat, and monitor health conditions during the conduct of clinical care (Fenstermacher, 2010; http://www.hhs.gov). Typically, CER starts with the biometric, or observational clinical data that are entered by the providers into the EHR, or de-identified and captured into a metadata system, to compare intervention outcomes with one or more modalities (e.g., surgery versus physical therapy for knee injury). This type of treatment outcome comparison differs from what would occur in laboratory-controlled RCTs (efficacy research). CER can include prospective clinical trials, or retrospectively gathered data from actual point-of-service records.

Recognizing that not every drug or intervention procedure has been or can be tested in the research laboratory, CER reports and outcome data are currently being used and increasingly will be used by public and private payers to assess the adherence to best practices and identify variations in care. CER data are used to compare costs and results between providers and organizations in conditions where the cost to the public is high. For example, as part of the American Recovery and Reinvestment Act (ARRA) of 2009 (HHS, n.d.), the federal government authorized $1.1 billion to support patient-centered outcomes research with $400 million for CER projects. In May 2010, Mathematica Policy Research, Inc. was given a $7 million grant to establish the Center of Excellence for Disability Research. This two-year project, also funded under the AARA, is creating a foundation and data infrastructure to support comparative effectiveness research on the care for adults with disabilities. The goal of the project is described in the HHS Web site as follows:

> Like all Americans, adults with disabilities seek affordable and effective care that maximizes their well-being and independence. The Center is organized to support that goal: we are collaborating with stakeholders in the health care and disability communities to ensure that our work is relevant and practical. The Center's research findings and publications will help consumers, family members, other caregivers, providers, and policymakers identify effective strategies for promoting and maintaining the quality of life of individuals with disabilities. Building a strong data infrastructure will allow researchers to address complex questions about the effectiveness of alternative ways of delivering long term support services and coordinating these services with medical services. (Health and Human Services, n.d., p. 1)

## ♦ Demand for Relevant Outcomes

The movement toward greater transparency and accountability in health care and education has led us to what Rao discusses in Chapter 8 of this text as the "consumer-centric" era (Boone, 2011). When the interests of the "person served" become the primary concerns, we are effectively required to focus our services on those outcomes that are most relevant, or *what matters*, to patients/clients, students, parents, administrators, and the general public. Increasingly, our outcomes, the ultimate result and consequence of the contributions we make in education, clinical service, and even research, must be logically aligned with what matters most to our consumer-constituents. If we are producing results that are perceived to be meaningful and impactful, the utility of our work will be valued.

## What Matters?

What matters to patients/clients is individualized care resulting in personally relevant improvements in quality of life and functional activities. What matters to public policy makers and the public and private funders of education and clinical services is cost-containment, without sacrificing quality standards, and improved status in the health and education of our citizens. What matters to our speech-language pathology graduate students (and their families) is a valid, relevant course of study that prepares them to enter their careers as fully qualified and competent practitioners, researchers, or educators within the profession (Baker, 2011). What matters to school administrators is the provision of effective services that align with educational policy mandates and district obligations and objectives, risk management concerns, and budget restrictions. What matters to parents is the social and academic success of their children. What matters to administrators in health care organizations is satisfied patients who have experienced services that are aligned with best practices that were provided in a safe environment and resulted in good health-related quality-of-life outcomes with the least financial burden to the organization. In health care today, patient satisfaction has become a top priority second only to patient safety. Patient-reported outcomes and satisfaction measures are taken into consideration during department budgeting, resource allocation, and salary determinations. **Figure 2.7** is an example of an actual graph from a medical center's quarterly patient satisfaction survey data showing the occurrence of the response "excellent" when the patients/respondents were surveyed and asked the question, "How would you rate the overall quality of care you received?" The line across the top represents this medical center's percentile scores compared

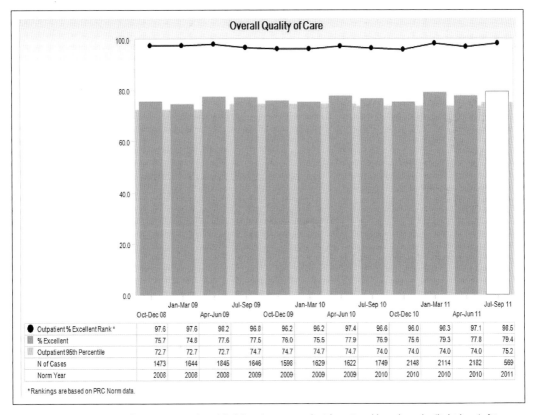

| | Oct-Dec 08 | Jan-Mar 09 | Apr-Jun 09 | Jul-Sep 09 | Oct-Dec 09 | Jan-Mar 10 | Apr-Jun 10 | Jul-Sep 10 | Oct-Dec 10 | Jan-Mar 11 | Apr-Jun 11 | Jul-Sep 11 |
|---|---|---|---|---|---|---|---|---|---|---|---|---|
| ● Outpatient % Excellent Rank * | 97.6 | 97.6 | 98.2 | 96.8 | 96.2 | 96.2 | 97.4 | 96.6 | 96.0 | 98.3 | 97.1 | 98.5 |
| ▒ % Excellent | 75.7 | 74.8 | 77.6 | 77.5 | 76.0 | 75.5 | 77.9 | 76.9 | 75.6 | 79.3 | 77.8 | 79.4 |
| ▒ Outpatient 95th Percentile | 72.7 | 72.7 | 72.7 | 74.7 | 74.7 | 74.7 | 74.7 | 74.0 | 74.0 | 74.0 | 74.0 | 75.2 |
| N of Cases | 1473 | 1644 | 1845 | 1646 | 1598 | 1629 | 1622 | 1749 | 2148 | 2114 | 2182 | 569 |
| Norm Year | 2008 | 2008 | 2008 | 2009 | 2009 | 2009 | 2009 | 2010 | 2010 | 2010 | 2010 | 2011 |

*Rankings are based on PRC Norm data.

**Fig. 2.7**  Outpatient satisfaction survey data (dark bars) compared with national benchmarks (light bars). [From Professional Research Consultants (PRC), Inc. 11326 P Street, Omaha, NE 68137–2316. Reprinted by permission.]

with the benchmarks of comparable hospitals within the national database of the surveyors (Professional Research Consultants, n.d.).

## Patient-Reported Outcomes and Standardized Assessment

The need to measure patient-reported outcomes (PROs) in health care has been supported for decades, and several instruments are published that are specifically designed to measure PROs for particular conditions and disorders, including communication disorders. Several PRO instruments related specifically to communication disorders are described in the first edition of this text by Frattali (1998b). Although speech-language pathologists (SLPs) report rarely using these instruments to measure intervention results (Simmons-Mackie, Threats, & Kagan, 2006) there is a rapidly escalating emphasis on PROs, also referred to as *patient-reported outcome measures* (PROMs). A demand, supported by CMS, has evolved for standardization of these assessments in health care outcomes. This growing emphasis on PROs and the application of psychometric methods to develop standardized patient assessment tools and improve measurement efficiencies across care settings collectively are another converging factor in service delivery today.

Patient-reported outcome tools include surveys of the perceptions of health-related status that are taken directly from the patient or a surrogate/proxy (parent or other family member or partner). Tools examining the level of perceived health-related outcome are becoming a primary index for determination of reimbursement in postacute rehabilitation and to index treatment effectiveness. Chapters 5 and 8 elaborate further on the Developing Outpatient Therapy Payment Alternatives (DOPTA) and the anticipated implementation of the Continuity Assessment Record and Evaluation (CARE) tool (Research Triangle Institute, n.d.).

### Minimally Important Difference

The clinician's experience and expertise and the client's preferences come into play when deciding if a significant performance improvement on a test score is *clinically significant* (Conture, 2011), that is, if evidence of a positive change in a test score or a behavioral or biometric measure is perceived to be of notable clinical or functional consequence to the client or the clinician provider. PRO surveys/rating scales are often included in the assessment methodologies for clinical research to answer this question: Do subjects perceive a difference from this (drug, surgery, rehabilitation) intervention? Surveys of patient-reported quality of life, functional status, perceived handicap, or pain scales, are appealing in clinical practice as well as clinical trials, but both researchers and clinicians struggle to interpret the data. This is particularly challenging in large-scale outcome studies. One way to address the problem in research is through a statistical treatment of PRO data to find the minimal important difference (MID) in the scaled scores. There are several terms used to refer to MIDs that vary with slightly nuanced differences: *clinically important difference, minimally detectable difference*, and *subjectively significant difference* (King, 2011). As King notes: "There is no universal MID, despite the appeal of the notion. Indeed, for a particular patient-reported outcome instrument or scale, the MID is not an immutable characteristic, but may vary by population and context" (p. 171).

The statistical treatment of PRO data to arrive at the MID typically involves one of four methods: paired *t*-tests, effect size statistic, clinical anchor-based methods, or standard error measurement (King, 2011; Walters & Brazier, 2003). Quality-of-life (QoL) scales, for example, the SF-36 and its variants (Ware, Gandek, & the IQOLA Project Group, 1994) and the Functional Assessment of Chronic Illness Therapy (FACIT) (Yost & Eton, 2005), have applied MID measurement to reveal the "tipping point" of positive effects in QoL outcomes (Jaeschke, Singer, & Guyatt, 1989; Yost & Eton, 2005). Some authors argue that when PROs are used in clinical practice to index the adequacy of treatment effects to inform decisions about discontinuing, continuing, or increasing a given intervention (e.g., analgesic dosage), the scales should be raised from a minimal difference level to a *really important difference* (RID) level for each individual (Wolfe, Michaud, & Strand, 2005). Lee, Hobden, Stiell, and Wells (2003) report an application of MID statistics to visual analog scale (VAS) data taken from patients' pain ratings, and they conclude that a minimally detectable difference was not a good indicator of analgesic control, recommending that the bar be raised to a minimally *clinically important* difference (MCID) level, because the perception of a clinically important difference may be more appropriate when evaluating the effect of treatment for acute pain.

### Item Response Theory and Patient-Reported Outcome Measurement

Patient-reported outcome survey questionnaires are routinely used in clinical trials and rehabilitation research, but researchers recognize that long questionnaires can be a burden for participants to complete, and different studies may ask essentially the same questions or study similar interventions but use different PRO instruments with different scaling properties, making the results difficult to compare. The application of *item response theory* (IRT) to assessments provides an answer to these challenges. IRT has been proposed as the preferred health outcomes measurement for the 21st century (Hays, Morales, & Reise, 2000). IRT is a psychometric theory in which generalized linear mathematic models are applied to test individual items to determine the probability of a particular response (item response function) as representative of a latent (nonobservable) trait (e.g., fatigue). The technique requires computing the values of individual test items as correlated with a particular trait, conducting a confirmatory factor analysis at an item-by-item level, and then linking scores from one instrument to the equivalent items and score from another instrument; for a comprehensive review of these methods see Hays, Morales, and Reise (2000).

Item response theory and *Rasch analysis* methodologies were introduced in the 1950s and 1960s and have been applied in large-scale educational and psychological testing and in the armed services for several decades (Baylor et al, 2011). IRTs are increasingly embraced by rehabilitation researchers and researchers involved in clinical trials using PROs as a way to improve standardization across instruments, allow for data pooling, and improve assessment efficiency (Batcho, Tennant, & Thonnard, 2012). And to further promote efficiencies, computerized IRT methods, *computer-adapted testing* (CT, CAT) are now a standard feature. CT is widely accepted outside of health care as a method for large-scale assessment (e.g., aptitude tests). The IRT-CT methodology involves drawing upon a large, calibrated item bank to identify those items that have been found to validly discriminate and reliably predict a response. When applying computerized IRT, the computer automatically determines the number of items required for administration, based on how the person responds to the initial items; thus, the entire survey or test is not administered to every respondent. Predictive models calculate the extent to which additional items need to be added to reliably identify a trait and determine the score. For example, an instrument with 36 items might require administration of only five or six items to validly quantify the score for an individual. IRT methodology with a CT adaptation is particularly useful for test validation studies, multicenter pharmaceutical studies, and other clinical trials. These methods are currently being used to validate the standardized patient assessment tool—the CARE Tool (Research Triangle Institute, n.d.) discussed in Chapters 5 and 8. The CARE tool is being developed as a way to measure status across time, at acute hospital discharge, at postacute care (PAC) admissions, and at the time of PAC discharge.

### Item Response Theory in Rehabilitation Intervention Research

The emergence of IRT in intervention research came on the back of decades of demonstrated value of IRT and Rasch analysis in large-scale testing and item analysis (Chang & Reeve, 2005), and these methods are a natural fit with the current demand to assess relevant outcomes in a manner that is reliable and valid, psychometrically sound, and sufficiently broad to encompass the entire episode of care. IRT addresses those challenges (Jette, 2010). The value of IRT in rehabilitation research gained particular notice following a symposium held at the Rehabilitation Institute of Chicago in 2009, on the topic of improving efficiency in health outcome measurement. That meeting leveraged outcome measurement away from traditional, conventional testing methods using a hodge-podge of paper-and-pencil, published and unpublished patient questionnaires, toward the use of item-response banks and IRT methods, with computer-assisted technology. Proponents refer to IRT as "modern test theory" (Gershon et al, 2011) and argue against the traditional testing methods of classical test theory, where standardized tests and measurements are indexed by how well individual items correlate with the sum of the remaining items in the instrument—Chronbach's α coefficient (Eadie et al, 2006). Since 2005, with the development of item banks, IRT-based assessment methods have evolved to offer improved standardization and efficiencies in situations requiring analysis of PRO scales. Applying IRT to PRO data and other questionnaire data is appealing because it is a marriage of test-taking efficiency with broad-based item banks that have face validity as a measure of "what matters" to the individual. IRT can be used to detect the minimal important difference (MID) point for individuals; thus, the use of IRT with PRO data has advantages over biometric health status measures and behavioral test change scores for making comparisons of effectiveness of intervention in rehabilitation research and for measuring the end points in clinical trials with certain conditions. It appears that IRT will be endorsed in measurement methods for reimbursement schemes in postacute rehabilitation.

### Item Response Theory in Speech-Language Pathology

Several communication sciences and disorders university research groups (principally allied with the University of Florida in Gainesville, the University of Pittsburgh, and the University of Washington in Seattle) are currently exploring the advantages of IRT and Rasch analysis in tests for communication disorders (for example, Baylor, Yorkston, Eadie, Miller, & Amtmann, 2009; del Toro et al, 2011; Hula, Austermann Hula, & Doyle, 2009; Hula, Donovan, Kendall, & Gonzalez-Rothi, 2010; Hula, Doyle, & Austermann Hula, 2010; Justice, Bowles & Skibbe, 2006; Kendall et al, 2011).

Baylor and her colleagues (2011) provide a tutorial on IRT and Rasch analysis tailored for SLPs. In this article they explain the theoretical basis, mathematical features, and definitions of IRT, with examples drawn from applications to communication disorder assessments. Using these examples, they describe the methods involved with single-parameter logistic (1-PL), two-parameter logistic (2 PL), and polytomous models (such as a Rasch-based partial credit model) (Baylor et al, 2009) to develop item banks from scaled or yes/no type instruments. An illustration of this methodology is found in a study by Baylor and colleagues (2009) describing the development of the communicative participation item bank (CPIB), drawn from a Rasch analysis of response data from patients with spasmodic dysphonia. IRT has been applied to one of the more widely used PRO tools for communication disorders, the *Communicative Effectiveness Index* (CETI), see Donovan, Kendall, Young, and Rosenbek (2008) and Donovan, Velozo, and Rosenbek (2007), and in patient reported cognitive impairment (Hula, Doyle, & Austermann Hula (2010).

### Item Response Theory and Rasch Analysis for Efficiencies in Speech-Language Pathology Clinical Testing

Along with considering ways to improve standardization and efficiencies in the collection and analysis of PRO data using IRT, IRT analysis is applied to enhance measurement efficiency and interpretation of test findings. For example, Hula, Donovan, Kendall, and Gonzalez-Rothi (2010) report an IRT analysis of the item fit within a standardized aphasia test, the *Western Aphasia Battery* (WAB). Applying IRT, Hula and his colleagues found that some items in the WAB did not contribute productively to the diagnosis of aphasia. Further, Rasch-based scores tended to be more normally distributed than traditional scores, and the reliability of WAB scores was found to vary across ability range.

### Testing the Tests

Before leaving the topic of testing efficiencies, let's remember that, as we seek to apply evidence to inform practice, we should also use EBP in our diagnostic testing and evaluation methods. In the book *Studying a Study and Testing a Test*, Riegelman (2005) makes the point that, in EBP, it is important for clinicians not only to be able to critique, analyze, interpret, and extrapolate clinically useful information from research, that is, "studying the study," but also to be able to assess the diagnostic efficiency and cost-effectiveness of the tests and assessment methods they use, or "testing the test." Even though standardized testing and clinical assessments are necessary tools for clinicians to *define* the disorder or disease (Riegelman, 2005), the use of lengthy and expensive diagnostic testing with multiple test batteries and redundant items measuring the same constructs is simply not defensible today in any setting. So the challenge is to arrive at an accurate diagnosis as efficiently as possible, with the fewest possible, or abbreviated, tests administered in the shortest possible time. Clinicians need to understand the fundamental principles of diagnostic testing and examine the tests they routinely use to determine "which questions they answer and which they do not, which tests increase the diagnostic precision and which merely increase the cost" (Riegelman, 2005, p. 128). Providing psychometric data about the *specificity* and *sensitivity* of a given test, diagnostic, or screening procedure can assist the clinician in achieving greater efficiencies or justifying more extensive testing when screening tests are not sufficiently definitive (Golper & Brown, 2007).

# ◆ Defining the End Points

## Models of Disablement

Models of disablement have for decades provided health service providers and researchers with a schema to conceptualize intervention in a manner that takes into account factors beyond the physical-medical diagnosis and its biological markers to encompass a broader perspective that includes functional activities, life participation, satisfaction, and quality of life. As Frattali noted in Chapter 1, disablement models provide a theoretical base for interventions across medical specialties and professional disciplines, particularly in geriatrics, rehabilitation medicine, rehabilitation therapies, and communication sciences and disorders. Disablement models are referenced in risk management literature (Bickenbach, Chatterji, Kastanjsek, & Ustün, 2003), in clinical research, and in best practices protocols for various groups of individuals with chronic illness, such as end-stage renal disease, cancer, depression, vision impairments, musculoskeletal disorders, stroke, traumatic brain injury, heart disease, and autoimmune diseases (Arthanat, Nochajski, & Stone, 2004; Bennett et al, 2001; Bruyère, VanLooy, & Peterson, 2005; Cieza et al, 2004; King, 2008; Sousa & Kwok, 2006).

Increasingly, models of disablement are providing a means to objectify and focus the treatment "end point" with chronic disease and disability. Stineman and her colleagues recognized well over a decade ago that disability outcome measurement has gradually shifted toward "participation" and quality-of-life measures and away from more "impairment-specific" measures, such as the Functional Impairment Measure (FIM) (Stineman, Jette, Fiedler, Granger, 1997; Stineman et al, 1996). If "quality of life" or "life participation" are defined as the targeted end points of intervention, then measurement of intervention outcomes must include tests with items that are logically linked to those constructs (Abresch, Carter, Han, & McDonald, 2009; Yorkston et al, 2008).

The three most commonly referenced classification schemes and models of health care quality and disablement are found in Chapter 1: the Nagi framework (see **Fig. 1.2**), Wilson and Cleary's model of health-related quality of life outcomes (HRQoL) (see **Fig. 1.3**), and the 1980 version of the World Health Organization's model of the consequences of disease and disorders (WHO, 1980; see **Fig. 1.1**). At the time of the publication of the first edition of this text, the WHO model was referred to as the International Classification of Impairment, Disability, and Handicap (WHO-ICIDH) framework. Since then, the WHO-ICIDH framework has undergone a couple of iterations of development, with the ICIDH II in 1999, and ultimately the current operating model, the International Classification of Functioning, Disability, and Health, or WHO ICF (described in Chapter 3 in greater detail). The current model (WHO ICF, 2001; WHO, 2002) is provided in **Fig. 2.8**.

### Why Are Disablement Models Important?

Disablement models help policy makers, researchers, and service providers recognize and acknowledge the following:

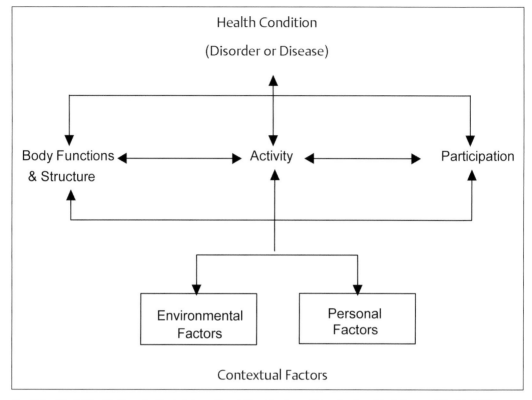

**Fig. 2.8** World Health Organization's International Classification of Functioning, Disability, and Health (ICF) Model. [From World Health Organization (WHO). (2002). *Towards a common language for functioning, disability and health, ICF.* Geneva: Author. http://www.who.int/classifications/icf/training/icfbeginnersguide.pdf. Reprinted by permission.]

- The relationship between pathology and any attendant functional impairment or limitations (Verbrugge & Jette, 1994);

- How characteristics of the individual and the environment interact to affect health-related quality-of-life outcomes (Üstün, Chatterji, & Kostanjsek, 2004); and

- The scope, multidimensionality, and interrelatedness of biological, psychological, social, personal, and environmental factors that need to be considered in interventions and their measurement (e.g., Jette, Tao, & Haley, 2007; Selkowitz et al, 2006).

### World Health Organization's International Classification of Functioning, Disability, and Health

The contextual frameworks of the three models mentioned above are described in greater detail in Chapter 1. In this section we focus on the WHO ICF model, as it continues to figure prominently in health care outcome research and has assisted us in achieving a common vocabulary for clinicians and researchers across disciplines and around the world. The WHO ICF provides a common language of disablement with internationally accepted classifications and a standardized language for coding that is consistent with the International Classification of Diseases, 10th edition (WHO, 2003). Consequently, the WHO ICF framework has emerged as the preferred model for conceptualizing and providing a vocabulary for rehabilitation intervention outcomes with adults and children (IOM, 2007;

Jette, 2009; WHO, 2007). In a 2007 report, the Institute of Medicine's (IOM) Committee on the Future of Disability in America explicitly recommended adopting the WHO ICF framework (IOM, 2007; Jette, 2009). Consequently, researchers and clinicians in the international community of rehabilitation sciences are opting for adoption of the WHO ICF model as a way to synthesize earlier models, provide a common language of disablement, and establish an operational theory for conceptualizing and evaluating the consequences of various health conditions and treatment outcome (Jette, 2009, 2010). In Chapters 3 and 5, both the conceptual basis of the ICF and the applications of these constructs specifically to speech-language pathology are examined. Here we will touch upon research in speech-language pathology intervention from an ICF approach in a couple of areas, but mainly the following section presents a broad overview of current concepts, definitional challenges, the impact of the ICF on rehabilitation intervention generally, and how these concepts are integrated into post-acute payment reform today.

## WHO ICF and Speech-Language Pathology Research

The WHO ICF is found in outcomes research in nursing, occupational therapy, physical therapy, pediatric and adult rehabilitative medicine, depression studies, and pain management clinical trials (Bruyère et al, 2005; Cieza et al, 2004; Haglund & Henriksson, 2003; Heerkens, VanDerBrug, Ten Napel, & Van Ravensberg, 2003; Kearney & Pryor, 2004; Peterson, 2005; Rauch, Cieza, & Stucki, 2008). Speech-language pathology and audiology intervention studies over the past decade reference the WHO ICF (e.g., Eadie, 2007; McLeod & McCormack, 2007; Rangasayee, Mukundan, Dalvi, Nandurkar, & Kant, 2010; Threats, 2002, 2007a,b, 2008; Threats & Worrell, 2004; Westby, 2007; Worrall & Hickson, 2008; Yaruss, 2007; Yaruss & Quesal, 2004). The importance of the WHO ICF framework in service delivery within communication disorders is also evident by its incorporation into the scope of practice of the American Speech-Language-Hearing Association (ASHA, 2001). In a recent WHO report on disability (WHO, 2011) strong recommendations are made and strategies are suggested for improving services to individuals with disabilities worldwide, including services for individuals with hearing, speech, and language disorders.

## Measuring Body Functions and Structure

In the WHO ICF framework the primary physical injury, disease, or impairment (e.g., stroke, hemiparesis, aphasia) is encompassed in the *body functions and structure* domain (WHO ICF, 2001; WHO, 2002). Measurement in this domain involves physical findings, biometric data, standardized tests, and instrumental assessments of body structures and functions. Even though, as emphasized earlier, there is growing interest in patient-reported outcomes, PROs do not index the body functions and structure assessment. Patients cannot "self-report" laboratory values or a score on a standardized speech-language assessment. They may report frustration and decreased independence due to their communication disorder. They may identify levels of fatigue or a degree of diminished activity that could be associated with certain blood chemistries, such as low blood sugar. And a physician may intervene with drug therapies and diet and exercise recommendations, aimed at effecting both an improvement in laboratory findings and a corresponding improvement in the perceived level of fatigue. But most intervention plans start with the body function and structure domain assessments. These assessments can verify or clarify the reasons for the symptoms the patient reports.

In speech-language pathology, our traditional (standardized, norm-referenced, and criterion-referenced) diagnostic testing procedures and instrumental assessments serve several essential purposes. Measures of the body functions and structure (impairment) domain, or what Frattali (1998b) referred to as *modality-specific* measures, are essential for treatment planning. These measures

1. reveal the physical, cognitive, communicative, and related pathologies contributing to the disorder;

2. enable the examiners to make a differential diagnosis of conditions;

3. provide a profile of strengths or residual abilities as well as deficits;

4. provide a comparison of an individual's performance against normal performance or typical expectations for similar cohorts; and

5. quantify the current severity of the disorder and, with some conditions, allow for a prognosis or prediction of the trajectory for improvement with and without intervention.

Doing the right thing, for the right person, at the right time involves first determining if a significant disorder exists and if the disorder is or is not likely to resolve without direct intervention. Reliable standardized tests of communication and swallowing disorders and other clinical, biometric, and behavioral assessment data are as important to SLPs in treatment planning as laboratory values, vital signs, imaging studies, and a physical examination are to physicians. With certain conditions, assessments that are limited only to measures of the degree of impairment (e.g., percent of intelligibility) may not be the best way to target the end point of intervention. A survey conducted by Nina Simmons-Mackie and her colleagues (Simmons-Mackie, Threats, & Kagan, 2006) found that few clinicians working with patients who are aphasic reported outcome measurements beyond impairment measures (i.e., standardized tests). Even though aphasia is generally acknowledged to be a chronic condition, apparently few clinicians use measures of quality of life or communication participation scales to define the impact of the intervention. Often a meaningful result from treatment for a given individual will not be captured by change scores on standardized tests, but rather by quality-of-life measures and PROs that query the extent to which the individual has assumed new activities, resumed previously enjoyed activities, or proceeded to *participate* socially with others in the exchange of knowledge, information, feelings, or ideas (Eadie et al, 2006).

### Measuring Functional Status, Activity, and Participation

An emphasis on an individual's ability to participate in society has been a central mandate for rehabilitation since the Americans with Disabilities Act of 1990 and remains a funding priority for the National Institute of Disability and Rehabilitation Research (NIDRR). The NIDRR priorities provide a powerful incentive for researchers to develop and refine reliable, objective measurements within the "activity" and "participation" domains. The constructs contained in these domains as described in the ICF (WHO, 2002) seem to share some ground with what are commonly referred to as "functional" abilities. Functional abilities usually refer to some measure of the independent performance of basic life skills (toileting, eating, dressing, ambulating, reading, writing, speaking, understanding others, etc.), with "100% independence" or a descriptive rating of normal/near-normal performance; see the discussion of the National Outcomes Measurement System (NOMS) in Chapter 5. A reference to measures of "functional status" usually takes into account the degree of independence or assistance provided by others in the environment. How well an individual performs functionally also depends on the motivation to perform certain activities, with or without help, and the extent to which that level of assistance is consistently available. Functional limitations are also defined by the individual and his or her expectations, priorities, goals, social supports, and other factors (Frattali, 1998b). Delineation of what we mean by functional status compared with performance areas that fall into the ICF activity and participation domains has been a challenge. In the WHO ICF model, as illustrated by **Fig. 2.8**, the activity and participation domains are qualified within a context of environment and personal factors. The WHO model links activity and participation into the same chapter, and the associated behavioral items listed there run the gamut from basic self-care to participation in civic life. Measuring social participation, the ultimate goal of rehabilitation, is a challenge, as social events occur outside of clinical control (domestic life, civic life, interpersonal relationships). Thus, measurements of activity and participation necessarily rely on self-reports or proxy reported observations, through interviews and survey questionnaires.

### Item Response Theory in Activity and Participation Measurement

The difficulty with the disambiguation of activity and participation in rehabilitation research using the ICF framework is discussed by Jette et al (2007), Dijkers (2010), and Batcho et al (2012). A special supplement issue of the *Archives of Physical Medicine and Rehabilitation*, titled "Measurement of Participation in Rehabilitation Research," published in 2010, specifically focused on these issues. In the introduction to this supplement, Heinemann, the director of the Center for Rehabilitation Outcomes Research (CROR) at the Rehabilitation Institute of Chicago, described several initiatives and projects, principally involving the application of IRT to evaluate self-reported outcome instruments, and highlights developments in the conceptualization and measurement refinement of the participation domain for research purposes (Heinemann, 2010).

This supplement on the measurement of participation also contains a series of related commentaries and reviews of potential interest to rehabilitation outcome researchers, with topics related to meta-analysis of contemporary participation measures by Magasi and Post (2010), applications of response shift theory to participation measurement methods (Schwartz, 2010), an examination of the intersection between the WHO ICF participation and environmental factors (Noreau & Boschen, 2010), and issues related to measurement of participation in clinical trials (Whiteneck, 2010).

With support from the NIDRR, colleagues at the CROR are currently focused on questions about reliable measurements of the *activity* domain. An example of a scale expressly measuring the activity domain in rehabilitation is the Boston University Activity Measurement for Post-Acute Care (AM-PAC) (Jette, 2010; Jette et al, 2012). The AM-PAC was validated for postacute care in 2000 with support from an NIDDR grant. The initial data were drawn from 1041 patients in skilled nursing facilities, inpatient rehabilitation facilities, home health programs, and outpatient clinics. The assessment has 269 core functional activity items across three domains (daily activities, basic mobility, and life skills/applied cognitive abilities). The AM-PAC is currently published in 20 languages and is designed to track activities across care settings. There are three versions currently available—an adaptive outpatient short-form version, a free-standing CT version, and a Web-based CT version—with all three calibrated to a common functional ability scale (Jette, 2010). This instrument has been chosen by CMS to be the assessment tool for prospective payments in outpatient settings and is endorsed by the National Quality Forum.

### Measuring Communicative Participation

The WHO ICF defines participation as involvement in life situations. This definition has challenged the measurement of *communicative participation,* as Eadie and her colleagues (2006) note. Those researchers examined 15 functional assessment and quality-of-life instruments with a focus on six self-report instruments purporting to be measures of *communicative participation.* They examined the psychometric properties relative to how well these tools addressed the "participation" component of the WHO ICF (2001), and found none of the instruments reviewed were strictly measures of communicative participation. They concluded that such instruments were extremely limited and recommended the application of IRT to develop item banks from these instruments: "Applications of item response theory (IRT) modeling have increased considerably in the past 10 years in medical rehabilitation because of its utility for instrumental development and evaluation, development of short and alternative forms of instruments, instrument, linking and computerized adaptive testing" (Eadie et al, 2006, p. 317; see also Streiner & Norman, 2003).

Yorkston, Baylor, and their colleagues in their research projects at the University of Washington have taken the lead in speech-language pathology and are addressing this challenge by operationally defining communicative participation and activity and applying IRT methods to these assessments (Baylor, Yorkston, Bamer, Britton, & Amtmann, 2010; Baylor, Yorkston, Eadie, Miller, & Amtmann, 2008; Baylor, Yorkston, Eadie, Maronian, 2007; Baylor et al, 2009; Yorkston et al, 2007, 2008).

### Measuring Quality of Life

Quality of life (QoL), or health-related quality of life (HRQoL), is the acknowledged objective for interventions with certain chronic or end-stage conditions, such as cancer, end-stage renal disease, and progressive neurologic diseases, as well as with palliative care and in clinical trials (Yost & Eton, 2005). The Wilson and Cleary model explicitly targets life quality as the end result, at the far right of the model. Abresch and his colleagues (2009) describe HRQoL as the "new clinical end point" in rehabilitation medicine. These authors provide a review of several assessment tools that run the gamut of physical (e.g., nutrition), psychological (e.g., body image), and social factors (e.g., ability to communicate), each contributing and assessing some aspect of QoL. QoL instruments are self-reports, and they address a range of life dimensions affecting life quality end points, which is why instruments such as the SF-36/SF-36v2 are so often included as outcome data in clinical trials. However, as we said earlier, researchers recognize the test-taking burden with some QoL instruments can be problematic for individuals with medical fragility. Thus, researchers have taken advantage of IRT to create valid, accessible measurements of HRQoL. For example, the Functional Assessment of Chronic Illness Therapy (FACIT) measurement system uses MID methods for group comparisons of HRQoL outcomes and IRT item banks and CT for several scales (Webster, Cella, & Yost, 2003). FACIT is an efficient and useful tool providing a collection of quality-of-life assessment questionnaire items with 50 scales and symptom indices. The FACIT is currently published in over 50 languages (http://www.facit.org/FACITOrg/Questionnaires).

In addition to the FACIT, another frequently used QoL tool in clinical practice and rehabilitation research is the SF-36v2. The SF-36, and the newer SF-36v2 version, is an instrument developed by the Rand corporation and the Medical Outcomes Study (MOS) (http://www.rand.org/health/surveys_tools/mos/mos_36 item_survey.html). The SF-36 provides a 36-item short interview survey (in person or over the telephone). The basic instrument contains items related to physical and mental health with responses across a 5-point scale ("all of the time" to "none of the time"). The items are psychometrically well designed, normed and standardized, and tested across a wide range of disorders; see Ware and colleagues (1994). Another IRT-based instrument available in the public domain is NeuroQoL, a health-related QoL instrument specifically designed to measure outcomes with neurological populations using item banks or scales for mental health, social health, and physical health with reference to relevant domains (such as pain, fatigue, and upper and lower extremity function scales in physical health rating). The NeuroQoL was developed and has been studied by Cella and colleagues at Northwestern University's Feinman School of Medicine since 2009 (Gershon et al, 2011). Research and development continues with this instrument. Currently, the NeuroQoL provides the platform to evaluate intervention outcome with traumatic brain injury, stroke, multiple sclerosis, Parkinson's disease, and brain tumors. An additional example of an HRQoL measure originally designed for use in Europe is the EQ-5D. The EuroQoL, now known as the EQ-5D, is used worldwide. This is a 15-item instrument, with a 0 to 100 rating scale for health and well-being.

## ♦ Data Capture Tools and Support

### Web-Based and Phone Survey Tools for Patient-Reported Outcomes

There have been several innovations and instruments developed over the past decade that enable computerized and Web-based data captures in outcomes research. Research projects and clinical programs can draw upon an array of instruments from paper-and-pencil questionnaires, to phone interviews and special-purpose online surveys available through various vendors and publishers. One well-known method for gathering survey data at a nominal cost is Survey Monkey (http://www.surveymonkey.com/). Online PRO surveys using Survey Monkey are a way to gather local PRO data for clinical practice or research purposes. As research tools, online and Web-based systems must include features to protect the respondent's identity and ensure secure data storage. Several online, Web-based applications, or telephone access methods are available for researchers and service providers who want to capture quality-of-life and functional or health status outcomes through PRO data collection. Some examples:

• *Bright Outcomes.* Bright Outcomes employs Web-based, telephone, or hand-held device systems for patient input and is designed to measure outcomes by tracking patient symptoms and side effects.

Bright Outcomes is intended to provide patient education and to alert care providers or clinical trial teams about a problem (http://www.brightoutcome.com).

- *Computer-Assisted Interview* (Ci3 2.6.16). Computer-Assisted Interview is a subscription software system (not Web based) for data entry by telephone. Another survey software product for online interviews available from the same vendor is *Survey Software for Online Interviewing* (SSI) (http://www.sawtoothsoftware.com).

- *Electronic Patient-Reported Outcomes* (e-PRO). A for-profit, Web-based, voice-interactive data collection system used for real-time data access and measures of compliance (http://www.perceptive.com/epro).

- *Focus on Therapeutic Outcomes* (FOTO). A functional outcomes database for neuromuscular, musculoskeletal, cardiopulmonary, industrial, and pediatric populations, used to provide a risk-adjusted national benchmark comparison (http://www.fotoinc.com).

- *Neuro-Quality of Life* (Neuro-QoL) and *Neuro-QoL Computerized Adaptive Testing* (CT). The Neuro-QoL, mentioned earlier, is a multisite, National Institute of Neurological and Communicative Disorders and Stroke (NINCDS)-sponsored project developed to provide a health-related quality-of-life assessment tool in English and Spanish for children and adults with neurological disorders (http://neuroqol.org).

- *Patient-Reported Outcomes Measurement Information System* (PROMIS®) (Riley et al, 2010). PROMIS® is a Web-based, research management tool, that is domain-focused (includes items referencing feelings, perception, or general health) rather than disease-focused (e.g., stroke, cancer, depression). PROMIS® provides item banks that can be administered as computerized-adapted tests, which tailor the questionnaires to the individuals. The PROMIS® item banks were developed through National Institutes of Health (NIH) support, drawn from a large collection of items, and available in the public domain. The essential purpose of PROMIS® is to provide uniformity and apply psychometric rigor to instruments and items assessing health-related quality of life. PROMIS® currently has physical health, mental health, and social health item banks that were created by psychometric methods applied to multiple instruments, based on the principles of IRT (discussed above). The IRT methodology has enabled the development of short forms out of a variety of instruments, yielding sets of items for each domain, as well as enabling researchers to tailor and select their own items. Currently, the PROMIS® network of 15 research sites provides support for researchers using patients' self-reported outcomes across domains of interest. The types of research potentially using PROMIS® include clinical, observational, comparative effectiveness, population surveillance, and health care delivery studies (http://www.NIHPROMIS.org).

## Web-Based Data Capture and Informatics Support for Translational Research

Web-based products that provide access to grant-supported IT teams are being used to provide informatics support to offer researchers more efficient data collection and searches, shared resources, collaboration, database development, center networking, and data pooling between research centers. Multicenter clinical trials typically collect data across large numbers of subjects that are managed by centralized, metadata repositories to allow data submission and retrieval by the participating research centers. This is made possible through IT initiatives built on metadata management. Here we will focus on a couple of prominent examples: REDCap, or Research Electronic Data Capture, (Harris et al, 2009) and the PROMIS® network (http://nihpromis.org; http://www.assessmentcenter.net), discussed briefly above.

### Research Electronic Data Capture (REDCap) Web-Based Support

REDCap is a Web-based, metadata initiative available to REDCap consortium member partners (research-funded institutions) at no charge. REDCap was developed in 2004 subsequent to an NIH assessment revealing a need among researchers for data capture and data management in small and medium-sized research projects. The impetus behind the initial study was the observation that although pilot projects and NIH RO1 projects are the "cornerstone of America's biomedical research program" (Harris et al, 2009, p. 377; see also Zerhouni, 2003), researchers often lack the financial resources and informatics support and expertise required to collect, store securely, and share data. Consequently, the REDCap project (http://www.project-redcap.org) was initiated within the Department of Biomedical Informatics at Vanderbilt University, under the direction of Paul Harris. In 2006, the REDCap consortium's primary partners were university medical center members at three institutions: Oregon Health and Science University, Mayo Clinic, and Vanderbilt University. By 2010, the REDCap project, with support from the National Center for Research Resources (NCRR) and NIH, was expanded and currently assists with data capture for over 9000 end-users, conducting several thousand research projects of varied sizes across consortium partners around the world. REDCap is not "open-source" software. It is available at no charge to its institutional partners, for noncommercial purposes, but the redistribution is restricted to Vanderbilt University. The objectives of REDCap are to provide a Web-based, metadata methodology to collect, store, analyze, and share data across clinical and translational studies that meet the data security and audit trail standards required by HIPAA and IRBs. REDCap provides the platform to structure Web-based data captures for research and has other features (such as a Survey Monkey–type survey instrument). REDCap's data capture system can also be used by consortium member research universities to conduct organizational internal performance improvement projects and quality and patient safety studies, which will be discussed by Bradham in Chapter 11.

### PROMIS® Web-Based Support

Another example of metadata management providing informatics research support specifically aimed at rehabilitation and disablement outcome research is PROMIS®, described earlier. This system is an initiative supported by the NIH and also available to researchers and clinicians at no cost. The PROMIS® network provides a Web-based method for researchers to collaborate and coordinate using the PROMIS® item bank (with several measures for children and adults). The system enables the creation of a study-specific URL. The user can select from a particular domain (e.g., physical functioning, global health, fatigue, depression, pain, and so forth) and designate the mode of data collection (online or computer and paper), the instrument type (computer-adapted testing, short form, or profile), and length (number of items). There are a dozen primary research sites currently funded by the NIH that are responsible for developing the item banks for PROMIS®. The initiatives and objectives of these collaborators are described by Bode, Hahn, DeVellis, & Cella (2010). The project involves collecting data, conducting validity studies on the PROMIS® instrument, and then facilitating the conduct of independent studies. In addition, PROMIS® provides IT support and research scientist consultation for its associated projects.

## ◆ Conclusion and Future Directions

Outcomes measurements in health care services, research, and education today are being shaped by a confluence of issues, trends, and developments: the worldwide economic crisis; burgeoning data storage capacity; consumer and policy-maker demands for meaningful results; and pressure to demonstrate "best practices" that are informed by evidence and provided in an efficient, accountable, and transparent manner (**Fig. 2.9**). Gerben DeJong describes this convergence as "positive and exciting," and predicts that the rehabilitation professions are entering what may be our "greatest period for innovation toward the development of best practices" (DeJong, 2010).

The world is changing. To borrow a phrase from Thomas Friedman (2011), if we want to succeed in a changing world, we have to "plan for the future and not the past." For those of us who are speech-

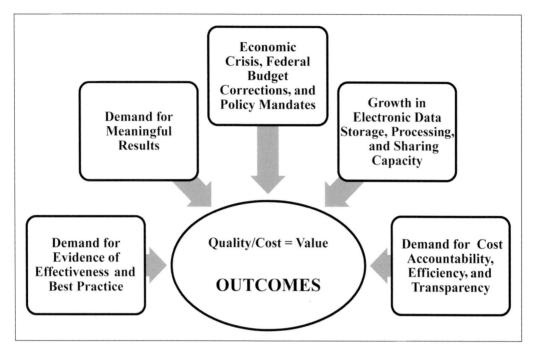

**Fig. 2.9** Contemporary issues and convergences in outcomes measurement.

language pathology researchers, educators, clinicians, and students preparing for careers in these areas, the future rests with our capacity to grasp and embrace the incentives for change that are in the wind today and to make the psychological and strategic adjustments needed to respond to those changes. It is important that we remain committed to adding weight to the quality side of the value equation through EBP as we reduce costs through efficiencies. If we do that, we will enhance the value of our work and worth, and will position our profession so that our best outcomes lie ahead of us.

# References

Abresch, R. T., Carter, G. T., Han, J. J., & McDonald, C. M. (2009, Dec). New clinical end points in rehabilitation medicine: tools for measuring quality of life. *American Journal of Hospice and Palliative Medicine, 26,* 483–492

Academy of Neurologic Communication Disorders and Sciences (ANCDS). (n.d.). *Practice guidelines project.* http://www.ancds.org

Agency for Healthcare Research and Quality (AHRQ). (n.d.). *Clinical quality measures: inclusion criteria.* http://www.qualitymeasures.ahrq.gov)

American Speech-Language-Hearing Association (ASHA). (2001). *Scope of practice in speech-language pathology.* http://www.asha.org/docs/html/SP2007-00283.html

American Speech-Language-Hearing Association (ASHA N-CEP). (n.d.) National Center on Evidence-Based Practice (N-CEP). *Systematic Reviews.* http://www.asha.org/members/ebp/EBSRs.htm

Arthanat, S., Nochajski, S. M., & Stone, J. (2004, Feb). The international classification of functioning, disability and health and its application to cognitive disorders. *Disability and Rehabilitation, 26,* 235–245 10.1080/0963828031000137063

Axelrod, R. C., & Vogel, D. (2003). Predictive modeling in health plans. *Disease Management & Health Outcomes, 11,* 779–787

Baker, K. F. (2011). Active learning: Relevancy matters. *Perspectives on Issues in Higher Education, 14,* 64–69 http://div10perspectives.asha.org/cgi/content/abstract/14/2/64

Batcho, C. S., Tennant, A., & Thonnard, J. (2012). ACTIVLIM-Stroke: A crosscultural Rasch-built scale of activity limitations in patients with stroke. *Stroke,* (43), 815–823

Baylor, C., Hula, W., Donovan, N. J., Doyle, P. J., Kendall, D., & Yorkston, K. (2011, Aug). An introduction to item response theory and Rasch models for speech-language pathologists. *American Journal of Speech-Language Pathology, 20,* 243–259 10.1044/1058-0360(2011/10-0079)

Baylor, C., Yorkston, K., Bamer, A., Britton, D., & Amtmann, D. (2010, May). Variables associated with communicative participation in people with multiple sclerosis: a regression analysis. *American Journal of Speech-Language Pathology, 19*, 143–153

Baylor, C. R., Yorkston, K. M., Eadie, T. L., & Maronian, N. C. (2007, Mar). The psychosocial consequences of BOTOX injections for spasmodic dysphonia: a qualitative study of patients' experiences. *Journal of Voice, 21*, 231–247

Baylor, C., Yorkston, K., Eadie, T., Miller, R., & Amtmann, D. (2008, Dec). Levels of Speech Usage: A self-report scale for describing how people use speech. *Journal of Medical Speech-Language Pathology, 16*, 191–198

Baylor, C. R., Yorkston, K. M., Eadie, T. L., Miller, R. M., & Amtmann, D. (2009, Oct). Developing the communicative participation item bank: Rasch analysis results from a spasmodic dysphonia sample. *Journal of Speech, Language, and Hearing Research: JSLHR, 52*, 1302–1320

Beeson, P. M., & Robey, R. R. (2006, Dec). Evaluating single-subject treatment research: lessons learned from the aphasia literature. *Neuropsychology Review, 16*, 161–169

Bennett, S. J., Perkins, S. M., Lane, K. A., Deer, M., Brater, D. C., & Murray, M. D. (2001). Social support and health-related quality of life in chronic heart failure patients. *Quality of Life Research, 10*, 671–682

Bernstein, J., MacCourt, D. C., Jacob, D. M., & Mehta, S. (2010, Oct). Utilizing information technology to mitigate the handoff risks caused by resident work hour restrictions. *Clinical Orthopaedics and Related Research, 468*, 2627–2632

Bickenbach, J. E., Chatterji, S., Kastanjsek, N., & Üstün, B. (2003). Ageing, disability and the WHO's international classification of functioning, disability and health (ICF). *The Geneva Papers on Risk and Insurance, 28*, 294–303

Blackboard Inc. (n.d.). http://www.blackboard.com

Bode, R. K., Hahn, E. A., DeVellis, R., & Cella, D.; Patient-Reported Outcomes Measurement Information System Social Domain Working Group (2010, Sep). Measuring participation: the Patient-Reported Outcomes Measurement Information System experience. *Archives of Physical Medicine and Rehabilitation, 91*(9, Suppl), S60–S65

Boone, B. J. (2011). Accreditation—a quality frame work in the consumer-centric era. In S. R. Flanagan, H. Zaretsky, & A. Moroz (Eds.), *Medical aspects of disability: A handbook for the rehabilitation professional* (4th ed., pp. 687–706). New York: Springer Publishing Company

Bowden, M. (2011). *Worm: The first digital world war*. New York: Atlantic Press Monthly, Inc.

Bruyère, S., VanLooy, S., & Peterson, D. (2005). The international classification of functioning, disability, and health (ICF): Contemporary literature overview. *Rehabilitation Psychology, 50*, 1–21

Campbell, J. M. (2004). Statistical comparison of four effect sizes for single-subject designs. *Behavior Modification, 28*, 234–246 doi: 10.1177/0145445503259264

Centers for Medicare and Medicaid Services (CMS). (2011a). Quality measures. http://www.cms.gov/QualityMeasures.asp

Centers for Medicare and Medicaid Services (CMS). (2011b). Definition of meaningful use. https://www.cms.gov/ehr incentiveprograms/30_Meaningful_Use.asp

Chang, C. H., & Reeve, B. B. (2005, Sep). Item response theory and its applications to patient-reported outcomes measurement. *Evaluation & the Health Professions, 28*, 264–282

Chartlinks. (2010). *Rehabilitation software*. www.chartlinks.com

Cieza, A., Stucki, A., Geyh, S., Berteanu, M., Quittan, M., Simon, A., et al. (2004, Jul). ICF Core Sets for chronic ischaemic heart disease. *Journal of Rehabilitation Medicine, (44*, Suppl), 94–99

Coleman, J. J., Hemming, K., Nightingale, P. G., Clark, I. R., Dixon-Woods, M., Ferner, R. E., et al. (2011, May). Can an electronic prescribing system detect doctors who are more likely to make a serious prescribing error? *Journal of the Royal Society of Medicine, 104*, 208–218

Congressional Budget Office, Office of Management and Budget (CBO). (March, 2011). *Preliminary analysis of the President's budget for 2012*. http://www.cbo.gov/doc.cfm?index=12103

Congressional Budget Office, Office of Management and Budget (CBO). (n.d.). *The White House: Historical Tables*. http://www.whitehouse.gov/omb/budget/Historicals/

Conture, E.G. (2011). What is translational research? Vanderbilt University, Department of Hearing and Speech Sciences' Speech-Language Pathology Grand Rounds presentation, September 26, 2011

Cousins, M. S., Shickle, L. M., & Bander, J. A. (2002). An introduction to predictive modeling for disease management risk stratification. *Disease Management, 5*, 157–167 10.1089/109350702760301448

Croskerry, P., & Nimmo, G. R. (2011, Jun). Better clinical decision making and reducing diagnostic error. *Journal of the Royal College of Physicians, 41*, 155–162

Dalton, W. S., Sullivan, D. M., Yeatman, T. J., & Fenstermacher, D. A. (2010, Dec). The 2010 Health Care Reform Act: a potential opportunity to advance cancer research by taking cancer personally. *Clinical Cancer Research, 16*, 5987–5996

DeJong, G. (2010). The focus on cost, quality and outcomes. Paper presented at the MediServ Rehabilitation Outcomes Conference, Phoenix, AZ, August 11–13, 2010

del Toro, C. M., Bislick, L. P., Comer, M., Velozo, C., Romero, S., Gonzalez Rothi, L. J., et al. (2011, Aug). Development of a short form of the Boston naming test for individuals with aphasia. *Journal of Speech, Language, and Hearing Research: JSLHR, 54*, 1089–1100

Dijkers, M. P. (2010, Sep). Issues in the conceptualization and measurement of participation: an overview. *Archives of Physical Medicine and Rehabilitation, 91*(9, Suppl), S5–S16

Dollaghan, C. (2007). *The handbook for evidence-based practice in communication disorders*. Baltimore, MD: Brookes

Donovan, N. J., Kendall, D. L., Young, M. E., & Rosenbek, J. C. (2008, Nov). The communicative effectiveness survey: preliminary evidence of construct validity. *American Journal of Speech-Language Pathology, 17*, 335–347

Donovan, N. J., Velozo, C. A., & Rosenbek, J. C. (2007). The Communicative Effectiveness Survey: Investigating its item-level psychometric properties. *Journal of Medical Speech-Language Pathology, 15*, 433–447

Eadie, T. L. (2007, Nov). Application of the ICF in communication after total laryngectomy. *Seminars in Speech and Language, 28*, 291–300

Eadie, T. L., Yorkston, K. M., Klasner, E. R., Dudgeon, B. J., Deitz, J. C., Baylor, C. R., et al. (2006, Nov). Measuring communicative participation: a review of self-report instruments in speech-language pathology. *American Journal of Speech-Language Pathology, 15*, 307–320

Eisenberg, J. (1997). *Testimony on healthcare quality*. http://www.ahrq.gov/news/test1028.htm

Elamin, M. B., Flynn, D. N., Bassler, D., Briel, M., Alonso-Coello, P., Karanicolas, P. J., et al. (2009, May). Choice of data extraction tools for systematic reviews depends on resources and review complexity. *Journal of Clinical Epidemiology, 62*, 506–510 [Review]

Evers, K. E. (2006). eHealth Promotion: The use of the internet for health promotion. *American Journal of Health Promotion, 20*(4, Suppl), 1–7, iii

Evers, K. E., Cummins, C. O., Prochaska, J. O., & Prochaska, J. M. (2005, Jul). Online health behavior and disease management programs: are we ready for them? Are they ready for us? *Journal of Medical Internet Research, 7*, e27

Execution Make It Happen. (n.d.) *What is meta data?* http://www.executionmih.com/metadata/definition-concept.php

Fenstermacher, D. (2010). *Metadata: The cornerstone for tomorrow's health care management.* http://www.youtube.com/watch?v=YCBLqLUi0BY

Fisher, W. P., Jr, & Burton, E. C. (2010). Embedding measurement within existing computerized data systems: scaling clinical laboratory and medical records heart failure data to predict ICU admission. *Journal of Applied Measurement, 11,* 271–287

Fox, S. (2007). *E-patients with a disability or chronic disease.* PEW Internet & American Life Project. http://www.pewinternet.org/

Frattali, C. M. (1998a). Outcomes measurement: Definitions, dimensions, and perspectives. In C. M. Frattali (Ed.), *Measuring outcomes in speech-language pathology* (pp. 1–27). New York: Thieme

Frattali, C. M. (1998b). Measuring modality-specific behaviors. In C. M. Frattali (Ed.), *Measuring outcomes in speech-language pathology* (pp. 55–88). New York: Thieme

Friedman, T. (2011). Interview: National Public Radio. Broadcast date: October 3, 2011

Geisser, S. (1993). *Predictive inference: An introduction.* New York: Chapman and Hall

Gershon, R. C., Lai, J. S., Bode, R., Choi, S., Moy, C., Bleck, T., et al. (2011). Neuro-QOL: quality of life item banks for adults with neurological disorders: item development and calibrations based upon clinical and general population testing. *Quality of Life Research.* http://www.ncbi.nlm.nih.gov/pubmed/21874314

Golper, L. (2001). ANCDS Practice Guidelines Coordinating Committee Report: Proceedings of the Academy of Neurologic Communication Disorders and Sciences. *Journal of Medical Speech-Language Pathology, 9,* ix–x

Golper, L., & Brown, K. A. (2007). Applying evidence to clinical practice. In R. Lubinski, L. Golper, & C. Frattali (Eds.), *Professional issues in speech-language pathology* (3rd ed., pp. 560–576). Clifton Park, NY: Thompson Delmar Learning

Haglund, L., & Henriksson, C. (2003). Concepts in occupational therapy in relation to the ICF. *Occupational Therapy International, 10,* 253–268

Harris, P. A., Taylor, R., Thielke, R., Payne, J., Gonzalez, N., & Conde, J. G. (2009, Apr). Research electronic data capture (REDCap)—a metadata-driven methodology and workflow process for providing translational research informatics support. *Journal of Biomedical Informatics, 42,* 377–381

Haynes, R. B., Devereaux, P. J., & Guyatt, G. H. (2002a, Aug). Clinical expertise in the era of evidence-based medicine and patient choice. *Vox Sanguinis, 83*(1, Suppl 1), 383–386 [Editorial]

Haynes, R. B., Devereaux, P. J., & Guyatt, G. H. (2002b). Physicians' and patients' choices in evidence-based medicine: evidences does not make decisions, people do. *British Medical Journal, 324,* 1350 [Editorial]

Hays, R. D., Morales, L. S., & Reise, S. P. (2000, Sep). Item response theory and health outcomes measurement in the 21st century. *Medical Care, 38*(9, Suppl), II28–II42

Health and Human Services (HHS). (n.d.). *Center of Excellence for Disability Research.* http://www.hhs.gov/disability research/)

Health and Human Services, Office of the Inspector General (HHS). (2009). *Adverse events in hospitals: National evidence among Medicare beneficiaries.* http://oig.hhs.gov/oei/reports/oei-06-09-00090.pdf

Heerkens, Y., van der Brug, Y., Napel, H. T., & van Ravensberg, D. (2003, Jun). Past and future use of the ICF (former ICIDH) by nursing and allied health professionals. *Disability and Rehabilitation, 25,* 620–627

Heinemann, A. W. (2010, Sep). Measurement of participation in rehabilitation research. *Archives of Physical Medicine and Rehabilitation, 91*(9, Suppl), S1–S4

Hilbert, M., & López, P. (2011, Apr). The world's technological capacity to store, communicate, and compute information. *Science, 332,* 60–65

Horn, S. D., & Gassaway, J. (2007, Oct). Practice-based evidence study design for comparative effectiveness research. *Medical Care, 45*(10, Suppl 2), S50–S57

Hula, W., Austermann Hula, S. N., & Doyle, P. J. (2009). A preliminary evaluation of the reliability and validity of self-reported communicative functioning item pool. *Aphasiology, 23,* 783–796

Hula, W., Donovan, N. J., Kendall, D., & Gonzalez-Rothi, L. (2010). Item response theory analysis of the Western Aphasia Battery. *Aphasiology, 24,* 1326–1341

Hula, W. D., Doyle, P. J., & Austermann Hula, S. N. (2010, Mar). Patient-reported cognitive and communicative functioning: 1 construct or 2? *Archives of Physical Medicine and Rehabilitation, 91,* 400–406

Institute of Medicine (IOM). (1999). *To err is human: Building a safer health system.* Washington, DC: National Academies Press

Institute of Medicine (IOM). (2001). *Crossing the quality chasm.* Washington, DC: National Academies Press

Institute of Medicine (IOM). (2007). *Future of disabilities in America.* Washington, DC: National Academies Press

Jaeschke, R., Singer, J., & Guyatt, G. H. (1989, Dec). Measurement of health status. Ascertaining the minimal clinically important difference. *Controlled Clinical Research Trials, 10,* 407–415

Jette, A. M. (2009, Nov). Toward a common language of disablement. *The Journals of Gerontology. Series A, Biological Sciences and Medical Sciences, 64,* 1165–1168

Jette, A. (2010). Changing the landscape of outcome assessment. Paper presented at the MediServ Rehabilitation Outcomes Conference, Phoenix, AZ, August 11–13, 2010

Jette, A., Pengsheng, N., Rasch, E. K., Appelman, J., Sandel, M. E., Terdiman, J., et al. (2012). Evaluation of patient and proxy responses on the Activity Measure for Postacute Care. *Stroke, (43),* 824–829

Jette, A. M., Tao, W., & Haley, S. M. (2007, Nov). Blending activity and participation sub-domains of the ICF. *Disability and Rehabilitation, 29,* 1742–1750

Justice, L. M. (2008, Nov). Evidence-based terminology. *American Journal of Speech-Language Pathology, 17,* 324–325

Justice, L. M., Bowles, R. P., & Skibbe, L. E. (2006, Jul). Measuring preschool attainment of print-concept knowledge: a study of typical and at-risk 3- to 5-year-old children using item response theory. *Language, Speech, and Hearing Services in Schools, 37,* 224–235

Kahol, K., Vankipuram, M., Patel, V. L., & Smith, M. L. (2011, Jun). Deviations from protocol in a complex trauma environment: errors or innovations? *Journal of Biomedical Informatics, 44,* 425–431

Kamhi, A. G. (2011, Jan). Balancing certainty and uncertainty in clinical practice. *Language, Speech, and Hearing Services in Schools, 42,* 59–64

Kearney, P. M., & Pryor, J. (2004, Apr). The international classification of functioning, disability and health (IFC) and nursing. *Journal of Advanced Nursing, 46,* 162–170

Kendall, D., del Toro, C., Nadeau, S., Johnson, J., Rosenbek, J. C., & Velozo, C. A. (2011). The development of a standardized instrument of phonology in aphasia: construct validity, sensitivity and test retest reliability. Paper presented at the 2011 Clinical Aphasiology Conference

King, D. L. (2008). Using the Revised Wilson and Cleary Model to explore factors affecting quality of life of persons on hemodialysis. Unpublished dissertation. http://libres.uncg.edu/ir/listing.aspx?id=185

King, M. T. (2011, Apr). A point of minimal important difference (MID): a critique of terminology and methods. *Expert Reviews: Expert Review of Pharmacoeconomics and Outcomes Research, 11,* 171–184

Kirklin, J. W., & Vicinanza, S. S. (1999, Sep). Metadata and computer-based patient records. *The Annals of Thoracic Surgery, 68*(3, Suppl), S23–S24

Leapfrog Group. (2008). *Factsheet: Computerized physician order entry.* http://www.yalemedicalgroup.org/stw/page.asp?patID=STW036289

Lee, J. S., Hobden, E., Stiell, I. G., & Wells, G. A. (2003, Oct). Clinically important change in the visual analog scale after adequate pain control. *Academic Emergency Medicine, 10,* 1128–1130

Magasi, S., & Post, M. W. (2010, Sep). A comparative review of contemporary participation measures' psychometric properties and content coverage. *Archives of Physical Medicine and Rehabilitation, 91*(9, Suppl), S17–S28

Marshall, J., Goldbart, J., Pickstone, C., & Roulstone, S. (2011, May–Jun). Application of systematic reviews in speech-and-language therapy. *International Journal of Language & Communication Disorders, 46,* 261–272

McLeod, S., & McCormack, J. (2007, Nov). Application of the ICF and ICF-children and youth in children with speech impairment. *Seminars in Speech and Language, 28,* 254–264

MediServe. (n.d.). *MediServe: Inpatient and outpatient solutions.* http://mediserve.com/rehab_medilinks_acute.php

Merrill, M. (2011). DoD joins with NIH to build TBI Data Base. http://govhealthit.com/news/dod-joins-nih-build-tbi-database\

Miller, M. R., Elixhauser, A., Zhan, C., & Meyer, G. S. (2001, Dec). Patient Safety Indicators: using administrative data to identify potential patient safety concerns. *Health Services Research, 36*(6 Pt 2), 110–132

Mish, F. C. (1983). *Merriam-Webster's new collegiate dictionary* (9th ed.). Springfield, MA: Merriam-Webster

National Institutes of Health (NIH). (2008). *Human genome project.* http://www.ornl.gov/sci/techrouces/Human_Genome/home.shtml

National Institutes of Health (NIH). (2011). *NIH database will speed research toward better prevention, diagnosis and treatment of traumatic brain injury.* http://www.nih.gov/news/health/aug20121/ninds-29.htm

Noreau, L., & Boschen, K. (2010, Sep). Intersection of participation and environmental factors: a complex interactive process. *Archives of Physical Medicine and Rehabilitation, 91*(9, Suppl), S44–S53

O'Mathúna, D. P. (2010, Aug). Critical appraisal of systematic reviews. *International Journal of Nursing Practice, 16,* 414–418

Pear, R. (2010). *Standards issued for electronic health records.* http://www.nytimes.com/2010/07/14/health/policy/14health.html

Peterson, D. B. (2005). International classification of functioning, disability and health (ICF): An introduction for rehabilitation psychologists. *Rehabilitation Psychology, 50,* 105–112

Professional Research Consultants (PRC) Inc. (n.d.). Vanderbilt University Medical Center Patient Satisfaction Survey, September, 2011. https://www.prceasyview.com/

Rangasayee, R., Mukundan, G., Dalvi, U., Nandurkar, A., & Kant, A. (2010). Invited tutorial: The International Classification of Functioning, Disability, and Health (ICF) for audiologists and speech-language pathologists. *Journal of the Indian Speech and Hearing Association, 24,* 1–23

Rao, P. (2011). *From the President: Evidence-based practice: the coin of the realm in CSD.* http://asha.org/Publications/leader/2011/110607

Rauch, A., Cieza, A., & Stucki, G. (2008, Sep). How to apply the International Classification of Functioning, Disability and Health (ICF) for rehabilitation management in clinical practice. *European Journal of Physical and Rehabilitation Medicine, 44,* 329–342

Research Triangle Institute Health Solutions. [RTI(h)(s)]. (n.d.). *Patient-reported outcomes: Capturing the patient's perspective.* www.rtihs.org/request/index.cfm?fuseaction=display&pid=5196

Riegelman, R. K. (2005). *Studying a study and testing a test: How to read the medical evidence* (5th ed.). Philadelphia: Lippincott, Williams & Wilkins

Riley, W. T., Rothrock, N., Bruce, B., Christodolou, C., Cook, K., Hahn, E. A., et al. (2010, Nov). Patient-reported outcomes measurement information system (PROMIS) domain names and definitions revisions: further evaluation of content validity in IRT-derived item banks. *Quality of Life Research, 19,* 1311–1321

Rogers, G., & Joyner, E. (n.d.). *Mining your data for healthcare quality improvement.* http://www2.sas.com/proceedings/sugi22/EMERGING/PAPER139.PDF

Sackett, D. L., Richardson, W. S., Rosenberg, W. M. C., & Haynes, R. B. (2000). *Evidence-based medicine: How to practice and teach EBM.* London: Churchill Livingstone

Sackett, D.L., Rosenberg, W.M.C., Gray, J.A.M., Haynes, R. B., & Richardson, W.S. (1996). Evidence-based medicine: What it is and what it isn't. *Article based on an editorial in the British Medical Journal, 312,* 71–72

Schaffner, W. (2011). *Interview: Growth, Change for Preventative Medicine Mission, Carol Bartoo, Vanderbilt University Reporter,* Thursday, June 2, 2011. http://www.mc.vanderbilt.edu/reporter/index.html?ID=10813

Schlosser, R. W. (2007). Appraising the quality of systematic reviews. *Focus: Technical Brief Number 17,* 1–8

Schwartz, C. E. (2010, Sep). Applications of response shift theory and methods to participation measurement: a brief history of a young field. *Archives of Physical Medicine and Rehabilitation, 91*(9, Suppl), S38–S43

Selkowitz, D. M., Kulig, K., Poppert, E. M., Flanagan, S. P., Matthews, N. D., Beneck, G. J., et al.; Physical Therapy Clinical Research Network (2006). The immediate and long-term effects of exercise and patient education on physical, functional, and quality-of-life outcome measures after single-level lumbar microdiscectomy: a randomized controlled trial protocol. *BMC Musculoskeletal Disorders, 7,* 70–85

Sibelius, K. (2009). *Congressional confirmation hearing,* April, 2009. http://www.advocacyed.com/Docs/Personalized_Medicine_Issue_Brief.pdf

Simmons-Mackie, N., Threats, T. T., & Kagan, A. (2006). Outcome assessment in aphasia: a survey. *Journal of Communication Disorders, 38,* 1–27

Solanas, A., Leiva, D., & Salafranca, L. (2010, Feb). Bias and standard error for social reciprocity measurements. *The British Journal of Mathematical and Statistical Psychology, 63*(Pt 1), 139–161

Solanas, A., Manolov, R., & Onghena, P. (2010, May). Estimating slope and level change in N = 1 designs. *Behavior Modification, 34,* 195–218

Source Therapy Net™. (n.d.). *Source Therapy™.* http://sourcemed.net/rehabilitation/

Sousa, K. H., & Kwok, O.-M. (2006, May). Putting Wilson and Cleary to the test: analysis of a HRQOL conceptual model using structural equation modeling. *Quality of Life Research, 15,* 725–737

Stewart, J. (2011). Global data storage calculated at 295 exabytes. *News Technology.* http://www.bbc.co.uk/news/technology-12419672

Stineman, M. G., Jette, A., Fiedler, R., & Granger, C. V. (1997, Jun). Impairment-specific dimensions within the Functional Independence Measure. *Archives of Physical Medicine and Rehabilitation, 78,* 636–643

Stineman, M. G., Shea, J. A., Jette, A., Tassoni, C. J., Ottenbacher, K. J., Fiedler, R., et al. (1996, Nov). The Functional Independence Measure: tests of scaling assumptions, structure, and reliability across 20 diverse impairment categories. *Archives of Physical Medicine and Rehabilitation, 77,* 1101–1108

Streiner, D. L., & Norman, G. R. (2003). *Health measurement scales: A practical guide to their development and use* (3rd ed.). Oxford, England: Oxford University Press

Sylvia, M. L., Shadmi, E., Hsiao, C. J., Boyd, C. M., Schuster, A. B., & Boult, C. (2006, Feb). Clinical features of high-risk older persons identified by predictive modeling. *Disease Management, 9,* 56–62

Threats, T. (2002). Evidence-based practice using the WHO-ICF. *Journal of Medical Speech-Language Pathology, 10,* xvii–xxiv

Threats, T. (2007a). Access for persons with neurogenic communication disorders: Influences of Personal and Environmental Factors of the ICF. *Aphasiology, 21,* 67–80

Threats, T. T. (2007b, Nov). Use of the ICF in dysphagia management. *Seminars in Speech and Language, 28,* 323–333

Threats, T. (2008). Use of the ICF for clinical practice in speech-language pathology. *International Journal of Speech-Language Pathology, 10,* 50–60

Threats, T., & Worrell, L. (2004). Classifying communication disability using the ICF. *Advances in Speech Language Pathology, 6,* 53–62

Tonelli, M. R. (2006, Jun). Integrating evidence into clinical practice: an alternative to evidence-based approaches. *Journal of Evaluation in Clinical Practice, 12,* 248–256

Tsapas, A., & Matthews, D. R. (2008, Jun). N of 1 trials in diabetes: making individual therapeutic decisions. *Diabetologia, 51,* 921–925

Tsapas, A., & Matthews, D. R. (2009, Mar). Using N-of-1 trials in evidence-based clinical practice. *Journal of the American Medical Association, 301,* 1022–1023, author reply 1023 [letter]

Unicharts™. (n.d.). *EMR.* http://www.unicharts.com

U.S. Federal Budget. (n.d.). *United States federal budget: Tax revenue and expenses as a percent of the GDP 1981–2012.* http://en.wikipedia.org/wiki/United_States-federal_budget

Ustün, B., Chatterji, S., & Kostanjsek, N. (2004, Jul). Comments from WHO for the Journal of Rehabilitation Medicine special supplement on ICF core sets. *Journal of Rehabilitation Medicine, 44*(44, Suppl), 7–8

Verbrugge, L. M., & Jette, A. M. (1994, Jan). The disablement process. *Social Science & Medicine, 38,* 1–14

Walters, S. J., & Brazier, J. E. (2003). What is the relationship between the minimally important difference and health state utility values? The case of the SF-6D. *Health and Quality of Life Outcomes, 1,* 4 10.1186/1477-7525-1-4

Ware, J. E., & Gandek, B., & the IQOLA Project Group (1994). The SF-36® Health Survey: Development and use in mental health research and the IQOLA Project. *International Journal of Mental Health, 23,* 49–73

Webster, K., Cella, D., & Yost, K. (2003). The Functional Assessment of Chronic Illness Therapy (FACIT) Measurement System: properties, applications, and interpretation. *Health and Quality of Life Outcomes, 1,* 79 10.1186/1477-7525-1-79

Westby, C. (2007, Nov). Application of the ICF in children with language impairments. *Seminars in Speech and Language, 28,* 265–272

Westfall, J. M., Mold, J., & Fagnan, L. (2007, Jan). Practice-based research—"Blue Highways" on the NIH roadmap. *Journal of the American Medical Association, 297,* 403–406

Whiteneck, G. G. (2010, Sep). Issues affecting the selection of participation measurement in outcomes research and clinical trials. *Archives of Physical Medicine and Rehabilitation, 91*(9, Suppl), S54–S59

Wolery, M., & Dunlap, G. (2001). Reporting on studies using single-subject experimental methods. *Journal of Early Intervention, 24,* 85–89

Wolfe, F., Michaud, K., & Strand, V. (2005, Apr). Expanding the definition of clinical differences: from minimally clinically important differences to really important differences. Analyses in 8931 patients with rheumatoid arthritis. *The Journal of Rheumatology, 32,* 583–589

World Health Organization (WHO). (1980). *International classification of impairments, disabilities and handicaps: A manual of classification relating to the consequences of disease.* Geneva: Author

World Health Organization (WHO ICF). (2001). *International classification of functioning, disability and health.* Geneva: Author

World Health Organization (WHO). (2002). *Towards a common language for functioning, disability and health, ICF.* http://www.who.int/classification.icf

World Health Organization (WHO). (2003). *International statistical classification of diseases and related health problems. 10th Revision (ICD-10).* Geneva: Author

World Health Organization (WHO). (2007). *Classification of functioning, disability and health Version for children and youth.* Geneva: Author

World Health Organization (WHO). (2011). *Report on Disabilities.* http://www.who.int/disabilities/world_report/2011/report/en/index.html

Worrall, L., & Hickson, L. (2008). Use of the ICF in speech-language pathology research: Towards a research agenda. *International Journal of Speech-Language Pathology, 10,* 72–77

Yaruss, J. S. (2007, Nov). Application of the ICF in fluency disorders. *Seminars in Speech and Language, 28,* 312–322

Yaruss, J. S., & Quesal, R. W. (2004, Jan-Feb). Stuttering and the International Classification of Functioning, Disability, and Health: an update. *Journal of Communication Disorders, 37,* 35–52

Yorkston, K. M., Baylor, C. R., Dietz, J., Dudgeon, B. J., Eadie, T., Miller, R. M., et al. (2008). Developing a scale of communicative participation: a cognitive interviewing study. *Disability and Rehabilitation, 30,* 425–433

Yorkston, K. M., Baylor, C. R., Klasner, E. R., Deitz, J., Dudgeon, B. J., Eadie, T., et al. (2007, Nov-Dec). Satisfaction with communicative participation as defined by adults with multiple sclerosis: a qualitative study. *Journal of Communication Disorders, 40,* 433–451

Yost, K. J., & Eton, D. T. (2005, Jun). Combining distribution- and anchor-based approaches to determine minimally important differences: the FACIT experience. *Evaluation & the Health Professions, 28,* 172–191

Zerhouni, E. A. (2003). A new vision for the National Institutes of Health. *Journal of Biomedicine & Biotechnology, 3,* 159–160

# 3

# WHO's International Classification of Functioning, Disability, and Health: A Framework for Clinical and Research Outcomes

*Travis T. Threats*

## ♦ Chapter Focus

This chapter references outcome measurement within the framework of the current World Health Organization's (WHO) International Classification of Functioning, Disability, and Health (ICF) (WHO, 2001). The ICF's holistic framework is described and proposed as a unifying classification system and coherent model for rehabilitation outcomes research and clinical outcome measurements in speech-language pathology. Outcomes with communication disorders can be studied and viewed through the lens of each component of the ICF framework as well as through the prism of synergies and correlations across these domains. The ICF challenges us to consider the importance of client-defined goals, the consequences of disabilities across activity and participation domains, and the perceptions of interventions from the perspective of the recipients of those services.

## ♦ Introduction

The 1980 publication by the World Health Organization (WHO) of the International Classification of Impairments, Disabilities, and Handicaps (ICIDH) (Frattali, 1998; Frattali, Thompson, Holland, Wohl, & Ferketic, 1995; WHO, 1980) sparked increased interest in the classification of disabilities. The ICIDH was the result the WHO's efforts at meeting the challenge of its original 1948 definition of health, which states, "Health is a state of complete physical, mental, and social wellbeing and not merely the absence of disease or infirmity" (WHO, 2006, p. 1). This definition suggests functional health and life participation are central to health and well-being. Currently, the WHO is advocating for combining the ICF codes with the International Statistical Classification of Diseases and Related Health Programs (ICD) (WHO, 1992, 2011) to produce a unified and multifactorial classification system to better define health.

In 1993, the WHO started work to improve the framework and to include more stakeholders in the process. Unlike the earlier ICIDH, the ICF includes operational definitions for all categories and individual items, a complete coding system, more neutral terminology, inclusion of environmental factors, and more input from socially oriented models of disability (WHO, 2001). In 2007, the WHO published the International Classification of Functioning, Disability, and Health for Children and

Youth (ICF-CY) (WHO, 2007). Whereas the ICF covers an age range of 18 and older, the ICF-CY ranges from birth to age 17. The ICF-CY has developmental codes such as "acquiring syntax." Because the ICF-CY extends up to age 17, nearly all of the codes that are in the ICF are also found in the ICF-CY. The ICF-CY and ICF coding enable disability classification across an individual's life span. This is especially important for lifelong congenital disabilities, such as cerebral palsy, and acquired, chronic conditions, such as traumatic brain injuries in childhood.

## ♦ International Classification of Functioning, Disability, and Health Applications in Speech-Language Pathology and Rehabilitation

The profession of speech-language pathology was one of the earliest adopters of the ICF framework. The ICF was used as the framework for the field by the American Speech-Language-Hearing Association (ASHA) in its 2001 Scope of Practice for Speech-Language Pathology, the same year that the ICF was published. The ICF has been referenced in cardinal documents of the ASHA since then. Frattali et al (1995) provided a strong voice in support of the importance of applying the WHO's ICF (ICIDH) principles in communication rehabilitation.

The ICF has been incorporated into other countries' scope of practice documents in speech-language pathology including Canada, United Kingdom, and Australia. Other professional organizations in the United States have also adopted the ICF framework in their policy documents, including the American Physical Therapy Association (APTA), the American Therapeutic Recreation Association (ATRA), the American Occupational Therapy Association (AOTA), the Association of Rehabilitation Nurses (ARN), and the International Society of Physical Medicine and Rehabilitation.

At a recent preconference symposium of the American Congress of Rehabilitation Medicine (ACRM) and the American Society of Neurorehabilitation, the focus was placed on one of the ICF's core concepts, *participation.* The September 2010 supplement to the ACRM's journal, *Archives of Physical Medicine and Rehabilitation*, was devoted entirely to the important topic of measurement participation in rehabilitation research. In his commentary on that meeting, Heinemann (2010) observed: "In the United States, participation is the hallmark of legislative and executive initiatives, including Healthy People 2010, the Americans with Disabilities Act, and the New Freedom Initiative" (p. S1). Another important application of the ICF model in international health and quality outcomes research is found in the development, validation, and application of the WHO's Disability Assessment Schedule (DAS) II (Garin et al, 2010).

### The ICF Model in Research in Communication Disorders

The ICF and the ICF-CY have received considerable attention in the speech-language pathology literature. There have been two special issues of journals in communication disorders that have discussed the specific applications of the ICF, its components, and the types of communication disorders. In an 2007 issue of the journal *Seminars in Speech and Language*, the use of the ICF with specific communication disorders was addressed and included articles pertaining to aphasia (Simmons-Mackie & Kagan, 2007), child articulation/phonological disorders (McLeod & McCormack, 2007), child language disorders (Westby, 2007), dementia (Hopper, 2007), acquired hearing disorders (Hickson & Scarinci, 2007), laryngectomy (Eadie, 2007), motor speech disorders (Dykstra, Hakel, & Adams, 2007), fluency disorders (Yaruss, 2007), dysphagia (Threats, 2007b), cognitive communication disorders (Larkins, 2007), and voice disorders (Ma, Yiu, & Abbott, 2007).

In 2008, the *International Journal of Speech-Language Pathology* published a special double issue that addressed the various components and applications of the ICF in relationship to communication disorders, including the following broad categories: body functions/structures (McCormack & Worrall, 2008), activities and participation (O'Halloran & Larkins, 2008), contextual factors (Howe, 2008), quality of life (Cruice, 2008), clinical practice (Threats, 2008), research (Worrall & Hickson, 2008), graduate education in rehabilitation (Doyle & Skarakis-Doyle, 2008), professional policy (Brown & Hasselkus, 2008), and epidemiology (Mulhorn & Threats, 2008), as well as describing the ICF for children and youth (ICF-CY) (McLeod & Threats, 2008). These two journals had the same guest editors, representing expertise across the global use of the ICF and ICF-CY in the profession, including assessment, intervention strategies, education, policies, research, and outcome measurement. Rangasayee, Mukundan, Dalvi, Nandurkar, and Kant (2010) provide a tutorial on the ICF and a review of audiology and speech-language pathology research based on this model.

## Standardization

The WHO developed the ICF and the ICF-CY to bring some standardization to functional health and well-being measurement. The specific aims of the ICF are stated as follows:

1. To provide a scientific basis for understanding and studying health and health-related states, outcomes, and determinants

2. To establish a common language for describing health and health-related states to improve communication between different uses, such as health care workers, researchers, policy makers, and the public, including people with disabilities

3. To permit comparison of data across countries, health care disciplines, services, and time

4. To provide a systematic coding scheme for health information systems (WHO, 2001, p. 5)

Each of these aims is outcomes-oriented, but the outcomes are not tied to a specific disease, disorder, or professional specialty. Rather, the WHO seeks to standardize and make easily accessible outcomes terminology that could be equally understood by researchers, clinicians, policy makers, and persons with disabilities. Furthermore, the ICF is not targeting any specific therapy approach, procedure, or service provider. The model is indifferent as to who or what has brought about positive changes in the lives of individuals with disabilities. For example, if caring for pets improves functioning among individuals residing in nursing homes more than direct rehabilitation services, then the ICF-derived outcome could be applied to endorse pet therapy as the better intervention. Within the ICF framework and descriptions, there is no specific mention of the professional titles or therapeutic disciplines.

## Terminology

The ICF is written in lay language as much as possible to make the descriptions and terminology accessible to the general public. As a result, the outcome objectives tend to be broad targets and may not strictly conform to the definitions found in professional textbooks. For example, there is a body function ICF code "Articulation" that roughly relates to intelligibility. If children with a phonological impairment were rated using an ICF-based measure, improvement on a specific phonological process would not necessarily indicate a meaningful change, unless that improvement resulted in improved overall intelligibility. Improving from 30% to as much as 80% on a specific therapy phoneme category, for example, would also not necessarily be detected using an ICF-based assessment of articulation, unless it led to an demonstrable overall improvement in intelligibility across communicative contexts.

## ♦ Developing a Functional Outcomes Philosophy

An outcome is simply a result—any result. An outcome can be confidently attributable to some action or intervention; it may be the by-product of some other factor (environment, personality), or merely the result of the passage of time.

The outcome of studying hard for a test, it is hoped, is to do well on it. The outcome of losing weight might be lowered blood pressure. In terms of communication disorders, an outcome could be any event, including specific therapy interventions, growth and development, and spontaneous recovery, that can be linked to a behavioral measurement taken across points in time. It is important to remember that an outcome is not necessarily *change*. Sometimes the best functional result may be *no change* or maintaining a current level of function.

The ICF is not an outcome measure; it is a classification system that takes into account many factors influencing disability, health, and well-being. The ICF provides a list of categories of behaviors that can be monitored, but offers no judgment or guidelines as to which codes to pick to evaluate. It does not prescribe therapeutic techniques or specify the best way to measure a given behavioral code. Essentially, the ICF is a classification philosophy or orientation for working with persons with disabilities.

The first tenet in that philosophy is that achieving the highest possible life functioning is the right of all human beings. This philosophical tenet places primacy on the achievement of personally relevant outcomes beyond those defined by good science or research verification that a given intervention works. In a professional-centric, top-down hierarchy, the trained professional decides what is best for a given client and the client merely complies with the therapy plan. The ICF maintains that the client and family are equal partners of the professional in the decision-making and planning processes, which is essential if their needs are to be best served. Only clients can tell you what they really want. The clinician can ascertain the principal disorders, can measure the degree or severity of that impairment, and can form a professional opinion about an optimal intervention plan, including what environmental or personal factors are most interfering with the client's functioning. But, ultimately, the universe of a communication disorder and its management is unique to the individual. For example, a speech-language pathologist's goal for a person with aphasia might be to enable the person to name pictures of family members, which certainly seems like a highly relevant and functional goal. But if the aphasic person rarely called people by name, that goal may not have much personal utility. There may be other skills that the aphasic person or the family can identify as more important and relevant to communicative activities. The ICF framework is applied in a client-centered approach to evaluation and treatment by emphasizing that the clients' and their families' roles must be involved in determining the desired outcomes. That emphasis is found in the ethical annex of the ICF, which states the following:

> Wherever possible, the person whose level of functioning is being classified (or the person's advocate) should have the opportunity to participate, and in particular to challenge or affirm the appropriateness of the category being used and the assessment assigned. . . . ICF information should be used, to the greatest extent feasible, with the collaboration of individuals to enhance their choices and their control over their lives. (WHO, 2001, pp. 244–245)

In the ICF framework, assessment should be an interactive process between the professional and the client. This process allows for the type of client and client family input needed to later determine the appropriate outcome goals. Hancock (2003) reported that the use of the ICF framework at an inpatient rehabilitation unit improved the client/family outcomes. The author compared interviews with clients and their families before and after the implementation of the ICF to ascertain any differences. Hancock found that the application of the ICF framework resulted in a notable increase in clients' understanding of the purposes of rehabilitation. Hancock also found that both the clinicians and the clients perceived better outcomes using the ICF as a framework. Hancock also observed an initial resistance among therapists to having the client and family so centrally involved in the outcomes setting process.

## Client-Centered Holistic Goals

A second philosophic tenet of the ICF is that behavior and personal goals are complex and thus must be viewed holistically. Thus, it can be artificial to isolate and address specific behavioral outcomes without consideration of the whole person. Traditional scientific inquiry emphasizes isolating and controlling the factors that influence discrete behaviors. Similarly, in intervention therapists separate and target discrete aspects of functioning differentially (short-term goals) with the objective of arriving at a more global, functional end result (long-term goals). However, for many clients with complex communication problems, the sum can be more than the total of the parts. For example, a person with aphasia demonstrates only mild problems across modalities, yet his or her overall communicative functioning might be moderately or even severely impaired in terms of that individual's level of participation in life.

The ICF framework considers communication interventions and outcomes as they contribute to that individual's universe of overall functioning and life participation. Children seen for speech and language therapy often have co-occurring difficulties in various areas, including cognitive, behavioral/emotional, social, and educational. Almost all communicatively impaired persons with congenital, acquired, or progressive disabilities encounter life difficulties beyond those that speech-language pathologists (SLPs) treat. Thus, as members of the team, we should be working toward the overall life participation outcomes for a given patient. Consider, for example, if the client's principal desired outcome is to be able to participate in religious services. A composite of many skills are required to achieve that outcome. The individual will need to be able to get dressed, to travel to and from the facility where the religious service is held, manipulate and understand reading materials, understand others and express verbal responses, and engage in conventional social interactions. Thus, achieving an array of interrelated subgoals is essential to achieving the client's primary desired outcome.

Attention to holistic, real-life outcomes must be given more attention in rehabilitation interventions and research. As will be discussed elsewhere in this text, policy makers and payers in the United States are concerned with results from specific speech-language therapy interventions if they can be measured within the context of life functioning and satisfaction of the individual. Policy makers and payers expect rehabilitation to be aimed at global outcomes such as enabling clients to return to their home, continue employment or leisure activities, achieve independence and self-sufficiency, and, most of all, function in such a way as to prevent or reduce further medical and functional health consequences. The activity/participation codes of the ICF consist of many broad codes that address interpersonal communication, work, leisure, and community involvement. The use of the ICF can not only elucidate effective outcomes for communication and swallowing but also support how these improvements are crucial to achieving broader life-functioning and healthy living outcomes.

## Outcomes for Rehabilitation

According to the WHO's recently published *World Report on Disability* (WHO, 2011), there are five broad outcomes for rehabilitation: (1) prevention of the loss of function, (2) slowing the rate of loss of function, (3) improvement or restoration of function, (4) compensation for lost function, and (5) maintenance of current function. Speech-language pathology rehabilitation contributes to all five of these broad outcomes but only in partnership with other professionals, the patient, and the family. Rehabilitation services need to combine forces to achieve meaningful benefits. Evidence has demonstrated that highly coordinated rehabilitation services are the most effective and efficient (WHO, 2011). As a result we need to use the ICF to promote transdisciplinary research and service delivery models to improve the quality of life in the persons we serve.

## Applications of the ICF Philosophy

Another key philosophic tenet of the ICF is found in the description of its functions. The WHO has intended for the ICF to have applications in five areas: statistics, research, clinical, social policy, and education. Thus, the WHO is proposing that a single classification tool can be used across diverse applications because the core objective should be to improve the functional lives of all of the world's citizens. The assumption is that the best way to achieve this aim is to have a common yardstick. Thus, the WHO suggests that research and clinical outcomes should be approached with the same framework and even the same agreed-upon operational definitions of specific behaviors. The belief here is that such a shared vision will have an added value and unifying effect on all. In that context, research based on the ICF will improve its clinical utility, and as a consequence clinical care coming from that body of research will be improved as clinicians can more readily understand and translate the constructs. In addition, if social policy is aligned with an overarching research and service philosophy, then social policy will better allocate rehabilitation resources and grant money in support of ICF constructs in disability rehabilitation research. Finally, if education of students across health disciplines also embraces the same philosophical constructs, then both transdisciplinary clinical care and research can be fostered in the classroom and among graduating service providers.

Within the ICF framework, research is holistic and *translational*, and thus intended to help clinicians determine whether the intervention studied is applicable to their setting or relatable to their patients. For example, SLPs in a rehabilitation hospital reading a study with ICF as the framework might determine that the body function descriptions of the patients in the study are applicable to their patients but that the personal factors and environmental factors of the participants are too dissimilar to be applied to their client.

Clinically relevant research acknowledging the complexity of questions that need to be addressed is greatly needed in all clinical fields. In Chapter 12, Olswang and Bain argue for increased effectiveness and implementation research in communication sciences and disorders. Clinicians who embrace the ICF model are asking for the translation of treatment research into a meaningful clinical context. The problem lies not only in the research-to-clinic disconnects but also with the lack of a coherent model of outcome assessment (Simmons-Mackie, Threats, & Kagan, 2005). If clinicians cannot tell researchers what they want and they are too idiosyncratic in how they record data or view outcomes, then researchers need to find ways to make a meaningful linkage and analysis of outcomes to actual rehabilitation or educational settings. A study by Simmons-Mackie et al (2005) surveyed aphasia therapists about their use of outcome measures and their views about outcomes in aphasia intervention. The authors observed:

> One interesting finding of this survey was the large percentage of respondents attempting to measure outcomes. Another finding of note was the variability in outcome assessment practices across respondents. As noted previously, inconsistency in relation to outcome assessment practices and apparent discontinuity of practices with public policy is a potential problem for our field. We need a coherent model of outcome assessment to guide the choice of outcome assessment tools and the management of outcome data. (p. 17)

This inconsistency in outcome definitions and practices is evident across interventions in the field. Although it is true that a wide variety of therapeutic approaches may be needed to help the unique and varied individuals the SLP serves, we need to have standardized objectives and ways to view the outcomes of these treatments. How can one reliably tell whether research treatment A is better than research treatment B if the studies examining both of these treatments use different outcome measures? How can one tell if rehabilitation hospital A is producing better outcomes than rehabilitation hospital B if there are no common outcome yardsticks? Further adding to the confusion, what if research in a given area consistently uses different outcome approaches and measures than are used in a related field? The application of the ICF could provide answers to these questions. Stucki, Reinhardt, and Grimby (2007) state the following:

> The professional rehabilitation sciences are operating at the cutting edge between rehabilitation research and practice. They are thus uniquely positioned to improve the transition from translational research to research translation. While it makes sense to differentiate between professional rehabilitation sciences (study how to provide best care) and professional rehabilitation practice (provision of best care), the distinction between professional rehabilitation scientists and professionals in rehabilitation is only of analytical value. Indeed, every rehabilitation professional should apply scientific standards to the accomplishment of his or her work, should contribute to the development of new research questions and interventions related to his practical experience, and should be a qualified partner for clinical or community-placed trials as well as outcome and validation studies in specific settings. In turn, every professional rehabilitation scientist should be rooted and experienced in a professional rehabilitation

discipline, such as PMR (Physical Medicine and Rehabilitation), rehabilitation nursing, occupational therapy, physiotherapy, or speech therapy. While biomedical rehabilitation scientists and engineers primarily concentrate on the efficacy of interventions, rehabilitation professionals should be interested in the scientific study of the interventions' effectiveness in their particular setting. (pp. 305–306)

An ICF-based outcome system raises the stakes for all rehabilitation disciplines. It demands more results and more *comprehensive* results beyond what we have traditionally considered as evidence of successful outcomes. However, we need to realistically look at the state of the rehabilitation sciences now. We are chronically underfunded in research, our reimbursement is constantly challenged, and our profile in the overall medical establishment is not as strong as it should be. Instead of being wary about the challenges the ICF presents, we should be enthusiastic if it challenges us to demonstrate the overall global positive health effects and the cost-effectiveness of providing therapy services. There are few things more central to being a functioning human being than communication and no life activity more vital and important physiologically and psychologically as the ability to swallow. By being an essential part of something greater, we expand our reach.

## Outcomes Across ICF Components

The ICF has five component sections, or domains, that should be considered when defining or targeting intervention outcomes: (1) body structures, (2) body functions, (3) activity/participation, (4) environmental factors, and (5) personal factors. Each component will be briefly described and then the possible areas of outcomes discussed (see **Fig. 2.8**).

### Body Structure and Body Function

Body *structures* are defined in the ICF as "the anatomical parts of the body such as organs, limbs, and their components" (WHO, 2001, p. 10). Body *functions* are defined as "the physiological functions of a body system, including psychological functions" (WHO, 2001, p. 10).

Although there are some instances when speech-language pathology intervention could directly change the body structure of a client (e.g., voice therapy to reduce or eliminate vocal nodules), more often SLPs are in a position to recommend the body structure–related procedures (such as surgeries) to facilitate speech and swallowing. Body function outcomes, however, are a common concern in our field. For communication, the body function codes cover speech and voice production and quality, fluency, hearing acuity and discrimination, reading and writing basics, oral and pharyngeal swallowing, memory, problem solving, attention, syntax, and semantics. They are the most discretely measurable aspects of the field and thus have the best standardized data. They are the building blocks of communication but do not constitute the actual ability to communicate with others. A person could be mildly impaired in many of the above skills yet their real-life communication ability may be at the moderate or severe level. On the other hand, a person could have a moderate specific body function disorder such as agrammatism as a feature of Broca's aphasia and still be a highly effective communicator. We cannot assume improvements in a body function level will directly equate to improvements in a person's social participation functioning or the person's perceived quality of communicative life. Body function skills related to speech, language, cognition, and swallowing are essential to communication and thus of primary concern to SLPs, but considered alone they do not define effective communication.

One area that needs further examination is the study of the effects of related body functions on communication and swallowing disorders (McCormack & Worrall, 2008). For example, what is the role of deficits in specific memory functions in aphasia? How does the regulation of emotion affect children's communication functioning with language disorders and stuttering? How does the perception of pain affect the communication of persons who have a cognitive communication disorder secondary to a traumatic injury? How does disruption of smell affect an individual's response to foods? What is the contribution of a body function impairment in one modality upon functioning in another (e.g., the deaf child with visual perception impairments)? Clinicians know that there are multiple interactive influences on their clients that affect their communication. However, outcomes research often controls for and excludes participants with other body function difficulties. For example, in aphasia research, participants with a history of alcoholism may be excluded from a study. Yet we know that there are persons with aphasia who are alcoholics, and clinicians need to consult the literature to help them better understand how these conditions interact.

### Activities/Participation

The ICF defines the activity/participation component as "including the executions of actions by individuals and these behaviors' relationship to their individual lives" (WHO, 2001, p. 10). The codes that are most directly related to communication disorders are the ones dealing with conversation, producing narratives, understanding language, using communication technologies such as email, using nonverbal communication, reading and writing for information and pleasure, recreation, involvement in community activities, involvement in education, interpersonal relationships, learning, managing self-care and household chores such as shopping, and work.

Outcomes have not been well studied in these areas. For example, there are many studies on increasing word-finding skills in persons with aphasia, defined by ICF as a body function, but less attention has been given to the ability of aphasic persons to participate in conversations including starting, sustaining, and terminating conversations. There is even less research on persons with acquired communication disorders function when they return to the workplace (Garcia, Barrette, & Laroche, 2000).

Within the activity/participation component are two important categorical qualifiers: *capacity* and *performance*. The capacity qualifiers have to do with behaviors exhibited in a structured setting such as during a therapy session, where, theoretically, the fullest possible "capacity" to perform a given behavior should be evident. By definition, a clinician is with the client and the clinician has set up the clinical interaction and provided support for the client's successful performance. The performance qualifiers reference what happens outside of a therapy setting and the behaviors in the clients' actual lives when the clinician is not present. Both research and clinical outcomes need to consider capacity and performance. For example, a group conversation training intervention with teenagers with Asperger syndrome may demonstrate significant positive clinical outcomes. However, this improvement would only constitute clinical outcomes on the capacity level of the activities/participation component. To demonstrate this improvement at the performance level, the researcher or clinician would need to gather ethnographic evidence (real-world observations) to determine if these conversational skills are being used in natural environments (for example, see Kagan et al, 2008). Since the researcher or clinician is not usually in a position to do naturalistic observations, reliable and valid self-report tools and patient-reported outcomes (PROs) need to be developed to measure outcomes at the performance level of activity/participation.

This paucity of research at this activity/participation level is detrimental to the discipline of speech-language pathology because these types of outcomes serve to justify the time, effort, and expense of therapy services to clients, families, payers, and policy makers. Clients do not come to us and say, "Please help me with my visual confrontation naming skills and my difficulties with understanding passive sentence structures." They bring complaints such as "I can't talk to my granddaughter about which college she should choose." "I can never understand the jokes that the other kids say at school, and that makes me stand out and other kids make fun of me." "I am the person who has earned a promotion but I can never get my ideas across to the group because I stutter." The outcomes that our clients and others care about achieving are often those measured with the activity/participation scale.

### Environmental Factors

Environmental factors are defined by the ICF as factors that are not within a person's direct control, such as social support, work, government agencies, laws, attitudes of others, and cultural beliefs. Unlike the other components of the ICF, the environmental factor qualifiers (severity measures) include both *facilitators* and *barriers*. Thus, a given environmental factor such as immediate family support could range from 4 (complete barrier) to +4 (complete facilitator). Philosophically, the ICF supports the WHO's contention that disability is an interaction of a person's inherent functional limitations and society. Persons with functional limitations are thus not expected to simply work hard enough to be "less disabled" but should expect society, governments, and other individuals to do their parts. Disabled individuals work hard to do things for themselves to the greatest extent they can, and a responsible society does its part by leveling the playing field as much as possible. Take the example of someone in a wheelchair trying to get through a door that automatically closes. It is reasonable for public buildings to have doors that persons in wheelchairs can manipulate, or for society to have responsible citizens who will hold the door open for them. Metaphorically, we should all be willing to "hold the door open" for persons with disabilities.

Of all the possible influences identified in the ICF model, environmental factors may end up having the greatest impact on provision of services to persons with disabilities and on rehabilitation research. This addition to the ICF framework emanated from disability advocacy agencies that complained effectively that the medical model puts the entire onus of functioning on the person with the disability (Hurst, 2003). The social model states that it is the environment that truly determines and often limits the functioning of persons with disabilities. For example, a person who uses a wheelchair may have the skills to do a particular job in a company, but his or her performance is hampered when the company's building is not fully wheelchair accessible. In that situation, it is the building that has to change to achieve the desired outcome.

If the goal is maximizing life participation outcomes, then both researchers and clinicians must consider the role of environmental factors equally to the role of body function in defining the disability. Only by developing appropriate measures for environmental factors can we determine if a given intervention is making a difference. There are some disorders such as dementia where it has been shown that intervention through environmental adjustments leads to better outcomes than direct behavioral intervention with clients (Hopper, 2007). Not all environmental factors are amenable to change and consequently should be considered in the prognosis for independent functioning.

In designing and evaluating the outcome of an intervention, it behooves us to consider the effects of environmental factor *facilitators* as well as *barriers*. Perhaps a beneficial outcome is not due entirely to the intervention, but to some unexamined or unappreciated environmental factor. For example, enrolling children in an early childhood literacy program may have the coincidental effect of encouraging parents to read to their children, effectively boosting language and literacy development opportunities at home. Enrolling a child in stuttering therapy may have the added advantage of bringing parents together in the waiting room as an informal support group. Oelschlaeger (1999) researched good examples of spouse conversational facilitators in aphasia. Persons living with people with disabilities may be untapped sources of successful intervention methods and models. Greater systematic study is needed to qualify features of naturally good facilitators of communication within the family context compared with those who are not such good examples (barriers), if we are to consider conversational partners as an environmental factor in successful therapy.

The reality of caseloads and clinician contact time often restricts the clinical service "dosage" (timing, frequency, length, and duration of sessions) to something far less than optimal or evidence based. Traditional individual therapy sessions, conducted in a manner supported by treatment research, can be effective, but may be difficult to achieve in a real world. All SLPs know the limitations of what they can achieve with the caseloads and time limitations they have. They know that the time they spend with teachers, family members, and caregivers can often be the most valuable part of their day, and that interaction may be the best avenue to extend the therapy session to other contexts. Clinicians need greater guidance to achieve desired outcomes by tapping facilitative environmental factors.

Research examining and manipulating environmental factors is regularly done by other fields such as public health. However, such research paradigms are not as common in communication disorders research. Greater acceptance of the ICF model to guide outcomes research, including research on environmental factors, may enhance acceptance of this line of research among funders and in refereed publications.

*Personal Factors*

Personal factors are defined as "the particular background of an individual's life and living that comprise features of the individual that are not part of the health condition or health states. These factors may include gender, race, age, other health conditions, fitness, lifestyle, habits, upbringing, coping styles, social background, education, profession, past and current experience, overall behavior pattern and character style, individual psychological assets and other characteristics, all or any of which may play a role in disability at any level" (WHO, 2001, p. 17). Personal factors are not coded in the ICF because of wide variability among cultures, but are included in the framework because they have a high likelihood of having an impact on functioning and on the outcomes of different interventions (WHO, 2001).

As with environmental factors, this is another area well studied in other fields, but often neglected in the communication disorders outcomes literature. Two of the very few areas within this construct that have been studied to any significant extent are race/ethnicity and communication functioning and disorders. This may be due to ASHA's increased emphasis on diversity and multicultural issues. This inclusion represents a significant advancement in the field.

Embracing the personal factors aspects of the ICF involves more than addressing strict demographic aspects of our clients, such as race, socioeconomic level, age, and educational levels. Our clients also have varied background influences, life experiences, and individual personalities that influence how their communication disorder affects their lives and how they respond to the disorder and the extent of engagement in intervention. All of these factors ultimately will influence clinical outcomes. Thus, children with autism may have different underlying personalities that influence the types of interventions that are the most effective. Two individuals with aphasia may have equivalent educational and socioeconomic status and language impairments, but very different life experiences, social interests, and temperaments, potentially affecting outcomes.

Consideration of personal factors in research and in the clinic could expand our knowledge of how these factors affect communication outcomes. We know that a child's temperament is an important factor in predicting which children with childhood dysfluency are more likely to develop a persistent stutter compared with those children who do not (Anderson, Pellowski, Conture & Kelly, 2003). The influences of temperament and personality-based responses to disabilities and intervention may be difficult for the practicing clinician to fully appreciate and circumvent. Research in temperament and personality characteristics across communication disorders would enhance our understanding of these important factors. SLPs bring technical knowledge and effectiveness research to bear upon our intervention, but we cannot treat a communication disorder the way a plumber fixes a drain. We treat dynamic and complex human beings who have diverse and unique life experiences and personalities. These factors combine to interact with the communication disorder and can influence the intervention outcome.

## ♦ Outcomes and the Components of the ICF

In the preceding sections, for instructional purposes, I artificially separated the different ways of looking at outcomes by different ICF components. The central tenet of the ICF, however, is that all components are synergistic—interconnected and interdependent. The personal factors of a given client may affect the willingness of others in their environment (e.g., family, coworkers, colleagues) to help them (Threats, 2007a). A person's body functions often directly affect their activity/participation, and an active activity/participation behavior may actually improve a specific body function. A college professor with mild anomic aphasia may prefer practice drills on the pronunciation of technical words in his or her profession to improve verbal fluency—a body function goal. Another person with anomic aphasia might prefer to be able to better manage social discussions at his or her weekly book club meetings—a goal within the activity/participation domain.

Embracing complexity and multidimensionality of communication and communication disorders is a monumental task for researchers and for therapy planning. That being said, no study can look at every factor at the same time. Thus, a balance needs to be struck between including more complex research designs while ensuring that the data from them can still be interpreted. McCormack and Worrall (2008) in their conclusion on an article on the ICF state the following:

> The ICF is a classification system, and while it provides SLPs with a holistic system by which to classify clients, this will only happen if it is used in its entirety. Focusing on the level of the impairment (i.e., considering only Body Functions and Body Structures) fails to acknowledge the full range of difficulties that may be experienced by individuals with communication and or swallowing disorders. However, considering the interactions of Body Functions and Body Structures with Activities and Participation, Environmental Factors, and Personal Factors could result in greater understanding of the many factors that contribute to health and the impact of health on life functioning. This would be an expansion of clinical thinking and an advance for the field. However, there are limitations to the practicality of the ICF in its current form and these limitations need to be addressed in the clinical and research literature and by the professional and advocacy communities. (p. 16)

## How Much Outcome Improvement Is Enough? Who Gets to Pick the Outcome?

If the ICF were merely a framework, then the sections of this chapter so far would capture the main ideas embodied in using the ICF to guide clinical and research outcome thinking. However, the ICF is also a classification system with specific operational definitions of behaviors, such as "starting a conversation," that need to be challenged in the research laboratory and the clinic, and future versions of the ICF adapted accordingly.

A notable difference between the ICF and most other classification systems is the inclusion of *severity qualifiers*, or rating scales. Qualifiers denote the severity of the problem and are represented by one or more numbers following a decimal point. The qualifiers represent the following levels of limitation or restriction: 0, no problem or within normal limits; 1, mild; 2, moderate; 3, severe; 4, complete or profound. The use of these severity ratings is not considered to be optional. They are considered a crucial aspect of the system. Specifically, the ICF states, "The ICF codes are only complete with the presence of a qualifier, which denotes the magnitude of the level of health (e.g., severity of the problem). . . . Use of any code should be accompanied by at least one qualifier. Without qualifiers, codes have no inherent meaning" (WHO, 2001, p. 21).

The challenges and possible implications for use of the ICF rating for determining outcomes are profound. If functioning is coded using the ICF in computerized health and educational records, then the only way to demonstrate improvement on a given behavior would be for there to be a change in the severity qualifier category (for example, a change score showing improvement from severely impaired on a given ability to a rating indicating a moderately impaired ability). The range of rating from mild to complete (profound) was adapted by the WHO because such qualifiers are conventionally used across clinical fields. The fact that most clinical fields use these qualifiers does not, however, mean that the fields really know what they mean (Threats, 2008).

In terms of interrater reliability, the agreements in rating a disability as "mild" versus "severe" would no doubt be high. However, rater agreement between response items such as "within normal limits" and "mild," or "mild" and "moderate," is more likely to vary. Add to this the task of ranking clients across a wide range of communication disorders of various etiologies and the situation is even more daunting. Is a ranking of moderate stuttering and moderate voice disorder an equivalent degree of severity? If most of the clients we treated became normal following treatment, these severity ratings would not be of consequence to the field. For example, persons with aphasia rarely fully recover their language skills, and thus an improvement from moderately impaired to mildly impaired is considered a good outcome.

One response to this challenge might be to simply decide that because these qualifiers do not have a reliably agreed upon meaning, we should just stop using them. This would not address the need to distinguish between quantitative improvement and qualitative improvement. Qualitative improvement is important to measure. Conversely, if we think that is not politically or administratively feasible, the field could simply pick some measurement tool appropriate for a particular communication disorder and designate a "mild" score range, and further define the severity score boundaries for moderate, severe, and complete (profound). In the ICF, the developers provide some general guidelines for determining the cutoffs for the severity levels, mainly via percentages. The boundary percentages in the ICF are as follows: 0 to 4%, within normal limits; 5 to 24%, mild impairment; 25 to 49%, moderate impairment; 50 to 95%, severe impairment; and 96 to 100%, complete (profound) limitation. Other suggestions provided are to qualify no problem as "none" or "absent," mild problems as "slight" or "low," moderate problems as "medium" or "fair," severe problem as "high" or "extreme," and complete/profound problems as "total."

The percentages suggested by the ICF could be problematic for supporting beneficial therapy outcomes in speech-language pathology. The severity qualifier 4 (severe) ranges from a decrease in performance from 50 to 95%, and thus a client who started at a skill level of 5% and improved to 50% would, according to this marker, have still remained severely impaired despite obvious improvements. Generally, in speech-language pathology a measured improvement from 5 to 45% would be considered significant change for the better. However, according to the criteria for qualifier 4 (severe), if the score for a given individual remained below 50%, then significant improvement would not be demonstrated.

As stated previously, WHO considers these percentages suggestions. Specifically, the ICF states:

> Appropriate qualifying words as shown in brackets below should be chosen according to the relevant classification domain. For this quantification to be used in a universal manner, assessment procedures need to be developed through research. Broad ranges of percentages are provided for those cases in which calibrated assessments instruments or other standards are available to quantify the impairment, capacity limitation, or performance or barrier. (WHO, 2001, p. 22)

The key phrase in this quotation is "assessment procedures need to be developed through research." Thus, it is left up to the rehabilitation professions to come up with standard measurements and consensual designations of severity levels. In the context of assessing improvement, we need to consider how much improvement the recipients of our services, our clients, consider worth the cost and effort of therapy. Clients may use an internal scale of their performance, such as the following: (1) I can never do that task; (2) I can do it some of the time; (3) I can do it about half of the time; (4) I can do it most of the time; and (5) I can almost always do that well. The challenge is thus at what point do clients perceive their levels of functioning to have reached a meaningful level of improvement, say, to have changed from "some of the time" to "half of the time"? Different individuals, due to personal factors, may view the same objective level of performance improvement differently based on their interpretation, expectations, or desired level of functioning.

In the field of psychology, it has long been recognized that humans do not perceive differences in physically measurable, absolute terms. An example coming from audiology is the decibel (dB) scale, which is a logarithmic scale. Humans do not perceive and differentiate sounds strictly on by the acoustic-physical properties. A sound pressure level (SPL) of 40 is not judged by the human ear as twice as loud as a SPL of 20. The decibel scale was designed to account for this perceptual phenomenon by using a "just noticeable difference" (1 dB) scale in which increments are defined and measured logarithmically. Thus, a 40-dB tone is not, in absolute acoustic terms, twice as loud as a 20-dB tone, but the human ear may perceive the difference as such. To add to the complication, the human ear responds to different frequencies with different relative scales in judgments of loudness.

The intent with this example from psychophysics is to make the point that even with the most basic of perceptual levels (differences in sounds), humans do not respond to absolute physical differences, but make relative, perceptual judgments. Thus, a patient-reported outcome judgment on the question, "How much have you improved?" is a complex decision. For a given area, is an improvement from 30% to 50% viewed as the same amount of change as to go from 60% to 80%? Maybe and maybe not. Both represent an improvement of 20%, which on paper and for a researcher would equate to similar progress or a similar outcome. But the individual might ask, "Compared to what?"

This question is not academic. The health care system is increasingly directed toward greater involvement of patients both in sharing the financial costs of their health care and in their engagement in decision making. We are increasingly relying on patient-reported outcomes to assess the value of medical and other interventions. In addition, there is increased attention given to evidence-based practice to determine where resources (health care and education dollars) are placed. An important aspect of evidence-based practice is patient preferences and perceptions of satisfaction. In short, patients are not better unless and until an improvement is perceived *by them* to have made a noticeable difference in some functional area.

One way policy makers can judge the evidence for rehabilitation services is to directly survey current or past clients of speech-language pathology services. If they used the ICF 1 to 5 qualifier scale, the surveyor could ask clients to rate themselves or their family member on specific performance areas at the beginning of therapy and at the end of therapy. Another method might to rate the amount of improvement on specific skills from a range of "no change at all" to "great change—independent in this area now." With either question, it is not a matter of absolutes but a matter of the change being of sufficient magnitude to be perceived as a qualitatively improved function. Thus, in terms of severity ratings, we must take our clients' views into consideration.

A study by Hettenhausen (2009) used the ICF-CY qualifiers and found that the severity ratings made by the parents of preschool children in an early childhood speech-language therapy program differed markedly from those of the service providers. Specifically, the SLP considered certain abilities of the child as "mild," whereas parents found the same areas "moderately" impaired. Results also demonstrated scaling differences where the SLP rated the child as more severely impaired on a given area than did the parents. It could be that the SLPs view severity within a range across the clients they have seen with a given disorder, comparing the least severe to the most severe clients they have seen, whereas the parents' judgments were based on the effects of a disorder on their child's level of functioning. Another possibility is that the SLP is judging the *capacity*, or level of performance observed within the clinic setting, and the parents were judging the skill at the *performance* (real-life) level. Again, raters (professionals versus the clients themselves) are likely to have different perspectives.

The difference between capacity and performance, discussed earlier, may also be evident in outcome measurements. As we said, capacity may be demonstrated within the therapy session, whereas performance is demonstrated in real life. It is possible for clients to believe that therapy is very beneficial because they perform so much better in the therapy room than they did before therapy started. A good example might be adult clients who have fluency disorders and become increasingly fluent in conversation in the therapy room as therapy progresses. Asked if therapy was working, such clients might answer affirmatively; however, if the question were couched in terms of public speaking specifically, the clients might not perceive any benefit. The outcome score can reflect both the content and psychometric qualities of items and how the questions are asked.

Psychometric analysis of test items is increasingly found in rehabilitation research applying *item response theory,* where issues in classical testing methods of given traits are being reconsidered to design more discriminating and efficient outcome assessment tools. We are finding applications of item response theory and Rasch analysis in speech-language pathology (Baylor et al, 2011; Hula, Donovan, Kendall, & Gonzalez-Rothi, 2010) and in rehabilitation therapies (Heinemann, 2010).

## ♦ Conclusion and Future Directions

According to the WHO's *World Report on Disability* (WHO, 2011), rehabilitation has long lacked a unifying conceptual framework. That report goes on to state that the ICF framework can be used for all aspects of rehabilitation to facilitate as full participation in life as possible for those persons with disabilities. This chapter discussed the advantages and challenges of using the ICF to expand the scope of outcomes measures in research and clinical practice in speech-language pathology. The ICF challenges us to (1) work collaboratively with clients and families to set desired outcomes, (2) look at global outcomes and how communication goals contribute to them, (3) evaluate the interaction of all functional impairments and limitations on communication, and (4) look at how the components of the ICF framework interact with each other. Special attention was given to clients' and their families' qualitative judging of their progress, which is ultimately the true test of the benefits of our services.

The WHO ICF is concerned with meeting the needs of persons with disabilities, which is the ultimate goal of rehabilitation. Thus, it should not be our preoccupation to evaluate how and if our services yield global, effective, meaningful communication improvements. Our primary concern is advancing the ability of the recipients of our services toward improving the quality of their lives and the fullest possible participation in society they desire. These broader aspirations require extending our notions of outcome assessment beyond the standard, classical clinical assessments of body structure and functions, and require expanding interdisciplinary research.

With all change, there is challenge. We are challenged to produce better outcomes. That challenge should be embraced. The challenges posed by the ICF described in this chapter can strengthen and solidify the profession and encourage us to "take it to the next level." As stated at the beginning of this chapter, our profession must take on this challenge because there is no other area more central to functional health than communication.

# References

Anderson, J., Pellowski, M. W., Conture, E. G., & Kelly, E. M. (2003). Temperament characteristics of young children who stutter. *Journal of Speech, Language, and Hearing Research, 46,* 1221–1233

Baylor, C., Hula, W., Donovan, M. J., Doyle, P. J., Kendall, D., & Yorkston, K. (2011). Item response theory: an introduction to Item Response Theory and Rasch models for speech-language pathology. *American Journal of Speech-Language Pathology,* 10.1044/1058-0360(2011/10-0079)

Brown, J., & Hasselkus, A. (2008). Professional associations' role in advancing the ICF in speech-language pathology. *International Journal of Speech-Language Pathology, 10,* 78–82

Cruice, M. (2008). The contribution and impact of the International Classification of Functioning, Disability, and Health on quality of life in communication disorders. *International Journal of Speech-Language Pathology, 10,* 38–49

Doyle, P., & Skarakis-Doyle, E. (2008). The ICF as a framework for interdisciplinary doctoral education in rehabilitation: Implications for speech-language pathology. *International Journal of Speech-Language Pathology, 10,* 83–91

Dykstra, A. D., Hakel, M. E., & Adams, S. G. (2007, Nov). Application of the ICF in reduced speech intelligibility in dysarthria. *Seminars in Speech and Language, 28,* 301–311

Eadie, T. L. (2007, Nov). Application of the ICF in communication after total laryngectomy. *Seminars in Speech and Language, 28,* 291–300

Frattali, C. M. (1998). Measuring modality-specific behaviors, functional abilities, and quality of life. In C. M. Frattali (Ed.), *Measuring outcomes in speech-language pathology.* New York: Thieme

Frattali, C. M., Thompson, C. K., Holland, A. L., Wohl, C. B., & Ferketic, M. M. (1995). *Functional assessment of communicative skills for adults.* Rockville, MD: American Speech-Language-Hearing Association

Garcia, L., Barrette, J., & Laroche, C. (2000). Perceptions of the obstacles to work reintegration for persons with aphasia. *Aphasiology, 14,* 269–290

Garin, O., Ayuso-Mateos, J. L., Almansa, J., Nieto, M., Chatterji, S., Vilagut, G., et al.; MHADIE consortium (2010). Valida-

tion of the "World Health Organization Disability Assessment Schedule, WHODAS-2" in patients with chronic diseases. *Health and Quality of Life Outcomes, 8,* 51 http://www.hqlo.com/content/8/1/51 10.1186/1477-7525-8-51

Hancock, H. (2003) Rehabilitation for enhanced life participation: A living well program. *Speech Pathology Online.* http://www.speechpathology.com/

Heinemann, A. W. (2010, Sep). Measurement of participation in rehabilitation research. *Archives of Physical Medicine and Rehabilitation, 91*(9, Suppl), S1–S4

Hettenhausen, A. (2009). Application of the International Classification of Functioning, Disability, and Health-Children and Youth (ICF-CY) to describe the communicative skills and functioning of children in an early childhood program. Unpublished master's thesis. St. Louis University

Hickson, L., & Scarinci, N. (2007, Nov). Older adults with acquired hearing impairment: Applying the ICF in rehabilitation. *Seminars in Speech and Language, 28,* 283–290

Hopper, T. (2007, Nov). The ICF and dementia. *Seminars in Speech and Language, 28,* 273–282

Howe, T. (2008). The ICF contextual factors related to speech-language pathology. *International Journal of Speech-Language Pathology, 10,* 27–37

Hula, W., Donovan, N. J., Kendall, D., & Gonzalez-Rothi, L. J. (2010). Item response theory analysis of the Western Aphasia Battery. *Aphasiology, 24,* 1326–1341

Hurst, R. (2003, Jun). The international disability rights movement and the ICF. *Disability and Rehabilitation, 25,* 572–576

Kagan, A., Simmons-Mackie, N., Rowland, A., Huijbregts, M., Shumway, E., McEwen, S., et al. (2008). Counting what counts: A framework for capturing real-life outcomes of aphasia intervention. *Aphasiology, 22,* 258–280

Larkins, B. (2007, Nov). The application of the ICF in cognitive-communication disorders following traumatic brain injury. *Seminars in Speech and Language, 28,* 334–342

Ma, E. P.-M., Yiu, E. M.-L., & Abbott, K. V. (2007, Nov). Application of the ICF in voice disorders. *Seminars in Speech and Language, 28,* 343–350

McCormack, J., & Worrall, L. (2008). The ICF body functions and structures related to speech-language pathology. *International Journal of Speech-Language Pathology, 10,* 9–17

McLeod, S., & McCormack, J. (2007, Nov). Application of the ICF and ICF-children and youth in children with speech impairment. *Seminars in Speech and Language, 28,* 254–264

McLeod, S., & Threats, T. T. (2008). Application of the ICF-CY to children with communication disabilities. *International Journal of Speech-Language Pathology, 10,* 92–109

Mulhorn, K., & Threats, T. (2008). Speech, hearing, and communication across five national disability surveys: Results of a DISTAB study using the ICF to compare prevalence patterns. *International Journal of Speech-Language Pathology, 10,* 61–71

Oelschlaeger, M. (1999). Participation of a conversation partner in the word searches of a person with aphasia. *American Journal of Speech-Language Pathology, 8,* 62–71

O'Halloran, R., & Larkins, B. (2008). The ICF activities and participation related to speech-language pathology. *International Journal of Speech-Language Pathology, 10,* 18–26

Rangasayee, R., Mukundan, G., Dalvi, U., Nandurkar, A., & Kant, A. (2010). Invited tutorial: The International Classification of Functioning, Disability and Health (ICF) for audiologists and speech-language pathologists. *Journal of Indian Speech Language and Hearing Association, 24,* 1–23

Simmons-Mackie, N., & Kagan, A. (2007, Nov). Application of the ICF in aphasia. *Seminars in Speech and Language, 28,* 244–253

Simmons-Mackie, N., Threats, T. T., & Kagan, A. (2005, Jan-Feb). Outcome assessment in aphasia: a survey. *Journal of Communication Disorders, 38,* 1–27

Stucki, G., Reinhardt, J. D., & Grimby, G. (2007, May). Organizing human functioning and rehabilitation research into distinct scientific fields. Part II: Conceptual descriptions and domains for research. *Journal of Rehabilitation Medicine, 39,* 299–307

Threats, T. (2007a). Access for persons with neurogenic communication disorders: Influences of Personal and Environmental Factors of the ICF. *Aphasiology, 21,* 67–80

Threats, T. T. (2007b, Nov). Use of the ICF in dysphagia management. *Seminars in Speech and Language, 28,* 323–333

Threats, T. T. (2008). Use of the ICF for clinical practice in speech-language pathology. *International Journal of Speech-Language Pathology, 10,* 50–60

Westby, C. (2007, Nov). Application of the ICF in children with language impairments. *Seminars in Speech and Language, 28,* 265–272

World Health Organization. (1980). *International classification of impairments, disabilities, and handicaps.* Geneva: Author

World Health Organization. (1992). *International statistical classification of diseases and related health problems,* 10th revision (ICD-10). Geneva: Author

World Health Organization. (2001). *International classification of functioning, disability, and health.* Geneva: Author

World Health Organization. (2006). *World Health Organization constitution.* Geneva: Author

World Health Organization. (2007). *International classification of functioning, disability, and health: children and youth version.* Geneva: Author

World Health Organization. (2011). *World report on disability.* http://www.who.int/disabilities/world_report/2011/report/en/index.html

Worrall, L., & Hickson, L. (2008). Use of the ICF in speech-language pathology research: Towards a research agenda. *International Journal of Speech-Language Pathology, 10,* 72–77

Yaruss, J. S. (2007, Nov). Application of the ICF in fluency disorders. *Seminars in Speech and Language, 28,* 312–322

# 4

# Outcomes Measurement in Federal Programs and Public Policy

*Kathleen Romanow and Janet E. Brown*

## ♦ Chapter Focus

This chapter familiarizes the reader with a wide array of federal programs, initiatives, key agencies, and regulatory bodies in which outcome measurements are integral. These programs are mainly aimed at oversight of large-volume, high-profile, high-risk medical interventions, and rarely address speech-language pathology or audiology services specifically. However, the requirements imposed by these broad mandates and initiatives establish quality standards and payer priorities and thus influence the manner in which speech, language, hearing, cognition, and swallowing services are provided. The types of and processes for data collection and the reporting requirements of the major federal programs and initiatives are highlighted in this chapter to illustrate the extent to which quality and cost performance data are being used to evaluate individual providers and provider organizations, and to inform payment policies.

## ♦ Introduction

By passing legislation establishing the Medicare and Medicaid programs in 1965, the federal government began a long-term commitment to support the health needs of elderly and low-income Americans. As the largest payer of health care services, the federal government wields significant influence on how health care is delivered, reimbursed, and evaluated. These federal programs have undergone continuous development of regulations and payment policies to control the mushrooming costs of this commitment and to monitor inappropriate and fraudulent billing of services under these programs. Despite all legislative and regulatory attempts to control costs, the number of Medicare beneficiaries and the cost of their health care have soared. By 2010, the Medicare program alone covered 47 million Americans and accounted for 12% of the federal budget (Henry J. Kaiser Family Foundation, 2010). Medicaid programs vary widely because coverage and payments policies are determined by each state with funding support from the federal government, but they also currently face severe challenges in providing health care to their neediest citizens with limited resources.

The concept of evaluating the cost and quality of services, called *value-based purchasing,* began with the efforts of pioneers in the private sector to take a data-driven approach to selecting health plans for their employees (Agency for Healthcare Research and Quality, 1997). By collecting data on the quality and cost of services, offering incentives to employees, and even working with providers to identify and adopt standards of care that would enhance outcomes, these employers became active partners in demanding quality improvement and accountability for the care being delivered. This approach has spread to the federal government, where agencies such as the Centers for Medicare and Medicaid Services seek tools and measures by which they can hold providers and systems accountable.

In its efforts to provide efficient and cost-effective services to the beneficiaries of its various programs, the federal government has identified quality measurement, including both process and outcome measures, as a means for objectively assessing the value of services and standardizing appropriate care. Quality measurement has engaged the expertise of federal agencies, legislatively appointed commissions, the health care research community, professional organizations, private industry, and public-private partnerships.

## ◆ Key Agencies and Organizations

### Centers for Medicare and Medicaid Services

Under the Department of Health and Human Services, the Centers for Medicare and Medicaid Services (CMS) (formerly the Health Care Financing Administration) is responsible for implementing legislative directives to regulate and reimburse providers for health care services delivered to beneficiaries of the Medicare and Medicaid programs. CMS contracts with private industry to conduct research and demonstration projects to develop tools that will provide reliable data for the analysis of resource utilization and payment. CMS's goal to obtain meaningful information to differentiate the cost and quality (e.g., patient health outcomes) of services, procedures, or providers has been elusive, particularly with respect to rehabilitation services. The tools and initiatives introduced by Medicare under its various programs are discussed later in this chapter.

### Agency for Health Care Research and Quality

The Agency for Health Care Research and Quality (AHRQ), formerly the Agency for Health Care Policy and Research (AHCPR), is an agency of the Department of Health and Human Services whose "mission is to improve the quality, safety, efficiency, and effectiveness of health care for all Americans" (AHRQ, 2011b). It encourages the application of research to practice to improve effectiveness and efficiency; it also promotes the use of evidence-based practice and disseminates clinical guidelines to improve health outcomes. The majority of its budget is devoted to grants and contracts to improve health care.

### Medicare Payment Advisory Commission

Established by the Balanced Budget Act of 1997 (BBA, 1997), the Medicare Payment Advisory Commission (MedPAC) advises Congress on Medicare issues, including payment, and conducts analyses of access to care and quality (MedPAC, 2011c). In its June 2011 report, MedPAC notes that the current fee-for-service reimbursement system (for outpatient services) rewards providers for the number of services they provide, not for their quality or value (MedPAC, 2011b). The report echoes the principles of *value-based purchasing* in the following recommendations: (1) requiring measures of quality care that are evidence-based, (2) increasing accountability to correct quality of low-performing providers, and (3) recognizing high-performing providers.

## National Committee for Quality Assurance

The National Committee for Quality Assurance (NCQA) was formed in 1990 as a nonprofit organization to improve health care quality (NCQA, 2011b). NCQA's consensus-based standards and performance measures are used to accredit private health plans and drive quality improvement. The Healthcare Effectiveness Data and Information Set (HEDIS) is the tool that is used to measure performance. Some HEDIS measures have subsequently been endorsed by the National Quality Forum.

## National Quality Forum

The National Quality Forum (NQF) was formed in 1999 as a nonprofit organization consisting of organizations from a broad spectrum of the health care stakeholders in the public and private sectors. Under the Medicare Improvements for Patients and Providers Act of 2008 (Public Law [PL] 110-275), Congress was directed to contract with an organization to "establish a portfolio of quality and efficiency measures for use in reporting on and improving healthcare quality . . . [that] will allow the federal government to more clearly see how and whether healthcare spending is achieving the best results for patients and taxpayers" (NQF, 2009). Measures endorsed by the NQF are viewed with a high degree of credibility and may be incorporated in national and private quality improvement initiatives, such as Medicare's Physician Quality Reporting System (PQRS), which is discussed later.

The NQF works closely with CMS on various projects in addition to the endorsement of consensus-based measures. Under the Patient Protection and Affordable Care Act of 2010 (PL 111-148), the NQF has contracted to coordinate additional activities related to safety and quality, which are discussed later in the chapter (see Public Policy) and elsewhere in this text.

# ♦ Medicare and Quality Initiatives

The Medicare program consists of several separate benefit programs that are administered and paid for in different ways. To understand how outcomes are incorporated into reimbursement for these different programs, it is important to understand the differences in the programs and their payment systems.

## Medicare Part A

Medicare Part A includes hospital, skilled nursing facility, and home health coverage using different eligibility criteria and payment systems.

### Acute Care Hospitals

Hospital costs are reimbursed by a lump sum payment established for the diagnosis-related group (DRG) based on the patient's condition or procedure. The hospital is responsible for managing all the services required for that hospitalization; the facility saves money when patients are discharged early, and loses money if patients develop complications or require a longer hospital stay than anticipated. To counterbalance the incentive to discharge the patient too soon, financial penalties are exacted if the patient is readmitted within 30 days of discharge or if the patient acquires other complications during hospitalization, such as pneumonia or other infections, which require additional treatment and length of stay.

### Home Health

Medicare Part A includes a home health benefit for beneficiaries discharged from the hospital who meet the criteria for being home bound. Under the Prospective Payment System for home health established by the Balanced Budget Act of 1997 (PL 105-33), Medicare pays a fixed amount for each 60-day episode of care; the amount is determined by data about the patient that is collected at admission. The data collection tool for home health is the Outcome Assessment and Information Set (OASIS), originally introduced by CMS as OASIS-B1 in 1999 and revised as OASIS-C in 2010. All Medicare-certified home health agencies must transmit OASIS data to CMS at prescribed times: the start of care, resumption of care (if an inpatient stay occurs during the home health episode), follow-up assessment (at the 60-day recertification period), transfer to an inpatient facility, and discharge from the agency. Although it was originally intended to measure patient outcomes, CMS acknowledges that the data serve multiple purposes, including payment, quality measures, case mix, and risk adjustment (CMS, 2009). Rather than describing OASIS as a patient assessment tool, CMS now describes it as "a dataset designed to collect information on the quality of home health care" (CMS, 2009, slide 15).

The 70-plus items on the OASIS-C administered at the start of care collect demographic information (e.g., name, address, gender, birth date, ethnicity, payment source); information about overall medical status (e.g., medical history, diagnoses and procedures, living information, hospitalization risks, etc.); and specific clinical items that are rated by the clinician who completes the tool (e.g., nurse, physical therapist, speech-language pathologist, occupational therapist). OASIS does not represent the comprehensive assessment of the patient; a discipline-specific assessment must also be included at the start of care to provide more detailed clinical information that will result in developing a plan of care.

A greater number of items on the OASIS are devoted to areas that may be of high risk to the patient's ability to function or likelihood of developing other complications, such as skin breakdown or wounds; elimination functions; medications; and activities of daily living. Items specifically addressing communication and swallowing function are extremely limited (**Table 4.1**). Of the 13 items addressing activities of daily living (ADL) and independent activities of daily living (IADL), only three involve functional areas directly addressed by speech-language pathologists (feeding or eating, ability to plan and prepare light meals, and ability to use the telephone). The rating descriptors for these items combine cognitive and physical factors as well as speech or swallowing, which limits their effectiveness as outcome measures for attributing change to treatment by one discipline.

According to CMS, the revision of the original OASIS was prompted by other agencies involved in health care quality (the Institute of Medicine, MedPAC, and the National Quality Forum) to increase the number and type of measures and to align OASIS measures with other postacute tools (CMS, 2011d). As a result, process measures have been added to the OASIS focusing on high frequency and risk conditions such as diabetes, pressure ulcers, and heart failure.

CMS's Home Health Quality Initiatives include outcome-based quality improvement (OBQI) and outcome-based quality management (OBQM) initiatives that must be reported by home health agencies on an annual basis to compare the agency's previous performance and national benchmarks. The OBQI Outcome Report consists of more than 40 risk-adjusted measures based on OASIS items, including improvement in eating, improvement or stabilization in speech and language, and improvement or stabilization in cognitive functioning. The OBQM initiatives include an Agency Patient-Related Characteristics Report and a Potentially Avoidable Event Report. An additional measure is the Home Health Care Consumer Assessment of Healthcare Providers and Systems (HHC CAHPS), part of a series of consumer surveys developed by the AHRQ.

CMS's Home Health Compare Web site reports scores on a variety of measures developed with the assistance of various stakeholders and quality organizations to assist consumers in their selection of a home health agency (CMS, n.d.). The NQF has played a key role in endorsing measures to be used for Home Health Compare. In the OASIS-C revision, NQF endorsed 13 process quality measures and 10 outcomes measures derived from OASIS-C items (CMS, 2011d). Outcome of care measures were divided into three categories: improvement measures, health care utilization measures (hospitalization and use of emergency department), and potentially avoidable events (e.g., pressure ulcers). The improvement measures include activities that are addressed by physical therapy and occupational therapy such as ambulation, bathing, and bed transfer, as well as nursing-related issues such as dyspnea and surgical wounds. Speech-language pathologists (SLPs) can contribute to the

**Table 4.1** OASIS-C Items Involving Communication, Cognition, and Swallowing

| Item Number | Item Description | Response Options |
|---|---|---|
| M1210 | Ability to hear (with hearing aid or hearing appliance if normally used) | 0: Adequate: hears normal conversation without difficult.<br>1: Mildly to moderately impaired: difficulty hearing in some environments or speaker may need to increase volume or speak distinctly.<br>2: Severely impaired: absence of useful hearing.<br>UK: Unable to assess hearing. |
| M1220 | Understanding of verbal content in patient's own language (with hearing aid or device if used) | 0: Understands: clear comprehension without cues or repetitions.<br>1: Usually understands: understands most conversations, but misses some part/intent of message. Requires cues at times to understand.<br>2: Sometimes understands: understands only basic conversations or simple, direct phrases. Frequently requires cues to understand.<br>3: Rarely/never understands.<br>UK: Unable to assess understanding. |
| M1230 | Speech and oral (verbal) expression of language (in patient's own language) | 0: Expresses complex ideas, feelings, and needs clearly, completely, and easily in all situations with no observable impairment.<br>1: Minimal difficulty in expressing ideas and needs (may take extra time; makes occasional errors in word choice, grammar or speech intelligibility; needs minimal prompting or assistance).<br>2: Expresses simple ideas or needs with moderate difficulty (needs prompting or assistance, errors in word choice, organization or speech intelligibility). Speaks in phrases or short sentences.<br>3: Has severe difficulty expressing basic ideas or needs and requires maximal assistance or guessing by listener. Speech limited to single words or short phrases.<br>4: Unable to express basic needs even with maximal prompting or assistance but is not comatose or unresponsive (e.g., speech is nonsensical or unintelligible).<br>5: Patient nonresponsive or unable to speak. |
| M1700 | Cognitive functioning: patient's current (day or assessment) level of alertness, orientation, comprehension, concentration, and immediate memory for simple commands | 0: Alert/oriented, able to focus and shift attention, comprehends and recalls task directions independently.<br>1: Requires prompting (cuing, repetition, reminders) only under stressful or unfamiliar conditions.<br>2: Requires assistance and some direction in specific situations (e.g., on all tasks involving shifting of attention), or consistently requires low stimulus environment due to distractibility.<br>3: Requires considerable assistance in routine situation. Is not alert and oriented or is unable to shift attention and recall directions more than half the time.<br>4: Totally dependent due to disturbances such as constant disorientation, coma, persistent vegetative state, or delirium. |
| M1740 | Cognitive, behavioral, and psychiatric symptoms that are demonstrated *at least once a week* (reported or observed). (Mark all that apply.) | 1: Memory deficit: failure to recognize familiar persons/places, inability to recall events of past 24 hours, significant memory loss so that supervision is required.<br>2: Impaired decision-making: failure to perform usual ADLs or IADLs, inability to appropriately stop activities, jeopardizes safety through actions.<br>3: Verbal disruption: yelling, threatening, excessive profanity, sexual references, etc.<br>4: Physical aggression: aggressive or combative to self and others (e.g., hits self, throws objects, punches, dangerous maneuvers with wheelchair or other objects).<br>5: Disruptive, infantile, or socially inappropriate behavior (excludes verbal actions).<br>6: Delusional, hallucinatory, or paranoid behavior.<br>7: None of the above behaviors demonstrated. |

(Continued on page 78)

**Table 4.1**   (*Continued*) OASIS-C Items Involving Communication, Cognition, and Swallowing

| Item Number | Item Description | Response Options |
|---|---|---|
| M1870 | Feeding or eating: current ability to feed self meals and snacks safely. Note: This refers only to the process of *eating, chewing,* and *swallowing, not preparing* the food to be eaten. | 0: Able to independently feed self.<br>1: Able to feed self independently but requires:<br>  (a) meal set up; or<br>  (b) intermittent assistance or supervision from another person; or<br>  (c) a liquid, pureed, or ground meat diet.<br>2: Unable to feed self and must be assisted or supervised throughout the meal/snack.<br>3: Able to take in nutrients orally and receives supplemental nutrients through a nasogastric tube or gastrostomy.<br>4: Unable to take in nutrients orally and is fed nutrients through a nasogastric tube or gastrostomy.<br>5: Unable to take in nutrients orally or by tube feeding. |
| M1890 | Ability to use telephone | 0: Able to dial numbers and answer calls appropriately and as desired.<br>1: Able to use a specially adapted telephone (i.e., large numbers on the dial, teletype phone for the deaf) and call essential numbers.<br>2: Able to answer the telephone and carry on a normal conversation but has difficulty with placing calls.<br>3: Able to answer the telephone only some of the time or is able to carry on only a limited conversation.<br>4: Unable to answer the telephone at all but can listen if assisted with equipment.<br>5: Totally unable to use the telephone.<br>NA: Patient does not have a telephone. |

measures by working on cognitive or language issues that may facilitate patients' comprehension and ability to comply with multistep instructions and safety precautions; however, such overarching measures would make it challenging for SLPs to demonstrate their specific contribution.

### Skilled Nursing Facilities

Medicare beneficiaries are also eligible for coverage of their stay in a skilled nursing facility (SNF) under Part A for up to 100 days following their hospitalization. As in home health, the Balanced Budget Act of 1997 created a Prospective Payment System that reimburses the SNF for the level of care needed by the patient according to their Resource Utilization Group (RUG). When the Part A benefit expires, Medicare beneficiaries are then covered by Part B, where services are reimbursed on a fee-for-service basis using the Medicare Physician Fee Schedule.

CMS has mandated several initiatives to measure quality in SNFs and to make that information available for public reporting and other analysis. The foundation of the data for quality reporting is the Minimum Data Set (MDS), which was implemented in 1996 and later revised as MDS 2.0 in 2000. According to CMS, the MDS assessment tool was primarily intended to identify SNF residents' problems that would lead to developing an individualized care plan; however, its use has been extended to include reimbursement by Medicare and by some state Medicaid programs, as well as for quality monitoring (CMS, 2011c). MDS data are collected at admission as well as on a quarterly and annual basis and when a change in status occurs. For residents covered by Medicare Part A, the assessments are also performed at frequent intervals to establish reimbursement rate.

The most recent iteration of the MDS was implemented in 2010 with significant changes to increase the reliability and validity of the clinical assessment and improve communication across the interdisciplinary team (CMS, 2011b). One of these changes in the MDS 3.0 is the implementation of a scripted patient interview component to increase attention to the resident's input. According to the

Rand Health Corporation, which developed the MDS 3.0 under contract to CMS, "The national trial for MDS 3.0 demonstrated the feasibility of giving NH [nursing home] residents voice by gathering MDS information directly from them and showed that MDS 3.0 improved the accuracy of the assessment items and increased the tool's efficiency. . . . Respect for the individual resident is fundamental to high quality care and quality of life" (Saliba & Buchanan, 2008, p. 2).

Other enhancements to MDS 3.0 include greater instruction about the need to identify and compensate for barriers to comprehension such as hearing loss, and the need for interpreters; however, individuals with significant cognitive or speech-language impairments who cannot respond to the patient interview must instead have information provided through staff interview. Information that is collected through the interviews includes cognitive patterns, mood, preferences for customary routine activities, pain, and goal setting. Although CMS solicited feedback from the American Speech-Language-Hearing Association (ASHA) and ASHA-recommended member experts, the MDS in all its versions has comparatively limited items for speech, hearing, language, cognition, and swallowing, reportedly due to the relatively small percentage of residents with these disorders and the burden of completing the already extensive assessment form (**Table 4.2**). Although a nurse may complete the entire MDS assessment, SLPs and other members of the interdisciplinary team may score the relevant portions or provide input to the nurse scoring the MDS.

Quality measures for nursing homes were established in 2003 in collaboration with the NQF. None of the current measures use items that directly relate to speech, language, swallowing, or cognition; the most directly related measure is the percent of residents who lose too much weight (compared with the previous 30 days). Examples of current measures include decreases in mobility and independence in daily activities, or increases in pressure sores, pain, depression, or bowel and bladder management. The reporting of these measures on Nursing Home Compare, a publicly available Web site, enables consumers to compare quality across available SNFs by examining separate qualities or examining the five-star quality rating, which includes health inspections, staff data, and quality measures.

### Inpatient Rehabilitation Facilities

The Inpatient Rehabilitation Facility–Patient Assessment Instrument (IRF-PAI) was implemented in 2002 to fill a role comparable to the OASIS and the MDS (CMS, 2011a). At the present time, there is no public reporting system for independent rehabilitation facilities; therefore, quality measures have not been developed that are analogous to the home health and SNF settings. Data from the IRF-PAI are used to establish payment for Medicare Part A patients.

Because the disorders and treatments for the patient populations in the IRF are more narrowly focused than for SNFs due to IRF admission criteria, the IRF-PAI is only three pages and 52 items long (**Table 4.3**). The majority of functional status assessment items come from the Functional Independence Measure (FIM™), a trademarked instrument developed by the University of Buffalo Foundation Activities. The IRF-PAI incorporates a few items adapted from other sources, including one item from OASIS; the Swallowing Functional Communication Measure adapted from ASHA's National Outcomes Measurement System; and one item from the Rehabilitation Institute of Chicago Functional Assessment Scale (RIC-FAS). The FIM instrument has been widely used in rehabilitation since it was developed in the mid-1980s, although it lacks comparable focus on areas relevant to speech-language pathology compared with the extensive number of items addressing activities of daily living such as toileting, dressing, and ambulation. In 1997 ASHA developed its own National Outcomes Measurement System with 15 functional communication measures modeled on the FIM seven-point scale to provide greater sensitivity and opportunity to analyze the different areas of focus treated by speech-language pathology (ASHA, n.d.). ASHA's NOMS is discussed in detail by Rogers and Mullen in Chapter 5.

## Medicare Part B

Unlike different programs under Part A, Medicare Part B does not have a prospective payment system that pays a lump sum for an episode of care. Instead, payment is made based on billed codes for

**Table 4.2** Sections of the MDS 3.0 Most Relevant to SLP Input for Scoring

| Section | Title | Question; Number of Response Options |
|---------|-------|--------------------------------------|
| A | Identification | |
| B | Hearing, speech, and vision | • Ability to hear (4); Hearing aid (2)<br>• Speech clarity (3)<br>• Makes self understood (4)<br>• Ability to understand others (4)<br>• Vision (5)<br>• Corrective lenses (2) |
| C | Cognitive patterns | • Could Brief Interview for Mental Status (BIMS) be conducted? (2)<br>• BIMS summary score: repetition of three words, temporal orientation, recall (0–15)<br>• Staff assessment if BIMS could not be administered (4 items)<br>• Signs and symptoms of delirium (4)<br>• Acute onset of mental status change (2) |
| D | Mood | |
| E | Behavior | • Includes psychosis, physical and verbal symptoms, rejection of care, wandering |
| F | Preferences for customary routine and activities | • Should interview for daily and activity preferences be conducted?<br>• Interview for daily preferences (8 items; 6 response categories)<br>• Interview for activity preferences (8 items; 6 response categories)<br>• Daily and activity preferences primary respondent<br>• Should the staff assessment of daily and activity preferences be conducted?<br>• Staff assessment of daily and activity preferences (21 items) |
| G | Functional status | • ADL self-performance (10 items; 7 response categories)<br>• Bathing self-performance (6)<br>• Balance during transitions and walking (5 items; 4 response categories)<br>• Functional limitation in range of motion (2 items; 3 response categories)<br>• Mobility devices (5 items)<br>• Functional rehabilitation potential |
| H | Bladder and bowel | |
| I | Active disease diagnosis | • Includes pneumonia, aphasia, cerebrovascular accident (CVA), dementia, Parkinson's, traumatic brain injury (TBI) |
| J | Health conditions | • Includes pain, falls, shortness of breath |
| K | Swallowing/nutritional status | • Swallowing disorder (5)<br>• Height and weight<br>• Weight loss (3)<br>• Nutritional approaches (5)<br>• Percent intake by artificial route |
| L | Oral/dental status | • 1 item; 8 responses |
| M | Skin conditions | |
| N | Medications | |
| O | Special treatments and procedures | |
| P | Restraints | |
| Q | Participation in assessment and goal setting | |
| V | Care area assessment (CAA) summary | • Includes cognitive loss/dementia, communication, and nutritional status as care areas that can be triggered and addressed in care plan |
| X | Correction request | |
| Z | Assessment administration | |

**Table 4.3**  IRF-PAI Selected Items Related to Function

| Item Number | Area Addressed | Number of Response Options |
|---|---|---|
| N25 A–C | Orientation to self, place, time | 2 (yes/no) |
| 27 | Swallowing status | 3 (regular, modified, tube feeding) |
| 33 | Tub transfer | FIM levels 1–7 |
| 34 | Shower transfer | FIM levels 1–7 |
| 35 | Distance walked | 4 options |
| 36 | Distance traveled in wheelchair | 4 options |
| 37 | Walk | FIM levels 1–7 |
| 38 | Wheelchair | FIM levels 1–7 |
| 39 | FIM instrument (self-care, sphincter control, transfers, locomotion, communication, social cognition, memory) | FIM levels 1–7 |
| N56 | Engagement (patient's cognitive and emotional resources) | 1–7 |

amounts set by annual adjustments to the Medicare Physicians Fee Schedule, which covers outpatient services delivered by all eligible providers, including SLPs, audiologists, physical therapists, and occupational therapists. Because this payment methodology rewards providers for delivering more care, the Balanced Budget Act of 1997 attempted to restrain escalating costs by establishing a combined therapy cap for speech-language pathology and physical therapy services, and a separate cap for occupational therapy services. These therapy caps are still in place despite protests from professionals and consumers that they arbitrarily restrict care without regard to need; however, an exceptions process has been approved annually in recent years by Congress for medically necessary services that exceed the cap. This reprieve does not address the overriding problem of demonstrating accountability for quality and efficiency in outpatient services.

## Physician Quality Reporting System (PQRS)

The Tax Relief and Health Care Act of 2006 (PL 109-432) required the Secretary of Health and Human Services (HHS) to establish a physician quality reporting system. In 2007, CMS established the program, called the Physician Quality Reporting Incentive (PQRI), which included an incentive payment for eligible professionals who satisfactorily reported on quality measures for covered professional services provided to Medicare beneficiaries. Originally, PQRI allowed eligible professionals to report on a claim form on at least three applicable measures for at least 80% of the Medicare Part B patients that they saw. Eligible professionals who reported correctly could receive an incentive payment of 1.5% for their allowable charges for the last 6 months of 2007.

The PQRI was modified by the Medicare, Medicaid, and SCHIP Extension Act of 2007 (PL 110-173), which extended the incentive payment for 2008 and 2009 and allowed the submission of data through clinical data registries (an organization approved by CMS that can submit PQRS data on behalf of the participating eligible professional). PQRI was made a permanent program under the Medicare Improvements for Patients and Providers Act of 2008 (PL 110-275) and incentive payments were set at 2% for 2010. The Patient Protection and Affordable Care Act (ACA) (PL 111-148) extended the incentive payments for the program through 2014. The bonus level was set at 1% for 2011 and 0.5% for 2012–2014. Starting in 2015, eligible professionals who do not satisfactorily report on quality measures will be subject to a penalty. This penalty will be a reduction in payments of 1.5% in 2015, and 2% in 2016 and each subsequent year. The ACA also changed the name of the program to the Physician Quality Reporting System (PQRS) to reflect that it was no longer an initiative; instead it was a permanent program.

The number of PQRS measures has increased throughout the years. In 2007, there were only 74 quality measures. By 2009, there were 153 quality measures, and in 2010 there were 175 measures. As of 2011, there were 190 approved PQRS quality measures, and it is likely this number will increase year by year. CMS prefers to approve measures that have been endorsed by a national consensus organization such as the NQF.

The PQRS measures are generally process measures (such as measuring whether care has been provided), although there are also some outcomes measures. CMS has indicated that it would like to see PQRS measures move toward more outcome measures.

### Speech-Language Pathology Measures

Speech-language pathologists were added in 2009 as eligible professionals who could report on PQRI measures. NQF-endorsed measures were approved for reporting as of 2010. The eight endorsed measures are Functional Communication Measures (FCMs) from the National Outcomes Measurement System (NOMS). NOMs is the data collection system developed by ASHA to illustrate the value of speech-language pathology and audiology services provided to adults and children with communication and swallowing disorders (ASHA, n.d.). Based on an individual's treatment plan, FCMs are chosen and scored by an SLP on admission and again at discharge to reflect the amount of change in communication or swallowing abilities after intervention. Comparing scores from admission and discharge demonstrates the amount of change and the outcome of treatment.

The eight PQRS measures that can be administered by SLPs to Medicare Part B beneficiaries who have had a stroke are in the following areas: attention, spoken language comprehension, spoken language expression, memory, motor speech, reading, writing, and swallowing. ASHA is an approved PQRS registry for reporting these measures. At the present time, only private practitioners are eligible for PQRS incentives; in addition, the provider does not need to demonstrate a prescribed amount of change to receive the incentive. As PQRS continues, penalties rather than incentives will be awarded to providers who do not meet benchmarks for improvement.

### Medicare Part B Research Projects

**Developing Outpatient Therapy Payment Alternatives**   Despite the therapy caps, Medicare B costs for rehabilitation services continue to grow (MedPAC, 2011a). Both Medicare and Congress have placed a priority on developing an alternative to the therapy caps. However, reports from MedPAC, the Government Accountability Office (GAO), and Computer Sciences Corporation (CSC) have indicated that Medicare needs more information about people who use therapy services and their outcomes to develop alternative payment policies (Ciolek & Hwang, 2006; MedPAC, 2006; U.S. GAO, 2005).

To collect more information, CMS awarded the Developing Outpatient Therapy Payment Alternatives (DOTPA) contract to Research Triangle Institute (RTI) in January 2008. This 5-year research project was designed to collect a large amount of demographic and clinical data concerning a beneficiary's need for and effectiveness of outpatient therapy services. RTI developed a tool to identify and collect demographic and clinical information related to beneficiary need for and effectiveness of outpatient therapy services. Different versions of the tool were developed for patients in nursing facilities or day rehabilitation settings and for those in community-based (outpatient) settings. Following the data collection period, RTI will analyze the data and recommend long-term payment alternative options. The effort to collect clinical information about functional abilities suggests that alternatives may focus on demonstrated outcomes of treatment.

**Short-Term Alternatives for Therapy Services**   CMS determined that additional study was needed to develop an alternative to the therapy caps, and awarded another contract in 2008: the 2-year Short-Term Alternatives for Therapy Services (STATS). This project, awarded to the CSC, was designed to develop alternatives that could be expected to be implemented within 2 or 3 years after approval by CMS. Specifically, CSC was tasked with updating data on the utilization of therapy services, developing a method for CMS to update utilization data quarterly, using these data and clinical expertise to identify characteristics of patients who need therapy services, and developing short-term alternatives to limit payment to medically necessary outpatient therapy services.

CSC conducted stakeholder work groups to solicit input, discuss potential revisions to outpatient therapy payment policy, and develop recommendations for alternatives. By September 2010, CSC completed its project and stated that in the long-term, "The most likely payment model for outpatients therapy services will be one based upon the episode of care. Provider payment will be influenced by beneficiary characteristics and the outcomes, or values, resulting from provider intervention" (CSC, 2010, p. 27).

To provide CMS with data to develop this model, short-term policy changes would need to be implemented to increase information on the claim form about patient characteristics, expected outcomes, and treatment progress. A long-term goal was to develop a single outpatient therapy function or an outcomes reporting tool to measure outpatient therapy quality.

CSC then presented three possible short-term policy options: (1) therapists report at the first session and at periodic intervals new Healthcare Common Procedure Coding System (HCPCS) codes reflecting patient function, and modifiers representing functional severity or complexity; (2) CMS applies an edit that would deny services when per-beneficiary expenditures reach a predetermined value; (3) CMS introduces new codes that would package the current version of the Current Procedural Terminology (CPT) billing codes into a single, per-session payment.

To date, CMS has not decided to implement any of CSC's suggested short-term policy options. However, based on CSC's assumption about long-term directions and suggested short-term policy changes, data collection and patient outcomes will play a role in future payment models. The DOTPA data collection tool may prove to be the basis of a single postacute tool mandated by Congress to determine the most appropriate cost-efficient postacute setting for patients and to track clinical information, functional needs, and progress from one setting to the next.

## Medicare Advantage (Part C)

The Medicare Advantage program is an alternative payment system to traditional Medicare Part A and Part B that covers the same services. Beneficiaries may opt to join a Medicare Advantage plan (such as a health maintenance organization, preferred provider organization, private fee-for-service plan) to receive all services. Medicare pays a monthly amount to the plan on behalf of the beneficiary, and the beneficiary also pays the Part B, Part D (prescription drugs), and supplemental benefits monthly premiums.

As discussed earlier, the National Committee for Quality Assurance (NCQA) developed and maintains the Healthcare Effectiveness Data and Information Set (HEDIS), a set of performance measures widely used by commercial health plans, as well as Medicare and Medicaid managed care plans. More than 90% of health plans in the United States use HEDIS to measure performance across different dimensions of care and service (NCQA, 2011c). The resulting data make it possible for consumers to compare the performance of different health plans.

HEDIS has a total of 75 measures across eight domains of care (NCQA, 2011a). Some of these domains are effectiveness of care, access/availability of care, use of services, and cost of care. Measures under effectiveness of care domain include glaucoma screening in older adults, care for older adults, breast and colorectal cancer screening, and controlling high blood pressure. Other examples of measures include relative resource use for people with diabetes (cost of care domain), inpatient utilization in a general hospital for acute care (use of services domain), and adults' access to preventive/ambulatory health services (access/availability of care domain). Some measures are applicable to commercial insurance, some to Medicaid, and some to Medicare. NCQA reviews the measure set each year to make sure it stays current and relevant (NCQA, 2011c).

As more Medicare beneficiaries joined managed care organizations in the mid-1990s, CMS began developing the Medicare Health Outcomes Survey (HOS) in 1996 (HSAG, n.d.; Jones, Jones, & Miller, 2004). It was the first patient-reported outcomes measurement tool used in Medicare managed care. Its purpose was to measure the quality of care and functional health status of Medicare beneficiaries enrolled in a managed care plan (HSAG, n.d.; Jones et al, 2004). By gathering data, CMS could use this information in quality improvement activities and pay for performance, as well as program oversight (CMS, 2010b). CMS partnered with NCQA by incorporating the Medicare population into the HEDIS measure set to create a measurement tool (the HOS) that examined the physical functioning and mental well-being of Medicare beneficiaries (Jones et al, 2004). In 1998, the HOS was first administered to a sample of Medicare beneficiaries participating in managed care; a follow-up survey was conducted 2 years later (HSAG, n.d.).

CMS still administers the HOS in this manner. The current version of HOS includes four HEDIS effectiveness of care domain measures, as well as additional questions (HSAG, n.d.). Each spring a random sampling of beneficiaries is drawn from each managed care organization participating in Medicare (CMS, 2010b). A baseline survey is administered to those beneficiaries, and then 2 years later, a follow-up survey is given to those same beneficiaries. Results of the HOS are part of the Medicare Advantage Five Star Ratings System. CMS developed this system to help beneficiaries compare managed care plans, to educate them about quality, and to make quality data transparent. There are other measures included in addition to the HOS measures. The six HOS measures that are part of the Five Star Ratings System include

- Improving or maintaining physical health
- Improving or maintaining mental health
- Osteoporosis testing
- Monitoring physical activity
- Improving bladder control
- Reducing the risk of falling

The CMS will use the 2011 Five Star Ratings as the basis for quality bonus payments in the Medicare Advantage program starting in 2012 (HSAG, 2011, August).

In regard to Medicare Advantage, the March 2011 MedPAC report stated that it "believes that outcome measures are better indicators of plan quality, and such measures (to the extent they are available) should be the most important factor in determining a plan's overall rating on quality" (MedPAC, 2011a, p. 294).

MedPAC has stated, "Resource-based payments do not adequately account for the relative effects of different services on clinical outcomes. In other words, a resource-based payment system values all services on an equal footing, regardless of their clinical efficiency." (MedPAC, 2011b, p. 14). In addition, during a discussion of technical assistance, MedPAC recommends that a provider's performance should be evaluated based on outcome measures (MedPAC, 2011b).

## ◆ Medicaid

Since Medicaid programs are administered at the state level, great variability exists in terms of whether quality measures are used or required to ensure accountability. Like Medicare managed care plans discussed above, some Medicaid managed care plans are required to submit data on HEDIS measures. In Maryland, for example, Medicaid managed care organizations must submit HEDIS data to the Department of Health and Mental Hygiene every year (Data Collection and Reporting, 2011; Quality Assessment and Improvement, 2011). Medicaid managed care organizations in New Mexico must also submit HEDIS data to the Human Services Department and are "expected to use HEDIS data as a measure of performance and to incorporate the results of each year's HEDIS data submission into its [quality improvement/quality management] plan (Quality Management Broad Standards, 2011).

# ◆ Children's Health Insurance Program

The Children's Health Insurance Program (CHIP) provides services to children whose families do not qualify for Medicaid but have low income. The Children's Health Insurance Program Reauthorization Act (CHIPRA) of 2009 (PL 111-3) reauthorized the program until 2013, and included requirements to strengthen health outcomes and quality of care for children receiving health care services under CHIP and Medicaid. As part of these requirements, the Secretary of Health and Human Services had to identify and publish an initial core measure set of children's health care quality measures. The measures were for voluntary use by Medicaid and CHIP programs. The bill called for measures that applied to treatment and management of acute and chronic conditions in children and care in integrated health settings, as well as other factors. Overall, the measures were to provide an estimate of the overall quality of care, facilitate analyses, and help identify disparities. In 2009, CMS collaborated with the AHRQ to develop these measures (CMS, 2010a). Both agencies worked together to create an initial set of measures that focused on prevention and health promotion services, management of chronic conditions, management of acute conditions, oral health, and family experiences of care (CMS, 2010a).

In late 2009, the Secretary of Health and Human Services published an initial core set of measures that were enhanced using feedback from public comments (CMS, 2010a; Medicaid and CHIP Programs, 2009). Under the domain of prevention and health promotion, the resulting measures include developmental screening the first 3 years of life (assessing the extent to which children at various ages up to 36 months were screened for social and emotional development with a standardized, documented tool or set of tools). Under the domain of management of acute conditions, a measure example is "otitis media with effusion (OME)—avoidance of inappropriate use of systemic antimicrobials in children–ages 2 through 12" (measuring the percentage of patients age 2 months through 12 years with a diagnosis of OME who were not prescribed systemic antimicrobials), and an example of a measure under the domain of management of chronic conditions is "annual number of asthma patients (2 through 20 years old) with one or more asthma-related emergency room visits" (CMS, 2010a). Most of the measures are process measures, but it is likely that CMS will want to add more outcome measures.

The initial set of core measures is just a first step in measuring and improving the quality of care provided to children under CHIP and Medicaid. These measures will be modified over the next several years to make them more easily collected by state Medicaid and CHIP programs and delivery models (such as managed care or fee-for-service), and to better reflect the quality of care.

CMS and AHRQ were required, as part of CHIPRA, to establish the Pediatric Quality Measures Program (PQMP) by 2011 (AHRQ, 2010). The purpose of PQMP is to refine the initial core set of measures, making them easier for data collection, and to develop more evidence-based, consensus pediatric quality measures (CMS, 2010a). In December 2010, AHRQ put out a request for public comments on PQMP because CHIPRA requires consultation with national stakeholders to establish priorities for development and advancement of measures (AHRQ, 2010). As of 2011, there have been seven cooperative agreement grant awards given to seven programs. These programs, known as PQMP Centers of Excellence, will work to find solutions to pediatric health quality measurement issues (AHRQ, 2011a).

In 2009, NQF convened a Child Health Outcomes Steering Committee in response to the initial set of core measures released under CHIPRA to complement the work being done by AHRQ and CMS (NQF, 2010). The mission of the committee was to identify gaps in existing outcomes measures, and identify, evaluate, and endorse additional child health outcome measures for public reporting and quality improvement. The committee has called for public comment on measures it recommends for NQF endorsement. Eventually, a certain number of child health measures will be endorsed by NQF and may be used as quality measures by CHIP and Medicaid.

# ◆ Public Policy

## Patient Protection and Affordable Care Act

Quality measurement can be addressed through legislation. The most recent and sweeping legislation that incorporated quality measures was the Patient Protection and Affordable Care Act of 2010 (ACA), which was signed into law on March 23, 2010. This legislation changed parts of the health care law and created new initiatives. Several provisions in the legislation focused on patient outcomes and improvement in care, including quality measures, that would encourage and quantify these priority areas. Some examples are discussed below.

### National Strategy for Quality Improvement in Health Care

Section 3011 of the ACA provides for a National Strategy for Quality Improvement in Health Care (National Quality Strategy). This section requires the Secretary of Health and Human Services to establish "a national strategy to improve the delivery of health care services, patient health outcomes, and population health." (Patient Protection and Affordable Care Act [ACA], 2010, § 3011(a)(1)). The Secretary is first required to identify national priorities to help develop the strategy, and these priorities must meet certain requirements. For example, the priorities must have the greatest potential for improving health outcomes (ACA, 2010, § 3011(a)(2)). The Secretary is also required to coordinate strategy efforts with state Medicaid agencies. There must also be a strategic plan to achieve the priorities, as well as a health care quality Web site.

  The Secretary presented a report to Congress in March 2011, outlining the initial National Quality Strategy and plan (HHS, 2011). After a collaborative effort with stakeholders, including individuals and organizations, the Secretary determined that the National Quality Strategy would focus on three aims: better care, healthy people and healthy communities, and affordable care. Priorities include making care safer, ensuring person- and family-centered care, promoting effective communication and coordination of care, and making quality care more affordable. To support these priorities, the report states that measurement of care processes and outcomes are needed. "In order to achieve the quality improvements envisioned by the National Quality Strategy, data on care delivery and outcomes should be measured using consistent, nationally endorsed measures in order to provide information that is timely, actionable, and meaningful to both providers and patients" (HHS, 2011, § III(6)). The report further states that HHS will continue to coordinate quality measurement efforts and develop national consensus on measures. There are likely to be several quality measures, including outcome measures, developed as a result of the National Quality Strategy.

### Medicare Shared Savings Program (Accountable Care Organizations)

In March 2011, the Department of Health and Human Services released a proposed rule regarding the shared savings program (Medicare Shared Savings Program, 2011) through accountable care organizations (ACOs). The proposed rule set forth potential governance and leadership requirements, suggested how to determine shared savings, and discussed other structural, legal, and financial arrangements. In addition, it also proposed 65 quality measures, grouped into the following domains: patient/caregiver experience, care coordination, patient safety, preventive health, and at risk population/frail elderly health (e.g., diabetes and heart failure) (Medicare Shared Savings Program, 2011, pp. 19571–19591). There are some outcome measures included in the mix of measures. For example, the measures of diabetes care require a patient's blood pressure to be less than 140/90, low-density lipoprotein (LDL) cholesterol levels to be less than 100, and hemoglobin $A_{1c}$ (measurement of average blood sugar level) to be less than 8% (Medicare Shared Savings Program, 2011, p. 19581).

### Measurement Development

The ACA demonstrates its commitment to measuring quality by assigning one section of the bill purely to measure development. Section 3013 allocates $75 million for each fiscal year 2010 through

2014 for quality measure development. The legislation requires that the Secretary of Health and Human Services, along with the director of the AHRQ and the administrator of CMS, identify gaps in quality measure development and existing measures that need updating or improvement. The Secretary must also award grants or contracts to eligible entities that will develop, improve, update, or expand quality measures. The legislation gives priority to certain areas of measure development, including "quality measures that allow assessment of health outcomes and functional status of patients" (ACA, 2010, § 3013(c)(2)(A)).

### Measure Applications Partnership

Section 3014 of the ACA requires a consensus-based entity to gather multi-stakeholder group input on the selection of quality measures. These measures are to be used for Medicare, reporting performance information to the public, and in other health care programs (ACA, 2010, § 3014(a)(B)). *Multi-stakeholder* is defined as "a voluntary collaborative of organizations representing a broad group of stakeholders interested in or affected by the use of such quality measures" (ACA, 2010, § 3014(a)(D)). The legislation allocates $20 million for each fiscal year 2010 through 2012 for these purposes (ACA, 2010, § 3014(c)). Called the Measure Applications Partnership, the NQF serves as the neutral convener of stakeholders, which includes a representative from ASHA, the American Physical Therapy Association, consumer groups, and many other health care organizations and measure experts.

### Hospital Value-Based Purchasing

Section 3001 of the ACA requires the Secretary to establish a hospital value-based purchasing (VBP) program that would reward hospitals that meet certain performance standards. In May 2011, CMS issued the final rule establishing the hospital VBP program (Medicare Program, 2011). Starting in October 2012, Medicare will provide incentive payments to hospitals based on how they perform on certain measures. The first set of initial measures consists of clinical process measures and patient experience of care measures (Medicare Program, 2011, p. 26495). However, for fiscal year 2014, CMS will use different measures to determine incentive payments, which include five outcome measures (Medicare Program, 2011, p. 26495). These outcome measures include three 30-day mortality measures for heart failure, pneumonia, and acute myocardial infarction. The measures track whether a patient who was admitted with a diagnosis of heart attack, heart failure, or pneumonia died 30 days from the admission date, regardless of whether the patient was still in the hospital or discharged (Medicare Program, 2011, p. 26497). The other two outcome measures look at mortality rates for selected medical conditions and complications that may arise from hospital care (Medicare Program, 2011, p. 26511).

## ◆ Conclusion and Future Directions

The measures approved to date represent early efforts to identify critical processes in high-profile, high-risk areas of medical intervention. Increasingly, outcome measures will be collected and reported not only to assure the government and private insurers of the quality of the services they are purchasing, but also to provide the public with information to select a provider or facility. While few of the measures adopted by federal programs currently address rehabilitation or specific speech-language or audiology outcomes, the trend for the future in the importance of quality measures for payment and public reporting has been clearly established.

The passage of the Patient Protection and Affordable Care Act in 2010 set the vision for initiatives that have not been fully implemented; while subsequent years will see changes and modifications to the vision, the use of outcomes measures as one aspect of quality measurement in health care is undoubtedly here to stay.

# References

Agency for Healthcare Research and Quality (AHRQ). (1997, Nov). (Formerly Agency for Health Care Policy and Research.) *Theory and reality of value-based purchasing: Lessons from the pioneers.* AHCPR Publication No. 98–0004. Agency for Health Care Policy and Research, Rockville, MD. http://www.ahrq.gov/qual/meyerrpt.htm

Agency for Healthcare Research and Quality (AHRQ). (2011a, March). *Pediatric Quality Measures Program (PQMP) Centers of Excellence Grant Awards.* http://www.ahrq.gov/chipra/pqmpfact.htm

Agency for Healthcare Research and Quality (AHRQ). (2011b, May). *At a glance.* http://www.ahrq.gov/about/ataglance.htm

Agency for Healthcare Research and Quality Priority Setting for the Children's Health Insurance Program Reauthorization Act (CHIPRA) Pediatric Quality Measures Program (AHRQ), 75 Fed. Reg. 75469. (2010).

American Speech-Language-Hearing Association (ASHA). (n.d.). *National outcomes measurement system (NOMS).* http://www.asha.org/members/research/NOMS/default.htm.

Balanced Budget Act of 1997 (BBA). (1997). Pubic Law 105-33, 111 Stat. 251

Centers for Medicare and Medicaid Services (CMS). (2009). *OASIS-C: Development and impact on agency operations. Medicare Learning Network.* https://www.cms.gov/HomeHealthQualityInits/downloads/HHQIOASIS_C20091022Call.pdf

Centers for Medicare and Medicaid Services (CMS). (2010a, Feb). *CHIPRA initial core set technical specifications manual.* https://www.cms.gov/MedicaidCHIPQualPrac/Downloads/CHIPRACoreSetTechManual.pdf

Centers for Medicare and Medicaid Services (CMS). (2010b). *Health Outcomes Survey (HOS) overview.* http://www.cms.gov/hos/

Centers for Medicare and Medicaid Services (CMS). (2011a). *IRF patient assessment instrument.* http://www.cms.gov/InpatientRehabFacPPS/04_IRFPAI.asp#TopOfPage

Centers for Medicare and Medicaid Services (CMS). (2011b, revised). *MDS 3.0 for nursing homes and swing bed providers.* https://www.cms.gov/NursingHomeQualityInits/25_NHQIMDS30.asp#TopOfPage

Centers for Medicare and Medicaid Services (CMS). (2011c). *MDS 3.0 RAI manual.* https://www.cms.gov/NursingHomeQualityInits/45_NHQIMDS30TrainingMaterials.asp#TopOfPage

Centers for Medicare and Medicaid Services (CMS).(2011d). *OASIS-C guidance manual.* http://www.cms.gov/HomeHealthQualityInits/14_HHQIOASISUserManual.asp

Centers for Medicare and Medicaid Services (CMS). (n.d.). *List of quality measures. Medicare.gov.* http://www.medicare.gov/homehealthcompare/(S(hefybrivamfbt345d5qnwuur))/Data/Measures/List.aspx

Ciolek, D., & Hwang, W. (2006). *Outpatient therapy services utilization and edit report.* http://www.cms.gov/TherapyServices/SAR/itemdetail.asp?filterType=none&filterByDID=99&sortByDID=3&sortOrder=descending&itemID=CMS1187930&intNumPerPage=10

Computer Sciences Corporation (CSC). (2010, July 9). *Final report on short term alternatives.* https://www.cms.gov/TherapyServices/downloads/STATS_Short_Term_Alternatives_Report.pdf

Data Collection and Reporting, MD. *Code Regs.* COMAR 10.09.65.15 (2011)

Health and Human Services (HHS). (2011, March). *Report to Congress: National strategy for quality improvement in health care.* http://www.healthcare.gov/center/reports/quality03212011a.html

Health Services Advisory Group (HSAG). (2011, Aug). *Survey results.* Updated August, 2011. http://www.hosonline.org/Content/SurveyResults.aspx

Health Services Advisory Group (HSAG). (n.d.). *Medicare health outcomes survey overview.* http://www.hosonline.org/Content/ProgramOverview.aspx

Henry J. Kaiser Family Foundation. (2010, Aug). *Medicare spending and financing* [Fact sheet]. http://www.kff.org/medicare/upload/7305-05.pdf

Jones, N., III, Jones, S. L., & Miller, N. A. (2004, Jul). The Medicare Health Outcomes Survey program: overview, context, and near-term prospects. *Health and Quality of Life Outcomes, 2,* 33

Medicaid and CHIP Programs. (2009). *Initial core set of children's healthcare quality measures for voluntary use by Medicaid and CHIP programs.* 74 Fed. Reg. 68846

Medicare Payment Advisory Commission (MedPAC). (2006, June). *Report to the Congress: Increasing the value of Medicare.* http://www.medpac.gov/documents/Jun06_EntireReport.pdf

Medicare Payment Advisory Commission (MedPAC). (2011a, March). *Report to the Congress: Medicare payment policy.* http://www.medpac.gov/documents/Mar11_EntireReport.pdf

Medicare Payment Advisory Commission (MedPAC). (2011b, June). *Report to the Congress: Medicare and the health care delivery system.* http://www.medpac.gov/documents/Jun11_EntireReport.pdf

Medicare Payment Advisory Commission (MedPAC). (2011c). *About MedPAC.* http://www.medpac.gov/about.cfm

Medicare Program. (2011). *Hospital inpatient value-based purchasing program.* 76 Fed. Reg. 26490 (To be codified at 42 C.F.R. pts. 422 and 480)

Medicare Shared Savings Program. (2011). *Accountable care organizations,* 76 Fed. Reg. 19528

National Committee for Quality Assurance (NCQA). (2011a). *2011 Summary table of measures, product lines and changes.* http://www.ncqa.org/Portals/0/HEDISQM/HEDIS%202011/HEDIS%202011%20Measures.pdf

National Committee for Quality Assurance (NCQA). (2011b). *About NCQA.* http://www.ncqa.org/tabid/675/Default.aspx

National Committee for Quality Assurance (NCQA). (2011c) *What is Hedis?* http://www.ncqa.org/tabid/187/default.aspx

National Quality Forum (NQF). (2009) *HHS performance measurement.* http://www.qualityforum.org/About_NQF/HHS_Performance_Measurement.aspx

National Quality Forum (NQF). (2010). *Funding.* http://www.qualityforum.org/About_NQF/Funding.aspx

Patient Protection and Affordable Care Act (PPACA), Pub. L. No. 111–148, 124 Stat. 119 (2010)

Quality Assessment and Improvement, MD. *Code Regs.* COMAR 10.09.65.03 (2011)

Quality Management Broad Standards, N.M. *Admin. Code.* NMAC § 8.305.8.11(B) (2011)

Saliba, D., & Buchanan, J. (2008). *Development and validation of a revised nursing home assessment tool: MDS 3.0.* Rand Corporation. https://www.cms.gov/NursingHomeQualityInits/25_NHQIMDS30.asp

U.S. Government Accountability Office (GAO). (2005, November). *Report to congressional committees: Little progress made in targeting outpatient therapy payments to beneficiaries' needs.* http://www.gao.gov/products/GAO-06-59

# II

# Clinical Services

# 5

# Outcomes Measurement in Health Care

*Margaret A. Rogers and Robert C. Mullen*

## ◆ Chapter Focus

This chapter continues the discussion of trends in outcomes measurement in health care, and rehabilitation in particular, with emphasis on large-scale, health care–related outcomes measurement in speech-language pathology. The central theme of this chapter is directed toward understanding *what works best for whom, in what circumstances and in what respects, and how,* and exploring how, through statistical approaches applied to large databases, the multiple factors that have been identified as relevant to outcomes can be modeled. As Frattali (1998) wrote in the first edition of this book, "outcome measurement . . . is meaningful only if linked to facility, client, and clinician characteristics (to allow comparison of 'apples to apples'), and the various processes of care (to allow us to make relational statements about the effects of specific interventions)" (p. 8). To this end, this chapter explores how multiple domains of functioning and health, and personal and service delivery factors, can and should be incorporated into the measurement of outcomes in speech-language pathology. The chapter illustrates this point by showing how two instruments, supported by large databases, are approaching the question of how best to predict the rehabilitation potential of patients, the benefits derived from rehabilitation, and how to model the resources and the potential costs associated with these services.

## ◆ Introduction

Outcomes measurement in health care has assumed a central role in considerations of future payment systems. Transformation of the infrastructure that currently supports health care in the United States is necessary to develop new payment systems that can sustain affordable and accessible quality health care. Health care spending continues to grow more precipitously than inflation in spite of initiatives that have been implemented in an attempt to curb this growth, such as health maintenance organizations, preferred provider organizations, and prospective payment systems (e.g., the Medicare Physician Fee Schedule). Accordingly, stakeholders from diverse interests have been intensely debating how to shape the future. Amidst much disagreement, interestingly, there are a few tenets upon which stakeholders seemingly concur, namely that future health care systems need to incentivize quality and accountability and be economically sustainable while also decreasing health disparities, and that health care decisions, regulatory policies, and the valuation of services should be based more solidly on valid and comprehensive data. The increasing reliance on cost-benefit analyses to determine which services should be covered in a health plan will require accelerated development of valid measures of the benefits associated with those services. The central role that data play in this envisioned transformation has raised national awareness of the need for increased support to advance clinical practice research, comparative effectiveness research, implementation and health services research, and cost-benefit analyses.

Central to the goals of cost containment and budgeting health care expenditures is the ability to predict that, based on the incidence of a given condition, *x* number of individuals will need *y* treatments for *z* cost annually. Payment systems based on predictive modeling need to be able to predict, based on historical data, the rehabilitation potential of individual patients and then, based on evidence about which approach to intervention is likely to be most effective for a given type of patient in a given circumstance, predict the resources that will be required to achieve pre-specified rehabilitation goals. According to Massof (2010), the primary goal for such modeling is to predict the probability of obtaining a specified outcome given a mix of patient-specific factors and the choice of interventions. Goulding revisits this topic in Chapter 7 in the context of long-term care. Because outcome measures, patient-specific factors, and service delivery factors are each critical components of the data needed to model the probability of obtaining a specified outcome for a particular patient-grouping receiving a given intervention, a large-scale data set containing information about all three components is required (i.e., as in an outcomes registry or electronic health record). So, at a minimum, the data elements that are needed to inform future payment systems based on predictive modeling approaches include information about patients (case-mix data), their outcomes, service delivery factors, and an accounting of the resources utilized to achieve these outcomes. As patient factors mediate the effects of services on outcomes, *case-mix adjusted* data are necessary to compare the effectiveness of different interventions and ultimately, to model the costs and benefits of providing services for specific patient groupings. Thus, as Pawson and Tilley (2004, p. 2) suggest, "The basic question asked, and hopefully answered, is thus multi-faceted . . . [so we should not ask] 'What works?' or, 'Does this program work?' but instead, 'What works for whom in what circumstances and in what respects, and how?'"

It is being increasingly recognized that a valid evaluation of patient outcomes cannot occur out of context. Case-mix factors (e.g., patient characteristics such as their health problems and the severity of those conditions, comorbidities, and demographic information), combined with information about service delivery (e.g., facility type, practitioner factors, type and dosage of treatment) and health care systems, must provide the broader context within which it becomes possible to validly interpret changes in health, function, and participation in life roles and situations as associated with specific health conditions and services. Speech-language pathology and other health care disciplines are advancing knowledge concerning *what works best for whom, in what circumstances and in what respects, and how,* but no discipline will be able to satisfactorily address this multifaceted question without large-scale data collection instruments that amass information across each of these critical data elements in a centralized repository so that adequately powered analyses can be conducted to examine the effects that case-mix and service delivery factors have on patient outcomes. Two such efforts are described in this chapter: the American Speech-Language-Hearing Association's (ASHA) National Outcomes Measurement System (NOMS) and the Center for Medicare and Medicaid Services' Developing Outpatient Therapy Payment Alternatives (DOTPA) initiative.

# ◆ International Classification of Functioning, Disability, and Health

The theoretical framework of disablement advanced in the International Classification of Functioning, Disability, and Health (ICF) is of central importance to outcomes measurement in health care.

Based on the World Health Organization's (WHO) ICF model (WHO, 2001), described by Golper in Chapter 2 and Threats in Chapter 3, outcomes can be considered across three domains: body functions and structures, activity, and participation. The 2001 model for the WHO-ICF is provided in **Fig. 2.8**. *Body functions and structures* refer to the anatomy and physiology of body structures and functions including cognitive and psychological functions. Difficulties of body structures and function are referred to as *impairments. Activity* occurs at the task level, and involves such activities as ordering food at a restaurant, talking over the phone, reading a book, and adhering to an appointment schedule. *Participation* occurs at the societal level and is an interaction between the person and the environment in social and life roles, involving such phenomena as engaging in life situations, interacting with family and friends, and fulfilling one's roles and responsibilities associated with being a spouse, parent, friend, student, employee, citizen, and so on. Difficulties in these latter two areas are referred to collectively as *activity limitations* and *participation restrictions.* In the ICF, the experience of disability is modeled as an interaction among these domains as well as *contextual factors. Contextual factors* include both *personal factors,* which encompass attributes of an individual and his or her background (e.g., gender, race, ethnicity, education, coping style, lifestyle, psychological characteristics), and *environmental factors,* which include the physical, social, and attitudinal environment in which people live and conduct their lives. According to ASHA (2004), the ultimate goal of intervention is "improving the lives of individuals with communication disorders in terms of sense-of-wellness and functional health through high-quality services which they consider important and valuable" (p. 7). Garrett and Pimentel (2007) argue that "this is best accomplished when the clinician carefully considers the disorder within a framework that acknowledges the communicator and his or her impairments, functional contexts, and communication partners, as well as desired activities and goals" (p. 29). ASHA's Scope of Practice for Speech-Language Pathology (ASHA, 2001) incorporates the ICF as it provides a useful framework to guide assessment and treatment decisions, supporting the idea that communication status and treatment goals be considered across the multiple ICF domains (i.e., impairments, activity limitations, participation restrictions, and personal and environmental barriers).

## Intervention and the ICF

Intervention services provided by speech-language pathologists (SLPs) for individuals in acute, post-acute, and long-term care can be provided to achieve a variety of goals, and these goals can be conceptualized using the ICF framework. Treatments targeting improved body functions or structures—such as increasing hyoid elevation during a swallow; increasing articulatory, lexical, and grammatical accuracy; or improving the physiological functioning of the vocal folds—aim to ameliorate one or more impairments. Approaches that support individuals in performing specific tasks and activities, such as using multiple modalities to receive and convey messages or using assistive devices to remember appointments, aim to decrease activity limitations. These approaches are not intended to reduce the severity of impairment, but rather, through the provision of compensatory strategies and techniques, to make targeted activities easier to perform or, by altering the task requirements, more achievable. Participation restrictions are also commonly addressed in speech-language pathology, in part because communication is predominantly a social activity as it typically involves at least two people. Social approaches to treating communication disorders, such as the Life Participation Approach to Aphasia Project Group (2001), group treatment, and community-based services, promote participation and engagement in life situations. Social approaches may also decrease impairments and activity limitations since specific behaviors and tasks can be reinforced and practiced in naturally occurring, authentic communication contexts such as are typically afforded in group therapy. Changes to environmental factors are also addressed by SLPs. For example, SLPs often counsel the families of individuals with aphasia and hearing loss, as well as other communication disorders, to make environmental adjustments such as limiting background noise and positioning oneself to face the conversational partner so as to improve comprehension. Additionally, efforts to increase national awareness or a spouse's or an employer's understanding of the nature of a given communication disorder can help greatly to reduce attitudinal barriers that can worsen the burden of a disability.

Thus, in speech-language pathology, both the approach to and goals of intervention often encompass multiple ICF domains and contextual factors. Furthermore, it is likely that patient outcomes are improved maximally if approached comprehensively, across the impairment, activity, and participation domains, as well as addressing personal and environmental factors.

## Outcomes Measurement and the ICF

Outcomes measurement can be similarly stratified across the ICF domains. Performance measures, such as percent correct information units (Nicholas & Brookshire, 1993) or tongue strength and endurance (Robin, Somodi, & Luschei, 1991), serve as surrogate measures of body function and structure. These types of dependent variables are used most commonly to measure outcomes associated with impairment-focused treatments, such as *semantic feature analysis* to treat anomia (e.g., Boyle & Coelho, 1995) and *oral motor exercise* to improve strength (e.g., Robbins et al, 2007). Examples of measures targeting communication activities include tools such as the Communication Effectiveness Index (CETI) (Lomas et al, 1989), the Functional Linguistic Communication Inventory (FLCI) (Bayles & Tomoeda, 1994), the Communication Activities of Daily Living-2 (CADL-2) (Holland, Frattali, & Fromm, 1999), ASHA's NOMS, and ASHA's Functional Assessment of Communication Skills for Adults (ASHA FACS) (Frattali, Thompson, Holland, Wohl, & Ferketic, 1995). There are also a few participation-oriented instruments available to evaluate how well adults with communication and related disorders (e.g., dysphagia) are engaging socially and participating in life situations. These include such tools as the ASHA Quality of Communication Life Scale (ASHA-QCL; Paul et al, 2004), the Code-Müller Protocols (CMP; Code & Müller, 1992), the Swallowing Quality of Life Questionnaire (SWAL-QOL; McHorney et al, 2000), and portions of the Burden of Stroke Survival Scale (BOSS; Doyle, McNeil, Hula, & Mikolic, 2003). Although an exhaustive accounting of the available outcome measures and their psychometric properties is not attempted here (see Garrett & Pimentel [2007] for a more detailed summary of outcome measures commonly used in speech-language pathology and Stiers et al, [2012] for a review of participation measures developed for use with individuals with traumatic brain injuries), it is evident that there are tools available to assess outcomes across the ICF domains of body structure and function, activity, and participation for individuals with communication and related disorders. However, the number of measurement tools specifically targeting participation outcomes is relatively limited.

### Measuring Participation

The ICF models the experience of disability as being influenced by multiple factors including health conditions (i.e., impairments of body structures and functions), activity limitations, participation restrictions, and contextual factors (i.e., environment and personal factors). Participation is defined in the ICF (WHO, 2001) as "involvement in a life situation," and the converse (participation restrictions) is defined as "problems an individual may experience in involvement in life situations." Participation in social, family, civic, vocational, and avocational roles is an ecologically important outcome, especially for individuals with communication impairments because communication is so often integral to the manner in which people engage in life situations. Development of an instrument, items, or protocols designed to measure the participation outcomes of individuals with communication impairments requires a conceptual model of communicative participation (Eadie et al, 2006). One important step in defining the concept of communicative participation is to differentiate participation from other related concepts. Dijkers, Whiteneck, & El-Jaroudi (2000) and Dijkers and Greenwald (2006) suggest that there is conceptual overlap between participation and other constructs such as activity, community integration, and social disability. Participation also has been linked conceptually to quality of life as well as to subjective measures of global life satisfaction. Stiers and colleagues (2012) add that there is uncertainty regarding whether self-reported measures of satisfaction with participation differ from self-reported measures of well-being, which has been conceptualized as encompassing both eudemonic concepts (e.g., purpose in life, personal growth, positive relationships with others, environmental mastery, self-acceptance, and autonomy), as well as hedonic concepts such as happiness and life satisfaction (Kahneman, Diener, & Schwarz, 1999).

Another challenge has been to differentiate the construct of "activity" from "participation," and, in fact, the authors of the ICF (WHO, 2001) merged activity and participation into a single construct in the ICF classification system, ostensibly to increase the reliably of clinicians' judgments (Eadie et al, 2006). Despite the fact that the ICF merges activity and participation into a single construct, many continue to argue that activity and participation should be distinctly conceptualized and independently measured (e.g., Whiteneck, Bogner, & Heinemann, 2011). To optimize rehabilitation outcomes, research is needed to model the independent effects as well as the interactions among the ICF domains; however, operationalizing "activity" separately from "participation," and even from "body functions and structures," has proven challenging (Perenboom & Chorus, 2003). Although participation restrictions and activity limitations may be correlated variables, they can also vary independently in part because each has multiple factors that independently influence them. For example, contextual factors like social support can greatly improve participation in family roles and positively influence adaptation to living with a communication-based disability (e.g., Burns, Dong, & Oehring, 1995), but may not necessarily affect one's ability to perform specific communicative activities such as using the telephone or independently communicating with unfamiliar people. Improved definition of the concept of communicative participation and further differentiating it from the construct of communicative activities would likely help elucidate how these constructs can be independently measured. Because of the conceptual overlap among the constructs of activity, community integration, social disability, well-being, quality of life, and participation, developing measures that can estimate the latent trait of "involvement in life situations" (i.e., participation) apart from these other concepts is challenging. However, the current state is not surprising because, in comparison to the number of studies that have focused on measuring impairment outcomes, the study of participation outcomes is clearly in the nascent but developing stage—a point that has been made previously in reference to the field of communication disorders (Eadie, 2001; Threats, 2000) as well as other rehabilitation disciplines (e.g., Dijkers et al, 2000), and mentioned elsewhere in this text. Over the past decade, research is increasingly focused on measuring participation outcomes, and greater clarity concerning the definition of communicative participation (as distinct from communicative activities, well-being, quality of life, etc.) is emerging in an iterative manner and helping us to refine these measures so that we will have valid data that can guide us to improve the participation outcomes of those who receive speech-language pathology services.

There are several trends supporting the development of ecologically and psychometrically valid outcome measures of participation. In the United States, participation plays a central role in both legislative and executive initiatives, including the Americans with Disabilities Act, Healthy People 2010, and the New Freedom Initiative. Growing appreciation of the ICF model may be influencing federal agencies, policy makers, researchers, clinicians, and other stakeholders to focus more on participation outcomes. There is a growing awareness that, in addition to the disabling effects of impairments and activity limitations, environmental factors, including social, attitudinal, and public resource barriers, also limit participation for people with disabilities. As depicted in the ICF, these environmental barriers can further exacerbate, or in some cases even cause, participation restrictions. Thus, the individual's impairments and activity limitations are not the sole source of participation restrictions, but instead stem from "a person–task–environment interaction arising from the individual's condition, the task in which they are engaged, and the environment in which they engage with the task" (Stiers et al, 2012, p. 142). Valid measures of participation for individuals with communication disorders would allow us to better: (a) assess the effects of impairments, activity limitations, personal factors, and environmental barriers on participation restrictions; (b) conduct intervention, implementation, and comparative effectiveness research; and (c) evaluate the value and improve the quality of speech-language pathology services.

One very significant challenge to addressing this pressing need for valid measures of participation outcomes is that, since participation is a person–task–environment interaction, it is difficult to attribute changes in participation to any single factor (e.g., choice of intervention, health care system, activity limitations, and impairment severity). Further, as participation is likely to continue to improve for many months after therapy has been terminated, consideration should be given to when participation outcomes are optimally measured. For example, participation measures obtained at discharge from a rehabilitation facility may not be valid estimates of how well the patient is going to adapt to living in the home environment. If it is not valid to assess participation at discharge, then measurement of this domain will be further complicated by the need to conduct assessments after the patient has undergone a period of adaptation in the home environment. Following-up some months after discharge to collect participation outcome data may be necessary to validly assess whether patients are successfully participating in life roles and situations. Thus, given that many factors affecting participation outcomes (i.e., person–task–environment interaction) and that measurement of participation outcomes probably should not be obtained immediately following discharge from therapy, directly associating the effects of therapy with participation outcomes is a complicated endeavor that, in all likelihood, can only be validly addressed if analyzed in the context of a large database so that the multiple sources of influence and variance can be modeled.

Participation in social role activities is challenging to measure. As Whiteneck and Dijkers (2009) discuss, objective indices such as counts or inventories of social activities can be used as simple surrogate measures of participation. However, as objective indices of participation, such as counting the number of social engagements within a defined period, are typically normed on nondisabled populations, it is unclear whether these are valid measures by which to assess participation among individuals with disabilities. Even if these measures were normed on individuals with communication disorders, it is not clear whether a single instrument with a single normative database collected from individuals with a variety of communication impairments could be used validly to interpret the participation outcomes across the wide array of etiologies that give rise to communication impairments (Baylor, Yorkston, Eadie, Miller, & Amtmann, 2009). Additionally, objective measures of participation have been criticized because they do not take into account individual variation, especially regarding individual preferences. It is also unclear whether more participation should be the target outcome as opposed to more diverse types of participation or a better quality of participation. Stiers and colleagues (2012, p. 142) hypothesize that "optimal participation, rather than maximal participation may be most important" to measure. Measures of optimal participation would take into account individual preferences regarding which social activities are important, the perceived quality of those interactions, and what specific aspects of participation are challenging for the individual. To identify the factors that significantly influence participation outcomes, it is important to identify, from the patient's perspective, what it means to participate "successfully" in life roles. It is also important to understand which factors influence, both positively and negatively, one's adaptation to living with a disability as concerns participation in life roles and situations. Thus, measuring "successful participation" from a patient-oriented perspective is likely to be critical to the development of a conceptual model of communicative participation and valid measures of communicative participation outcomes (Eadie et al, 2006).

### Integrating Outcomes Measurement Across the ICF Domains

The importance of measuring outcomes across ICF domains is underscored by the notion that, for individuals as well as populations, one cannot infer that the severity of the impairment will necessarily predict the extent of activity limitations, and even less so, participation restrictions. The notion that activity limitations and participation restrictions are not wholly determined by impairment severity is integral to the ICF model as well as to principles of rehabilitation underlying compensatory and social approaches to treating communication and related disorders (e.g., Rogers, Alarcon, & Olswang, 1999). From a clinical perspective, decisions have to be made about what domain(s) to treat and what measure(s) to use. It could be argued that outcome measures should be selected that match the ICF domain(s) targeted in treatment (e.g., impairment outcomes applied to assess progress associated with impairment-directed treatments). Despite the parsimonious appeal of this "matching" approach to selecting outcome measures, it can be argued that if treatments directed at impairments are successful, the effects ought to be observable in terms of functional improvements performing everyday activities, and accordingly, the activity domain (e.g., tasks associated with functional communication) would be the most critical to measure. In the next section, ASHA's NOMS is described, in part, to better elucidate measurement of the activity domain.

Although assessing changes in functional communication is clearly important, others have argued that since improved function does not necessarily result in improved participation, specific measures of participation ought to be obtained in addition to measures of function (Kagen & Gailey, 1993; Stiers et al, 2012). Furthermore, although the activity domain is probably the most common focus of speech-language pathology services, especially in rehabilitation, participation is probably more often the focus of concern for patients, their families, and their friends. For example, concerns about being able to go out to eat with friends, interacting with unfamiliar people, and otherwise continuing to engage in familial and societal roles are frequently conveyed by those receiving rehabilitation services from SLPs. Accordingly, participation is arguably the most clinically meaningful and ecologically valid domain by which to assess the enduring effects of rehabilitation. Unfortunately, Simmons-Mackie, Threats, and Kagan (2005) found that only 8% of the SLPs who responded to their survey reported that they included caregivers in their assessment practices, and by far the most frequently used outcome measures were standardized tests of communication impairment. Unfortunately, standardized tests do not tend to be sensitive indices of change due to the fact that they typically sample a wide variety of abilities and skills, and thus are not usually good candidate outcome measures as sensitivity and specificity are diminished with composite scoring. The DOTPA instruments developed for the Centers for Medicare and Medicaid Services (CMS) for use as an outcomes measurement tool in rehabilitation include separate sections designed to document the presence and severity of patients' impairments, their activity limitations, and also include patient-reported measures of their activity limitations and participation restrictions. This initiative is described in more detail to explicate how the ICF framework can be incorporated to measure patient outcomes more comprehensively.

Of particular relevance to outcomes measurement is the notion that, just as the experience of disability is an interaction of impairments of body structure and function, activity limitations and participation restrictions, and factors specific to the person and his or her environment, patient outcomes are likely to result from similar interactions across the ICF domains. Accordingly, it may be difficult to attribute a given outcome to only one variable, such as the effects of an intervention or the severity of impairment. Although this point may be self-evident, the implications for measurement and intervention research are important. The presence of a given factor from one ICF domain, such as the severity of impairment, may account for a portion of the variance observed across patients, but in all likelihood, greater explanatory power would be derived from models capable of accounting for the interaction among factors from each of the ICF domains as well as contextual factors. This logic suggests that relying on a single outcome measure, which may be tied to just one ICF domain, is unlikely to yield as precise an assessment of outcomes as a measurement tool that includes items designed to sample behaviors and perspectives across all ICF domains. To improve the quality of services provided to individuals with communication and related disorders, and thus to advance the discipline, it is not enough to simply know that positive changes were observed on a given set of measures for a given individual. Rather, it is critical to know how a given patient's progress compares to similar cases in similar environments. These types of analyses need to be based on large representative samples, which can only be obtained through the use of large-scale data collection instruments that amass data in a centralized repository such as exemplified by ASHA's National Outcomes Measurement System.

## ◆ The National Outcomes Measurement System

In the late 1980s and early 1990s, the need for more than anecdotal evidence of the gains made by clients receiving speech-language pathology services grew increasingly apparent. Payers, administrators, and clients and their families called upon SLPs to be explicit about what progress could be expected under what circumstances. State-level health insurance reform initiatives in Florida crystallized the need for empirical data there, and these reforms were soon evident in all states. In 1994, ASHA established a task force on treatment outcomes and cost-effectiveness. A major goal of the task force was to establish at ASHA a clearinghouse of outcomes data collected by ASHA member clinicians. These data could then be aggregated into a national database (or databases) to inform the development of ASHA policy positions related to reimbursement schemes and other issues, respond to the increasing number of queries from Medicare and Medicaid for national-level data, and to establish national benchmarks that individual programs and facilities could use for comparison with their own data.

The clearinghouse never came to be. One reason was that few programs were collecting outcomes data on any formal basis. Another reason was that, of the programs and facilities that were collecting outcomes data, most were using inappropriate tools, for example, the *Functional Independence Measure* (FIM™), a widely used tool intended for measurements in the *impairment* domain, as Stineman and her colleagues describe (Stineman, Jette, Fiedler, & Granger, 1997; Stineman et al, 1996). Unfortunately, the items on the FIM were developed by and for other disciplines and were inappropriate for speech-language pathology (http://www.udsmr.org/WebModules/FIM/Fim_About.aspx). Consequently, the Task Force recommended that ASHA establish the National Center for Treatment Effectiveness in Communication Disorders (NCTECD). This later became the National Center for Evidence-Based Practice in Communication Disorders (NCTECD). The NCTECD, or N-CEP, was formed in 1997 to develop functional outcomes measures specific to speech-language pathology, and oversee nationwide collection of data on these measures.

The measures developed by ASHA members and staff are known as the Functional Communication Measures (FCMs). Each FCM is a disorder-specific seven-point ordinal scale describing clients' functional communication from a least-functional level, level 1, to full functionality, level 7, as exemplified in **Table 5.1**.

The initial focus was on adults receiving SLP services in health care settings, so the initial set of FCMs to be developed consisted of:

- Attention
- Fluency
- Memory
- Motor speech
- Pragmatics
- Reading
- Spoken language comprehension
- Spoken language expression
- Swallowing
- Voice
- Writing

In subsequent years, four additional FCMs have been added:

- Alaryngeal communication
- Augmentative-alternative communication
- Problem solving
- Voice following tracheostomy

**Table 5.1**   Sample Functional Communication Measure

| Spoken Language Comprehension |
| --- |
| **Level 1:** The individual is alert, but unable to follow simple directions or respond to yes/no questions, even with cues. |
| **Level 2:** With consistent, maximal cues, the individual is able to follow simple directions, respond to simple yes/no questions in context, and respond to simple words or phrases related to personal needs. |
| **Level 3:** The individual usually responds accurately to simple yes/no questions. The individual is able to follow simple directions out of context, although moderate cuing is consistently needed. Accurate comprehension of more complex directions/messages is infrequent. |
| **Level 4:** The individual consistently responds accurately to simple yes/no questions and occasionally follows simple directions without cues. Moderate contextual support is usually needed to understand complex sentences/messages. The individual is able to understand limited conversations about routine daily activities with familiar communication partners. |
| **Level 5:** The individual is able to understand communication in structured conversations with both familiar and unfamiliar communication partners. The individual occasionally requires minimal cuing to understand more complex sentences/messages. The individual occasionally initiates the use of compensatory strategies when encountering difficulty. |
| **Level 6:** The individual is able to understand communication in most activities, but some limitations in comprehension are still apparent in vocational, avocational, and social activities. The individual rarely requires minimal cuing to understand complex sentences. The individual usually uses compensatory strategies when encountering difficulty. |
| **Level 7:** The individual's ability to independently participate in vocational, avocational, and social activities is not limited by spoken language comprehension. When difficulty with comprehension occurs, the individual consistently uses a compensatory strategy. |

## Building the Functional Communication Measures

To develop the FCMs, the first step was for the committee of member volunteers and N-CEP staff to identify the disorders most frequently treated by ASHA member clinicians. Upon identifying those disorders, the committee queried clinicians in informal discussions as to the characteristics of the most and least severe clients they encounter with those disorders, and identify the pertinent aspects of functional communication that change and in what order. This first step was deliberately targeted to generalist clinicians rather than specialists or researchers, as the intent was to develop measures that could be understood and used by generalists. The committee took this feedback and developed the first drafts of the seven-point scales. These drafts were then sent for review to generalist clinicians, as well as to specialists and researchers, to comment on the construct, or face, validity of the draft measures. Reviewers were asked to comment on whether the appropriate dimensions of functional communication (in the context of that particular disorder) were included and whether the progression through the levels in that order made sense from a clinical perspective. When possible, clinicians were encouraged to score a sample of their patients on the measures to see what, if any, difficulties arose. The committee utilized this feedback to make changes to the measures. There were typically several iterations of review, revision, more review, and so on, for each FCM.

Once face validity was established through the multiple iterations of review and deliberation by experts, the committee developed a series of patient scenarios and solicited more from volunteers. These scenarios were utilized to test the inter-rater reliability of the measures. The scenarios were sent to groups of clinicians to score, and the reported scores were analyzed to assess reliability. The committee established a threshold of 80% inter-rater reliability for scoring each of the seven levels of each FCM before an FCM was considered to have acceptable inter-rater reliability. Revisions were made to each of the FCMs based on the reported scores. In some cases, revisions were made to the patient scenarios instead of or in addition to revisions of the FCMs themselves if it was determined that a scenario contained missing of contradictory information or if the scenario was found to be unrealistic. Again several iterations of scoring, revision, and more scoring were necessary to develop the FCMs to the point where each level of each FCM yielded acceptable reliability. An early version of the problem-solving FCM was among those initially developed, but its inability to demonstrate sufficient reliability led to its being dropped from the initial group of FCMs, and only resurrected and further refined years later. Face validity and inter-rater reliability were the necessary criteria for the committee and ASHA as a whole to release the first FCMs. After three years of data collection, additional analyses of convergent and discriminate validity were further undertaken to ensure the validity of the measures.

With the initial set of 11 FCMs having demonstrated good face validity and inter-rater reliability, data collection instruments were developed to capture FCM scores and data elements that were thought likely to have an impact on outcomes. These instruments, and the databases that eventually were created to house the data, were known under the umbrella term of the National Outcomes Measurement System for Speech-Language Pathology (NOMS). This was again done through an iterative process of querying members, drafting instruments, sending them out for review, and using the review feedback to revise the instruments. There is inevitably a tension between the abundance of questions on which researchers, including those on the ASHA staff, would like to have data, and the importance of developing data collection instruments that keep to a minimum the reporting burden placed on busy clinicians, particularly in a voluntary system such as NOMS. An important aspect of the review of and feedback on the instruments, then, was the amount of time involved in completing them. What emerged in 1997 has changed only slightly from what is in use today, with the notable exception of the transformation of NOMS data collection from a paper-form–based system to one that is entirely Web-based.

### Functional Communication Measures Endorsed by the Centers for Medicare and Medicaid Services as Quality Measures

In recent years, the eight FCMs most frequently used with stroke patients (i.e., spoken language production, spoken language comprehension, motor speech, swallowing, reading, writing, attention, and memory) have been endorsed by the National Quality Forum (NQF), which is the preferred preliminary step to obtaining endorsement by CMS for measures to be included in the Medicare Physician Quality Reporting System (PQRS) (see Chapter 4 by Romanow and Brown for an overview of NQF and PQRS, and additional discussion in Chapter 8 by Rao and Chapter 10 by Swigert). In 2007, CMS established the PQRS program to incentivize providers to report quality measures for Medicare-covered services provided to Medicare beneficiaries. In 2012–2014, incentive payments of 2% of allowable charges are currently given as bonuses to eligible providers who report on at least three relevant measures for at least 80% of the applicable Part B beneficiaries to whom they provide services. Penalties, as opposed to bonuses, are currently imposed on eligible providers that do not satisfactorily report on quality measures. Currently, these eight FCMs are the only speech-language pathology measures included in the Medicare PQRS, and ASHA's FCMs are among the very first outcomes measures from any field to be adopted into systems that historically focused solely on process measures as quality indicators. *Outcome* measures focus on functional gains, whereas *process* measures are typically checklists of procedures to be performed, such as assessment, treatment, and referral procedures (see Chapters 8 and 11 for additional elaboration of the National Quality Measures). ASHA also is an approved PQRS registry for reporting these eight FCMs. In addition, these eight and all other FCMs have been included in the Agency for Healthcare Research and Quality's National Quality Measures Clearinghouse.

### Data Collection

At the conclusion of the first SLP treatment session, ostensibly after the treatment goals for a given patient have been identified, the SLP submits an admission form. The purpose of the admission form is to describe the patient. Basic demographic (age, race, sex) and diagnostic (International Classification of Diseases [ICD]-9 codes and SLP diagnoses) information is reported, and the clinician scores the patient on whichever of the FCMs relate to that patient's treatment plan. The latter provides a baseline of the patient's functional communication status. Clinicians new to NOMS take on average 3 to 4 minutes for the completion of an admission form for a single patient. Clinicians who have participated in NOMS for 6 months or more on average require only 2 to 3 minutes.

At the conclusion of the final speech-language pathology treatment session for the patient during that episode of treatment, the clinician submits a discharge form. The purpose of the discharge form is to describe the services provided to that patient. The discharge form includes the amount of treatment, the frequency and intensity of sessions, the service delivery model, the primary payment source, and in patients treated for more than one speech-language pathology disorder, the relative amount of treatment time devoted to each. It also captures whether treatment goals were met, whether additional speech-language pathology services are recommended, and the patient's destination (e.g., inpatient rehabilitation, skilled nursing, home) upon discharge from this episode of care. Finally, the clinician must score the patient on those FCMs that were originally scored on the admission form for which the patient has been treated. It is important to note that, with the Web-based reporting format, clinicians do not have access to their original scores (unless they have written them down outside of the system) and thus are ostensibly blinded to their original scores. The extent to which a patient made or failed to make progress in terms of FCM levels is the primary outcome measure utilized in NOMS.

Participation in NOMS is voluntary. It is limited to ASHA members, and there are no costs to participants beyond their membership dues. To participate, all ASHA-certified SLPs in a facility must participate, and all must pass what is known as a *User Test*. The user test contains 20 patient scenarios similar to those used in the development of the FCMs. Prospective participants (upon completion of an online training module) score those scenarios with what they feel to be the appropriate FCM level for that patient. Their scores are compared with the "correct" answers as determined by the scores submitted in the development of these scenarios to ensure inter-rater reliability. Clinicians must have a score of at least 85% (17 of 20) to pass the User Test before they are allowed to participate in NOMS.

Participating facilities and programs have access to a Web site that allows them to download a standard report of their data and national benchmark data for comparison. In addition, the site contains a tool that enables them to undertake customized analyses of any aspect of their data. At the facility level, the data are used most frequently for quality improvement and for patient education. One inpatient rehabilitation facility in Texas, for example, found that their patients seemed to make considerably less progress on the memory FCM than did comparable patients in comparable settings nationwide. A further review of their data showed that they were providing far less treatment to their memory-disorder patients than were comparable facilities. They developed a "care pathway" for patients with memory disorders, which involved increasing the amount of memory-specific treatment they provided. Within a year, their patients were demonstrating progress similar to that found nationwide.

## Data Analysis

At the national level, the data are used to detect trends in service delivery and patient characteristics, to develop hypotheses related to treatment outcomes and their determinants for use in other research endeavors, and to inform ASHA's position on policy and reimbursement issues. One of the key questions is, What are the factors that predict how much treatment is needed for a patient? Episodes of treatment reported to NOMS, illustrated in **Fig. 5.1**, ranged from less than 1 hour to over 2000 hours of SLP treatment, with a mean of 8.8 hours (standard deviation = 16.1).

Given this enormous range, regression analysis can be used to identify those variables captured by NOMS that can help to explain why the hours of service received by some patients are at the low end of the range, and why others receive much more treatment. Regression analyses show that over 60%

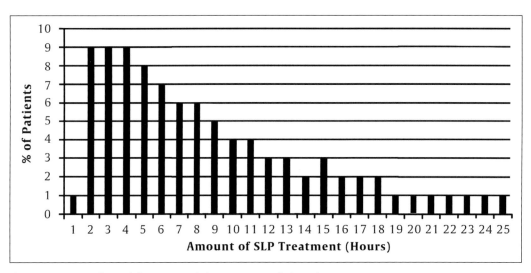

**Fig. 5.1**    Amount of speech-language pathology treatment (in hours).

of the variability in the amount of treatment can be explained by four factors: medical diagnosis, speech-language pathology diagnosis, severity, and complexity (**Fig. 5.2**).

*Medical Diagnosis*

As **Fig. 5.2** demonstrates, medical diagnosis explains 3% of the variability in the number of hours of treatment. Patients with a head injury or stroke tend to receive the most hours of treatment; those with respiratory diseases the least.

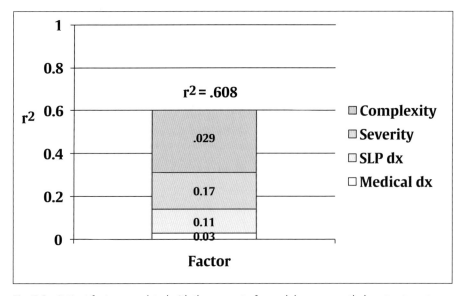

**Fig. 5.2**    Patient factors correlated with the amount of speech-language pathology treatment.

## Speech-Language Pathology Diagnosis

Accounting for 11% of the variability, the speech-language pathology diagnosis explains more of the variability in the number of hours of treatment than does medical diagnosis. Patients with apraxia or aphasia receive the most treatment; patients with fluency, voice, and swallowing the least.

### Severity

Patient severity explains 17% of the variability. Patients' FCM levels at the beginning of the episode serve as the proxy for severity. Level 1 represents the lowest level of functional communication up to a high of level 6 (a patient at an FCM level 7 at the beginning of the episode would not require treatment). In analyzing severity, two characteristics of the FCMs should be kept in mind. One, the FCMs are ordinal, rather than interval, scale measures. That is, level 6 is higher than level 5, but one cannot assume that the magnitude of the difference between levels 5 and 6 is similar to the difference between, for example, levels 5 and 4. Two, although all of the FCMs were constructed in a similar vein, enough differences persist across FCMs such that a level 5 on one FCM cannot be equated with a level 5 on another. Despite these caveats, the data on severity do illustrate some patterns of influence upon the amount of treatment that is provided.

As can be seen in **Fig. 5.3**, patients scored at a level 1 (i.e., the most severe), receive the most treatment. Patients at levels 2 through 5 receive amounts of treatment fairly similar to each other but less than level 1. Patients at level 6 receive more treatment that those at levels 2 through 5, albeit still not as much as level 1. This suggests that perhaps it is more difficult to move from a level 6 to a level 7 (full functionality) than in one-level increments of progress lower in the scale.

### Patient Complexity

The greatest single contributor to the amount of treatment provided is *patient complexity*. Just as a motor vehicle accident victim who sustains a fractured ankle is a less "complex" patient than another passenger who sustained a fractured ankle and a fractured femur, so too are some speech-

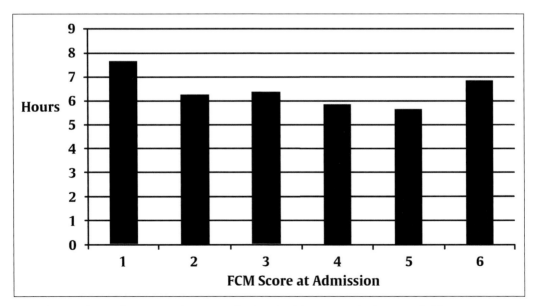

**Fig. 5.3** Mean hours of motor speech treatment by Functional Communication Measures (FCM) score at admission.

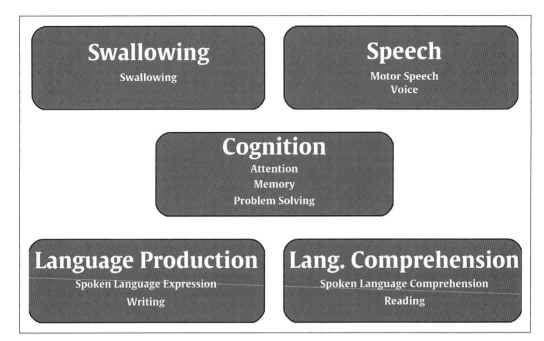

**Fig. 5.4** Domains of speech-language pathology disorders.

language pathology patients more complex than others. Patient complexity, as used in the context of NOMS, is informed by the designation of different domains of communication/swallowing disorders, illustrated in **Fig. 5.4**.

Each domain is defined by the set of FCMs for which speech-language pathology treatment is thought to have a synergistic effect and is likely to be subserved by interrelated systems (e.g., cortical or subcortical regions, biomechanically interrelated structures). For example, for some patients, treatment of a motor speech disorder might be expected to have some impact on a voice disorder, but would not be expected to improve their memory. Therefore, the addition of a treatment goal related to voice for these patients might not necessitate as much additional treatment as would be the case were they not already being treated for motor speech. Conversely, adding a voice-related treatment goal (or one involving attention, or reading, or spoken language) to a patient who until that point was being treated only for dysphagia would likely require a larger amount of voice treatment than if some other treatment in the speech domain was already ongoing. Returning to the car crash analogy, a patient with a fractured right ankle and a fractured right femur is likely to be less complex in terms of rehabilitation needs, and the amount of treatment required, than if the right ankle fracture were accompanied by a fracture of the femur in the other leg. The treatment of the fracture in one leg not only would be unlikely to help the recovery in the other leg, but may actually hinder progress.

Complexity, then, involves the number of FCMs scored as well as the number of domains involved. This way of grouping the FCMs has proved useful in analyzing the data and accounting for the variance regarding the number of hours of treatment. For example, data confirm that treatment of memory and language comprehension requires more hours than treatment of memory and attention, which in turn requires more hours than treatment of memory alone. Thus, when several different domains are involved, the number of hours of treatment is likely to be more than when a comparable number of FCMs are being treated within a single domain. Not surprisingly, the highest amounts of treatment are found among patients with complexity scores of 1 or above in multiple domains. A complexity score for each patient can be derived by enumerating the number of FCMs being treated in each of the domains for that patient.

# ◆ Potential for Building a Payment Mechanism

All of the patient episodes reported to NOMS can be categorized according to the four factors described above (i.e., medical diagnosis, speech-language pathology diagnosis, severity, and complexity), and the data can be analyzed to identify expected amounts of treatment with even more precision than shown in **Fig. 5.2**. As a result of such an analysis, it is possible that, at the conclusion of the first speech-language pathology treatment session, patients could be matched with the appropriate profile, and an expected amount of treatment could be identified. These patient groupings, or profiles, could then be used as the basis upon which to predict the amount of treatment that will be needed. Using the NOMS data in this manner could support the development of a data-based payment system for speech-language pathology that uses case-mix adjusted data (i.e., information about the patient's diagnoses, impairments, the severity of those impairments, and other demographic information) to estimate the resources (e.g., hours of treatment) needed for a given episode of care.

A variety of policy alternatives can be supported with this approach. There are at least three major considerations that need to be resolved to develop a payment model based on this approach. The first decision concerns how one operationally defines a "successful" episode of care. The data used in **Fig. 5.3**, for example, were based on those patients who progressed by at least one FCM level. If patients were scored on more than one FCM, then they were included only if they progressed by at least one FCM on each of the FCMs on which they were scored. This is only one of a myriad of alternatives that could be used in operationalizing the definition of a successful episode of care. Policy makers could choose, for example, to define success as progress on at least one FCM even if multiple FCMs were involved. Or, they could choose to define it more stringently, with multiple levels of FCM progress required for "success." A successful episode of care could be defined as patients reaching a certain FCM level, such as a level 6 or 7, without regard to where they started (though this alternative is clearly unrealistic). Success might even be defined without specifically referring to FCM progress. It could be defined as meeting treatment goals as reported by the clinician, or perhaps moving from one level of care to a less restrictive level upon discharge (e.g., from a skilled nursing facility to home health).

Once the definition of a successful episode of care has been established, the data can be analyzed to identify the target amount of speech-language pathology treatment associated with those episodes for each of the patient profiles. Homing in on this target amount, though, is again open to a variety of alternatives. Specifically, the second consideration that would need to be resolved to develop a payment system using such a data-based approach is to establish the target as the amount of treatment at which some percentage of the patients in that profile have a successful episode (e.g., the 80th, 90th, 100th percentile). Clearly, the 100th percentile would yield an unreasonably large amount of treatment dictated by the most treatment ever received by a patient with that profile. Basing a reimbursement target on that most extreme case would be hugely inefficient and unrealistic. On the other hand, setting the target at the 50th percentile might be too low. The 50th percentile would mean that half of the patients who had a successful episode of care had that amount of treatment or less, but the other half of successful episodes involved more treatment. To limit reimbursement based on the 50th percentile would likely preclude half of the patients from achieving success. A more reasonable approach might be to set the target somewhere closer to 80 to 90%. This would identify the level at which most patients would have a successful episode, but there would likely be a small number of outliers, or exceptions, who would need more treatment.

The issue of exceptions leads to the third major consideration for policy makers, and that is what happens with patients who need more than the targeted amount of treatment associated with their profile. One alternative might be to treat the targeted amount of treatment as a "hard cap" (i.e., a fixed financial limitation or capitation of payment), above which reimbursement would not be provided. A second alternative might be to treat the target as a "soft cap." Providers who perceive a need to exceed the target would be reimbursed for the additional treatment only upon successful completion of an exceptions process. This soft cap approach has been utilized in Medicare Part B reimbursement since 2000. Notably, the target amount of treatment could be used not as a cap but rather as an audit flag. Under such an approach, payers who identified providers with a pattern of exceeding the target levels of treatment might choose to undertake an audit of that provider to ensure that the amount of treatment being provided is clinically appropriate.

An important advantage of NOMS, then, is that it is not tied to a specific policy or reimbursement approach, but can be used to provide supporting data for a variety of approaches. Should future payment systems be designed to set reimbursement rates based on episodes of care, rather than the currently prevalent fee-for-service model, information about a patient's health condition and other important case-mix data will undoubtedly play a more prominent role in determining payment. Currently, the Medicare Part B therapy cap does not distinguish among the different health conditions of patients or their rehabilitation needs (and even worse, combines speech-language pathology and physical therapy services under a single cap). Thus, the current payment model used by CMS, and other payers, limits the annual amount of therapy services patients can receive regardless of their condition or need. This approach has likely had a disproportionate impact on vulnerable populations (Olshin, Ciolek, & Hwang, 2002) and on those who need more extensive therapy services. As NOMS captures information regarding medical and speech-language pathology diagnoses, severity, complexity, and demographic data, NOMS is well positioned to provide supporting case-mix data that could be used to develop an episodic payment scheme that sets reimbursement rates based on patient factors (as opposed to arbitrary reimbursement limits based on rehabilitation discipline). Additionally, NOMS is well suited to support the development of a payment system consistent with the tenets of value-based purchasing (described below and referenced in other chapters) as the value of the services provided can be estimated in terms of patient outcomes. These are the data elements that are likely to be central to the development of future payment systems modeled on the value-based purchasing framework.

## ◆ Value-Based Purchasing

As Romanow and Brown explained in Chapter 4, value-based purchasing is a payment model that uses case-mix adjusted data and the quality and cost of services to predict resource utilization, and, ultimately, to determine reimbursement rates. In other words, value-based purchasing is a payment system model that allocates resources based on value, measured by outcomes, as opposed to volume (e.g., the number of sessions, tests, procedures), and incentivizes or penalizes to ensure quality services, improvement, and accountability. Under the value-based purchasing framework, rehabilitation providers and facilities would be reimbursed for managing patients to achieve specified functional improvements rather than simply for providing some number of treatment sessions.

The use of outcomes measures and other quality indicators to document initial function and progress is integral to value-based purchasing, but certainly not unique to that model. The notion that reimbursement should be tied to functional improvements that are objectively measured has been stipulated by CMS for many years even though it is not incorporated into the fee-for-service payment model that CMS currently uses. Although there is an explicit expectation that functional improvement will be objectively documented, payment is not tied to functional outcomes. For example, the CMS's Medicare Benefit Policy Manual states, "Therapy services must be provided with the expectation . . . that the condition of the patient will improve materially in a reasonable and generally predictable period of time. Improvement is evidenced by objective successive measurements" (CMS, n.d., p. 59). So certainly the focus on outcomes is not new, but in the value-based purchasing context it is likely to assume heightened significance as new payment systems are developed that no longer operate within a volume-based, fee-for-service framework. In the future, payments are more likely to be based on the effectiveness of the services in helping patients achieve functional gains and to improve their participation in life roles.

Value-based purchasing is appealing, if not intuitive, from a patient's perspective. Undoubtedly, consumers of health care would view the value-based purchasing proposition of receiving quality services that enable predetermined goals to be realized in a predictable time frame as a very positive result. It is hypothesized that, across most health conditions, there are two themes that likely underlie many of the questions posed by patients undergoing rehabilitation and their families: What improvements can be expected due to your services? And how long will it take? Depending on the patient's health care plan and health condition, a third common question is likely to be: How much will it cost? Of course, these are also the same questions and data points that policy makers, payers, health care economists, health service researchers, and other stakeholders need to develop new payment systems that simultaneously promote quality while containing costs—two aims that are not typically considered symbiotic. The critical importance of a large-scale data repository that can be used to model outcomes and cost, as well as test and ultimately predict which approach is most likely to work best with which patients, has been recognized for many years (e.g., Warren, 1998). However, thus far, no single instrument captures all of these critical data elements (i.e., outcomes, treatment type and dosage, case-mix data and cost) in one data set at a national level. Additionally, further research is needed to determine which types of measures provide the best estimates of value and quality.

# ♦ Patient-Reported Outcomes

How patients experience the quality of the care provided to them is another important quality indicator. Patient-reported outcome measures (PROMs), or patient-reported outcomes (PROs), provide a means of measuring the way patients experience their health, their disability, and the effects that treatment and lifestyle adjustments have on their quality of life (http://phi.uhce.ox.ac.uk/home.php). PROMs have high ecological validity, and arguably provide data from the perspective of "what matters most" to the consumers (see Chapter 2). PROMs, such as the World Health Organization Quality of Life Assessment instrument (WHOQOL), are commonly used to assess quality of life (WHOQOL Group, 1994), health-related quality of life, such as the SF-36 (Ware, Gandek, & IQOLA Project Group, 1994), and satisfaction with life, such as the Quality of Life Index (Ferrans & Powers, 1992). They have also been used to measure patients' perceptions of their participation restrictions, such as the Participation Objective-Participation Subjective Scale (POPS) (Brown et al, 2004) and the ASHA-Quality of Communication Life Scale (ASHA-QCL) (Paul et al, 2004). Typically, proxy and surrogate measures are used when self-report is not feasible or the reliability of self-reported measures is questionable due to such factors as language barriers, cognitive impairments, or the age of the patient (i.e., very young children). For some individuals with communication disorders, such as aphasia and traumatic brain injury, the reliability of self-reported measures may be a concern. As it is generally more desirable to collect data from the patient directly, tools such as the ASHA-QCL have been developed to minimize the language demands of the reporting tool for individuals with communication disorders. The ASHA-QCL uses visual analog scales, instead of linguistically encoded response formats, wherein patients draw a line across a vertical scale to indicate how positive or negative they feel about an item. The ASHA-QCL includes 18 items designed to address three domains: socialization/activities, confidence/self-concept, and roles and responsibilities. Although only 36% of the patients who participated in the validation protocols required no clinician assistance, the instrument has been validated for use as a PROM with adults with aphasia, cognitive-communication disorders secondary to traumatic brain injury or right-hemisphere stroke, and dysarthria.

Outcomes can be measured using a variety of methodologies including practitioner ratings of specific or global behaviors, standardized tests and instrumental assessments, and, as just described, PROMs. Each of these three approaches (i.e., instrumental and standardized tests, practitioner-reported outcomes, and PROMs) must be examined in terms of how sensitive a particular measure is to change, as that is of central importance when selecting or developing an outcome measure. Instrumental assessments are considered highly objective, though typically the data obtained still require interpretation by a professional. Instrumental assessments are not always feasible or appropriate, especially to measure cognitive functions such as language, executive functions, and memory. Standardized tests can be useful to obtain fairly objective, surrogate measures of cognition, though they often require much time to administer and may present too much of a response burden in clinical settings where only 10 to 15% of time is allocated to documentation, reports, and other professional communications. Reducing the response burden of persons documenting outcomes is an important concern for those developing outcome measurement tools because increased burden decreases the likelihood that the tool will be used. An important concern regarding the use of standardized tests as an outcome measure concerns the sensitivity to change that can be afforded by global measures that typically sample across several performance domains. Alternatively, using practitioner-reported outcome measures is highly practical because these types of measures are typically quick to score, can be incorporated easily into the documentation that is done routinely, and may be more sensitive to change than standardized tests. However, one perceived drawback of using practitioner-reported measures of patient outcomes is the concern that these measures may be subject to bias or, worse yet, falsification.

Within a value-based purchasing framework, as opposed to a fee-for-service model, the potential for conflict of interest with respect to practitioner-reported outcome measures is heightened because payment would no longer be based straightforwardly on volume (e.g., the number of sessions or procedures) but rather on the perceived value or effectiveness of the services, which is a far more subjective and multifaceted measurement construct than units of time. Although concerns about bias and fraud are not endemic to practitioner-reported measures, and although there is likely to be a way to "scam the system" regardless of the type of measure used, nonetheless this concern is one factor accounting for the importance now being placed on PROs. The importance being placed by policy makers, payers, researchers, and other stakeholder groups on PROs is exemplified by the data collection project sponsored by CMS—Developing Outpatient Therapy Payment Alternatives. In each of the four data collection instruments that were developed for this project by the CMS subcontractor, Research Triangle Institute (RTI), approximately a third of the measures are dedicated to items requiring *patient*, or when necessary, *proxy* report.

## ◆ Developing Outpatient Therapy Payment Alternatives

In Section 545 of the Benefits Improvement and Protection Act (BIPA) of 2000 (Public Law 106-554), Congress required the Secretary of Health and Human Services to report on the development of standardized assessment instruments for outpatient rehabilitation therapy. As part of the response to this requirement, CMS envisioned a new method of paying for outpatient therapy based on classifying beneficiary needs as well as the effectiveness of services; however, CMS could not implement this type of payment system because the data collected by CMS from providers (i.e., the claims data) do not include critical data elements such as health and functional status pre- and post-outpatient therapy services. In 2007, CMS established a research project titled *Developing Outpatient Therapy Payment Alternatives* (DOTPA) to identify, collect, and analyze therapy-related information tied to beneficiary need and the effectiveness of outpatient therapy services. This effort was undertaken to develop a new payment system that would provide an alternative to the financial cap, and exceptions process, on outpatient therapy services. The 5-year contract was awarded to RTI in January 2008.

The DOTPA project was designed, in part, to address information gaps in the claims data, including case-mix factors such as the etiology of the patient's health condition, impairment severity, extent of activity limitations, and extant comorbidities. These are important case-mix data for classifying beneficiary needs and evaluating outcomes such as the number and types of comorbidities, which has been shown to affect patients' functional status and course of rehabilitation (Groll, To, Bombardier, & Wright, 2005). Notably, there is no information in the claims data concerning the severity of the patient's condition(s) or functional status at admission and discharge; and therefore, currently no means of measuring outcomes or the effectiveness of therapy services. The DOTPA project was designed to provide data elements that would allow for case-mix adjusted analyses of patient outcomes across both impairment and activity domains so that resource utilization could be considered relative to the value of the services provided (i.e., to support cost-benefit analyses).

Research Triangle Institute, which developed the *Continuity Assessment Record and Evaluation* (CARE) tool currently in use (discussed in Chapters 2, 7, and 8), developed four new data collection instruments, all with similar items, that were designed to be used in the diverse settings in which outpatient rehabilitation therapy services are provided: hospital-based outpatient facilities, long term care (LTC), skilled nursing facilities (SNFs), comprehensive outpatient rehabilitation facilities (CORFs), outpatient rehabilitation facilities (ORFs), and private practice. The CARE-C was designed for use in community-based settings and the CARE-F for day rehabilitation programs and SNFs. Each tool has a version for use at admission and another for use at discharge so that outcomes can be assessed pre- and post-rehabilitation. In order for beneficiary needs and outcomes to be compared across settings and disciplines (i.e., physical therapy, occupational therapy, and speech-language pathology), one requirement in developing these instruments was that the data had to be collected using similar items across settings and disciplines. This requirement included the use of a common rating scale, a requirement that, unfortunately, precluded the use of NOMS. Accordingly, ASHA staff and ASHA members worked with the RTI team to develop items that sampled aspects of communication, swallowing, and cognitive function. The four DOTPA instruments can be viewed in their entirety on the RTI homepage under the Assessment Tool tab (http://optherapy.rti.org). Communication, cognition, and swallowing impairments and function are assessed in several sections by the clinician, but in addition there are sections that contain patient-reported items. Two examples of practitioner-rated items designed to assess the severity of the patient's communication impairment are shown in **Table 5.2**. In a section labeled "Life Skills" shown in **Table 5.3**, patient-reported items are employed to measure the patient's perspective of his or her activity limitations. In addition, there is also a section shown in **Table 5.4** designed to measure the patient's perspective of his or her participation restrictions.

As previously mentioned, one of the charges to RTI was to develop instruments that would be used by all three rehabilitation disciplines (i.e., physical therapy, occupational therapy, and speech-language pathology). To be able to equate severity of impairments and activity limitations across each of these rehabilitation disciplines, it was deemed important to use comparable scales where possible. A four-point equal interval scale (**Table 5.2**) was chosen that divided the severity range, based on an assumption of a normal distribution, into the following categories: (1) *never or rarely* (less than 20% of the time); (2) *sometimes* (20 to 49% of the time); (3) *usually* (50 to 79% of the time); and (4) *always* (at least 80% of the time). Whether the distribution of severity across the many health conditions for which these instruments will be used is in fact normally distributed cannot be determined yet. However, in all likelihood, the distribution of severity scores will not prove to be normally distributed for most disordered populations, but until the shape of these distributions is known it is most logical to divide the range into roughly even quartiles as opposed to arbitrarily carving up the range in some other manner.

The SLPs and researchers who provided input to the item and scale development suggested that the sensitivity of the scale to severity and change might be improved if two additional factors were incorporated. The first factor is a division based on how demanding or complex the activity is, and so, for example, a division of basic versus complex information is made for the cognitive construct of attention; for intelligibility, a division of short versus long utterances is employed; and for assessing voice, a division of low vocal demand versus high vocal demand situations is used. It was reasoned that a scale that included consideration of the level of task demand or complexity would likely be more sensitive to change and to severity, especially for high-functioning individuals. The second factor that was incorporated into the scale was a division regarding how well an individual functions with and without assistance. Functioning with assistance includes performing the activity with cuing, assistive devices, or other compensatory or augmentative communication strategies. Thus, as can be seen in **Table 5.2**, there are two sections for every item wherein the clinician can indicate how well the patient does without assistance versus with assistance. Incorporating information about the effects of assistance is in keeping with the ICF qualifiers for activity limitations as both performance

**Table 5.2**   Impairment Measures: Sample Items from the Developing Outpatient Therapy Payment Alternatives (DOPTA) Instrument

| III. Provider Information | | | | |
|---|---|---|---|---|
| **H.11a Spoken Language Expression**<br>Answer only if you answered "Yes" to H.9–13, "Does the patient have any signs or symptoms of a possible communication problem?" and if you have the skills, knowledge, or training to provide a response; otherwise, leave this section blank. | | | | |
| **The Patient Conveys:** | Always<br>At least 80%<br>of the time | Usually<br>50–79%<br>of the time | Sometimes<br>20–49%<br>of the time | Never/Rarely<br>Less than 20%<br>of the time |
| **Without Assistance** | Patient performance **without** cuing, assistive device, or other compensatory augmentative intervention. | | | |
| **H.11b Basic Information:** Basic information regarding wants/needs or daily routines; using 1 or 2 words or short phrases without assistance. | | | | |
| **H.11c Complex Information:** Thoughts/ideas using sentences; in conversations about routine daily activities or a variety of topics. | | | | |
| **With Assistance** | Patient performance **with** cuing, assistive device, or other compensatory augmentative intervention. | | | |
| **H.11d Basic Information:** Basic information regarding wants/needs or daily routines; using 1–2 words or short phrases without assistance. | | | | |
| **H.11e Complex Information:** Thoughts/ideas using sentences; in conversations about routine daily activities or a variety of topics. | | | | |
| **H.12a Motor Speech Production**<br>Answer only if you answered "Yes" to H.9–13, "Does the patient have any signs or symptoms of a possible communication problem?" and if you have the skills, knowledge, or training to provide a response; otherwise, leave this section blank. | | | | |
| **The Patient's Speech Is:** | Always<br>At least 80%<br>of the time | Usually<br>50–79%<br>of the time | Sometimes<br>20–49%<br>of the time | Never/Rarely<br>Less than 20%<br>of the time |
| **Without Assistance** | Patient performance **without** cuing, assistive device, or other compensatory augmentative intervention. | | | |
| **H.12b Intelligible in Short Utterances:** Spontaneous production of automatic words, predictable single words, or short phrases. | | | | |
| **H.12c Intelligible in Longer Utterances:** Spontaneous production of multisyllabic words in sentences. | | | | |
| **With Assistance** | Patient performance **with** cuing, assistive device, or other compensatory augmentative intervention. | | | |
| **H.12d Intelligible in Short Utterances:** Spontaneous production of automatic words, predictable single words, or short phrases. | | | | |
| **H.12e Intelligible in Longer Utterances:** Spontaneous production of multisyllabic words in sentences. | | | | |

*Note:* This instrument was developed by Research Triangle Institute and this section was designed to assess impairment severity of spoken language expression and motor speech production. These items are designed to be rated by the clinician before therapy and again at discharge.

**Table 5.3** Activity Limitation Measures: Patient-Reported Items from the Developing Outpatient Therapy Payment Alternatives (DOPTA)

| II. Patient Information | | | | | |
|---|---|---|---|---|---|
| **E.4 Life Skills** Do you have difficulty with communicating, remembering, organizing, or planning in your daily life? | | | | | |
| Yes ☐ | If "yes," please answer the rest of this section. | | | | |
| No ☐ | If "no," please skip to section F, Participation. | | | | |
| **How much DIFFICULTY do you currently have...** (If you have not done an activity recently, how much difficulty do you think you would have if you tried?) | Unable | A Lot of Difficulty | A Little Difficulty | No Difficulty | I Don't Know/ Unknown |
| a. Understanding instructions involving several steps (e.g., how to prepare a meal or following directions)? | | | | | |
| b. Following/understanding a 10- to 15-minute speech of presentation (e.g., lesson at a place of worship, guest lecture)? | | | | | |
| c. Answering yes/no questions about basic needs (e.g., "Do you need to use the restroom?" "Are you in pain?")? | | | | | |
| d. Making yourself understood to other people during an ordinary conversations? | | | | | |
| e. Telling someone important information about yourself in case of an emergency? | | | | | |
| f. Explaining how to do something involving several steps to another person? | | | | | |
| g. Reading and following complex instructions (e.g., directions to operate a new appliance or for a new medication)? | | | | | |
| h. Telling others your basic needs (e.g., need to use the restroom, have a drink of water or request help)? | | | | | |
| i. Planning for or keeping appointments that are not part of your weekly routine (e.g., a therapy or doctor appointment, or a social gathering with friends)? | | | | | |
| j. Reading simple material (e.g., a menu or the TV or radio guide)? | | | | | |
| k. Filling out a long form (e.g., insurance form or an application for services)? | | | | | |
| l. Writing a short message or note? | | | | | |
| m. Remembering where things were placed or put away (e.g., keys)? | | | | | |
| n. Keeping track of time (e.g., using a clock)? | | | | | |
| o. Putting together a shopping list of 10 to 15 items? | | | | | |
| p. Remembering a list of four or five errands without writing them down? | | | | | |
| q. Taking care of complicated tasks like managing a checking account or getting appliances fixed? | | | | | |

*Note:* This instrument was developed by Research Triangle Institute and this section was designed to assess the patient's perspective regarding how well he or she is able to perform common life skills associated with cognitive and communication functioning.

**Table 5.4** Participation Restriction Measures: Patient-Reported Items from the Developing Outpatient Therapy Payment Alternatives (DOPTA)

| II. Patient Information | | | | | | |
|---|---|---|---|---|---|---|
| **F. Participation** | | | | | | |
| **F1. Even with help or services, tell us how much you are limited in...** | Extremely Limited | Very Much Limited | Somewhat Limited | A Little Limited | Not At All Limited | I Don't Do This/I Don't Know |
| a. Keeping your home clean and fixed up? | | | | | | |
| b. Providing personal care to yourself? | | | | | | |
| c. Getting groceries or other things for your home? | | | | | | |
| **F2. How much are you currently limited in...** | Extremely Limited | Very Much Limited | Somewhat Limited | A Little Limited | Not At All Limited | I Don't Do This/I Don't Know |
| a. Going to movies, plays, concerts, sporting events, museums, or similar activities? | | | | | | |
| **F3. Think about how you currently get together or do things with others, like going out or visiting with family and friends. Which of the following best describes you? (Check one box.)** | | | | | | |
| ☐ I do not have difficulty doing things with other socially. | | | | | | |
| ☐ Even though it's hard, I keep doing things with people as usual. | | | | | | |
| ☐ I no longer can do as much or the same kind of things with others. | | | | | | |
| ☐ I hardly ever do the types of things I used to do, or I hardly ever get together with others. | | | | | | |
| ☐ I do not see family or friends, and I only see those who take care of me. | | | | | | |
| ☐ I don't know/unknown. | | | | | | |

*Note:* This instrument was developed by Research Triangle Institute and this section was designed to assess the patient's perspective regarding how well he or she is able to participate in life situations, roles, and social relationships.

and capacity are to be considered relative to the provision of assistance in the ICF. By incorporating the task complexity dimension and the comparison of functioning with and without assistance, the four-point scale becomes a 16-point scale, which is more likely to be sensitive to change, especially changes in function due to the use of augmentative and alternative communication and the use of assistive devices to support cognitive, sensory, and motor impairments.

The patient-reported measures depicted in **Table 5.3** also use a four-point scale (i.e., unable, a lot of difficulty, a little difficulty, no difficulty). These items in the Life Skills section are only responded to if the patient answers yes to having difficulties with communicating, remembering, organizing, or planning. These items will be subjected to Item Response Theory (IRT) and Rasch analyses, mentioned in Chapter 2, after the data have been collected, to determine how well these items represent the latent traits that the item was constructed to assess (see Baylor et al, 2011 for a tutorial of IRT and Rasch modeling).

## Developing Alternative Payment Systems

Once the data using these new CARE-C and CARE-F instruments have been collected and analyzed, RTI will develop a set of alternative payment model options for CMS that could be used as the basis for developing a new payment system for outpatient therapy services. There are four elements that are likely to be incorporated into an alternative payment model as they served to motivate item development. These elements include case-mix classification, bundling, patient-level payment limits, and pay-for-performance.

Case-mix classification will likely determine patient-level payment limits such that payment limits will be assigned based on case-mix classification. Bundling or bundled payments is an approach to paying for care where providers collaborate to manage multiple procedures and services as part of a single episode with a single payment (http://innovations.cms.gov/areas-of-focus/patient-care-models/). There are four models for bundling payments being considered by the Center for Medicare and Medicaid Innovation (CMMI). In the first model, an episode of care is defined as the acute hospital stay only. The second model includes not only the acute care hospital stay but also the postacute care. The third model includes only the postacute care. The fourth model includes all services. Under the latter model, CMS would make a single prospective, bundled payment, based on patient-level payment limits as determined by case-mix classification and historical data, to cover all services provided during the episode of care.

Practitioners would be paid for their services using a fee-for-service system (just like the current reimbursement system). At the conclusion of the episode, there could be a positive or negative balance, and if expenditures were less than the bundled payment, providers could share in those savings. One way to interpret these models is explained on the CMS Web site as follows, "Through the Bundled Payments initiative, providers have great flexibility in selecting conditions to bundle, developing the health care delivery structure, and determining how payments will be allocated among participating providers" (http://innovations.cms.gov/areas-of-focus/patient-care-models/).

One likely consequence of bundling, regardless of the specific model, is that providers who increase costs without demonstrating value will be less and less likely to receive referrals (i.e., value-based purchasing). On the positive side, bundling and value-based purchasing are expected to (1) lead to "better health, better care, and lower costs through continuous improvement" (a concept that is referred to as the "three-part aim outcomes"); (2) shorten the time it takes practitioners to adopt evidence-based practices; and (3) accelerate the development of new evidence-based knowledge (http://innovations.cms.gov/documents/payment-care/BundledPaymentsnewFAQscombinedfor posting_09-20-11.pdf).

## ♦ Conclusion and Future Directions

Fourteen years ago, Frattali's (1998) discerning and prescient thoughts on quality improvement capture the essence of the challenge that still lies ahead:

> Methods to improve quality can lead directly to greater efficiency and cost reduction. And, if predictions are accurate, competition in service delivery will shift away from a pure price basis to a combination of price and quality. As a result, the issue of quality will become fundamental to the survival of any service organization, and become the basis for competition over the next decade and beyond. (p. 184)

The considerable challenge associated with developing outcome measures that are sensitive to change across the severity continuum, that can be reliably used in clinical practice, and that yield clinically meaningful indices of the quality and value of the services provided is actually only half of the battle. The other half concerns how best to amass the data needed to support quality improvement efforts at the facility level and, at the national level, to develop and maintain payment systems based on case-mix stratification (i.e., the clinical need), which can be continuously refined as more clinical data are amassed. The concept that payment and quality improvement systems could be developed and continuously updated based on data that includes case-mix information, outcomes, and resource utilization has been addressed extensively by the Institute of Medicine's Learning Health System Series (IOM, 2011). They report on existing initiatives and resources that are contributing to the digital infrastructure that will support a new learning health system:

> Health and health care are going digital. As multiple intersecting platforms evolve to form a novel operational foundation for health and health care—the nation's digital health utility—the stage is set for

fundamental and unprecedented transformation. Most changes will occur virtually out of sight, and the pace and profile of the transformation will be determined by the stewardship that fosters alignment of technology, science, and culture in support of a continuously learning health system. In the context of growing concerns about the quality and costs of care, the nation's health and economic security are interdependently linked to the success of that stewardship. Progress in computational science, information technology, and biomedical and health research methods have made it possible to foresee the emergence of a learning health system that enables seamless and efficient health delivery of best care practices and the real-time generation and application of new knowledge. Increases in the cost and complexity of care compel such a system. (p. 1)

Continued development and utilization of outcome measures and databases in speech-language pathology will be critical to meeting the many challenges posed by the changing landscape in health care. It is crucial that we remain vigilant and keep up with the growing digital infrastructure that is rapidly emerging by developing, testing, and refining outcome measures and by contributing our measures to electronic health records, personal health records, health information portals, and other health information databases. It is hoped that these current and future efforts will sustain the profession as well as accelerate the development of evidence-based knowledge, quality improvements, and enhanced patient outcomes.

# References

American Speech-Language-Hearing Association (ASHA). (2001). *Scope of practice in speech-language pathology.* http://www.asha.org/policy

American Speech-Language-Hearing Association (ASHA). (2004). *Evidence-based practice in communication disorders: An introduction* [Technical report]. http://www.asha.org/policy

Bayles, K. A., & Tomoeda, C. K. (1994). *Functional Linguistic Communication Inventory.* Austin, TX: Pro-Ed

Baylor, C., Hula, W., Donovan, N. J., Doyle, P. J., Kendall, D., & Yorkston, K. (2011, Aug). An introduction to item response theory and Rasch models for speech-language pathologists. *American Journal of Speech-Language Pathology, 20,* 243–259

Baylor, C. R., Yorkston, K. M., Eadie, T. L., Miller, R. M., & Amtmann, D. (2009, Oct). Developing the communicative participation item bank: Rasch analysis results from a spasmodic dysphonia sample. *Journal of Speech, Language, and Hearing Research: JSLHR, 52,* 1302–1320

Boyle, M., & Coelho, C. A. (1995). Application of semantic feature analysis as a treatment for aphasic dysnomia. *American Journal of Speech-Language Pathology, 4,* 94–98

Brown, M., Dijkers, M. P., Gordon, W. A., Ashman, T., Charatz, H., & Cheng, Z. (2004, Nov-Dec). Participation objective, participation subjective: a measure of participation combining outsider and insider perspectives. *The Journal of Head Trauma Rehabilitation, 19,* 459–481

Burns, M. S., Dong, K. Y., & Oehring, A. K. (1995). Family involvement in the treatment of aphasia. *Topics in Stroke Rehabilitation, 2,* 68–77

Centers for Medicare and Medicaid Services (CMS). (n.d.). *Medicare benefit policy manual.* http://www.cms.gov/manuals/Downloads/bp102c07.pdf

Code, C., & Müller, M. (1992). *The Code-Müller protocols: Assessing perception of psychosocial adjustment to aphasia and related disorders.* London, United Kingdom: Whurr

Dijkers, M. P., & Greenwald, B. (2006). Functional assessment in TBI rehabilitation. In N.D. Zasler, D. Katz, & R. Zafonte (Eds.), *Brain injury medicine* (pp. 225–245). New York: Demos Publishers

Dijkers, M. P., Whiteneck, G. G., & El-Jaroudi, R. (2000, Dec). Measures of social outcomes in disability research. *Archives of Physical Medicine and Rehabilitation, 81*(12, Suppl 2), S63–S80

Doyle, P. J., McNeil, M. R., Hula, W., & Mikolic, J. M. (2003). The Burden of Stroke Scale (BOSS): Validating patient-reported communication difficulty and associated psychological distress in stroke survivors. *Aphasiology, 17,* 291–304

Eadie, T. L. (2001). The ICIDH-2: Theoretical and clinical implications for speech-language pathology. *Journal of Speech-Language Pathology and Audiology, 25,* 181–200

Eadie, T. L., Yorkston, K. M., Klasner, E. R., Dudgeon, B. J., Deitz, J. C., Baylor, C. R., et al. (2006, Nov). Measuring communicative participation: a review of self-report instruments in speech-language pathology. *American Journal of Speech-Language Pathology, 15,* 307–320

Ferrans, C. E., & Powers, M. J. (1992, Feb). Psychometric assessment of the Quality of Life Index. *Research in Nursing & Health, 15,* 29–38

Frattali, C. M. (1998). Outcomes measurement: Definitions, dimensions and perspectives. In C. Frattali (Ed.), *Measuring outcomes in speech-language pathology* (pp. 1–27). New York: Thieme

Frattali, C. M., Thompson, C. K., Holland, A. L., Wohl, C. B., & Ferketic, M. M. (1995). *The American Speech-Language-Hearing Association Functional Assessment of Communication Skills for Adults (ASHA FACS).* Rockville, MD: American Speech-Language-Hearing Association

Garrett, K. L., & Pimentel, J. T. (2007). Measuring outcomes of group therapy. In R. Elman (Ed.), *Group treatment of neurogenic communication disorders: The expert clinician's approach* (2nd ed., pp. 25–61). San Diego, CA: Plural

Groll, D. L., To, T., Bombardier, C., & Wright, J. G. (2005, Jun). The development of a comorbidity index with physical function as the outcome. *Journal of Clinical Epidemiology, 58,* 595–602

Holland, A. L., Frattali, C. M., & Fromm, D.(1999). *Communication Activities of Daily Living (CADL-2)* (2nd ed.). Austin, TX: Pro-Ed

Institute of Medicine (IOM). (2011). *Digital Infrastructure for the Learning Health System: The Foundation for Continuous Improvement in Health and Health Care: Workshop Series Summary*. Washington, DC: The National Academies Press

Kagen, A., & Gailey, G. F. (1993). Functional is not enough: Training conversation partners for aphasic adults. In A. L. Holland & M. M. Forbes (Eds.), *Aphasia treatment: World perspectives* (pp. 199–225). San Diego, CA: Singular

Kahneman, D., Diener, E., & Schwarz, N. (Eds.). (1999). *Well-being: The foundations of hedonic psychology*. New York: Russell Sage

Life Participation Approach to Aphasia Project Group. (2001). Life participation approach to aphasia: A statement of values for the future. In R. Chapey (Ed.), *Language intervention strategies in aphasia and related neurogenic communication disorders* (pp. 235–245). Baltimore, MD: Lippincott Williams & Wilkins

Lomas, J., Pickard, L., Bester, S., Elbard, H., Finlayson, A., & Zoghaib, C. (1989, Feb). The communicative effectiveness index: development and psychometric evaluation of a functional communication measure for adult aphasia. *Journal of Speech and Hearing Disorders, 54*, 113–124

Massof, R. W. (2010). A clinically meaningful theory of outcome measures in rehabilitation medicine. *Journal of Applied Measurement, 11*, 253–270

McHorney, C. A., Bricker, D. E., Kramer, A. E., Rosenbek, J. C., Robbins, J., Chignell, K. A., et al. (2000). The SWAL-QOL Outcomes Tool for Oropharyngeal Dysphagia in Adults: I. Conceptual foundation and item development. *Dysphagia, 15*, 115–121

Nicholas, L. E., & Brookshire, R. H. (1993, Apr). A system for quantifying the informativeness and efficiency of the connected speech of adults with aphasia. *Journal of Speech and Hearing Research, 36*, 338–350

Olshin, J., Ciolek, D., & Hwang, W. (2002). *Study and report on outpatient therapy utilization: Physical therapy, occupational therapy, and speech-language pathology services billed to Medicare Part B in all settings in 1998, 1999, and 2000* [CMS Contract Number 500–99–0009 Task Order: 0002]. http://www.cms.gov/TherapyServices/SAR/

Paul, D. R., Frattali, C. M., Holland, A. L., Thompson, C. K., Caperton, C. J., & Slater, S. C. (2004). *Quality of Communication Life Scale (ASHA QCL)*. Rockville, MD: American Speech-Language-Hearing Association

Pawson, R., & Tilley, N. (2004). *Community matters*. http://www.communitymatters.com.au/RE_chapter.pdf

Perenboom, R. J. M., & Chorus, A. M. (2003, Jun). Measuring participation according to the International Classification of Functioning, Disability and Health (ICF). *Disability and Rehabilitation, 25*, 577–587

Robbins, J., Kays, S. A., Gangnon, R. E., Hind, J. A., Hewitt, A. L., Gentry, L. R., et al. (2007, Feb). The effects of lingual exercise in stroke patients with dysphagia. *Archives of Physical Medicine and Rehabilitation, 88*, 150–158

Robin, D. A., Somodi, L. B., & Luschei, E. S. (1991). Measurement of tongue strength and endurance in normal and articulation disordered subjects. In C. Moore, K. Yorkston, & D. Beukelman (Eds.), *Dysarthria and apraxia of speech: Perspectives on management* (pp. 173–184). Baltimore, MD: Brookes

Rogers, M. A., Alarcon, N. B., & Olswang, L. B. (1999). Aphasia management considered in the context of the World Health Organization model of disablements. In I. R. Odderson & E. M. Halar (Eds.), *Physical medicine and rehabilitation clinics in North America* (pp. 907–924). Philadelphia: Saunders

Simmons-Mackie, N., Threats, T. T., & Kagan, A. (2005, Jan-Feb). Outcome assessment in aphasia: a survey. *Journal of Communication Disorders, 38*, 1–27

Stiers, W., Carlozzi, N., Cernich, A., Velozo, C., Pape, T., Hart, T., et al. (2012). Measurement of participation outcomes in the rehabilitation of persons with traumatic brain injury. *Journal of Rehabilitation Research and Development. 49*, 139–154

Stineman, M. G., Jette, A., Fiedler, R., & Granger, C. V. (1997, Jun). Impairment-specific dimensions within the Functional Independence Measure. *Archives of Physical Medicine and Rehabilitation, 78*, 636–643

Stineman, M. G., Shea, J. A., Jette, A., Tassoni, C. J., Ottenbacher, K. J., Fiedler, R., et al. (1996, Nov). The Functional Independence Measure: tests of scaling assumptions, structure, and reliability across 20 diverse impairment categories. *Archives of Physical Medicine and Rehabilitation, 77*, 1101–1108

Threats, T. T. (2000). The World Health Organization's revised classification: What does it mean for speech-language pathology? *Journal of Medical Speech-Language Pathology, 8*, 13–18

Ware, J. E., & Gandek, B., & the IQOLA Project Group. (1994). The SF-36® Health Survey: Development and use in mental health research and the IQOLA Project. *International Journal of Mental Health, 23*, 49–73

Warren, R. (1998). Overcoming barriers to outcomes measurement. In C. Frattali (Ed.), *Measuring outcomes in speech-language pathology* (pp. 309–225). New York: Thieme

Whiteneck, G. G., Bogner, J. A., & Heinemann, A. W. (2011, Apr). Advancing the measurement of participation. *Archives of Physical Medicine and Rehabilitation, 92*(4), 540–541

Whiteneck, G., & Dijkers, M. P. (2009, Nov). Difficult to measure constructs: conceptual and methodological issues concerning participation and environmental factors. *Archives of Physical Medicine and Rehabilitation, 90*(11, Suppl), S22–S35

WHOQOL Group. (1994). The development of the World Health Organization Quality of Life Assessment instrument (the WHOQOL). In J. Orley & W. Kuyken (Eds.), *Quality of life assessment: International perspectives*. Heidelberg, Germany: Springer-Verlag

World Health Organization. (2001). *International Classification of Functioning, Disability and Health: ICF*. Geneva: World Health Organization

# 6

# Outcomes Matter in School Service Delivery

*Jean Blosser*

## ◆ Chapter Focus

This chapter explores outcomes measurement for speech-language services in the school setting from a broad range of perspectives. The importance and benefits of measuring student outcomes is explained. The link between the types of outcomes schools value and outcomes for speech-language services is discussed. Three specific types of outcomes measurement are explored: student outcomes, partnership outcomes, and program change outcomes. Examples of processes and tools for systematic data collection and analysis are provided. Finally, readers are encouraged to participate in and advocate for outcomes data collection to demonstrate the benefits and results of speech-language services.

## ◆ Introduction

School speech-language pathologists (SLPs) may wonder: "Does the therapy I provide really make a difference to the children on my caseload? Do their parents see changes in their child's communication skills during home and leisure activities? Is my intervention really educationally relevant and will my students improve their academic performance as a result of the intervention approaches I implement? What is the most effective system for speech-language service delivery in the school setting? Does collaboration with teachers decrease the amount of time students spend enrolled in the therapy program? Is a pull-out model of service delivery as effective as integrating services into the classroom? Would combining models be even more effective? Can we really measure treatment outcomes in school-based service delivery? Will anyone care if we do? Can gathering data and reporting our outcomes to administrators lead to greater support for our therapy program?" SLPs, school leaders, family members, education team colleagues, and students with communication disorders hope the answer to all these questions is a resounding *yes*. Questions such as these stimulate us to investigate the efficacy of our intervention and service delivery methods and to define the outcomes we are accomplishing.

Schools are confronted with unprecedented challenges to meet constituents' demands and expectations. Difficult economic times place a burden on school leaders to demonstrate that they can deliver high-quality services but with limited resources. For decades, community and education leaders have called for proof that the education and special education services students receive is of high quality and results in positive outcomes. Many constituent groups including community leaders, school administrators, taxpayers, families, and others seek proof that the education children receive will enable them to succeed in school, graduate, get good jobs, and contribute to society. Schools, teachers, and professionals (including SLPs) must be accountable for the decisions they make and educational services they offer.

## ♦ Outcomes in the Schools

*Outcomes* is a term that means the results of care or intervention. Outcomes are the benefits for participants during or after their participation or involvement in a program. Outcomes may be related to documented changes in knowledge, skills, attitudes, values, behaviors, conditions, or status. The indicators of success or outcomes are observable, measurable, and represent achievement. When measuring outcomes we engage in data collection, analysis, and interpretation of the effectiveness of interventions. Spady (1994) suggested, "A system based on outcomes gives top priorities to ends, purposes, learning accomplishments, and results."

The public is very concerned about the quality of education in America's schools today. Constituents from many different perspectives say that they are not convinced that the education provided in our schools is at the level of quality that it should be. Students across the country take state standardized tests to measure their progress and performance in academic curricular areas including reading and math. The test results of many schools in the United States demonstrate that students are not making adequate progress. The scores are reported as *adequate yearly progress* (AYP). When AYP scores are not adequate, schools must take steps and implement strategies to indicate how they will improve students' performance on standardized tests over time. Unfortunately, students in subgroups including special education, African-American and Hispanic heritage, and those receiving free and reduced-price lunches are among the students who frequently fall below the benchmarks set for AYP. Examples of strategies that some schools implement when gaps are revealed are special tutoring, extra "doses" of reading and math time, and specialized instructional or intervention approaches.

The call for improved instruction, for measuring outcomes in our schools, and for data analysis and improvement strategies in education has never been greater. Communities dissatisfied with the outcomes of their local schools are in revolt and taking steps to make sure that change in educational practices occurs. Schools that perform poorly are subject to community scrutiny. In fact, when schools fail today, several very critical actions may be implemented by local leaders as part of an overall strategy to dramatically reduce the dropout rate and improve graduation rates. In 2010 the Obama administration made a historic commitment to support state and local education leaders in turning around America's lowest achieving schools. Funding was provided under the Title I School Improvement Grant Program. To qualify, states had to identify their lowest performing schools in economically challenged communities and transform those schools using one of four intervention models. The overarching goal of each of the intervention models is to improve student outcomes. The intervention models are as follows:

- Turnaround model: Replace the principal and teachers. Rehire no more than 50% of the staff. Grant the new principal sufficient operational flexibility to fully implement a comprehensive approach to substantially improve student outcomes.

- Restart model: Convert or close schools and then reopen them under an education management organization or charter school operator selected through a rigorous review process.

- School closure: Close schools and enroll students in other schools in the district that are higher achieving.

- Transformation model: Implement one of four strategies: (1) replace the principal and take steps to increase teacher and school leader effectiveness; (2) institute comprehensive instructional reforms; (3) increase learning time and create community-oriented schools; and (4) provide operational flexibility and sustained support.

As one can see, the new models are designed to promote achievement of a higher standard and a focus on student outcomes. Simply stated, there is a belief that students should complete school able to use information to function in society, to achieve goals, and to develop knowledge. Education reformers suggest that schools should prepare students to meet very specific education standards. The belief is based on the premise that by raising the standards, school achievement will also increase and students will be better prepared to enter college and the world of work. In addition, they will participate as citizens in a democratic and global society.

The adoption of the national Common Core Curriculum standards (National Governors Association and Council of Chief State School Officers of Education, 2010) has been one of the most significant national initiatives to improve education in the nation's schools in recent years. This initiative clearly defines the outcomes that schools seek. The national Common Core Curriculum standards serve as a vehicle for ensuring that students are prepared for advanced education and future employment. The Common Core Curriculum standards explicitly state the knowledge and skills that all students are expected to master. The standards describe what students should know and be able to do. In other words, they define what the outcomes of education should be. Positive outcomes for schools are defined by the numbers of high school students who stay in school, graduate, and successfully pursue college and work.

The Common Core Curriculum standards for English/language arts recommend that students should learn to read a variety of texts (fictional, nonfictional, informational, historical, political, and social/cultural). Students should learn to read visual texts such as film, television, photographs, graphics (charts and illustrations), and technological texts, such as via the Internet. Students are expected to learn to write for a variety of purposes and audiences. They should know the various purposes of writing as well as the technical and mechanical aspects. Thus, students are expected to be able to speak, listen, view, and visually represent language to self-reflect, communicate with others, and learn.

The core curriculum standards provide clarity about the content and skills that should be taught at each grade. Educational standards also define the "benchmarks" or key points along the learning path from kindergarten through twelfth grade. The intent is for the curriculum and formal instruction to consistently line up with the expectations for learning indicated by the standards.

# ◆ Curriculum, Outcomes, and the School-Based Speech-Language Pathologist

One might ask, "What do academic outcomes, low AYP scores, and the Common Core Curriculum have to do with SLPs and school services delivery?" The question arises because some individuals may still hold the perception that SLPs focus only on improving speech-language production, expression, and reception. The answer is simple; speech-language services can and should have a major impact on students' ability to succeed within classroom academic and functional literacy. The SLP's role has evolved (ASHA, 2010a). School-based SLPs are now an integral part of the education system. The national education agenda impacts the way speech-language services are now delivered and will continue do so even more in the future. School districts' focus on academic goals and outcomes will influence the interpretation of eligibility for services and perceptions of the effectiveness of intervention. The ultimate outcome of SLP services is the contribution SLPs can make to preparing students for success in school, graduation, advanced education, and future employment. Positive outcomes provide the evidence of our intervention and program effectiveness.

For these reasons, the SLP should be familiar with the Common Core Curriculum standards, expectations, and processes in place for measuring academic outcomes for each of the content areas but especially for the language arts, literacy, math, and science areas. They should know how the students they serve perform on state standardized tests and how their performance contributes to the district's AYP. Knowing this information enables SLPs to align their speech-language program and intervention goals with educational expectations and to identify and measure students' functional communication skills in that context. SLPs are expected to recommend goals for the individualized education program (IEP) that will enable students to access the curriculum. They are also expected to contribute to their students' academic outcomes, especially in the areas of communication, language arts, and functional literacy.

## ♦ Outcomes for Students with Disabilities

School programs for children with disabilities are regulated by the Individuals with Disabilities Education Act (IDEA). The 1997 amendments of IDEA placed emphasis on accountability of outcomes for services provided to students with disabilities with a mandate to "assess and ensure the effectiveness of efforts to educate children with disabilities" (IDEA, 1997). Schools must be able to ensure that all students, including students with disabilities, are equipped with the knowledge, competence, and qualities needed to be successful after they leave the educational system. To generate the desired outcomes, schools must be structured and operated so that outcomes can be achieved by all students. Parents, educators, legislators, and other constituents seek verification of the results of education and special education efforts.

Outcomes measurement and reporting enables educators to be accountable and responsible for providing appropriate educational programs (including intervention) to meet the individual needs of students. The efficacy of special educational programs, including speech-language programs, can be verified by describing, measuring, and documenting students' functional performance in high- and low-demand learning situations and by measuring and documenting their progress toward specific educational goals over time.

Outcomes measurement in the schools is not a new concept. In fact, schools have struggled with how to measure outcomes for decades. Through the years efforts to measure outcomes for students with disabilities have focused on improving student success through effective teaching methods, improving school culture, providing accommodations and modifications for students with disabilities, and gathering data through compliance reporting processes. Information gathered from measuring outcomes provides school-based professionals with knowledge to make decisions about teaching, intervention, and program planning. Data collected from outcomes measurement can describe intervention effectiveness in real-life learning situations and provide school administrators, funding agencies, community constituents, and consumers with information related to cost analysis, efficiency of services, impact of a specific disability on school performance, and quality of life.

Schools measure student success by their classroom performance, grades, scores on district and state standardized tests, and school completion (graduation) rates. Educational results are as important for students with disabilities as they are for students without disabilities. For this reason, they are included in the overall system of educational accountability measurement in schools. Unfortunately, the school completion picture for students with disabilities has not been a very positive one. When students with special needs do not perform well on school-based assessments such as state standardized testing, the results of the entire school can be depressed. As described earlier, schools must report their student population's performance annually on reports to their constituents including communities, families, taxpayers, and legislators. In these AYP reports, schools report outcomes related to how students performed in academic areas such as literacy, math, and science. Many districts report that the scores of students with disabilities lower the average yearly progress scores for the district (Council for Exceptional Children, 2004). Dropout rates for students with disabilities, as well as high school students in general, continue to soar. Students with disabilities may not be fully integrated into their communities, and their unemployment rates are very high. Because the cost of educating students with disabilities is significantly higher than that of students without disabilities, there is great pressure on special education providers to demonstrate program effectiveness by considering outcomes, especially student outcomes.

Of all of the areas of the curriculum, the greatest link between the educational standards and the services SLPs offer are in the English/language arts standards. The standards expect that students will increase their vocabulary, be prepared for 21st-century careers, and use formal English in writing and speaking. A compelling argument can be made for the need for speech-language intervention for a student who is unable to perform to the highest expectations of the standards due to communication impairment.

Effective instruction, including instructional support such as speech-language services, is expected to improve students' academic performance. This expectation has led to major changes in SLPs' goals and service delivery practices in the school setting. Of course SLPs must be proficient at identifying and explaining communication impairments. They and their education teammates must also be able to describe a student's present level of educational performance and explain how the communication impairment impacts his or her school performance. The description of the student's present level of education performance provides a profile from which to launch discussion about the student, including his or her strengths, capabilities, interests, and needs displayed in school, in the community, or at home. In addition, scores achieved on state standardized tests are included, especially scores on language arts, social science, history, listening, speaking, reading, and writing. SLPs must be aware of how to meaningfully discuss this educational impact with their educational counterparts and to make a case for how and why speech-language intervention and services will lead to improvements. Further, when reporting progress in speech-language treatment, they must be able to describe how treatment has contributed to the student's academic performance.

As a result of services provided in schools, speech-language pathologists, families, and educators want students to be able to participate to the greatest extent possible in school, home, and community activities. We want students to be able to communicate and perform in the classroom. They should be able to raise their hand and be understood when they answer the teacher's question; pay attention throughout a whole lesson; and follow instructions to complete classroom learning activities. They should be able to demonstrate improved literacy skills as a result of improved functional communication skills. SLPs would like to observe them socially interact with peers during extracurricular activities such as gym class, social groups, playground, science fairs, music class, and so on.

Speech-language pathologist must be able to measure their outcomes in the larger context of students' performance in the academic environment using the Common Core Curriculum standards as a benchmark and guide. In other words, the SLP's outcomes measures should be aligned with educational standards and expectations. Following this perspective, some outcomes SLPs can and should strive for their students to achieve are as follows:

- Competence in interactive communication and communication for learning
- Competence in problem-solving strategies and critical thinking skills
- Competence in communication for math, language arts, reading, and writing

## ◆ Benefits of Outcomes Assessment in School Speech-Language Programs

Learning outcomes are statements that specify what learners will know or be able to do as a result of a learning activity. Outcomes are usually expressed as knowledge, skills, or attitudes. In the case of speech-language services in the schools, outcomes provide information about how a student is able to function as a result of speech-language treatment. In the school setting, outcomes demonstrate how intervention changes the ability of students with communication impairments to access the school curriculum, function within the school environment, and meet the demands of the learning situation. School practitioners as well as our multiple constituents and education partners value accountability and evidence that demonstrates that our broad range of speech-language services yield positive outcomes. Further, if desired outcomes are not achieved, we value having data to help make improvements to ensure that positive results are achieved.

Some school-based SLPs believe that administrators and educators do not understand the contributions they make to students' school success. Unfortunately, many SLPs struggle with how to obtain, describe, and document the outcomes of their intervention and services. Understanding the processes for collecting and reporting treatment outcomes data in the school setting will promote consistent practices across clinicians within a school district. It will also permit consistent descriptions of students' communication status and needs as well as documentation of treatment that is provided (Blosser, Subich, & Ehren, 2000). Importantly, this chapter describes outcomes that schools value.

There are increasingly complex challenges that face SLPs and other educators in the current school environment. The roles and responsibilities of school-based SLPs have shifted in response to the challenges and trends in education and special education (ASHA, 2010a). Some challenges that have led to changes in our roles in the school setting are personnel shortages, growing numbers of children who present severe disabilities and communication impairments, diverse student needs, financial constraints, and cultural diversity.

There are inconsistent practices among services providers in terms of determining students' eligibility for services, defining impact of disabilities on educational performance, matching students to service delivery options, caseload planning and scheduling, workload management, and more. Challenges such as these have led to increased demands for greater accountability, efficiency, and cost-effectiveness. These trends in special education and speech-language pathology service delivery create a need for more clearly linking speech-language services to student learning as well as requiring greater consistency in and accountability for service delivery decisions. Consequently, school-based practitioners seek better methods of describing the populations they serve, selecting service delivery models for intervention, and determining the effectiveness of treatment.

Interests in determining outcomes in the school setting are fueled by competing educational goals and priorities. School administrators, fellow educators, and families seek proof that speech-language services make a difference. There are diverse opinions about the nature and value of special education services (including speech-language services), especially in view of concerns about inefficiencies, ineffectiveness, and spiraling costs. Constituent groups are demanding effective and relevant practices in special education, including speech-language services. There is an urgent call for professionals to develop plans and mechanisms for defining, measuring, and reporting outcomes.

Ongoing processes are needed to determine if speech-language outcomes are achieved. Collecting and reporting outcomes need not be considered as an imposition or as a useless exercise. Rather, outcome data can be used to shape intervention and reframe service provision. School-based SLPs must accurately describe students' functional communication to others and make a case for improving students' outcomes by managing key variables such as frequency, intensity, and duration of services. They must be able to demonstrate changes in students' functional communication skills as a result of treatment. They must be prepared to modify goals, interventions, and service delivery approaches when progress is limited or outcomes not achieved.

It is critical that SLPs contribute data so that appropriate services can be provided. In addition to being able to provide students with the right type, intensity, and level of services, SLPs can benefit by informing administrators and others of caseload and workload needs as well as potential personnel and resource needs.

# ♦ Framework for Outcomes Measurement

To determine speech-language outcomes processes that will be relevant and important in the school setting, one must understand the context for school-based service delivery. Speech-language services are considered "related services" or "instructional support services." They fall within the special education realm of educational opportunities provided to students. As such, schools and their constituents hold expectations for those services. They expect that services will be provided by highly qualified professionals who are sensitive to the school's vision, goals, limits, challenges, and initiatives. They expect that school practitioners will ensure compliance with district, state, and federal mandates. They also expect that services will be efficient and effective.

Collecting outcomes data in the school setting enables practitioners to engage in systematic, consistent, and thoughtful decision making, planning, and service delivery for students with communication disabilities. Outcomes data are used for IEP decision making and planning, to document progress on goals, to support team decisions to increase or decrease services or to modify intervention approaches, and to develop educational supports. In addition, outcomes data can be used to monitor program effectiveness as well substantiate the need for programmatic, organizational, and systemic changes that will yield more efficiency and effectiveness.

School-based SLPs focus their efforts on obtaining positive outcomes in three key areas of service delivery. These three SLP outcomes—student outcomes, partnership outcomes, and program and system outcomes—provide a relevant, interrelated framework for documenting outcomes in the school setting. Below is an overview of the components of each of these three outcomes areas within the school speech-language services outcomes framework.

## School Speech-Language Services Outcomes

- Student Outcomes

  - Improved functional communication in low- and high-demand communication situations

  - Improved educational performance including academic performance and participation in school activities as a result of improved communication goals

- Partnership Outcomes

  - Improved relationships with education partners and families

  - Increased understanding by education partners and families of communication impairments and the impact of those impairments on academic and social performance

  - Increased team coordination and competency to provide assistance and support to students by implementing recommended accommodations and modifications that will result in improved communication interactions

- Program and System Outcomes

  - Changes and improvements within the speech-language program or the education organization and system that result in greater efficiency, effectiveness, and services for students with communication disabilities

  - Improved school climate and culture to promote positive attitudes and conditions that support students

Each aspect of the school speech-language services outcomes framework is explained below, and examples of representative measurement tools and processes are described.

*Student Outcomes*

The Individuals with Disabilities Education Act (IDEA), the federal law that regulates school-based services for children with disabilities, mandates that professionals assess and ensure the effectiveness of efforts to educate children with disabilities. Although IDEA mandates assessment and effectiveness, there are only a few documented tools designed to measure the outcomes of students who receive speech-language therapy services in school. Common terminology and processes for determining treatment outcomes would be valued by clinicians as well as their education partners. Having information about student outcomes as a result of speech-language treatment and services would enable clinicians and their education counterparts to make meaningful clinical decisions about intervention approaches and service delivery recommendations. There are two aspects of student outcomes to consider in schools, and they must be considered together. One aspect is the change in students' *functional communication skills for low- and high-demand communication situations* as a result of treatment. The other is the effect of changes in communication on students' *academic performance as a result of improved communication skills*. Both aspects should be the focus of outcomes measurement and reporting in the school setting. To complete student outcomes measurement, SLPs should obtain input from many sources including student records, assessment data, and other team members. The intention is to collect, aggregate, and describe data of students who receive speech-language intervention to identify outcomes for treating and serving this population and subgroups within the population, such as students who present specific types of learning disabilities or specific types of communication impairments.

Outcomes enable professionals to determine the quality and effectiveness of various treatment approaches and service models. Student outcomes in speech-language programs are determined by measuring the change in functional communication performance that takes place between the time treatment is initiated and the time it is completed. Outcomes measures can be used to structure the assessment and intervention process. Outcomes can be described as the results that we want students to demonstrate at the end of a significant treatment period. Functional communication is critical to students' success in the learning situation. Outcomes collection and measurement can also lead to greater consistency in clinical decisions and service delivery as well as implementation of more effective and efficient intervention methods. Professionals acquire their education and knowledge of intervention and service delivery practices in many different ways during their pre-service education, externship experiences, work in different districts, continuing education training, peer-to-peer resource sharing, independent learning activities, and more. Consequently, teams of clinicians may demonstrate inconsistent clinical decision-making practices. They may use different terminology to describe the severity of impairments. They may recommend different types and amounts of treatment. Some of the inconsistencies that may be observed from clinician to clinician, program to program, or school district to school district are in the following areas:

- Terminology used to describe students' communication skills and their functional communication status at the initiation of therapy (or admission for services) and the point of discharge (or completion of services)

- Description of the level of severity

- Demonstration of how communication and educational performance are linked

- Determination of priorities for treatment (where to begin)

- Intervention approaches and dosage of treatment provided

- Matching students with appropriate service delivery variables

- Families' perceptions of the value and need for services

- Teachers' reporting of how disabilities may be impacting student classroom performance

- The type of information and data needed to make informed clinical decisions

Using outcomes data collection instruments can promote more consistent practices among SLPs and their education team colleagues.

### Data Collection and Analysis

*Student Outcomes and the Individualized Education Program*    In school-based practice, student's outcomes are measured by a student's ability to achieve the educational goals specified in the IEP. There is great pressure for SLPs to demonstrate the effectiveness of their intervention and services. Educators within the district, including the SLP, must establish what it is that the student will master at given points in time as they progress through school. In addition, systems must be established for measuring students' performance to confirm if those skills have been accomplished. Outcome results can help clinicians demonstrate the effectiveness of services. They can also provide insights about the prognosis for successful treatment.

The IEP goals for improving student's communication skills are written as outcomes in the context of learning. For example, instead of writing a speech-language goal that states, "The student will improve expressive language skills," the goal would be written to reflect the application of the skills in the *context of the curriculum*. For example, "The student will use language to ask the teacher questions when he does not understand how to complete an assignment," or "The student will follow directions to complete a math assignment," or "The student will improve the adequacy of explanations by increasing his or her understanding of the need to provide explanations of math problems." This approach can be applied to other speech-language domains as well; for example, "The student will initiate effective strategies to gain fluent speech production when experiencing a dysfluent situation while giving a report in the classroom."

Students' functional communication performance in the school setting means that they can perform the required low- and high-demand communication-related tasks in the classroom. To be accountable for outcomes, SLPs need tools and processes to measure outcomes of intervention for students, and use data to improve services. The tools and processes must be uncomplicated and identify change over time in the students they serve.

*Instruments for Measuring Functional Communication Outcomes*    The American Speech-Language-Hearing Association (ASHA, 2011) developed the National Outcomes Measurement System (NOMS) to provide an instrument that would enable communication disorders professionals to accomplish the following objectives (ASHA, 2003, 2011):

• Create a national database of information about communication disorders

• Offer a mechanism for benchmarking clinical progress

• Help clinicians benchmark the progress of clients in their caseload

The NOMS instruments have been designed to provide a standardized method for documenting the effectiveness of treatment procedures, for reflecting changes in clients' functional communication skills from admission to discharge, for providing information about the number of treatment sessions and amount of time required for intervention of specific communication impairments, and for soliciting consumer satisfaction. The NOMS has been used extensively in health care settings. It describes low-demand communication skills as initiations and responses that primarily require content and form that are acquired at a young age. High-demand communication skills are initiations and responses that primarily require more recently acquired language and content. Students should be able to communicate as independently as possible in low- and high-demand communication-related situations with the appropriate type and intensity of support to ensure that they achieve the greatest potential possible. Communication goals that are established for students who are eligible for speech-language services must relate to real-world communication demands and expectations in learning environments and contexts because communication forms the basis for most daily encounters, and certainly for learning and literacy.

A version of the NOMS was also designed to collect data for speech-language services for children in school and early intervention settings. The key to NOMS is the application of the functional communication measures (FCMs). In the NOMS, the FCMs are a series of disorder-specific, seven-point rating scales designed to describe the change in a student's functional communication ability over time. The 7 on the rating scale represents "consistently appropriate" whereas the 1 represents "rarely appropriate." The FCMs in the school-age NOMS include composition, fluency, emergent literacy, intelligibility, pragmatics, reading comprehension, speech sound production, spoken language comprehension, spoken language production, voice, word recognition, and writing accuracy. Based on a student's existing IEP, FCMs are chosen and scored on the seven-point scale. By examining the scores from year to year or time period to time period, clinicians can assess the amount of functional change and thus the benefits of treatment.

In the NOMS, students are entered into the data collection process at the time of the initial IEP when they are identified as eligible for services and at key milestones such as each annual or triennial IEP review. Data are then also entered at the time of discharge or service completion. In addition to rating the FCMs again, data on several other factors are indicated, including predominant service delivery model, percentage of treatment time allocated for each FCM, number of sessions per week, average length of sessions, and disposition. The NOMS is designed as the minimum data set (MDS), which is a standardized set of outcome measures that can be used to collect data across individuals to identify outcomes for people with particular characteristics and interventions. The MDS includes the fewest number of items possible to provide the information that is being sought. This enables clinicians to gather comprehensive data while considering efficiency for data collection and time factors. By having fewer items, clinicians are able to complete the tool quickly and gather relevant functional information on the students for whom they provide services. The availability of a quick assessment assists clinicians in gathering data about their students without taking extended time away from their daily activities. The time it takes to complete the data collection varies with the clinician's familiarity with the student and the student's IEP. Those familiar with the student and the IEP are able to complete the data collection form tool in about 10 minutes.

Unfortunately, the use of the NOMS and contribution to the database by school practitioners were lower than desired. Therefore, in 2010, the school version of the NOMS was suspended so that a team of practitioners could review the tool and its applicability for the school setting. It is anticipated that a revised version that is more reflective of current trends in school practice will be forthcoming. At about the same time, a team of SLPs who specialize in early intervention were asked to serve on a task force to help develop a version of the NOMS to measure the effectiveness of early intervention services for infants and toddlers.

The pediatric version of the Functional Independence Measure (SUNY, 1993), the WeeFIM, is another example of an MDS outcomes measurement tool. It too is a pediatric version of an adult outcomes measurement instrument. The WeeFIM was not developed to measure outcomes of school-based therapy. Rather, it is generally used in health care settings to assess outcomes in children who have sustained acute injuries or surgery. The types of services, goals, and anticipated functional changes in the health care environment differ greatly from the services, goals, and expected outcomes for children receiving services in schools. However, some schools use the WeeFIM as a tool for measuring and reporting outcomes for students who receive Medicaid.

Neither the NOMS nor the WeeFim includes data points for recording students' academic performance or for determining if improvements noted in speech language skills were related to changes in academic performance. Consequently, SLPs practicing in the school setting have to look to data provided by other avenues for academic performance changes as a result of therapy.

*Progress Monitoring*   Progress monitoring is a process by which educators assess students' performance on a regular basis to determine whether they are profiting appropriately from the instructional or intervention programs and to build more effective programs for students who struggle (Fuchs & Fuchs, 2011; Rudebusch, 2011). Schools across the country use several tools to monitor student progress and measure students' acquisition of literacy skills. SLPs, like their education colleagues, must monitor and report on student progress on a regular basis with the intention of making modifications in intervention if progress is limited. Theoretically, if intervention becomes more appropriate, students' progress will be notable and they will achieve desired academic and communication outcomes.

As previously described, to be eligible for speech-language services, students must demonstrate a speech-language impairment that adversely affects their academic performance. An adverse effect must be verified and documented using results of standardized achievement tests, grades, curriculum-based or criteria-based assessments, and other academic performance measures. SLPs must access data from these sources and be able to discuss them with their education team members. Recommendations for intervention and collaboration must be based on linking data about the speech-language disability with education information. It is that step that makes service delivery in the schools educationally relevant.

Because early literacy is a language-based skill, SLPs in schools should be able to use the results of educators' progress measures to determine if the intervention they provide is having a direct effect on students' performance in school. Thus, the relationship of therapy to school performance becomes more objectively evident to school colleagues, and SLPs can demonstrate the positive impact their services can have on students' school success. Even better, the opportunity for the teacher and the SLP to collaborate and share intervention and instruction strategies with one another is increased.

Two instruments that hundreds of schools have adopted are the Dynamic Indicators of Basic Early Literacy Skills (DIBELS) (University of Oregon, 2011) and the AIMSWeb Assessment (AIMSWeb Assessment and Measurement for RTI, 2011). The DIBELS is used to assess students' skills in three of the five major areas of early literacy, which are also referred to as the "big ideas in early reading." The five big ideas are phonemic awareness, alphabetic principle, accuracy and fluency with text, vocabulary, and comprehension. The measures are linked to one another, both psychometrically and theoretically, and have been found to be predictive of later reading proficiency. SLPs who target these skills in their speech-language intervention approaches will be able to collaborate and coordinate with their education partners to track students' progress.

AIMSWeb Assessment and Data Management for Response-to-Intervention (RTI; AIMSWeb.com) is a Web-based system that hundreds of districts use to benchmark and monitor students' performance on the curriculum. It is structured to enable schools to capture data on a continuous basis, manage the data, and prepare reports that document students' progress. Students' progress on the general education curriculum can be monitored. Students who struggle in school can be identified. In addition, the school's AYP can be monitored. The system provides monthly results and reports on students' progress that can lead educators to implement changes in their instructional and intervention strategies. Because AIMSWeb is geared toward strategy planning and modifications in instructional strategy, teams of teachers and SLPs can determine what changes in instruction and intervention may be required. The data would reveal students' progress and outcomes as a result of implementing more effective strategies.

*Partnership Outcomes*

Service delivery in the schools encompasses a broad range of activities. Many descriptions of service delivery models discussed in the literature consider collaboration to be a separate service delivery option. In contrast to that widely held opinion, this author suggests that collaboration is essential to successful service delivery. SLPs are expected and required to collaborate with their education partners and families every step of the way, including when assessing, planning, and treating students (Blosser, 2011a). Educators must gain an understanding of the nature of students' disabilities, the impact on school performance, and intervention strategies that can be implemented in the classroom to support students with communication disabilities. Integrating intervention strategies into classroom instruction increases the frequency and intensity of intervention and enhances the quality of the interactive communication between the teacher and student (Blosser, 2011a; Blosser & DePompei, 2003; Blosser & Kratcoski, 1997; Hanft & Shepherd, 2008). Clinicians engage with parents to provide similar information and guidance. Engagement and collaboration with education team members and families are required and essential in the school setting. However, providing this level of support to teachers and families requires organized effort, time, and resources. Unfortunately, there has been limited research to date to provide evidence of the value and benefits of collaboration (Cirrin et al, 2010). Thus, it would be beneficial to collect outcomes data on a wide variety of aspects related to collaboration. It is hoped that these findings could lead to improvements in processes for nurturing and developing collaborative relationships, building SLPs' capabilities for facilitating collaborative efforts, determining the type of information that should be exchanged between collaborative partners, and developing recommendations for key service delivery variables such as preferred provider, location, and dosage. For example, if the intensity of therapy can be increased through collaborative efforts and the time in therapy can be decreased, SLPs could make a compelling case for modifying their workload and responsibilities to enhance collaboration and coordination with their education partners and families.

Clinicians may consider collaboration with educators and families worth the effort but often indicate that they are unable to devote the time and resources necessary to establish meaningful relationships or to provide the level of training needed to build educators' knowledge and skills. Due to many competing challenges and priorities, it is difficult for school-based SLPs to integrate collaborative activities such as frequent meetings, training sessions, and co-teaching into their complex workload. Unfortunately, many clinicians lack the confidence, time, and resources to facilitate high-quality collaborative relationships. They frequently resort to distributing "strategy tip sheets" to teachers rather than engage on a more comprehensive level.

Given that premise, a project was undertaken to determine the efficacy of a model of service delivery in which a student received no direct therapy (Blosser, 2011b). Instead, the SLP collaborated with and coached reading instructors, helping them recognize when a communication breakdown had occurred and the strategies they could implement to improve student's communication skills. The NOMS and reading achievement tests were the instruments applied to determine outcomes. Results indicated that excellent outcomes were achieved after only 20 to 30 hours of reading instruction with the SLP coaching the reading instructors. The project and outcomes are summarized in **Table 6.1**.

### Data Collection and Analysis

*Efforts to Collaborate*   Many schools and professionals acknowledge the power of collaboration and strive to increase the amount and quality of parent and teacher involvement and engagement in special education and speech-language programs. Often reports of the type of engagement efforts that work, successes, and impact on student outcomes are only anecdotal. To determine the effectiveness of efforts to collaborate more frequently and at a higher quality level with families and teachers, SLPs are invited to follow the steps provided in the illustrations found in **Table 6.2** and **Table 6.3**. **Table 6.2** describes ways to measure the effect of efforts to obtain greater family and teacher engagement.

*Teacher Feedback*   Speech-language pathologists often report that they provide their education partners with tips and strategies for supporting and assisting students with communication impairments in the classroom. In addition, many SLPs provide in-service training to school colleagues as a method for conveying information about communication impairment and accommodations and strategies that can be implemented. The SLPs often do not know if their teacher audiences grasp the information shared, nor do they know if their efforts will make a difference in achieving student outcomes. Obtaining feedback prior to and following a full year of one-on-one collaborative exchanges or group in-service training and collaborative efforts would enable clinicians to report the outcomes of their efforts and potentially gain support for allocating additional time, effort, and resources to specific collaborative training efforts.

To measure outcomes, teachers of students served in the speech-language program are asked to complete a simple survey at the beginning of the school year and again at the end of the school year or when the student is discharged from service. Their responses can provide insights into the effectiveness of collaborative efforts and changes in their understanding and perception as a result of

**Table 6.1**    Outcomes of a Collaborative Speech-Language Intervention Model

An indirect collaborative approach was implemented to provide speech-language services to 97 middle school students who attended school in an urban school district. The SLP did not work directly with the students. Instead, she collaborated with four reading instructors and coached them to modify their instructional communication during daily reading lessons and activities. Students demonstrated improved communication and reading performance after 20 to 30 hours of indirect collaborative services. The SLP coached reading instructors to use proven intervention strategies. Following are highlights of the findings.

**Student Population**

Ninety-seven students in grades 6–8 in a large urban school district who had active IEPs; 47.4% were designated as learning disabled, 21.6% were designated as speech-language impaired, and 31% were in the lowest quartile for their grade.

**Services Provided**

The model included three major components:

*Individualized mastery reading instruction*
• Small group, intensive supplemental reading instruction using a 1:4 ratio (instructor to students)

*Indirect speech-language intervention*
• Targeted speech-language intervention with one SLP working *indirectly* with all of the students, but *directly* with the reading instructors, classroom teachers, and parents

*Parent involvement*
• Outreach to parents by a parent liaison in collaboration with the reading instructors and SLP

**Program Highlights**

A highly qualified intervention team was identified (consisting of an SLP, four reading instructors, and a parent liaison). The program provided students with comprehensive reading remediation strategies. Speech-language intervention was integrated into all instructional communication. Students did not receive traditional speech-language therapy services.

**Results**

77.32% of students participating in the reading program received at least 20 hours of instruction.

60.8% of students participating in the reading program received at least 30 hours of instruction.

After only 20 to 30 hours of indirect speech-language intervention and reading instruction, students demonstrated progress on the following measures:
• National Outcomes Measurement System for Speech-Language Pathology (NOMS)
• Burns/Roe Graded Word Tests
• Catapult Learning Reading Diagnostic Test (RDT)
• California Achievement Test/5 (CT/5)

**Measurement System**

The National Outcomes Measurement System (NOMS) measures change in students' functional communication abilities using seven-point rating scales that have been developed to describe the different aspects of a student's functional communication. The rating scales range from 1, least functional, to 7, most functional.

Students with 30 or more hours of instruction showed the following changes:
• 39% increased by one level on the Pragmatics subscale of the NOMS.
• 59% increased by one level on the Spoken Language Comprehension subscale of the NOMS.
• 57% increased by one level on the Word Recognition subscale of the NOMS.
• 56% increased by one level on the Reading Comprehension subscale of the NOMS.

**Reading Performance**

60% of the students with 20 or more hours of instruction made gains of at least one instructional level on the Burns/Roe Graded Word List.

Students who were designated as speech-language impaired (only) demonstrated the greatest gains on the Reading Diagnostic Test, gaining more than 78 percentage points on the following five subtests:
• Long vowel, double vowel, r-control vowel, vowel diagraphs, and diphthongs and syllabication.
• They also achieved mastery on five of the RDT subtests.
• The students in the lowest quartile achieved mastery (80% or better) on the following eight subtests of the RDT: consonant blends, short vowels, consonant diagraphs, long vowels, double vowel, r-control vowel, vowel digraphs and  diphthongs and syllabication.

**Table 6.1** (*Continued*) Outcomes of a Collaborative Speech-Language Intervention Model

Of the three classifications of students (speech-language impaired, learning disabled, and students in the lowest quartile) served by this program, the 31 students who were designated as learning disabled showed the greatest gains on the CT/5, gaining 3.19 normal curve equivalents (NCEs) overall and 3.65 NCEs on the comprehension subtest.

Students who attended at least 20 hours of instruction in reading achieved average total reading gains of 2.64 NCEs.

They produced gains on both subtests of the reading assessment and comprehension gains of 2.62 NCEs. In addition, they achieved vocabulary gains of 2.75 NCEs.

**SLP Responsibilities**

In this model, the SLP's goals were to:

Identify the specific speech-language impairments and learning disabilities that would interfere with reading success.

Recommend individualized communication modification strategies to promote learning.

Facilitate the teachers', parents', and the parent liaison's understanding of key information about the impact of communication and learning disabilities on reading.

Train team members to implement instructional accommodations and strategies that would improve performance.

Monitor implementation of prescribed instructional accommodations and modification strategies.

Observe and use dynamic assessment procedures to evaluate student communication performance throughout all phases of the reading instruction program to monitor progress and change.

The methods the SLP used:
- Construct a student profile summary.
- Review the student's academic portfolio.
- Assess speech and language demands and expectations.
- Consult and collaborate with reading instructors, parent liaison, and parents.
- Summarize the program activities weekly.
- Observe and document the student communication performance on an ongoing basis.
- Recommend intervention strategies and modification of instructional method, communication, and materials.

*Source:* From Blosser, J. (2011b). Outcomes of a collaborative approach: Improved communication, improved reading. American Speech-Language-Hearing Association Annual Convention. San Diego, CA. Data are drawn from the results of a project conducted by the author in affiliation with Progressus Therapy and Catapult Learning.

training or sharing information and recommending strategies. Results would also lead to the development of best practices for working with educators. **Table 6.3** is a survey designed by Blosser (2011a) that SLPs can use to obtain feedback from teachers about their knowledge of the SLP's role, communication impairments, impact on learning, strategies for supporting and assisting students, and changes as a result of treatment.

## Program and System Outcomes

As mentioned previously, school administrators are responsible for taking steps in their schools to increase graduation rates, improve the AYP scores of students enrolled in special education programs, and facilitate effective education practices. To that end, they are also interested in lowering the percentage of students who are removed from general education classes to receive special education services or enrolled in special charter and private schools because parents are not confident that the public school can provide the same quality of services. To reduce litigation and the high cost of penalties for noncompliance, school administrators also focus on monitoring compliance with IDEA requirements such as accuracy of documentation, timeliness of determining eligibility, and execution of pertinent aspects of the IEP, the individualized family service plan (IFSP), or the individualized transition plan (ITP). Schools value maintaining students in educational settings with typically

**Table 6.2** Measuring Outcomes of Efforts to Increase Family and Teacher Engagement

Establish a rating of family and teacher engagement. This can be accomplished through consideration of previous experience in the school, records review, or interviews with school administrators or education colleagues. The rating would be subjective, but it would at least provide a base for understanding.

Rate family and teacher engagement at three predetermined times throughout the school year; for example, fall, midyear, and end of year.

- Seek information about the type of activities that families and teachers have been engaged in in relation to the speech-language program.
- Establish simple categories such as IEP-related meetings, open houses and invited events, strategy tip sheets, homework or class assignments, training or in-service sessions, contact (phone, e-mail, or mail contact), etc.
- Rate the level of engagement as "high," "moderate," or "low." Establish a goal for increasing the participation and quality of engagement (for each group: families and teachers).
- Rate the level of family and teacher engagement every 3 months. If families' and teachers' engagement and collaboration increases, then the outcome of those efforts would be positive.
- If the children of those families and teachers who were highly engaged showed more improvement than those children with the same disability whose parents were not highly engaged during a designated time period, then the link between family and teacher engagement and improved student success would be supported.

Implement simple efforts to engage families and teachers in speech-language program activities. Collect data to document family and teacher engagement efforts throughout the year by creating a simple chart of collecting data.

- Track phone, mail, or e-mail contacts.
- Track attendance and participation in meetings, open houses, or invitational events.
- Document the type of resources provided to families and teachers.
- Track the frequency of providing resources.
- Track questions and requests by families and teachers and your response to requests.
- Develop and share resources on a regularly scheduled basis.

Summarize and share your findings and successes with school administrators and colleagues. They need to hear about the outcomes of your efforts.

Replicate efforts that were successful.

developing peers, referred to as the *least restrictive environment* (LRE). In schools, the LRE is the general education classroom, and IDEA requires that children with disabilities be educated, to the maximum extent appropriate, with children who are nondisabled, that is, in the least restrictive environment. Special classes, separate schooling, or removal of children with disabilities from the regular education environment occurs only if the nature and severity of the disability is such that education in regular classes with the use of supplemental aids and services cannot be achieved satisfactorily. The LRE for students with communication impairments and other disabilities is stated in the individualized education program. Therefore, when the program is created, care must be taken by the SLP and other educators to determine the most appropriate learning environment, the rationale for the recommendation, and how the environment should change over time depending on the student's acquisition of skills and performance.

Consequently, school administrators encourage school-based clinicians and educators to provide instructional and intervention services using service delivery models that do not result in decreased time in the classroom. Trends in special education currently encourage educators and special educators to implement supports within the general education setting in two ways: first, to implement *universal design instruction* (UDI) methods (CAST, 2011); and second, to implement *response-to-intervention* (RTI) strategies to meet students' needs as soon as they begin to struggle with the general education curriculum. Although not all schools are currently fully invested in these approaches, the U.S. Department of Education is strongly in favor of their application, so both approaches will be a part of the future trends for serving students; thus, anything SLPs can do to align their programs and services with initiatives using RTI and UDL in their district will be perceived as appropriate and

**Table 6.3**  Teacher Feedback on Collaboration

**Teacher Feedback Survey**

Instructions: Teachers of students served in the speech-language program are asked to complete a simple survey at the initiation of service for the school year and again at the end of the school year or when the student is discharged.

Teacher's Name _____     SLP's Name _____

School_____     Grade/Special Education Placement _____

Number of students in the speech-language program _____

Teacher: Please respond to each statement below by indicating if you:
(1) strongly agree (2) agree (3) are not sure (4) disagree (5) strongly disagree

|  | 1 | 2 | 3 | 4 | 5 |
|---|---|---|---|---|---|
| I understand the school speech-language pathologist's role and responsibilities. |  |  |  |  |  |
| I understand the purpose and goals of the speech-language program within the school organization |  |  |  |  |  |
| I can describe the speech-language impairments that the students in my class demonstrate. |  |  |  |  |  |
| I can explain the impact of speech-language impairments on the academic performance of the students in my class (adverse effect). |  |  |  |  |  |
| I am aware of the speech-language related IEP goals established for each of the students in my class who demonstrate speech-language impairments. |  |  |  |  |  |
| I know several speech-language improvement techniques and strategies to assist students in my class. |  |  |  |  |  |
| I understand how to integrate the speech-language improvement strategies into my classroom instruction. |  |  |  |  |  |
| I try to use the speech-language improvement strategies during my classroom instruction on a regular basis. |  |  |  |  |  |
| I would like to learn more strategies and how to integrate them into my teaching. |  |  |  |  |  |
| My students' speech-language skills improved when I've used the strategies. |  |  |  |  |  |
| Comments or questions: |  |  |  |  |  |

*Source:* From Blosser, J. (2011a). School programs in speech-language pathology: Organization and service delivery. San Diego: Plural Publishing.

*Note:* At the end of the school year, questions can be provided to elicit teachers' perceptions of changes in students' speech-language performance and improvements in student's academic performance as a result of the intervention and the speech-language services.

aligned with initiatives to improve services for students with communication disabilities. School-based SLPs can begin by modifying the intensity of services from high-intensity direct services to distributed or reduced levels of direct service support and integrated models.

Outcomes assessment processes can be implemented to evaluate the efficiency and effectiveness of our school-based speech-language programs as well as how we are meeting the goals and the objectives of the educational organization in which we work. When SLPs gather data on programmatic aspects, they can be empowered to propose solutions and improvements. For example, outcomes measurement, analysis, and reporting can be structured to provide data for programmatic decision making regarding steps the SLP team can take to do the following:

- Ensure improved compliance monitoring systems to reduce of due process events
- Standardize eligibility and dismissal criteria
- Introduce new service options to decrease the length of treatment for mild and moderate communication impairments
- Initiate intervention programs that parents seek from alternative sites
- Improve the quality of teacher referrals
- Integrate services into the classroom
- Facilitate consistent practice at home
- Utilize clinicians' time and talent more efficiently

Service delivery refers to how services will be provided for children. School-based SLPs can and should engage in outcomes measurement to determine the most appropriate type of service delivery options to offer students with disabilities within their school district. Doing so will enable SLPs and their teammates to determine if the range of options should be expanded or if modifications can be made in existing options to increase efficiency and effectiveness.

Decades ago Richard Flower suggested that there are five essential characteristics of good service delivery (Flower, 1984): efficacy, coordination, continuity, participation, and economy. These characteristics are still relevant today. Although the definition of "efficacy" as compared with "effectiveness" of service delivery have been widely discussed and refined since this seminal 1984 paper (see Chapters 1, 2, 12, and 13 for elaborations), Flower's discussion of good service delivery continues to challenge us to ask essential questions:

*Efficacy*—Does the service make a difference?

*Coordination*—When multiple services are provided, are they coordinated and are all providers working toward the same end?

*Continuity*—Is the sequence of services uninterrupted, and is each phase of service implemented according to an established planned approach or protocol?

*Participation*—Is the individual receiving the service actively engaged and motivated? Does he or she demonstrate that the purpose of treatment and intervention strategies are understood?

*Economy*—Are the time, energy, funding, personnel, and other resources used as efficiently as possible to accomplish goals?

Service delivery options must be determined in collaboration with other members of each student's IEP team. The laws regulating special education are very clear on several major points. First, services must be delivered in the LRE. Second, regardless of the model implemented, the school district should make available a continuum of service delivery options for providing services. Third, the service delivery model selected should be appropriate for the student's unique characteristics and needs. Fourth, all services must be educationally or functionally relevant and help children make progress and achieve their educational goals.

The decisions about how services are delivered can only be made after the education team has jointly identified and addressed what the student's impairments are, the resulting impact on school performance, whether the expertise of an SLP is required, and what specialized interventions will be necessary to support the student and meet his or her needs. SLPs and special educators have vigorously debated the effectiveness or efficiency of many of the service options. There is not always complete agreement among communication disorders professionals on the appropriate approach, nor is there always agreement about how to match service delivery options with specific communication disabilities. However, there is consensus agreement that the approach selected must be designed to meet each individual student's needs.

Unfortunately, there is limited consensus concerning the definitions of many of the service delivery models used by SLPs in the schools. It is even more unfortunate that there are not many commonly shared definitions of service delivery models among educators and administrators. This presents a problem for educators, parents, administrators, and third-party payers. There is often confusion and misperception about the type of service to be provided, the reason that a particular model is selected, and the appropriateness for the student. Also, unfortunately, many parents and teachers are led to believe that one option is better than another and that more time with the SLP directly providing the majority of the services is preferable to incorporating other people (such as teachers) or providing services in different environments (including the classroom). This "more is better" concept has restricted the acceptance of expanded or alternative service delivery models. It has also limited the involvement of others who are significant in the student's life and who can contribute to improving the student's communication skills.

Numerous models for delivering speech-language pathology services are practiced in schools. Service delivery models are designed based on the specific needs of the population to be served, federal and state requirements, the resources and capabilities of the school district, the unique demographics of the community, and the insights and qualifications of professionals. School service delivery models vary from school district to school district. Differences may be due to the populations served, intervention goals, funding capabilities, administrative support (or nonsupport), and professional expertise and energy. Service delivery options may range from no service, to monitoring students' behavior, to engaging educators and parents in implementing strategies, to structured therapy in the classroom or therapy room, to special education placement. Service delivery models may be combined to meet the student's needs. To participate in speech-language intervention, services must fit into the school day. They may be integrated into classroom learning activities or woven into the students' academic and extracurricular schedule. Over 85% of clinicians report employing a "pull-out" model whereby students are removed from their classrooms to receive services (ASHA, 2010b). Unfortunately, many students may miss valuable academic lessons and class time to participate in therapy sessions. This poses a great dilemma for SLPs and educators. Many models have historical roots; with patterns of service delivery being passed from clinician to clinician through the ages. The literature on school-based service delivery provides some insights about some common models that are in place. Research is needed to define and create service delivery models that are proven to be efficient and effective. Thus, determining the outcomes that result from various service delivery models is essential.

Over the past several years, there have been many discussions of models for delivering speech-language services. An evidence-based systematic review of the effects of different service delivery models on communication outcomes for school-age children was completed by an ASHA-appointed team of experts in school service delivery (Cirrin et al, 2010). This expert panel reviewed peer-reviewed articles from the past 30 years that addressed the effect of various service delivery models and intervention outcomes. They followed explicit procedures and criteria defined in the evidence-based systematic review (EBSR) process. The results of the team's review indicated that the current evidence base does not support any particular service delivery model as preferable over another for meeting the communication needs of elementary school-age children. They indicated that the services for each student must be based on the specific needs of each student and that SLPs and their education colleagues must rely more on informed reason and expert consensus than research evidence (class III evidence) to make decisions about service delivery for individual students. The researchers concluded that further research is needed to determine effective service delivery options for school-age children. Although Cirrin and colleagues concluded that research-based evidence favoring one service delivery option over another is largely lacking, they identified three key areas that are in need of further study: the effectiveness of a wide range of specific service delivery options; the optimal combination of service delivery variables to fit the varied needs of individual students; and the effects of the frequency, number or length of treatment sessions, treatment intensity, and different schedules on communication performance.

Trying to sort through and understand service delivery options can be a difficult task. The task can be simplified by understanding the key service delivery variables that can be manipulated to meet a particular student's needed. Among the most important variables that an SLP must consider when recommending services are the following:

- The type and severity of the student's communication disability, including amount of assistance needed and impact on performance
- The dosage of services (frequency, intensity, amount, and duration of the services)
- The roles performed by the clinician
- The roles others play and the ways they can support speech-language development and improvement
- The location of the service (therapy room, classroom, resource room, community)
- The purpose of the service (screening, assessment, intervention, generalization)
- The presence of peers and the number of peers who participate (individual, small or large group, peers within the classroom)
- The scheduling format (weekly sessions throughout the school year; blocks of time within the school calendar; cycles throughout the year; a 3:1 model with 3 weeks of direct service and 1 week of indirect student support services such as observing, testing, consulting).

**Table 6.4** lists the key service delivery variables that SLPs consider when recommending services for students with communication disabilities (Blosser, 2011a). An individualized plan can be crafted by identifying the aspects that will best meet each student's individual needs. Measuring outcomes of various models of service will enable SLPs to confidently confirm the rationale for their recommendations.

### Data Collection and Analysis

Data for measurement of program and organizational outcomes can be obtained through uniquely designed and targeted surveys or retrospective summary reviews of data captured in school district student information systems (**Table 6.5**).

## ◆ Using Outcomes Data to Improve Programs and Systems

Calls for changes in the way that speech-language services are offered in schools will continue to increase as resources and funding decrease. With loss of funding associated with the ability to generate revenue in some regions, school boards may direct school administrators to find ways to cut or change programs or services. Following are three examples of how outcomes data can be gathered or used to recommend changes in programs and education systems.

### District Administrator's Request for Data

Meline and Kauffman (2010) describe a study they conducted to depict an evidence-based investigation of ways to maximize delivery of student services while reducing resources. The clinical question they asked was, "What is the most effective system of speech-language intervention service delivery in a school-based setting?" They implemented a scenario review method for their investigation. In their scenario, the SLP team in a school district had experienced a 25% revenue reduction and loss of funding associated with property taxes. The team examined service delivery options offered in the speech-language program in the district with a goal to recommend ways to (1) improve outcomes, (2) shorten times to dismissal, and (3) reduce costs. Their findings led to the recommendation that the education team needs to better align students' needs with service delivery models, vary the point

**Table 6.4**   Key Variables to Consider When Planning Services

| Key variables | Options |
| --- | --- |
| What activities are to be delivered? | Observation<br>Assessment<br>Planning<br>Intervention<br>Evaluation |
| Who will provide the services? | Therapist<br>Teacher<br>Family member<br>Other educators or specialists |
| What is the environment or location for intervention? | Away from the classroom (therapy room)<br>Classroom (general education, special education, unique program)<br>Other school contexts (lunch room, playground, extracurricular)<br>Community<br>Home |
| What other students should be included? | No other students<br>Students with similar disorders (2+)<br>Peers/ nondisabled (2+)<br>Family members |
| How intense should the services be? | Frequency (how many times per week, month, year)<br>Amount of time for each session (hours per week, month, year)<br>Duration (amount of time the services should last: week, month, year)<br>Identify the intensity for each environment and provider<br>* Identify ways to vary the intensity based on student's needs and progress |
| What is the context for the therapy? | Therapy treatment (different than classroom learning activities)<br>Classroom curriculum or lesson (including teacher instructing lesson, joint instruction therapist/teacher, center activity, individual learning activity)<br>Alternative augmentative communication or technology |
| What steps need to be taken to integrate services? | Identify additional providers (teacher, parent, aides)<br>Train providers<br>Coach providers |

*Source*: Blosser, J. (2011a). School programs in speech-language pathology: Organization and service delivery. San Diego, CA: Plural Publishing.

Note: The range of speech-language services, including prevention, assessment, intervention, and collaboration, must be delivered in a way that most effectively and efficiently meets each student's needs and enables the student to reach his or her highest potential. There are several variables that should be considered in developing the most appropriate service delivery plan for each student. In this model, collaboration is not considered a unique model of service delivery. Collaboration should be an integral part of all therapy.

**Table 6.5**   District-Level Student Information for Program Analysis and Decision Making

| |
| --- |
| Student identification |
| District student identification number |
| Disability (primary and secondary) |
| Individualized education program (disability, goals) |
| Prescription (amount of service, frequency, duration) |
| Attendance |
| Progress monitoring |

of intervention, implement programs that are related to student outcomes, and consider practical aspects such as time of day, curriculum, and the SLP's full workload. Their conclusion was that SLPs should gather their own data and develop local solutions.

## Technology as a Service Delivery Model

School districts are seeking service delivery models that will help them address personnel shortages. In addition, as mentioned previously, they are also seeking mechanisms for offering services in ways that will not increase students' time away from class. Clinicians are also seeking methods for increasing the frequency and intensity of intervention. *Telepractice* is a model of service delivery that offers solutions to all three challenges. Telepractice is a service delivery model that has gained professional and discipline acceptance in recent years. The ASHA position is that "the quality of services delivered via telepractice must be consistent with the quality of services delivered face-to-face" (ASHA, 2010b). ASHA's reports provide representative examples of telepractice services and the knowledge, skills, and competencies needed by professionals to provide telepractice. ASHA has developed official policies that support and provide guidance for the delivery of services via telepractice.

The literature in the field of communication disorders reports several studies that demonstrate the efficacy and benefits of telepractice as a viable method for delivering speech-language services to children in home and school settings. Several telepractice researchers have recommended using telepractice to reach children in rural school districts or urban settings where the access to services is limited due to the shortage of speech-language pathologists (Brown, Juenger, & Forducey, 2007).

Proponents of telepractice indicate that services provided via technology can yield the same treatment outcomes as face-to-face service delivery models if key elements are held consistent. In addition, supporters indicate that several challenges schools face with trying to provide services can be resolved by introducing telepractice as an alternative model. Outcomes research can provide evidence to determine if telepractice is an effective delivery format for assessment and intervention. Below is a list of several key aspects of service delivery that can be changed as a result of telepractice. Each can be measured to examine for the specific outcomes of telepractice. Simple tracking and data gathering methods can be established for each aspect.

*Key Aspects that Can Be Changed with Telepractice Service Delivery*

- Access to speech-language services can be increased by eliminating geographic and site-based barriers.
- Students with communication impairments can achieve clinical and educational outcomes, including improved literacy skills and school performance.
- The intensity and frequency of service delivery can be increased.
- Common scheduling challenges can be reduced.
- Costs for services can be reduced by introducing telepractice.
- Compensatory services can be provided.

## Breaking with Traditional Service Delivery Practices

Cirrin et al (2010) concluded that evidence supporting one service delivery option over another is largely lacking. They suggested that "clinicians must rely on reason based practice and their own data until more (scientific) data becomes available" (p. 250). Therefore, SLPs and their teammates in school districts should explore service delivery options, monitor students' progress, and take steps to determine the outcomes of various models. Cirrin and his fellow investigators recommended that controlled studies that examine the range of service models are needed. Reference was specifically made to the need for research on the effectiveness of *classroom-based* and *collaborative service* models.

**Table 6.1** highlights the design and results of a collaborative project implemented in a large urban school district. Ninety-seven middle school students demonstrated improved reading scores and communication skills after only 20 to 30 hours of indirect collaborative services. The SLP did not work directly with students. Rather, she very systematically coached reading instructors to use proven intervention strategies to elicit, modify, and reinforce speech-language skills.

## ◆ The Importance of Training

It is important that SLPs understand the value and benefits of outcomes measurement and reporting. They should also be prepared to administer tools systematically, reliably, and according to standardized procedures. Regardless of the outcomes collection instrument and process used, appropriate implementation can only be ensured by training clinicians to use the instruments and implement the processes properly. Training helps create the infrastructure necessary to support and sustain new practices and to ensure that the outcome data are being captured reliably. Training also enables team members to adopt common language for describing students, implementing services, discussing outcomes, and making clinical and programmatic decisions. Finally, team training helps build commitment to ensure that executing the process is a priority among team members. It also confirms that the organization is committing resources to ensure that the program will be a success.

Training should not be a single-session event. Because there are multiple occasions during the year when data may be collected or new projects undertaken, training should be provided for each significant aspect. Further, training should also be provided for new members of the school therapy team or education team as they join so that they can become familiar with the processes and procedures in place. Multiple media should be used to deliver the training, including face-to-face, written instructions and practice using case studies. Where there are teams of clinicians and educators who will use the tools, group training is advisable. That way the likelihood that they will use the tool appropriately and interpret the elements similarly will be increased.

In training and in written communication about the assessment instrument and measurement process, SLPs should do the following:

- Define the outcomes.
- Identify the outcomes data collection instrument to be used.
- Explain the purpose and value of collecting specific data to determine outcomes.
- Identify how collecting and reporting data fits into the speech-language program and school's goals and initiatives.
- Define specific competencies needed to administer the instrument and carry out the necessary steps.
- Emphasize the importance of functioning as an integrated, collaborative team.
- Provide guidance regarding how to incorporate the data collection into everyday service delivery practice by using the designated instruments to describe and create a profile for each child during the assessment, IEP, enrollment, and discharge processes.
- Explain how to administer, score, and interpret the instrument and follow step-by-step instructions.
- Specify methodology, tasks, and forms to be completed.
- Project the amount of time it will take to complete data forms for each student.
- Review outcomes data collection forms to ensure familiarity with procedures and terms as well as ease of administration.

- Provide timelines to follow, and stress the importance of adhering to the required methodology and guidelines.

- Explain how to integrate explanations of students' functional status profile and intervention outcomes into IEP discussions and meetings with parents and teachers.

- Identify potential challenges that may be encountered.

- Describe how to discuss outcomes with education partners.

- Explain how to respond to questions that may arise from others about outcomes or data collection.

# ♦ Achieving Administrator Understanding and Buy-In

Speech-language pathologists and school administrators must work together to execute the outcomes data collection process. Principals, general educators, special educators, and special education case managers/coordinators are familiar with instruments that document students' learning progress. For example, many districts implement the DIBELS instrument, which was mentioned earlier. It provides a database for schools to enter and report on student performance results for early literacy identified.

It is surprising to note that some school administrators may be reluctant for SLPs to introduce a new outcomes data collection process and instruments into the special education and related services process. Blosser, McCloskey, and Krupkin (2010) found that several administrators initially refused to let SLPs gather outcomes data for a treatment outcomes project using the NOMS, which was perplexing because there is so much emphasis in schools on data gathering, proving outcomes, and accountability. The administrators who expressed concern were contacted by phone and asked to express their concerns. The one reason consistently given was that they did not want to introduce new evaluation processes into the school system and speech-language service delivery, fearing litigation if new processes are introduced. They assumed that the NOMS was an assessment process and did not seem to understand that it was simply a method for gathering functional outcome data and reporting changes in functional communication status as a result of intervention. They did not want to step outside of the usual IDEA and IEP processes. Many thought that parents would have to sign a permission form for additional testing. Unfortunately, administrators' reluctance may actually be reflective of a lack of understanding of the goals of the speech-language disabilities and programs in general and the contributions SLPs make to the overall learning situation. Administrators may also lack awareness of methods for gathering and documenting outcomes data for the speech-language program. This lack of information presents an opportunity to increase administrators' awareness and understanding of the SLP's role, responsibilities, and capability for contributing to students' education success.

To conduct a successful outcomes measurement system, administrators and fellow education team members must be brought onboard so they understand the purpose and goals of outcomes measurement. Results should be explained so that their knowledge and appreciation for outcomes measurement in school-based speech-language services increases. Therefore, a recommended solution is to engage in discussions with administrators to determine the nature of their concern and to seize the opportunity to help them recognize the benefits of determining outcomes as a result of speech-language intervention. Steps should be taken to help them make the connection between their desire for accountability and the offer of a process and method for providing data. Ultimately we want administrators and education partners to realize the relationship between positive treatment outcomes and quality service delivery to the school's overall goals and initiatives. In most cases, the administrators do not understand that the tools used for data collection are simply tools that enable clinicians to describe students' functional performance and service delivery using available data.

Once the purpose is understood, administrators are generally very supportive of outcomes data collection, appreciating that these instruments are not a new assessment instrument or method outside of the IEP process, but are in support of the IEP process. Laying the groundwork with key administrators to guarantee buy-in prior to the implementation of outcome assessments is a logical and important first step in any new measurement methods. In addition to training the SLP team to implement outcomes data gathering processes, administrator and teacher training to increase awareness is also advisable.

## ◆ Conclusion and Future Directions

Schools are confronted with unprecedented challenges to meet constituents' demands and expectations. There is national consensus that students should complete school capable of using information to function in society, achieve goals, and develop knowledge. The national Common Core Curriculum standards serve as a vehicle for ensuring that students are prepared for advanced education and future employment. Constituents and advocates call for proof that the education and special education services students receive are of high quality and yield positive outcomes. They seek improved instruction, methods for measuring outcomes, and strategies for improving education. Speech-language pathologists can and should embrace this awesome responsibility to contribute to students' ability to access the curriculum, succeed within the educational context, and pursue productive lives. Doing so will ensure that the value and relevance of speech-language services are recognized.

This chapter presented a framework for considering the outcomes of three key aspects of school service delivery: student outcomes, partnership outcomes, and program outcomes. The three aspects are interconnected. The efficacy of the speech-language program can be verified in three ways: (1) by describing, measuring, and documenting students' functional performance in high- and low-demand learning situations and by measuring and documenting their progress toward specific educational goals over time; (2) by measuring and documenting changes in educators' and families' understanding and engagement in the intervention process; and (3) by observing and documenting changes in school organization practices and procedures to better support students with disabilities. This perspective encourages school-based practitioners to take a comprehensive perspective on their roles, responsibilities, and accomplishments.

Examples of the types of tools that can be used to gather and report pertinent data were provided. These tools serve as representative examples of the simple steps practitioners can take to better understand and manage the school work environment so that effective therapy can be implemented, significant people can be engaged, and systems can be modified. Students with disabilities will ultimately benefit.

## References

AIMSWeb Assessment and Measurement for RTI. (2011). PsychCorp. Bloomington, MN: Pearson Publishing. http://www.aimsweb.com

American Speech-Language-Hearing Association (ASHA). (2003). *National Outcomes Measurement System* (NOMS). Rockville, MD: Author

American Speech-Language-Hearing Association (ASHA). (2010a). *Roles and responsibilities*. http://www.asha.org

American Speech-Language-Hearing Association (ASHA). (2010b). *2010 Schools survey*. http://www.asha.org

American Speech-Language-Hearing Association (ASHA). (2011). *National outcomes measurement system (NOMS)*. http://www.asha.org/members/research/NOMS/default.htm

Blosser, J. (2011a). *School programs in speech-language pathology: Organization and service delivery.* San Diego: Plural Publishing

Blosser, J. (2011b). *Outcomes of a collaborative approach: Improved communication, improved reading.* American Speech-Language-Hearing Association Annual Convention, San Diego, CA

Blosser, J., & DePompei, R. (2003). *Pediatric traumatic brain injury: Proactive intervention* (2nd ed.) Clifton Park, NY: Delmar Learning

Blosser, J., & Kratcoski, A. (1997). PACS: A framework for determining appropriate service delivery options. *Language, Speech, and Hearing Services in Schools, 28,* 99–107

Blosser, J., McCloskey, L., & Krupkin, E. (2010). *Outcomes matter in school-based services.* Philadelphia: American Speech-Language-Hearing Association Annual Convention

Blosser, J., Subich, L., & Ehren, T. (2000). *Reliability and validity of data collection instruments in school speech-language pathology programs.* American Speech-Language-Hearing Association Task Force on Treatment Outcomes and Cost Effectiveness. Funded by the American Speech-Language-Hearing Foundation

Brown, J., Juenger, J., & Forducey, P. (2007). *Addressing shortages in schools via telepractice.* Rockville, MD: American Speech-Language-Hearing Association

CAST (Center for Applied Special Technology). (2011). *Universal design for learning guidelines,* version 2.0. Wakefield, MA: Author

Cirrin, F. M., Schooling, T. L., Nelson, N. W., Diehl, S. F., Flynn, P. F., Staskowski, M., et al. (2010, Jul). Evidence-based systematic review: effects of different service delivery models on communication outcomes for elementary school-age children. *Language, Speech, and Hearing Services in Schools, 41,* 233–264

Council for Exceptional Children. (2004). *Public policy update. Summary of regulations and guidance on accountability for academic achievement of students with significant cognitive disabilities.* http://www.sec.sped.org/Content/Navigation menu/PolicyAdvocacy/CECPolicyResources/AYP.pdf

Flower, R. M. (1984). *Delivery of speech-language and hearing services.* Baltimore, MD: Williams & Wilkins

Fuchs, L. S., & Fuchs, D. (2011). *What is scientifically-based research on progress monitoring?* www.aimsweb.com

Hanft, B., & Shepherd, J. (2008). *Collaborating for student success: A guide for school-based occupational therapy.* Bethesda, MD: The American Occupational Therapy Association

Individuals with Disabilities Education Act (IDEA). (1997). Public Law 1105-17, 20 U.S.C. 1400 *et. seq.*

Meline, T., & Kauffman, K. (2010). Evidence-Based Practice Briefs. A Speech-Language Pathologist's Dilemma: What is the Best Choice for Service Delivery in Schools? Pearson: Bloomington, MN. Retrieved from: http://www.speech andlanguage.com/ebp/pdfs/EBPV5A4.pdf

National Governors Association and Council of Chief State School Officers of Education. (2010). *The Core Curriculum State Standards.* Retrieved from: www.corestandards.org.

Rudebusch, J. (2011). *Measuring progress in SALSA.* Webinar, Louisiana Department of Education

Spady, W. G. (1994). *Outcomes-based education: Critical issues and answers.* Arlington, VA: American Association of School Administrators

State University of New York at Buffalo Research Foundation (SUNY). (1993). *Guide for the use of the uniform data set for the functional independence measure.* Buffalo: Author

University of Oregon College of Education, Center on Teaching and Learning. (2011). *DIBELS data system.* www.DIBELS .uoregon.edu

# 7

# Outcomes in Long-Term Care Settings

*William P. Goulding*

## ♦ Chapter Focus

This chapter amplifies the review of federal programs and policies discussed in Chapter 4 by looking at the effects of those programs and policies within the long-term care (LTC) setting. The unique nature and challenges of this setting are discussed in reference to both the positioning of LTC within the care continuum and the populations served. The impact of changes in regulation and reimbursement within LTC are discussed and how both federal and private attention to outcome measurement has caused the industry to move toward a more patient-centric, valued-based model of care.

## ♦ Introduction

Clinical outcomes have many potential uses besides simply measuring change in function. Outcomes can drive clinical decision making, help to identify clinical strengths and weaknesses, help to determine appropriate resource allocation, drive marketing initiatives, fuel patient advocacy efforts, provide a foundation for quality management, help to predict cost of care, and demonstrate value. Oftentimes, the setting in which the outcomes are used will determine the primary purposes that drive the need for an effective outcomes measurement initiative in that specific environment. That environment is made up of many, often conflicting, influences. In the LTC or skilled nursing facility (SNF), as in other settings, the critical driving forces that have shaped how outcomes are used include the ever-evolving *regulatory* and *reimbursement* forces, which have created a simultaneous evolution in priorities, patterns, and processes used in patient care by skilled rehabilitation providers. Because of this dynamic, outcomes have become a primary way to evaluate and demonstrate value. Outcomes in the LTC setting have and will continue to be used for a variety of purposes related to quality and patient safety oversight. Functional outcomes, particularly, are proving to be essential in measuring the value of skilled rehabilitation services in LTC and demonstrating the value of rehabilitation in the LTC setting within the care continuum.

# ♦ The LTC Setting

Before delving in detail into how outcomes are used in LTC settings, it may be helpful to discuss what makes this setting so unique. For it is only in understanding the distinctive nature of this setting that the evolution and usage of outcomes in LTC begin to make some sense. The primary LTC setting is the SNF. These two terms (LTC and SNF) will be used interchangeably throughout this chapter. The patient population in an SNF is typically composed of a certain percentage of residents who are admitted directly following discharge from the acute (hospital) setting after an acute or emergent intervention for an accident, surgery, acute illness, or significant exacerbation of an existing condition. In most SNFs the most frequent form of coverage for "room and board" and therapy services for those residents is Medicare (Part A). In some areas of the country, a growing percentage of coverage falls under a Medicare Advantage (Part C) policy (managed Medicare plan or a private managed care plan) that includes postacute services. The rest of the patient population in the SNF typically includes individuals whose therapy services are covered by Medicare (Part B) or "Medicare plus" policies, but the room-and-board portion of their costs are covered by Medicaid (a federally funded but state-administered medical assistance program) or by private insurance.

In the United States, the LTC setting lies smack in the middle of the continuum of care bridging the acute setting and multiple postacute intervention settings. For example, some patients are discharged from the hospital to an inpatient rehabilitation facility (IRF), some go to an SNF, and others go to their home or community setting with Home Health Agency services. As these settings have evolved from the 1990s up to the present, SNFs have taken a more prominent role in rehabilitation, and more and more patients have followed the path from hospital to SNF to home. The placement of the SNF in the center of the continuum means that the SNF therapists and care coordinators need to coordinate across settings. Although coordination across care settings has long been understood to be a central tenet of quality health care, regulatory and reimbursement processes are now mandating and monitoring care coordination across settings, as essential to "accountable care." Several factors are contributing to heighten the focus on better coordination across the care settings. One major factor is the pressure within acute care hospitals to minimize the length of stay (LOS) for hospital admissions; consequently, SNFs are accepting more patients who are sicker or less medically stable. As we will explore, this shift in the medical acuity status of patients admitted into SNFs has necessitated different treatment approaches and therapy utilization patterns. For postacute patients, it has become far more likely today than previously that they will be at the nursing facility only for their course of treatment and then they will be discharged back into a community setting. The SNF has, effectively, become a preferred subacute rehabilitation setting for those patients who are still too ill to go home, to be managed by home health services, or to be admitted directly into an inpatient or outpatient rehabilitation program, but who still require rehabilitation.

The provision of skilled therapy services in the SNF setting is increasingly viewed as a prudent approach to rehabilitation therapy in that rehabilitation intervention potentially decreases the SNF length of stay, increases the rate of successful facility discharges back to the community setting, and reduces the number of readmissions to the hospital. As was discussed in Chapters 4 and 5, hospitals receive financial penalties for readmissions occurring within 30 days of discharge. Even if the patient remains a resident in the SNF after skilled therapy has concluded, evidence suggests that the provision of skilled rehabilitation services during the postacute phase reduces the future "burden of care" to the facility. That burden can be measured by several objective indicators: the amount of staff time necessary to assist residents due to their deficits, medication use, and the extent of supplies and equipment usage necessary. As the burden of care decreases so does the cost of care. Outcomes in terms of cost data metrics and quality-of-life indicators for LTC residents support the provision of therapies within LTC settings aimed at increasing patients' functional status and independence as early as possible. Everyone benefits when patients become more independent.

In LTC one of the most important variables in treatment planning and outcome assessment is the age of the patient, as older patients tend to have more associated comorbidities and be more "medically complex." Comorbidities are one or more disorders or diseases that occur or are present in addition to the primary admitting condition. An example of the typical diagnostic and treatment scenario for a speech-language pathologist (SLP) might be a patient who presents with a cerebrovascular accident (CVA) with a secondary aphasia and dysphagia. The patient may have other preexisting conditions, such as late-stage parkinsonism and chronic obstructive pulmonary disease (COPD). These comorbid conditions present both a clinical intervention challenge for the SLP and an outcomes measurement challenge. Whether discussing the current burden of care or the rehabilitation potential of a patient, the LTC therapy provider cannot ignore the impact of comorbid conditions. Does the patient's parkinsonism include cognitive impairments along with the movement disorder, and how are those factors interacting with the language impairment and swallowing disorder? How do these combined deficits affect the patient's ability to benefit from restorative techniques? What additional risks will the COPD bring to the dysphagia and its management? Considering these factors, any attempt to measure outcomes needs to account for the impact of comorbid conditions.

## ◆ Outcomes Research on Rehabilitation in Long-Term Care

One of the factors that make it so difficult for LTC therapists to argue with key stakeholders (physicians, nurses, families, and clients) about the value of communication and swallowing therapy is that there has been relatively little effectiveness research looking at speech, language, cognitive, and swallowing treatment involving populations in an LTC setting. The recent attention given to outcomes research in rehabilitation is promising. However, there is not a lot of research involving nursing residents per se, and the cumulative total of studies in communication disorders associated with aging is limited. Clinicians who work in LTC facilities rely on research that is focused on the impact of "normal" aging on various functions, or on studies that have looked at specific diseases (parkinsonism, progressive neurological diseases) or disabilities (aphasia, dysarthria, dementia, traumatic brain injury, dysphagia, etc.). Unfortunately, often studies of these conditions have not controlled for the very comorbidities that are typically encountered in LTC settings.

## ◆ A Review of Outcomes Usage in Long-Term Care

A brief review of the history of outcomes in this unique care setting will help to provide some context for a discussion of the present and future state of outcomes usage. There is a long history of interest in outcomes measurement in the LTC setting. Health care as a "product" is an elusive entity to capture in objective terms, and yet it is critical to do so in a setting where dollars are limited and highly scrutinized prior to issuance; that is especially the case in LTC. Although that may seem to be a cold and calculated way of describing the situation, "limited resources" often means "limited dollars" and limited access to care for those who could benefit from services.

Since at least the 1950s, there have been scales that attempt or purport to measure physical function. In most cases, these early scales focused on activities of daily living (ADL) such as bathing, dressing, grooming, and toileting. Some examples of some of the very early leaders in this arena include the **P**hysical condition, **U**pper limb function, **L**ower limb function, **S**ensory components, **E**xcretory function, and emotional or mental **S**tatus (PULSES) Profile (Moskowitz and McCann, 1957) and the Barthel Index (Mahoney, Wood, & Barthel, 1958). However, with the possible exception of measuring eating (feeding) abilities, these scales do not typically encompass areas of concern to SLPs. It was not until the 1980s that tools were developed that attempted to measure communication skills for outcomes purposes. Early pioneers in this area included the Functional Status Rating System (Forer, 1981), the Patient Evaluation Conference System (PECS) (Harvey & Jellinek, 1981) and the Functional Independence Measure (FIM™) (Hamilton, Granger, Sherwin, Zielezny, & Tashman, 1987). The FIM, largely because of its popularity in the acute (hospital) setting, was perhaps the most widely used functional ability measure in LTC in the mid-1980s and 1990s. As of 2011, over 1400 facilities subscribed to FIM via the Uniform Data System for Medical Rehabilitation (UDSMR), and their databases included over 16 million patient assessments. Because of its early primacy on the outcomes landscape, the FIM remains the most widely used functional outcomes measure in clinical studies related to rehabilitation.

The American Speech-Language-Hearing Association (ASHA) developed the National Outcomes Measurement System (NOMS) (American Speech-Language-Hearing Association, 2003, n.d.), which is a data collection system that measures the impact of intervention services delivered to both adults and children with various communication and swallowing disorders. If there has been limited usage of the NOMS system in the LTC setting, it is only because it is a "single-discipline" tool. An outcomes measurement tool that only looks at the impact of a single discipline in a multidisciplinary treatment environment has limited applications. It is certainly useful from an internal clinical and quality management standpoint. In a setting that is increasingly being asked to focus more on demonstrating patient-centered value, however, the more useful measures are those that cross all rehabilitation disciplines. Because of the unique nature of the LTC patient and the LTC treatment environment, many rehabilitation providers in the 1990s looked for tools that could measure performance across all treatment disciplines and across a broader range of function. SNF-based providers need to be able to treat (and measure) the functions that are most important to the subacute patient, such as following basic commands, answering basic questions, and safely consuming nutrition. However, in the very same treatment day, they may be working with patients who are focusing on high-level executive functions such as balancing a checkbook or reading bus schedules and deciding on routes in preparation for a potential return to the community. Such a wide range demands a tool or tools that can represent the impact that speech-language services can have across that broad functional spectrum.

This led many providers in LTC to use multiple instruments in the same therapy practice. It also resulted in many "homemade" measurement tools in an effort to fill a perceived gap that was not met in commercially available tools. Although this made it increasingly difficult to compare across facilities or establish any sort of industry benchmarks, this was not seen as a critical need in the 1990s, because at that time outcomes were used for two primary purposes: internal quality improvement measures and external marketing. Most providers were content to be able to compare their clinicians' performance to each other and occasionally create a graph that demonstrated "measurable impact" on a specific patient or group of patients that could be used in a mailer or flyer to the local community. By the time the regulatory world for postacute patients turned upside down in 1999 with the advent of the Prospective Payment System (PPS), many providers had to reassess the importance of their outcomes programs. PPS is described in the next section, but suffice it to say here that to survive financially, non–revenue-generating clinical activities needed to be scrutinized, scaled back, and often eliminated. In an effort to make their departments as efficient as possible, many providers simply stopped or significantly curtailed such activities as screening, providing in-service training, and collecting functional outcomes measurements.

## ♦ Evolving Patterns of Regulation and Reimbursement in Long-Term Care

To truly understand outcomes in LTC settings, it is important to understand how rehabilitation services are paid in these settings. However, to understand how services are paid in LTC settings, we must begin with how services are paid in the setting that refers the most patients for LTC admissions—the acute hospital. For the most part, hospitals are paid via a system called "prospective payment." Prospective payment takes many different forms in the various settings in which it is now used. However, all prospective payment systems attempt to identify certain key predictors of cost so that the payer can calculate or negotiate the appropriate amount of payment with the provider of the services before they are actually provided. In the case of the hospital setting, the predictors that are used are the geographic location of the hospital (and its associated labor and supply costs) and diagnosis-related groups (DRGs). The DRG system was developed with material support from the Health Care Financing Administration (HCFA), which is now called the Centers for Medicare and Medicaid Services (CMS), discussed in greater detail in Chapter 4. The Department of Health and Human Services (DHHS) administers the Medicare program. In this chapter, we will use references to the "Medicare program" and "CMS" interchangeably.

In October 1983 the DRG system began to be phased in as the method by which hospitals are paid by the Medicare program. In essence, DRGs are a "per case" payment system that places a patient in a diagnostic category, such as "spinal disorders and injuries" or "degenerative nervous system disorders." The premise is that patients in those groupings will need similar services (physician fees, rehabilitation services, medications, supplies, etc.) during their hospital stay. Therefore, a flat per-case reimbursement fee is associated with each DRG in each different geographic region. Because of this kind of prospective payment system, hospitals know exactly what they will be paid to care for a given inpatient, based on his or her diagnoses. They also know that it will not matter if that patient ends up needing to stay more than the typical number of days or needs more than the typical amount of rehabilitation services or medications or supplies. Regardless of the services that the patient actually uses, the hospital will receive only the dollar amount associated with the DRG in that specific geographic area. This creates incentives for hospitals to be as efficient as possible in their care decisions. However, this system also creates an incentive for hospitals to discharge patients to the next (presumably less expensive) care setting sooner than they would have in the past. As a result, postacute care (PAC) settings such as inpatient rehabilitation facilities (IRFs), home health agencies (HHAs), and skilled nursing facilities (SNFs) were quickly beginning to see patients with a higher level of acuity. The short-hand (and somewhat cynical) way to refer to this phenomenon was that the PAC settings began to receive patients "quicker and sicker." It is no surprise, therefore, that each of these settings would eventually see the advent of cost containment by way of their own prospective payment systems.

In the SNF setting, payment reform came in 1997 with the passage of the Balanced Budget Act (BBA, 1997). Prior to this reform, nursing facilities were reimbursed for therapy services based on how much cost they associated with the services. If the patients that were being treated were in a distinct part of the building that was set aside to treat newly admitted patients who had recently been discharged from an acute hospital, much of the cost for running that distinct part of the building (utilities, nursing staff wages, etc.) was used to determine how much the facility would bill for the therapy services. This is an example of a form of retrospective or after-the-fact payment that CMS wanted to phase out in favor of prospective or before-the-fact payments. The BBA of 1997 introduced an enormous change in how SNF services would be paid for patients who were admitted after a hospital stay. Beginning July 1, 1998, SNF facilities were no longer paid on a reasonable cost basis, but rather on the basis of their own version of a prospective payment system. This new system was somewhat similar to the DRGs used in the hospital system, in that SNF PPS payment rates are adjusted for geographic variations in wages and cover all costs of furnishing covered SNF services. However, in this system, per diem (daily) payments for each patient are based on a classification system that attempts to predict the amount and type of resources that patients will use during their skilled stay. Based on data gathered from a resident assessment called the minimum data set (MDS), the patient is placed in a resource utilization group (RUG). The premise is that if the payer (CMS) knows the likely amount of resources that will be needed, it can set a daily fee that will be paid to the SNF as long as the SNF is able to justify that the patient needs that level of services, up to a maximum of 100 days per year. Once again, the provider of the care (the SNF) knows how much it will receive to care for that patient every day and also knows that this reimbursement rate will not change if the patient ends up needing more than the typical services, supplies, or equipment during that time period. At certain scheduled intervals (or if there is a significant change in the patient's status), the SNF is able to do a reassessment of the resources needed by the patient and has an opportunity to receive a different daily rate going forward from that time. Clearly, the incentive that is created by such a system is to get as clear and accurate a measure of the patient's status as possible and then to be as efficient as possible in the provision of care.

Although it may seem unusual for a text on outcomes to explain in detail the evolution of payment systems, it is not possible to separate the evolution of outcomes from the necessity of dealing with payment systems. How providers are paid has driven a need for them to revisit their models for care provision. They have been constantly looking for ways to be more efficient. In other words, they must ask, "Can we maintain our level of *effectiveness* but do so in a more cost-*efficient* manner?" Put another way, "How can we get quality clinical outcomes for less?" That is where the drive to accurately demonstrate the *value equation* as objectively as possible began.

As previously mentioned, in the health care world, delineating that value equation is a difficult process. If we envision the equation as "cost vs. benefit," we can see the problem. Cost is easily measured in any health care environment. The "weight" of that cost is obvious to the payers and consumers of health care as soon as they receive the bill for services and is often the primary focus because it is so eminently measurable. The "benefit" side of the equation is less tangible and the one that has always been difficult to define in objective terms. This is where functional outcome measures serve an invaluable purpose. It gives health care providers an objective measure against which to weigh the cost of care. However, because the rehabilitation industry has struggled for so long to develop and use a consistent measure of functional performance, the task has now been taken up and mandated by those who pay for the services.

## Centers for Medicare and Medicaid Services Initiatives to Define Value

The CMS has been in search of valid measures of value for many years so that it can shift from a fee-for-service (FFS) payment model to a value-based purchasing (VBP) model. CMS has already begun to pay for reporting of quality data for hospitals, home health agencies, and physicians. For example, the Tax Relief and Health Care Act of 2006 (TRHCA) (Public Law 109-432) required the establishment of a quality reporting system for eligible professionals, including an incentive payment for eligible professionals who satisfactorily report data on quality measures for covered professional services furnished to Medicare beneficiaries. CMS named this program the Physician Quality Reporting Initiative (PQRI). In the 2010 version of the PQRI, there were a total of 153 clinical quality measures from which eligible professional could select to report.

According to CMS's Roadmap for Implementing Value Driven Healthcare in the Traditional Medicare Fee-for-Service Program, the agency

> has begun to transform itself from a passive payer of services into an active purchaser of higher quality, affordable care. Further future efforts to link payment to the quality and efficiency of care provided would shift Medicare away from paying providers based solely on their volume of services. The catalyst for such change would be grounded in the creation of appropriate incentives encouraging all health care providers to deliver higher quality care at lower total costs. (CMS, n.d.)

In essence, this is what VBP is all about. Any VBP system in the health care setting must be founded upon some clinical measures that have been generally agreed upon as being effective measures of function, as well as resource utilization. The lack of consensus on that point has, of course, been the proverbial "thorn in the side" for the rehabilitation community. However, CMS is clearly looking for some measure by which care is evidence-based and outcomes-driven to better manage diseases and prevent complications from them.

Along these lines, CMS conducted several versions of VBP pilot programs that focused on different measures and incentives. In the SNF setting, the pilot program focused upon four domains: staffing (staffing levels and turnover rates), hospitalizations (rate of potentially avoidable hospitalizations), MDS outcomes (select outcomes from the already available resident MDS assessment), and survey deficiencies (from state survey inspections). CMS then awarded points to each nursing home based on how it performed on each measure. These points led to an overall quality score. For each state, nursing homes with scores in the top 20% and homes that are in the top 20% in terms of improvement in their scores were eligible for a share of that state's savings pool. This concept of shared risk and shared benefits is essentially the model for *accountable care organizations* (ACOs), which are discussed below (see Shared Risk and Care Coordination) and elsewhere in this text (see Chapters 4, 5 and 8).

## Post Acute Care Reform

Another initiative that CMS undertook to change the culture in PAC settings was to contract with the Research Triangle Institute (RTI) to develop a standardized patient assessment tool for use at the acute hospital discharge and at all PAC settings' admission and discharge. The concept is that this tool, the Continuity Assessment Record and Evaluation (CARE) tool, would measure the health and functional status of Medicare acute discharges and measure changes in severity and other outcomes for Medicare PAC patients across the various settings that a patient may utilize. This initiative began in November 2006 with input from the scientific communities, including each of the health care provider communities and experts in health services research and information technology.

This CARE tool uses informatics technology to develop interoperable, Web-based data reporting systems for the Medicare program. Most pertinent for this topic, it was designed to measure outcomes in physical and medical treatments while controlling for factors that affect outcomes, such as cognitive impairments and social and environmental factors. The assessment tool is being developed to eventually replace similar items on the existing Medicare assessment forms, including the Outcome and Assessment Information Set (OASIS) (home health), MDS (SNF), and Inpatient Rehabilitation Facility Patient Assessment Instrument (IRFPAI) (IRF) tools. For additional discussion of the CARE tool, see Chapters 2, 5 and 8.

## Managed Care Initiatives to Define Value

Managed care entities have long been far ahead of CMS in their efforts to move toward a "pay for performance" (sometimes abbreviated as P4P) reimbursement system. Unlike a federally administered program like those under CMS, there is no single model or representative entity that we can call "managed care." Managed care is essentially insurance organizations whose goal is to oversee the care decisions for their members (the patients) in such a way as to ensure efficiency and cost-effectiveness. The basic principles of managed care mirror many of the value equation concepts that are becoming increasingly more central in reimbursement for services in the PAC settings.

Because managed care organizations (MCOs) are varied and numerous (and growing every day) and unaffiliated with one another, there have been many variations on the theme to achieve the effectiveness versus efficiency balance. In general, however, the systems tend to depend on someone in a *case manager* role. That individual is responsible for granting initial and ongoing access to the member/patient. The case manager also (often after consultation with physicians and other team members) determines the amount of access that will be granted to the member/patient. For example, upon initial evaluation, an SLP might project getting the patient to a point that he or she could respond to and effectively convey simple one-step messages within 30 treatment sessions. The case manager will usually have some sort of a library of benchmark data against which to compare that goal and the estimated length of stay (LOS).

This example demonstrates how the informatics and data oversight within managed care entities are clearly ahead of CMS in the search for the value equation. MCOs typically require that specific data be submitted for billing purposes. These data will often include demographic information and clinical data that can be cross-referenced with functional measures and treatment patterns. Often, MCOs will have a specific tool or tools that they will expect the rehabilitation provider to use to measure function. For example, the FIM (mentioned previously) is utilized frequently in this manner. The data from these tools create the benchmarks that will carry weight in the case manager's decision-making process. That case manager can look at LOS data for patients with a similar diagnosis and, sometimes, even similar goals when making a determination as to how many sessions an SLP can have to treat one of the organization's patient/members with a given diagnosis and stated therapy goal.

Although this may seem restrictive at times, the MCOs have also been leading the way in helping to identify ways in which rehabilitation professionals can add value to the equation. One enormous area of focus has been on determining the best setting in the acute and postacute continuum in which to treat patients. Each setting has a different cost structures. For example, the acute care hospital setting is the most expensive setting for rehabilitation services compared with an inpatient rehabilitation facility setting, which is more expensive than the SNF setting, which is more expensive than a home health setting. If it can be confirmed that *outcomes* (for example, the rate of discharge back to a community setting without readmissions or the amount of functional return following intervention) are similar between two different settings, then the less expensive setting offers the better value. In the same manner, there has been increased focus on recidivism, which refers to patients who "recede" from a less restrictive (and less expensive) setting such as a SNF to a more restrictive (and more expensive) setting such as a hospital. Rehospitalizations that are thought to have been avoidable have become one of the primary markers of poor quality. Accordingly, if SLPs can demonstrate (for example) that improved cognition can lead to better safety and judgment and, therefore, to a lower likelihood of an accident that would lead to a hospitalization, or if they can diminish aspiration and the postdischarge pneumonia risk, they have added value to the value equation that can be understood by a case manager.

# ◆ The Future of Outcomes in Long-Term Care

## Predictive Modeling

Although it is quite difficult to accurately predict the future role of outcomes in LTC settings, there are clearly two trends that are in play to shape that role. Those that pay for LTC services want demonstrated value for their dollars. In addition, they prefer to have the financial commitment determined prospectively. Therefore, in order for providers of skilled therapy services to compete for patient access, they will employ a statistical methodology called predictive modeling that will allow them to predict for the payer the expected outcome as well as the cost to achieve that outcome with sufficient certainty to obtain approval for services. The subsequent challenge is to provide those services in an efficient manner, so as to maintain some profit margin in an increasingly competitive atmosphere.

In its simplest form, predictive modeling is a process by which a model is created to try to predict the probability of an outcome. That prediction is most often based on some form of regression analysis, in which unknown values are predicted based on known values of one or more variables. For example, the prospective payment model that was introduced in the LTC setting beginning in 1999 was based on gathering a "minimum data set" of information regarding the patient and using it to predict what resources the patient will utilize during an upcoming period of time. Predictive modeling is not an especially new analytic approach; some form of it has been used for decades by actuaries in the insurance industry and in financial services, by pharmacists, and by personnel in other areas of health care. However, its application is relatively new in the LTC rehabilitation world due to the relative paucity of foundational data that are available with respect to patient outcomes. It is difficult to do the sort of data mining that is necessary to make cost versus benefit predictions when there is relatively little data to be mined. Fortunately, the growing foundation of outcomes research in LTC rehabilitation and the even larger foundation of collected outcomes via commercial tools and industry instruments such as the MDS in SNFs has enabled several entities (both public and private) to begin to reliably predict the value equation (cost versus benefit) that payers and providers will need going forward. A commercial example of the application of predictive modeling within MCOs to improve efficiencies in LTC is found in the statistical tools developed and outcomes reported by SeniorMetrix (SeniorMetrix, n.d.). SeniorMetrix applies predictive modeling statistics to identify "at risk" members, decrease the length of stay in SNFs, and objectively quantify burden of care outcomes. The driving innovators behind this corporate product are Rick Ganz, CEO, and Reg Warren, chief science officer (an SLP and collaborator with the Health Disability Research Institute at Boston University's Sargent College). SeniorMetrix provides MCO health plans and disease management organizations with standards of care, objective measurements, and rehabilitation services for medically fragile elders, and is serving as a model for the LTC industry.

### Shared Risk and Care Coordination

Another trend that will almost certainly drive the future of outcomes in LTC is the movement toward "shared risk." One such endeavor falls under the umbrella that is sometimes referred to as an accountable care organization (ACO), mentioned earlier and discussed elsewhere in this text in Chapters 4, 5 and 8. An ACO is essentially a collaboration among physicians, hospitals, and other providers (such as rehabilitation specialists) that is held clinically and financially accountable for health care delivery for a given group of patients. These collaborators have a common goal: to improve quality and decrease costs across episodes of care. The reason that they have this goal in common is that they will share extra profit for care that is more efficient and results in cost savings to the payer. Conversely, they also share the risk that care could be more expensive than expected. It is easy to see how those entities that have reliable predictive analytics will be better able to participate as a member of such collaborative efforts.

The Medicare program ventured into this realm beginning in 2010, when it introduced its own ACO program pilot. It represents yet another attempt on the part of CMS to pay prospectively for proven value rather than retrospectively for services that have little to no measurable or reportable impact on reducing the burden of care on the health care industry. It also supports the primacy of coordination of care across PAC settings, to ensure that care is provided with a *patient-centric focus,* rather than from a provider-centric or a payer-centric focus.

## ♦ Conclusion and Future Directions

Perhaps ironically, the advent of the Prospective Payment System (PPS) in the LTC setting brought the potential uses of clinical outcomes full circle. Although PPS places a heavy emphasis on demonstrating value, to navigate and survive in an environment of increasing costs and decreasing reimbursement, providers of rehabilitation services will need to be able to know their costs, their clinical strengths and weaknesses, and the market value of their services, to continue to advocate for a fair cost-benefit balance as they strive to provide quality services.

The lessons for the LTC rehabilitation practitioner are clear. To be an efficient and effective provider for your patients, you will need to

- know the costs of providing care to various patient types;

- know how to predict outcomes and costs by patient types (i.e., by diagnostic group) and account for the impact of comorbidities; and

- know your clinical capabilities (i.e., the treatment areas you can reliably address and still provide meaningful outcomes).

But most importantly in LTC, considering the challenges of a largely geriatric patient population, you must be able to advocate for those individuals who do not have a sufficient voice in the discussion to advocate for themselves. The best resource for that advocacy is clinical outcomes data.

## References

American Speech-Language-Hearing Association. (2003). *National outcomes measurement system (NOMS): Adult speech-language pathology user's guide.* Rockville, MD: Author

American Speech-Language-Hearing Association. (n.d.). *National outcomes measurement system (NOMS).* http://www.asha.org/members/research/NOMS/default.htm

Balanced Budget Act (BBA). (1997), Public Law 105-33, 111 Stat. 251 (1997)

Centers for Medicare and Medicaid Services (CMS). (n.d.). *Roadmap for implementing value-driven health care in the traditional Medicare fee-for-service program.* https://www.cms.gov/QualityInitiativesGenInfo/downloads/VBPRoadmap_OEA_1-16_508.pdf

Forer, S. K. (1981). *Revised functional status rating instrument.* Glendale, CA: Rehabilitation Institute, Glendale Adventist Medical Center

Hamilton, B. B., Granger, C. V., Sherwin, F. S., Zielezny, M., & Tashman, J. S. (1987). A uniform national data system for medical rehabilitation. In: M. J. Fuhrer (Ed.), *Rehabilitation outcomes: Analysis and measurement* (pp. 137–147). Baltimore: Paul H. Brookes

Harvey, R. F., & Jellinek, H. M. (1981, Sep). Functional performance assessment: a program approach. *Archives of Physical Medicine and Rehabilitation, 62,* 456–460

Mahoney, F. I., Wood, O. H., & Barthel, D. W. (1958, May). Rehabilitation of chronically ill patients: the influence of complications on the final goal. *Scientific Medical Journal, 51,* 605–609

Moskowitz, E., & McCann, C. B. (1957, Mar). Classification of disability in the chronically ill and aging. *Journal of Chronic Diseases, 5,* 342–346

SeniorMetrix. (n.d.). http://www.seniormetrix.com/)

# III

# Organizational Performance

# 8

# Outcomes in Health Care: Achieving Transparency Through Accreditation

*Paul R. Rao*

## ♦ Chapter Focus

Health care in the United States is provided in a variety of venues, across severity and acuity levels of care, with a plethora of payment practices and a patchwork quilt of oversight policies and accrediting and licensing bodies. This chapter focuses on accreditation processes and accrediting programs that intersect with settings and services provided by audiologists, speech-language pathologists (SLPs), and other medical rehabilitation professionals. The chapter considers how health care and accreditation have been buffeted in recent decades by public policy priorities, yet the one constant and essential contribution of accreditation across all settings of care is the emphasis on *transparency*. This chapter argues for greater transparency, engendered by accreditation and demanded by the current consumer-centric era of health care services, as essential to the future of rehabilitation services.

## ♦ Introduction

A 2009 study by the Organization for Economic Cooperation and Development (OECD) found that spending on health care in the United States far outpaced that in other industrialized countries (Levey, 2011). Health care spending in the U.S. accounted for 17.4% of the nation's total economic output, nearly twice the average of the 34 OECD member countries. The next biggest health spender, the Netherlands, spent just 12% of its gross domestic product on medical care. Despite the level of spending, most other OECD countries have made far greater progress in recent decades in reducing child mortality and extending life expectancy (Levey, 2011). If there is one overarching lesson that can be drawn from outcome data in health care over the past three decades it is that increased spending does not necessarily translate to improved health outcomes. Bridging that disparity by engendering greater transparency of performance outcomes against quality standards is the essential purpose and challenge of accreditation programs in this country. Accreditation processes are principally aimed at ensuring the organization's compliance with quality of care and patient safety standards across settings and levels of care.

The settings and levels of care found in the U.S. are wide ranging, and include emergent care (emergency departments); intensive/critical care services (intensive care units); acute care settings (hospitals); acute and subacute rehabilitation (inpatient rehabilitation facilities); skilled nursing facilities and long-term care (nursing homes); long-term acute-care hospitals; observation beds, day hospitals, or day surgery (less than 24-hour admissions); home health agencies; specialty clinics, such as ambulatory outpatient care centers; comprehensive outpatient rehabilitation facilities; and private practice. It is not unusual for a patient who has suffered a traumatic head injury or stroke to pass through the hands of a half dozen different care teams, providing services across several different levels of care during the course of their rehabilitation intervention. Each level of care is under some type of accreditation microscope to oversee and vouch for the quality of care and to continuously scrutinize health outcomes data. Within this network, the professional disciplines of audiology and speech-language pathology are caught between "a rock and a hard place" with the challenge of demonstrating medical necessity and candidacy for treatment, while at the same time attempting to provide access to care for persons with disabilities within the least costly and the most effective and appropriate milieu.

## ◆ Accreditation in Rehabilitation

One way to appreciate the value of accreditation in health care as the beacon of quality via its quality framework is to examine the history of accreditation in rehabilitation and the evolution of accreditation to the broader industry of health care. Rehabilitation services have been "preaching and teaching" notions about functional outcomes and patient-centric care since the dawn of the professions. Many decades before other health care entities (medicine and surgery) formally recognized the importance of communication and teamwork in preventing medical errors, rehabilitation services were advocating for multidisciplinary communication, a "team" approach to service delivery, and standards built around the patient. According to Boone (2011), accreditation as a quality framework was constructed by the rehabilitation industry in response to environmental pressures to demonstrate a commitment to quality.

Since its inception in 1966, as the only rehabilitation-specific accrediting body, the Commission on Accreditation of Rehabilitation Facilities (CARF) has been setting quality standards for the broad rehabilitation industry, including medical rehabilitation (CARF, 2011). CARF's quality standards have changed through the years to meet the demands of the broader and changing health care environment. CARF has pioneered standards development and evaluation by making the process consumer-centric and always focusing on the needs of the person served. CARF surveyors come from the rehabilitation trenches and from organizations that have earned CARF accreditation. The CARF surveyors are somewhat unique in the accreditation industry, as they place the person served as their focus and bring that underlying principle to the survey of each organization seeking CARF accreditation. Other quality management frameworks include the Malcolm Baldridge National Quality Program (2011), the International Organization for Standardization (2000), and the Joint Commission (TJC, 2011), to be discussed later.

### Facility and Staff Licensure

Each state in the U.S. and the District of Columbia has a set of laws and regulations that provide health care institutions within that state guidance on the Certificate of Need (CoN), if applicable. For example, Texas and Louisiana have no CoN process, whereas in the District of Columbia, to open up a new program or purchase a piece of capital equipment that exceeds $100,000, the provider must complete a lengthy application and a CoN explaining the rationale for the request and vouching that the purchase would add value, not be duplicative within D.C., and would have a return on investment (ROI), and comply with the rules and regulations for the provision and operation of health care units and facilities. In Maryland law (Annotated Code of Maryland, 2001), under Health–General Article, a CoN is required for establishment of an open heart surgery, organ transplant surgery, or burn or neonatal intensive care service. In addition, an inpatient rehabilitation facility requires a CoN with criteria to expand licensed rehab beds in a 50-bed unit or less, and the average occupancy must be 80% to be considered.

The District of Columbia has a lengthy set of regulations that address the environment of care, patient care processes, infection control procedures, medical staff credentialing, human resources, administration, pharmacy, dietary, medical records, quality and performance improvement, and other areas such as risk management, privacy, and compliance. All licensed practitioners must hold current licenses. Failure of a health care provider to possess a current state license is grounds for immediate notice of failure to protect consumers, and could be grounds to close the facility. With respect to audiology and speech-language pathology, local requirements vary among jurisdictions but frequently have significant impact on the occupancy license involving such areas as fire safety, infection control, and the parameters of employees' entitlement to family and medical leave. State licensure requirements for audiology have been adopted in 50 states and the District of Columbia and been adopted in 49 states and the District of Columbia for speech-language pathology, although specific exemptions to these requirements sometimes exist. For example, school SLPs in Colorado, which currently has no SLP licensure, must possess the Certificate of Clinical Competence (CCC) from the American Speech-Language-Hearing Association (ASHA) or demonstrate equivalent completion of the CCC requirements to provide for and bill Medicaid services. Many states are also enacting laws to deal with speech-language pathology assistants (SLP-As). All such state and local requirements must be incorporated into the department's preparation for not only the state licensure survey but for the Joint Commission (TJC), when applicable.

In D.C., each licensed provider/facility must be licensed annually by the health department's regulatory arm to continue operations. For example, the National Rehabilitation Hospital (NRH; Washington, D.C.) facility's license expired on August 31, 2011. Hence the facility was expecting an unannounced visit from the D.C. Department of Health (DoH) Survey Team some time before the expiration date of its health care license. The DoH sends seven surveyors (nurses, an administrator, a sanitarian, a radiology technician, and a pharmacist), who conduct, over a period of 3 days, file reviews of closed and open medical records and of medical affairs and human resources files, data inspections including unusual occurrence reports, environmental inspections, and visits to and interviews within each department of the hospital. Each facility or hospital license visit itinerary is predictable, beginning with an opening session when the facility's administration provides the survey team an update of the facility (see example in **Table 8.1**), any important staffing or other changes that have occurred since last year's visit, any significant financial variance, data about the average length of stay, year-to-date metrics, as well as a review of major accomplishments and challenges. The survey team then branches out to the facility to conduct its review of all of the standards and regulations under its purview as well as checking to ensure the corrections recommended and approved from last year's DoH hospital license visit were in fact implemented. At the conclusion of the licensure visit, administration meets with the DoH survey team, and the surveyors report their list of findings, recommendations, and deficiencies. The survey report is expected to be received by the facility within 10 working days. The facility then has 45 calendar days to provide a plan of correction for each recommendation/deficiency. Once the DoH approves the plan of correction, an annual occupancy license is granted. The DoH in Washington, D.C., performs several other regulatory duties besides its annual licensure survey, and these will be illustrated in the discussion that follows with regard to the state of Maryland.

Not all state health departments conduct annual license/occupancy reviews. For example, by statute in the state of Maryland, all nursing homes must be surveyed annually by the health department, but hospitals are surveyed only at the time of opening for initial occupancy and afterward for cause (e.g., a serious safety incident or patient complaint), or as a part of a Centers for Medicare and Medicaid Services (CMS) validation survey. A for-cause health department survey may take days or weeks depending on the seriousness of the incidents or complaints. Once the DoH completes its for-cause survey at a Maryland facility, a report of findings and recommendations is compiled and brought to the facility for an in-person license review and summary of findings. The outcome of a for-cause survey by the DoH may result in at least one of four potential outcomes: (1) the complaint

**Table 8.1**   Template for the National Rehabilitation Hospital's 2011 Update to the Department of Health's Annual Survey for License for Occupancy

National Rehabilitation Hospital (NRH)
Annual Update
March 2011
NRH's silver anniversary year; opened 25 years ago on February 6, 1986

| | |
|---|---|
| Number of licensed beds | 128 adult, 9 pediatric |
| Average daily census (2010): | 101.9 |
| Average length of stay (2010): | 17.21 days |

**Programs:**

| | |
|---|---|
| 2 East | Orthopedic and stroke |
| 2 West | Spinal cord injury and cardiac rehabilitation |
| 3 East | Traumatic brain injury |
| 3 South | Stroke recovery |
| 3 West | National center for children's rehabilitation/pediatrics |

**Leadership:**
**Recognition:**
**Business Development:**
**Research:**
**Environment:**
**Satisfaction/Patient Experience:**
**Safety:**
**Publications:**
**Emergency Preparedness:**
**Information Systems:**
**Human Resources:**
**Community Outreach and Education:**
**Governance:**
**Performance Improvement:**
**Compliance:**
**Department of Health:**
**Accreditation:**

or report of harm was not sustained and there are no required actions on the part of the surveyed facility; (2) the complaint or report of harm was sustained, and the facility is fined and cited and given an opportunity to provide a plan of correction within a specified time frame and is revisited by DoH for compliance within a prescribed interval; (3) the complaint or report of harm was sustained and of such a serious nature that the facility is fined and put on conditional licensure and revisited by DoH within a prescribed period of time in order to remain open for services; and (4) the complaint or report of harm was sustained and of such a severe nature that the facility loses its license as a health care facility and is shut down pending an appeal.

Another DoH survey role is to conduct a validation survey. When a hospital receives a survey outcome from the TJC accrediting body, TJC has what is called "deemed status," effectively meaning it *accredits on behalf of and with the authority of CMS*. The CMS, however, must validate these non-CMS surveys. To validate these non-CMS accreditation surveys that provide deemed status to the surveyed hospital, CMS must sample and survey *10% of all accreditation surveys* that occur within a given year and that provide deemed status to the facility. If a given facility loses accreditation or deemed status, that facility can no longer admit Medicare or Medicaid beneficiaries or be reimbursed by CMS for Medicare or Medicaid services. NRH's inpatient case mix, for example, is 40% Medicare and 20% Medicaid; thus, 60% of the facility's reimbursement is tied to CMS. The loss of CMS approval would be devastating to most health care facilities. So the odds of a facility in Maryland receiving a validation survey within 30 days (the interval within which CMS requires the follow-up validation survey) by TJC are 1 in 10. The health department, which acts on behalf of CMS, must review all of the CMS conditions of participation (to be discussed later) and compare the validation results with the deemed status TJC survey. The director of CMS is required to report back to the congressional oversight panel the results of its validation surveys on an annual basis. This report to Congress is typically a very stressful and sometimes acrimonious hearing for the director, who must explain why a deemed status accrediting body such as TJC missed so many serious issues. As a result of such scrutiny, CMS has added greater oversight and review of current health care accrediting bodies such as TJC with deemed status, and has authorized deemed status to other accrediting bodies, allowing them to compete with the accreditors such as TJC.

## ◆ Centers for Medicare and Medicaid Services Conditions of Participation and Conditions for Coverage

The CMS develops *conditions of participation* (CoPs) and *conditions for coverage* (CfCs) that health care organizations must meet to begin and continue participating in the Medicare and Medicaid programs. These minimum health and safety standards are the foundation for improving quality and protecting the health and safety of beneficiaries. CMS also ensures that the standards of accrediting organizations recognized by CMS (again, through a process called "deeming") meet or exceed the Medicare standards set forth in the CoPs/CfCs.

The CoPs and CfCs are the minimum health and safety standards that providers and suppliers must meet to be Medicare and Medicaid certified. CoPs and CfCs apply to the following health care organizations:

- Ambulatory surgical centers
- Comprehensive outpatient rehabilitation facilities
- Critical access hospitals
- End-stage renal disease facilities
- Federally qualified health centers
- Home health agencies
- Hospices
- Hospitals
- Hospital swing beds
- Intermediate care facilities for persons with mental retardation (ICF/MR)
- Nursing facilities
- Organ procurement organizations
- Portable x-ray suppliers
- Programs for all-inclusive care for the elderly (PACE) organizations

**Table 8.2**   Chapter IV: Centers for Medicare and Medicaid Services, Department of Health and Human Services (Continued): Part 482—Conditions of Participation for Hospitals

| | |
|---|---|
| 482.22 | Condition of participation: Medical staff |
| 482.23 | Condition of participation: Nursing services |
| 482.24 | Condition of participation: Medical record services |
| 482.25 | Condition of participation: Pharmaceutical services |
| 482.26 | Condition of participation: Radiologic services |
| 482.27 | Condition of participation: Laboratory services |
| 482.28 | Condition of participation: Food and dietetic services |
| 482.30 | Condition of participation: Utilization review |
| 482.41 | Condition of participation: Physical environment |
| 482.42 | Condition of participation: Infection control |
| 482.43 | Condition of participation: Discharge planning |
| 482.45 | Condition of participation: Organ, tissue, and eye procurement |
| 482.51 | Condition of participation: Surgical services |
| 482.52 | Condition of participation: Anesthesia services |
| 482.53 | Condition of participation: Nuclear medicine services |
| 482.54 | Condition of participation: Outpatient services |
| 482.55 | Condition of participation: Emergency services |
| 482.56 | Condition of participation: Rehabilitation services |
| 482.57 | Condition of participation: Respiratory care services |
| 482.60 | Special provisions applying to psychiatric hospitals |
| 482.61 | Condition of participation: Special medical record requirements for psychiatric hospitals |
| 482.62 | Condition of participation: Special staff requirements for psychiatric hospitals |
| 482.66 | Special requirements for hospital providers of long-term care services ("swing-beds") |

*Source:* From Centers for Medicare and Medicaid Services (CMS), 2011 [42 CFR 482].

- Providers of outpatient services (physical and occupational therapists in independent practice; outpatient physical therapy, occupational therapy, and speech-language pathology services)
- Psychiatric hospitals
- Religious nonmedical health care institutions
- Rural health clinics
- Skilled nursing facilities
- Transplant hospitals

See **Table 8.2** for a list of CMS conditions of participation.

## Deemed Status

According to CMS (2011), section 1865(a) of the Social Security Act permits providers and suppliers accredited by a national accredited body to be *deemed* to meet Medicare's CfCs or CoPs. To receive approval, an accreditation organization must demonstrate to CMS that its requirements match or exceed the Medicare conditions. With respect to a recent decision of Approval of Deeming Authority that affects audiology and speech-language pathology, CMS announced on May 6, 2011, that the American Association for Accreditation of Ambulatory Surgery Facilities, Inc. (AAAASF, 2011) was granted deeming authority and is thus a national program for providers of outpatient physical therapy and speech-language pathology services seeking to participate in the Medicare or Medicaid programs (see CMS AAAAS memo #11–27-AO posted on May 6, 2011, for more details).

In the area of hospital accreditation, since the 1960s TJC (2011), formerly known as the Joint Commission on Accreditation of Healthcare Organizations (JCAHO), has enjoyed "deemed status" with the inauguration of what was originally the Medicare arm of the government—the Health Care Finance Administration (HCFA). HCFA later became known as the current Centers on Medicare and Medicare Services (CMS). Perhaps "enjoy" is not quite the right word for this is not a cozy relationship. Periodically over the years, when some atrocious incident occurred in a hospital and was reported by the press, the public and often Congress would ask why this situation was not prevented by the country's foremost health care accrediting body, the JCAHO (now TJC). These situations created opportunities for finger pointing from both CMS and TJC trying to deflect responsibility. Congressional concerns about the occurrences of the TJC accreditation lapses eventually resulted in CMS being required to conduct the aforementioned "validation surveys" to demonstrate that the deemed status is warranted and that the accrediting body is being held accountable to conduct credible and reliable compliance reviews.

With the above-described political push and pull, CMS has also granted an organization called DNV Healthcare (DNV Healthcare, 2011) authority to accredit U.S. hospitals. CMS, thus, has given an outside organization, aside from TJC, the ability to accredit U.S. hospitals for the first time in over 40 years. This organization has been granted accreditator status from September 26, 2008, until September 26, 2012. DNV Healthcare is a division of Hovik, the Norway-based Det Norske Veritas, which was established in 1864 as an inspector of ships, but now conducts accreditation reviews for many industries.

## Accrediting Bodies with Deemed Status

Voluntary accrediting organizations such as TJC and CARF offer health care facilities the opportunity to earn accreditation that they may present as a quality "seal of approval" to the consumer (Golper & Brown, 2004). Accreditation means that the facility has met accrediting organizations' standards based on rigorous review of documentation and a periodic on-site survey. Failure to earn or maintain accreditation may have a significant impact on a facility's public image, marketing, and financial viability. Besides the benefit of being able to be an approved Medicare and Medicaid provider and be reimbursed for the services provided to Medicare and Medicaid beneficiaries, providers also must seek and maintain accreditation to qualify for the various health plans throughout the country. For example, as the vice president for inpatient operations and compliance at the NRH, this author must provide to our corporate contract office, evidence of our hospital occupancy license as well as validation of our current hospital accreditation from TJC and CARF. This annual process is required in order for our insurance contracts with other non-CMS payers to be renewed annually. A small segment of the members of the discipline of audiology and speech-language pathology, approximately 2% of ASHA members, are in private practice or in the outpatient arena. In that capacity, they have chosen to accept private pay only and not go through the accreditation process or insurance verification and enrollment process. Consumers may receive a given speech-language pathology service from a licensed SLP or audiologist, pay out of pocket, and then submit the invoice to their insurance company for payment. The service may or may not be reimbursed by the insurance company. Finally, while discussing accrediting bodies, we should also mention that there is a national organization, the National Committee for Quality Assurance (NCQA), that accredits health plans/insurance plans (NCQA, 2003, 2011). NCQA has also been accrediting managed care organizations (MCOs) since 1991, in response to a demand for standardized, objective information about MCO performance. The NCQA evaluates all types of health plans using a common set of standards. Today, more than 100 million individuals in the U.S. (70.5% of all health plan members) are covered by a NCQA-accredited health plan. NCQA accreditation is reportedly a rigorous, comprehensive, and transparent evaluation process through which the quality of the systems, processes, and results that define a health plan is assessed, including the care and service that plans deliver in important health promotion and prevention areas, such as diabetes, childhood immunizations, and mammograms. Hence health care providers can now rightly ask their insurance plans if they are accredited just as the insurance plans require health care accreditation.

## ◆ The Joint Commission

The Joint Commission (TJC) (2011), an independent not-for-profit organization, as discussed earlier, has CMS deemed status to accredit the following entities:

• Ambulatory health care

• Behavioral health care

• Critical access hospitals

• Home care

• Hospital

• International accreditation

• Laboratory services

• Long-term care

As has been suggested above, TJC is a dominant player in accreditation, as it is the oldest health care accrediting body, the first organization to be granted "deemed" status accrediting body, and a major health care market stakeholder. According to TJC (2011), it accredits and certifies over 19,000 health care organizations and programs in the U.S., and it has an international arm as well. Finally TJC has a for-profit subsidiary, Joint Commission Resources (JCR, 2011) (see Resources, below, for contact information on JCR) that sells manuals, updated standards information, survey preparation and resource materials, and other publications, and also provides experienced surveyors for consultation and to conduct mock surveys. TJC's evolution over the past half century closely tracks the evolution of the pursuit of quality, moving from a quality assurance model to a performance improvement model to a continuous quality improvement model. TJC has moved progressively, starting from an inspection survey process wherein the survey team would arrive with the survey date known well in advance and the survey team spending most of the site visit going through reams of notes, policy binders, and paper documents to verify that the organization had all of the necessary policies and procedures in place and also possessed the necessary supporting documentation that would be required if needed for review in an unannounced survey. In the past, the survey process focused on a site visit inspection of the facility and meetings with administrators and organizational leaders. Now TJC's survey is more consultative, almost exclusively engaged in hands-on verification of compliance by tracking, or "tracing," care processes across the continuum of care, and looking for evidence of a culture of continuous quality improvement. The surveyors look for evidence of an organizational structure that gathers and uses outcomes to maintain quality and patient safety.

The Joint Commission has identified 14 priority focus areas, which are related to processes, systems, and structures that significantly impact safety and or quality of care provided. These focus areas constitute the accreditation survey umbrella, for example, assessment and care/services, infection control, patient safety, and staffing (CAMH, 2011). The accreditation decision categories are as follows:

• Preliminary accreditation

• Accredited

• Accredited with follow-up survey

   —Requires a follow-up survey usually within 30 days to 6 months

- Contingent accreditation

  —Requires follow-up survey in 30 days

- Preliminary denial of accreditation

- Denial of accreditation

The Joint Commission publishes several newsletters and periodicals that summarize preparation, survey process, and survey outcomes. TJC (2010) published "Top Standards Compliance Issues for the First Half of 2010" for all of its accreditation lines. Referencing the percent that a given standard was found to be noncompliant, a list from the Hospital and Home Health programs are provided in **Table 8.3** and **Table 8.4**.

As the reader can see, there is virtually no correlation between the most cited deficiencies in these two settings. This should not be surprising because four of the top five hospital standards dealt with the environment of care (physical plant standards and staff safety practices), which would not be evaluated in home care. SLPs and audiologists in hospitals and hospital-based clinics, and other health care settings are usually very familiar with the TJC survey process. One area where the two professions are drawn into participation directly with the accreditation process is the application of "tracer methodology." Tracer methodology requires surveyors to track, or trace, an individual patient's episode of care from preadmission to discharge, and in some cases into the follow-up services in the organization's outpatient clinics. Tracer surveys essentially follow the events of care and identify all of the care providers that are documented in the medical record. Surveyors identify the service units, personnel, and procedures and services that the patient encountered through an admission (and beyond). The surveyor looks at the ways in which each member and service within the organization contributed to ensuring quality care and patient safety through that admission. Surveyors interview the individuals who provided care to the patient; inspect the physical plant and verify the infection control and safety processes; ensure that the patient's rights to informed consent and confidentiality are protected; ensure that the diagnostic and intervention procedures are consistent with evidence-based standards of practice, and are provided by appropriately credentialed, competent, and qualified individuals; and ensure that the staff members working in the facility are knowledgeable about emergency and disaster procedures. TJC provides the organization a copy of its preliminary survey results as part of the exit conference. The final survey document is available to the public online within 48 hours of the completion of the survey.

**Table 8.3** The Top Compliance Issues in Hospitals in 2011

| Prevalence | TJC Standard | Description |
|---|---|---|
| 62% | RC.01.01.01 | The hospital maintains complete and accurate medical records for each individual patient. |
| 50% | LS.02.01.20 | The hospital maintains the integrity of the means of egress. |
| 44% | LS.02.01.10 | Building and fire protection features are designed and maintained to minimize the effects of fire, smoke, and heat. |
| 38% | EC.020305 | The hospital maintains fire safety equipment and fire safety building features. |
| 37% | LS.02.01.30 | The hospital provides and maintains building features to protect individuals from the hazards of fire and smoke. |
| 31% | MM.03.01.01 | The hospital safely stores medications. |
| 31% | PC.01.02.03 | The hospital assesses and reassesses the patient and his or her condition according to defined time frames. |
| 31% | RC.02.03.07 | Qualified staff members receive and record verbal orders. |
| 30% | IC.02.02.01 | The hospital reduces the risk of infections associated with medical equipment, devices, and supplies. |
| 30% | MM.04.01.01 | Medication orders are clear and accurate. |

**Table 8.4**   The Top Compliance Issues in Home Care in 2011

| Prevalence | TJC Standard | Description |
| --- | --- | --- |
| 31% | PC.02.01.03 | The organization provides care, treatment, or services in accordance with orders or prescriptions, as required by law and regulation. |
| 23% | HR.01.06.01 | Staff members are competent to perform their responsibilities. |
| 21% | NPSG.09.02.01 | Reduce the risk of falls. |
| 20% | HR.01.02.05 | The organization verifies staff qualifications. |
| 19% | IC.01.03.01 | The organization identifies risks for acquiring and spreading infections. |
| 17% | PC.01.02.01 | The organization assesses and reassesses its patients. |
| 16% | RC.02.01.01 | The patient record contains information that reflects the patient's care, treatment and services. |
| 16% | IC.01.04.01 | Based on the identified risks, the organization sets goals to minimize the possibility of spreading infections. |
| 16% | PC.01.03.01 | The organization plans the patient's care. |
| 15% | EM.03.01.03 | The organization evaluates the effectiveness of its Emergency Operations Plan. |

## National Patient Safety Goals

An important component of the TJC *standards set* is the National Patient Safety Goals (NPSGs), which were developed by TJC 5 years ago as a result of the public uproar and subsequent CMS scrutiny regarding medical errors in hospitals. The discipline of audiology and speech-language pathology should be very familiar with the NPSGs and take a leadership role in complying with them, as several of these goals relate to ensuring effective communication, infection control, and patient safety. The 2010 NPSGs are as follows (TJC, 2011):

1. Improve the accuracy of patient information.

2. Improve the effectiveness of communication among caregivers.

3. Improve the safety of using medications.

4. Reduce the risk of health care–associated infections.

5. Accurately and completely reconcile medications across the continuum of care.

6. Reduce the risk of patient harm resulting from falls.

7. Encourage patients' active involvement in their own care as a patient safety strategy.

8. Identify safety risks inherent in the patient population.

9. Improve recognition and response to changes in a patient's condition.

10. Apply the Universal Protocol for conducting an invasive procedure.

   Audiologists and SLPs perform some clinical procedures that might be deemed "invasive" (for example, endoscopies) but do not perform surgery or dispense medication. Audiologists participating in intraoperative monitoring during cochlear implant surgery will, as a member of the team, observe "time out," part of the Universal Protocol, in which a responsible individual, usually a nurse, checks to ensure that the team has the right patient, the right equipment, and is performing the right surgery on the right site. Also, the NPSG standard related to *fall prevention* is directly addressed by audiologists working with balance-disordered patients.

What appears to be the simplest and most obvious method of infection prevention, handwashing, is absolutely paramount to controlling the hospital and facility rates of infection. Like all other providers, SLPs and audiologists are compliant with handwashing before and after entering patient contact. Facilities are highly concerned with handwashing practices and have placed handwashing stations and disinfectant solution dispensers inside or outside of all patient and clinic examination rooms. Facilities conduct *handwashing audits* on hospital wards and in clinics to confirm compliance, and department managers are regularly provided with outcome data from those audits. Also as a result of the NPSGs, all providers are expected to check for two patient identifiers to make sure they are treating the correct patient. They are expected to inform patients of their rights and responsibilities, and conduct interventions in a manner that will ensure good between-provider communications, and engender the patient and the patient's family or advocates to be actively engaged in their own health care and safety protection. We can actively participate in a continuous preparation mode for an accreditation visit by complying with all of the NPSGs that are applicable.

### The Joint Commission's Emphasis on Communication Needs

Another way our profession plays a crucial role in the accreditation processes is seen in TJC's newly revised standards, which include a requirement that organizations identify and address patient communication needs (Standard PC.02.01.21), while emphasizing the need to be aware of and responsive to the variety of sociocultural perspectives within an environment that does not tolerate discrimination. This standard specifically refers to identifying and addressing the needs of patients with *speech, language, hearing, vision,* and *cognitive impairments,* as well as those who have limited English proficiency, limited literacy skills, little knowledge about health care, or cultural, sexual identity, or religious differences (TJC, 2010). Using the best available statistics, at least 168 million people in the U.S. fall into one or more of those demographics, and a significant percentage of them will be admitted to hospitals, especially in areas where hospitals treat a large number of patients who do not speak English (ASHA, 2008; Berke, 2010; Diamond, Wilson-Stronks, & Jacobs, 2010; Hasnain-Wynia, Yonek, Pierce, Kang, & Greising, 2006; NIDCD, 2011; Pleis & Lethbridge-Cejku, 2006). According to Sarah Blackstone, a noted specialist in augmentative and alternative communication (AAC) technology within our profession (Blackstone, 2011), the need to improve health care outcomes and reduce health care costs in the U.S. is an important national health policy goal. Research suggests that improving patient-provider communication is a critical step toward those goals. SLPs and audiologists are uniquely educated and clinically prepared to lead in this effort. Blackstone advocates for professionals from our discipline to become involved in implementing new standards and regulations that address the need for "effective communication, cultural competence, and patient- and family-centered care." In our discussions about our professional roles and the accreditation and CMS rules in this area, she sees a convergence of communication challenges faced by four groups with communication vulnerabilities, namely those with (1) speech, language, hearing, vision, and cognitive impairments; (2) limited English proficiency; (3) little knowledge about health care (poor health literacy); and (4) cultural, sexual identity, or religious differences. Blackstone feels SLPs and audiologists must advocate for the use of key assistive technologies and strategies that help individuals who are communication vulnerable, to interact more effectively with their health care providers. And, consistent with another NPSG ("Encourage patients' active involvement in their own care" [TJC, 2011]), we also must encourage (advocate for) active and systematic collaborations among professions representing groups currently at high risk for health disparities.

### DNV Healthcare

Given DNV Healthcare's international base, industry observers expect it to bring an increased focus on meeting international standards, particularly ISO 9001, into hospitals in the U.S. DNV has a system in place already, in fact, to combine CMS's conditions of participation with ISO 9001's quality management (DNV Healthcare, 2011). The program is known as the National Integrated Accreditation for Healthcare Organizations (NIAHO). To date, nearly 200 U.S. hospitals have switched from TJC and are now accredited by NIAHO. DNV accreditation requires an annual survey and the organization's continual compliance with the DNV accreditation process. At present, DNV accredits three program types:

- Hospital accreditation
- Primary stroke center certification/accreditation
- Critical access hospital accreditation

In a testimonial on the DNV website, Sara Phillips, the quality director of the Jordan Valley Medical Center in Utah, is quoted as saying, "DNV is a framework perfectly suited to the complex, variable world of health care delivery. But when it is fully integrated with the Medicare Conditions of Participation, and battle tested by the nation's top hospitals, you have something truly unique in the world of accreditation" (Phillips, 2011, accreditation Web page).

### Community Health Accreditation Program

The Community Health Accreditation Program (CHAP, 2011) accreditation process utilizes the CHAP standards of excellence that are driven by considerations of management, quality, client outcomes, adequate resources, and long-term viability. SLPs and audiologists in home health care will potentially encounter a CHAP survey during their career; however, TJC is the predominant accrediting body in the home health care arena. CHAP (2011) provides accreditation reviews for the following nine service areas:

- Home health (deemed and non-deemed)
- Hospice (deemed and non-deemed)
- Home medical equipment
- Pharmacy
- Private duty nursing
- Infusion therapy
- Public health
- Community nursing centers
- Supplemental staffing services

## ◆ Commission on Accreditation of Rehabilitation Facilities

The Commission on Accreditation of Rehabilitation Facilities (CARF) has a pending application for CMS deemed status for all of its customer service units that it accredits. CARF accredits the following business units:

- Aging services
- Behavior health
- Child and youth services

- Durable medical equipment prosthetics
- Orthotics and supplies
- Employment and community services
- Medical rehabilitation
- Vision rehabilitation services

CARF has developed its own set of standards for rehabilitation organizations that wish to obtain CARF accreditation. Evidence that these standards are met must be present at the organizational level and also at the individual program level (e.g., brain-injury program), if the organization seeks specialty program accreditation. To the extent that audiology and speech-language pathology departmental policies and procedures may complement or reinforce organizational or specialty program policies and procedures in meeting the standards of this and other accrediting bodies, these policies and procedures should be considered for inclusion in a departmental policy and procedure manual. The CARF standards (2010) as reflected in the requested survey resource documents that may have relevance for the audiology and speech-language pathology departmental policy and procedure manual include, but are not limited to:

- Documentation of the program's or department's role in the continuum of care
- Measurable criteria for the initiation and termination of specific treatments
- Policies and procedures that promote safety and security
- Procedures for filing grievances and appealing decisions
- Policies for advance directives and resuscitation orders
- Admission, continued stay, discharge, and exit criteria per department and program
- Policies that address confidentiality of records, release of records, records retention, records storage, and protection of records from fire and water damage
- Policies for electronic records that address protection of records, privacy of records, and security of records
- Policies concerning ethical conduct
- Policies and procedures related to taking and reporting disciplinary actions against practitioners
- Procedures for handling motor vehicle accidents and road emergencies
- Administrative policies and procedures
- Policies and procedures that identify the functions and the responsibilities of rehabilitation physicians providing treatment

CARF surveyors are rehabilitation professionals who work in CARF-accredited facilities and are trained to survey other rehabilitation organizations. This author has served as a CARF program and administrative surveyor for 15 years. CARF standards (CARF, 2011) are scored by the surveyors in terms of the following four levels of conformance with the standards: exemplary conformance (3), full conformance (2), partial conformance (1), and no evidence of conformance (0). On balance, the survey team assesses the organization's performance with all of the relevant sections of the standards manual for which the organization is seeking accreditation. Section 1 (Aspire to Excellence) and Section 2 (The Rehab Process of the Person Served) of the CARF standards must be assessed with each survey. Section 1 includes assessing the environment, setting a strategy, obtaining input from the person served, implementing the rehabilitation plan, reviewing results, and effecting change. Organizations, for example, in addition to seeking to be accredited by meeting the basic program requirements that all rehabilitation providers seeking CARF accreditation must meet, the Comprehensive Integrated Inpatient Rehabilitation Program (CIIRP) may also choose to seek other specialty program accreditations. These specialty accreditations include the spinal cord system of care, the stroke specialty program, and the brain injury program. CARF requires four accreditation conditions:

1. A 6-month track record of employing the appropriate CARF standards while providing services at each site or service seeking accreditation

2. All records and reports as requested by CARF

3. A quality improvement plan submitted within 90 days following notice of accreditation

4. For organizations achieving a 3-year accreditation, the submission of a signed Annual Conformance to Quality Report in each of the 2 years following the 3-year accreditation

CARF's accreditation decisions are as follows:

• 3-year accreditation

• 1-year accreditation

• Provisional accreditation

• Nonaccreditation

• Preliminary accreditation

Because CARF does not yet enjoy CMS deemed status, several prominent rehabilitation organizations have elected to no longer seek CARF accreditation. However, according to CARF (2011), most rehabilitation units and free-standing rehabilitation facilities throughout the country are indeed CARF accredited for the basic CIIRP level of accreditation. CARF still offers a combined survey with TJC if a free-standing rehabilitation facility elects to invite both accrediting bodies to conduct a survey at the same time.

## ♦ Evolution of Accreditation and Transparency

According to Boone (2011), the evolutionary phase of accreditation as a rehabilitation industry-specific quality management framework can be illustrated against the dynamic characteristics of the broader health care environment (**Fig. 8.1**). As Boone observes, one characteristic is the degree to which the environment is closed or exclusive versus open and inclusive. An inclusive environment would purposefully include and optimize the involvement of diverse stakeholders or those who participate in its accrediting processes. A second characteristic is the transparency of outcomes and how providers are held accountable as a result. Examples of this trend toward transparency are initiatives taken by CMS in displaying a variety of quarterly outcome data on several sectors of the health care industry in major urban newspapers as well as on its Web sites: Hospital Compare (2011) or Nursing Home Compare (Medicare.gov/NHCompare/Home.asp). This outcome transparency in health care has evolved over the past decade as a result of consumer, business, and congressional demands for greater accountability from CMS, the largest health care payer in the country. In **Fig. 8.1**, one can see the evolutionary history of accreditation moving from a more *exclusionary* "professional" era in the 1960s, to a more *participatory* phase in an "economic" era well established by the 1990s, and still prominent today, to a more *inclusive* "quality" era framework over the past decade and into the foreseeable future.

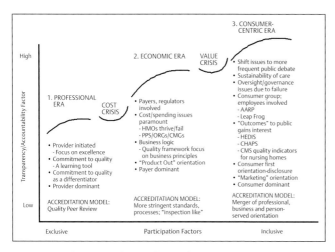

**Fig. 8.1**  Evolutionary phases of accreditation. CHAP, Community Health Accreditation Program; CMG, Case Mix Group; CMS, Centers for Medicare and Medicaid Services; HEDIS, Healthcare Effectiveness Data and Information Set; PPS, Prospective Payment System. [From Boone, B. J. (2011). Accreditation—A quality frame work in the consumer-centric era. In S.R. Flanagan, H. Zaretsky, & A. Moroz (Eds.), *Medical aspects of disability: A handbook for the rehabilitation professional* (4th ed., pp. 687–706). New York: Springer Publishing. Reprinted by permission.]

## The Professional Era (1960–1980)

In the early 1960s, rehabilitation professionals considered quality to be not only in their purview but also their primary ethical and professional responsibility. There was much debate within the rehab industry as to what to measure and what constituted quality. Such discussion and debate was not yet on the table of other health care accrediting bodies, providers, or insurers, but quality was increasingly on the rehab menu. The rehabilitation professions were also far ahead of the "outcomes curve" focusing on "pursuit of excellence" with a commitment to quality as a market differentiator and as a learning tool. In the 1960s there was little evidence of the use of benchmarks, a national data repositories, evidence-based practice standards, or outcome measures that were known to make a difference. Providers and their professional associations were scrambling to organize service delivery in a fashion that was coherent and comprehensive if not yet reliably efficient and effective. During this era, CARF (formed in 1963) and other accrediting bodies formed expert consensus panels with the resultant standards endorsed by the community of providers.

The American Speech-Language-Hearing Association (ASHA) entered into the accreditation fray at the tail end of the professional era. In 1980, ASHA's Legislative Council established the Professional Services Board (PSB) to accredit audiology and speech-language pathology clinical providers and programs. The PSB standards were continuously updated (ASHA, 1992) and broadly disseminated and promulgated. In fact, ASHA partnered with CARF in the 1990s to survey PSB programs jointly with the CARF surveyor teams. Finally, with the demise of the professional era, ASHA sunsetted the PSB in January 2001 due to the exorbitant expense of maintaining such a singular and anachronistic accrediting body and also due to decreased subscription and adherence to service-specific accreditation standards. In short, ASHA, along with the reminder of the service delivery sector, came to the inexorable and inevitable conclusion that the economic and consumer eras were upon us, and consumers were more interested in accountable and transparent accrediting bodies that enhanced quality without increasing cost. During the professional era, CARF and PSB surveyors would descend upon a health care organization when the survey dates were known months in advance and where the on-site review was intended to measure a given provider's degree of compliance with and conformance to required standards. Providers prepared far in advance to document, with reams of files and streams of notebooks, that each standard was documented and met. This professional era was marked by a peer review quality assurance approach to rehabilitation and health care. Consumers were rather passive, by today's standards, in their view of health care and standards and economics had not yet overshadowed the provision of health care. However, the pendulum was steadily swinging toward both greater accountability and rising costs due to a variety of factors: new technologies, a plethora of new pharmaceuticals, demand for more care, greater use of technologies in facility operations, more modern equipment and physical plants, and a movement away from professional-centric care to more consumer-centric care.

## The Economic Era (1990–Present)

### Cost Containment Tactics

Beginning in the early 1990s, it became clear that the fee-for-service model of paying for health care was not sustainable. Insurance companies were rethinking their business model, and employers could ill-afford the escalating cost of health insurance for their employees. We were and still are facing a crisis with health care economics. It was during this period that regulators and payers became more engaged and attuned to the environment as service provision concerns and escalating costs became more obvious not only to the number crunchers at CMS but to the general public as well. The era of managed care was upon us, and providers saw annual contracting as a duel over rates, carve outs, and other efforts to curb health care spending. Managed care approaches evolved to control costs during this period while trying to maintain access to appropriate care (Eccleston, 1995). Personnel, equipment, new technology, and compliance and regulatory costs continued to climb, and CMS and managed care efforts were aimed squarely at controlling costs. According to Boone (2011), the mantra of "doing more with less" was and remains a predominant theme in health care, much like the oft-repeated phrase "funding dictates form." With an increasing sensitivity to costs, accreditation became a prerequisite in the procurement of services by some payers. Some insurers used accreditation as a contract management and cost-containment tool to ensure that rehabilitation was explicitly included in their extended specialty-service provider networks (e.g., spinal cord injury services). Insurers would only pay providers if they were accredited in the claimed specialty in rehabilitation. Insurers used accreditation to verify that those claiming to provide specialty rehabilitation were qualified and that they managed those programs according to quality accreditation standards.

Regarding the above discussion of "funding dictates form," payment changes, and accreditation adaptations, when the Prospective Payment System (PPS) was begun in acute rehabilitation (CMS, 2004), a paradigm shift occurred as the rehabilitation industry moved from a fee-for-service model to a model where the reimbursement was determined on admission based on a variety of factors including diagnosis and functional assessment. The industry was forced to make dramatic changes in processes and personnel staffing to comply with this perspective (funding change) and consequent changes in CMS rules and regulations. Another important management mantra in this economic era is "no margin, no mission." So the health care industry adapted greater efficiencies while staying focused on the quality patient care that is required by providers to avoid losing market share, accreditation, and reputation.

### Employees Enter as New Participants

According to Boone (2011), in response to the cost crisis and the new business logic being employed, accreditation quality standards adjusted accordingly. Standards became lengthier with greater interpretive guidelines. Standards became much more stringent, more objective, and in some cases more prescriptive. Quality standards relating to performance outcomes were also added by accrediting bodies requiring providers to have in place a documented system of performance improvement that was broadly based and accountable to leadership with regularly reported results and plans of corrections. With the landmark publication of the incredible but accurate Institute of Medicine report (IOM, 1999), *To Err Is Human,* the 21st century ushered in an era of accountability and accreditation action on patient safety. With 44,000 to 100,000 Americans dying annually in hospitals due to medical errors, the health care industry went into an organizational behavior management frenzy aimed at preventing errors in health care. Surveys also became more stringent. Accreditation survey results began to find more serious flaws and unsafe practices in hospitals, and as a result the accreditation outcomes were given very serious attention. Because surveyors tended to find more problems, in some cases the intervals between accreditations became shorter and there was an increase in non-accreditation decisions. Congressional hearings were held, defensive articles were written, and interviews and speeches were given attempting to explain the inexplicable data. In 2001, the IOM published its follow-up study, *Crossing the Quality Chasm*, in which, unfortunately, no improvement was noted in the incidence of medical errors in health care. A culture of safety and continuous performance improvement was then demanded. According to Cebul, Rebitzer, Taylor, and Votruba (2008), the large, fragmented U.S. health care system, its structures, and its processes lead to disruptive service experiences, poor information flows, and misaligned incentives that degrade the quality and safety of care.

*Employer Advocacy*

According to Goldberg and Young (2011), the fiscal landscape of acute rehabilitation today remains severely overburdened by a litany of varying payment schemes, preadmission certification criterion, and regulatory mandates. The fee-for-service insurance option is hardly in evidence, and employers are beginning to join the discussion. The Leap Frog Group (leapfroggroup.org) is perhaps the most often referenced voice in this discussion. The Leap Frog Group (2004), with a decade of growth and credibility under its wings, has four simple and objective aims:

1. Reduce preventable medical mistakes and improve the quality and affordability of health care

2. Encourage health providers to report their quality and outcomes so that consumers and purchasing organizations can make informed health care choices

3. Reward doctors and hospitals for improving the quality, safety, and affordability of health care

4. Help consumers reap the benefits of making smart health care decisions

The Leap Frog Group (2011) and other business forces understand the economics of quality and safety and have become forces for patient safety advocacy with or without the accrediting bodies. Another example of employer advocacy is the National Business Group on Health (NBGH, 2009), a not-for-profit organization representing a large employer group dedicated to finding innovative and forward-thinking solutions in health care policy and practice issues such as cost control, patient safety, quality of care, and best practices. The NBGH, located near Capitol Hill, has recently established several initiatives and institutes to promote its cause to improve outcomes, enhance quality, and manage costs. Today it is clear that employers have reached their cost and quality threshold and have now demanded providers and government to provide relief from the annual double-digit increases in health insurance. Referring again to the NRH as an example, the increases passed on to the employer from our insurance provider were 11% in 2009, 12% in 2010, and 14% in 2011. Why should employer/businesses pay higher premiums when harm still happens in health care and even good accreditation review outcomes do not guarantee a good health outcome for your employee?

Boone (2011) describes another phenomenon seen in this era: an increase in public discussion and debate prompted by increased transparency demonstrating health care costs continuing to spiral upward despite cost-containment efforts across the board. One prominent and important example of this trend was the President's Advisory Commission on Consumer Protection and Quality in the Health Care Industry (1998), which investigated health care quality and recommended improvement strategies to enhance the national health care system's responsiveness and effectiveness. Health care was being pushed and prodded to take responsibility for the reforms necessary to reduce medical errors and improve quality outcomes more efficiently. Because the answer to the Advisory Commission mandate was not to be found in the health care industry, wiser health care leaders began investigating best practices and lessons learned from other industries. Acute care and acute rehab began embracing quality frameworks from outside of their industry (Counte & Meurer, 2001), such as the International Organization for Standardization (ISO 9000) (2000), Malcolm Baldridge National Quality Program (2011), total quality management, continuous improvement, quality control circles, statistical process control, balanced score cards/reports, re-engineering, management by results, Outcomes Management Century, Lean and Lean Six Sigma, and others.

### Cultural Coaching

Most health care organizations have gone through redesigns over the past decade, and many have contracted with "culture" coaching companies, such as the Studer Group (2011), which is considered the leading company in assisting organizations to achieve their desired results, and the Disney Institute (1999, 2009), which was adopted at the NRH (Rao, Ellis, & Douglas, 2002) due to the Disney program's emphasis on and approach to service with four simple priorities: safety, courtesy, care, and efficiency. Over the past decade, the NRH has seen a significant cultural transformation with outstanding employee satisfaction scores (>70% compared with the health care norm) over four separate surveys conducted over the past 10 years (Towers Watson, 2010), improved employee retention, excellent accreditation survey results, improved ratings on best hospitals lists (U.S. News and World Report, 2011), and the best financial performance in our quarter century of existence in fiscal year 2011. In addition, Lean Six Sigma (Buell, 2010) has become a routine quality application in health care today as well, addressing both patient safety on the one hand and waste and inefficiency on the other. At NRH this past year, we were able to find savings of over $1 million using the Lean Six Sigma approach, from reducing laundry supplies to par levels and monitoring for supply hoarding, to reducing length of stay by 1 day in the Medicare population. An organization that wishes to excel in patient safety and quality will always challenge itself to advance its customer service approach while at the same time discover cost-effective methods of delivering quality services. All of the above-listed "quality" techniques, are outcomes databased, and if used consistently, effectively, and appropriately, will assist the provider to "do more with less" without sacrificing quality.

## Consumer-Centric Era (2000 and Beyond)

A prevailing countertrend to cost-containment was described by Boone (2011). What we are seeing today are more outspoken, vigilant, autonomous, and empowered consumer groups. Health care consumers are rebelling at the apparent restrictions of access to care and the escalating copayments and pharmaceutical costs imposed by managed care. The payers, regulators, and providers will need to adjust to the new era of consumer-driven health care. The pendulum appears to be swinging in a circular motion. There are more patients eligible for care, more cuts across the board at all levels of care, more consumer self-advocacy and demands, more data, and greater transparency.

The health and human service industry is beginning to experience the early signs of a yet another fundamental paradigm shift of its environment. The person served is beginning to exercise choice, control, and with greater frequency being asked to bear the financial cost for services received. What are the symptoms of this consumer centric era? **Figure 8.1** lists at least eight indicators that inexorably point to a new day in health care and a new day in health care accreditation. Social media have the potential of becoming the unlicensed accreditor of choice in the marketplace; consider the impact of Angie's List, Facebook, Twitter, My Space, and YouTube. Families are blogging their satisfaction levels with health care services.

Did your care provider forget to wash his hands before treatment? Has your loved one been placed in a soiled patient room? Read the blog or see the video on YouTube. Yes, the new century welcomed an era when the Internet will strongly influence and create new demands, public oversight, and redefined performance measures in the health care system. Out of frustration, anger, or futility, patients and patient advocates are posting material on the Web that rightly or wrongly puts patient care on public trial. Consumers are transitioning from relatively uninformed passive recipients of services to highly engaged and demanding participants. Informed consumers will begin to advocate for improvements in the dimensions of all the levels of health care such as timely and friendly access to care, practice patterns consistent with evidence, and clinical and functional outcomes that exceed national or regional benchmarks (Goonan, 1994). Boone (2011) suggests that the future is now. This shift in social influence already can be observed in the growing number of consumer-directed health plans, personal spending accounts, and service options that have become instituted with greater frequency in the marketplace. Drug companies have also recognized the power of consumer authority as they begin marketing directly to consumers, often via television commercials, and bypassing the traditional physician-only marketing.

## Health Equity

An example of consumer driven accountability and transparency absent any regulatory or licensing authority is the Human Rights Campaign Foundation's (HRCF) Health Equality Index (HEI) (HRCF, 2011). The HRCF conducts an annual survey (HEI) of all health care providers to determine compliance with its criteria and standards that reportedly improve the quality of health care for the lesbian, gay, bisexual, and transgendered (LGBT) population. According to HRCF, the absence of clearly stated visitation and advance directive policies, for example, as well as having a definition of family that is more inclusive will determine a provider's rating and score as supportive of the HRCF's goal of greater acceptance and promotion of human rights. The completed HEI 2011 survey will be promulgated and disseminated nationally with press releases and media tool kits and will reportedly provide a report card, as it were, to the LGBT community and the community at large in selecting a health care provider. The seven binary choice criteria on the HEI 2011 survey are listed in **Table 8.5**.

Providers received a score of 1 to 7 on the HEI 2011 survey in mid-July, with provider comments available under each heading. This external health care HRCF initiative is a perfect illustration of a given community's harnessing its human resources and capital in deploying a health care survey and then holding providers accountable for the results of the survey.

An example of a *within* health care initiative to increase transparency and accountability is found in the story of Covenant Health (Bush, 2008). When Covenant Health's board members signed a pledge to lower mortality rates, the organization's information technology department leapt into action. With major investments in infrastructure and training, Covenant now tracks core measures on patients when they present to the emergency department and publishes 100% of its core measures in a quarterly system-wide quality data report on a newly formatted, cutting-edge Web site. Testifying to the need for change, the Chief Information Officer Ward stated, "The needs of the organization and the consumers have changed" (Bush, 2008, p. 10). Chief Financial Officer Geppi said, "From the outset, we knew that improving quality would demand relentless measurement and reporting. Otherwise, it would be difficult to convince the board that the hospital's efforts were paying off" (Bush, 2008 p. 11). Today, Covenant Health has a separate site for quality data, www.covenantquality.com,

**Table 8.5**   Health Equity Index Criteria

| Criteria | Credit y/n |
| --- | --- |
| Patients' bill of rights/nondiscrimination policy inclusive of sexual orientation | |
| Patients' bill of rights/nondiscrimination policy inclusive of gender identity | |
| Visitation policies grant same-sex couples (partners/spouses/significant others) the same access as different-sex couples and next of kin | |
| Visitation policies grant same-sex parents the same access as different-sex parents for visitation of their minor children | |
| Cultural competency training that addresses health care issues related to the LGBT community | |
| Employment nondiscrimination policy inclusive of sexual orientation | |
| Employment nondiscrimination policy inclusive of sexual gender identity | |

*Source:* Human Rights Campaign Foundation (HRCF). (2011). Healthcare Equality Index 2011. hrfc.org. Printed with Permission from Human Rights Campaign Foundation, Thomas Sullivan, Deputy Director, HRC Family Project, 1640 Rhode Island Avenue, NW, Washington, CD, 20036.

where consumers can access quarterly reports on each hospital as soon as the reports are delivered to Covenant's board, months before the data are released by CMS and TJC. The site also provides updates on Covenant's quality initiatives, information on topical issues like infection rates and the hospital's infection control policy, as well as details about the latest technological innovations. Chief Executive Officer Spezia said, "Getting ahead of the curve on transparency back in 2001 was a deliberate decision because the hospital recognized that consumers would eventually demand quality reporting from their providers" (Bush, 2008 p. 12).

# ♦ Quality Challenges in Accreditation and Service Delivery: The Future

We have spent a fair amount of space in this chapter emphasizing Medicare and Medicaid and health care reform. Readers might ask, What does CMS and health care reform have to do with accreditation? Much like the auto industry in the 1960s, when it was said that "as GM goes, so goes the nation," in health care we can say that as CMS goes, so goes accreditation! All accrediting bodies strive to achieve deemed status, which means that CMS recognizes its authority and standards and the effectiveness of its review processes. Just as accreditation is a seal of approval, achieving deemed status from CMS is a coveted endorsement. Providers must meet the CMS CoPs on an annual basis, and rather than invite the CMS survey team or the state licensing agency, most providers prefer to be surveyed by an accrediting body that has deemed status or acts on behalf of CMS. For that reason, we look further at the conditions of participation and health care reform in the context of whatever CMS does, all other accrediting and licensing bodies eventually will and must follow.

## Bundling

Recently, Gerben DeJong (2010) led a panel discussion at the American Congress of Rehabilitation Medicine to discuss the challenges in measuring and reporting quality in rehabilitation programs. When the landmark health care reform act passed, CMS moved forward with its agenda to develop *accountable care organizations* (ACOs), which included employing *bundling* (prospective payment) as a payment model not only to achieve cost savings but also to transform care delivery to become safer and more efficient. In July 2010, CMS released its final rule on bundling for renal dialysis providers (Walsh, 2010). The rehabilitation industry is now similarly confronted with addressing what outcomes to measure and how to measure them, and once that is settled we need to agree on what data to report and how to report them. With the multiple complex diagnoses and comorbidities to account for in the care continuum, how can the health care system successfully stratify case-mix and risk adjustment so that all providers and payers are on a level playing field? While plotting and attempting to engineer or, more accurately, re-engineer all of the above, how do we also avoid unintended consequences such as advantaging one sector over another or risk having insufficient resources for the most severe acuity? How do we engender coordinated levels of care that will function in a patient-focused fashion?

## CARE Tool

Health care measurement and quality outcome reporting thus require a 2011 and beyond context. We are clearly now operating on two converging tracks: advances in patient assessment and outcome measurement, and changes in payment system design. In a CMS initiative, *pay for performance* (P4P), payers are demanding value-based purchasing and improved outcomes quite simply by paying for performance. To reach this point in our quality and outcomes gestation where we crawl before we walk, one must refer to the legislative enablers that actually set the stage for this convergence of value-based purchasing in health care reform: the Deficit Reduction Act (DRA) (CMS, 2005) and the Patient Protection and Affordable Care Act (PPACA, 2010). The DRA, signed into law in February 2006, spawned the much debated and piloted Continuity Assessment Record and Evaluation (CARE) tool, which is to be finally implemented by CMS in October 2013. This assessment methodology is designed to capture, document, and navigate every Medicare beneficiary's health and functional status through the entire continuum of care beginning with the acute care admission and disposition. The CARE tool includes measurements of severity (scaled) and outcomes across medical, physical/functional, cognitive/functional, and environment domains. CARE has been criticized as too unwieldy and too time-consuming to complete. However, the CARE tool is the mechanism CMS vetted and selected to assist providers in placing patients into and through the most appropriate and least expensive level of care. In short, the CARE tool has won the beauty contest, and providers must court her with single-mindedness. The other enabler of CMS moving in the direction of value-based purchasing is PPACA, increasingly referred to as the ACA, whose title belies its intent—to protect patients and make health care affordable for all. The law is already in the early stages of implementation. Parents will be able to carry dependents up to the age of 26 on their insurance policies, and measures are underway to protect beneficiaries from being rejected for insurance coverage because of medical preconditions. The real tsunami of change will come later when 32 million individuals in the U.S. who are currently uninsured will become eligible for health care coverage in 2014.

This convergence will greatly accelerate measurement and reporting of quality and outcomes. As noted in **Fig. 8.2** (DeJong, 2010), a patient assessment track is initiated with the acute CARE tools now in place, such as the admitting history and physical and a discharge summary for a person with stroke. These assessments today are "handed off" to the next level of care. The next level of care might be home care, where the stroke patient is assessed using the Outcome Assessment and Information Set (OASIS) (CMS, 2010a), the assessment methodology that CMS has required of all home care providers as a condition of participation since October 1, 2000. If the patient requires more intense nursing and medical rehabilitation, the patient might be referred to an inpatient rehabilitation facility (IRF) where the interdisciplinary team collects data on the Patient Assessment Instrument (PAI) including capture of functional performance with the Functional Independence Measure (FIM) (CMS, 2004), also required by CMS as a CoP. If the person with stroke is unable to tolerate 3 hours of therapy at least 5 days per week, then the patient might be referred to a skilled nursing facility (SNF), where rehabilitation services may be provided, depending on the patient's tolerances and comorbidities (see Chapter 7), and a team will complete a Resident Assessment Instrument–Minimum Data Set (RAI-MDS) (CMS, 2010a). These postacute, setting-specific measures now in use to capture quality and functional outcomes will form the basis of CMS's prospective payment to each postacute provider. As has already been announced, the race is over, the data are in, and these tools are intended to be replaced by the CARE tool (CMS, 2005) by October 2013. For further discussion of current practices and the future of functional outcome measurement in health care, see Chapters 2 and 5.

Referring back to **Fig. 8.2**, a parallel payment track history is reviewed beginning with cost-based reimbursement in play, termed the Tax Equity and Fiscal Responsibility Act (TEFRA), which was signed into law by President Reagan to modify the payment system for health care that had been in place for two decades (TEFRA, 1982). This Public Law 97–248 was a sweeping revision of payment policy and had a major impact on health care until the Balanced Budget Act (BBA) of 1997. Another significant payment change was implemented in the late 1990s, when CMS moved away from TEFRA and diagnosis-related groups (DRGs) used as the payment formula for acute care to a more so-called equitable payment system called the Prospective Payment System (PPS) for postacute care. With BBA, the postacute industry braced for PPS, which CMS implemented in long-term care shortly after BBA, in home care in 2000, and in the acute rehab industry in 2004. Finally, coincident with the implementation of the CARE tool, CMS plans to implement a bundled payment system, discussed above, for all postacute care. The specifics or logistics have yet to be worked out by CMS, but the end game assumes that an entity such as an acute care hospital will complete the CARE tool on a patient prior to discharge from the facility and then also control/manage a bundled payment for the same patient's postacute care. The economic assumption underlying this payment reform is that the bundle owner will be more fiscally prudent in referring on to the next level of care because the bundle

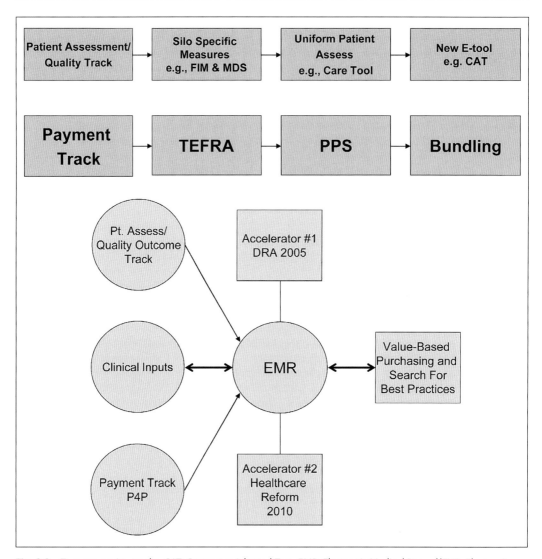

**Fig. 8.2**  Two converging tracks. CAT, Computer Adapted Test; EMR, Electronic Medical Record/EHR, Electronic Health Record; FIM, Functional Independence Measure;  MDS, minimum data set; PPS, Prospective Payment System; P4P, pay for performance; TEFRA, Tax Equity and Fiscal Responsibility Act; [Adapted from DeJong, G. (2010). *Challenges in measuring and reporting quality in rehabilitation programs, a measure for rehab programs.* American Congress of Rehabilitation Medicine-American Society of Neuro Rehabilitation: Joint Educational Conference, Montreal, Quebec, CA. Reprinted by permission.]

owner will be responsible for paying the downstream cost for the subsequent levels of care during the patient's episode of care. As **Fig. 8.2** illustrates, a tectonic shift is expected to occur in 2013 with the nexus of a single functional outcome measure and accountable payment system. Change will occur within the context of two converging forces, one leading to the development of the CARE tool and the other leading to payment bundling. The alphabet soup of functional assessments currently used (OASIS, FIM, MDS) will be replaced in 2013 with an assessment methodology that has no comparative archival outcome data. And postacute care providers will be expected to embrace CMS's new worldview: one uniform postacute payment and a comprehensive outcomes measure. As CMS goes, so go other payers, particularly if there will be a cost savings. In whatever form the "other players and payers" aside from CMS will take in health care reform, all non-CMS payers are likely to adopt the CMS model because it is predicted to cut billions of dollars out of Medicare and Medicaid costs in less than a decade.

Also notable in **Fig. 8.2** at the intersection of two converging tracks are the earlier-described legislative accelerators, the Patient Protection and Affordable Care Act (2010) and the Deficit Reduction Act (CMS, 2005). Coincidental to and preceding these acts is yet another federal initiative related to electronic management of medical/health records.

### Meaningful Use of the Electronic Health Record

A separate federal initiative that predated recent health care reform and deficit reduction acts of Congress is the current push by the Department of Health and Human Services (DHHS) to have all clinical health records managed in an electronic format (CMS, 2010b). The electronic health record (EHR) must meet certain data management, content, and control specifications that include measures referred to as a *quality data set* (QDS). Providers are now reaping federal windfalls when their EHR meets the electronic specification and the "meaningful use" requirements. The meaningful use requirement requires providers not only to have and to make use of electronic technologies, but also to demonstrate that their EHR *has advanced the quality of care* in the organization. Each provider must have three quality measures within the EHR and must apply those measures to improve care. By putting $27 billion behind this initiative, DHHS has incentivized health care providers to use electronic documentation technology and data management as a way to make meaningful changes in the provision of care. Hence the government is now jump-starting the health care industry's e-conversion in an effort to expedite the journey to the best of all possible outcomes in health care: *value-based purchasing* and the pursuit of *best practices* on the way to the gold standard, *evidence-based practice*. Achieving high value for patients must become the overarching goal of health care delivery, with value defined as the "health outcomes achieved per dollar spent" (Porter & Teisberg, 2006, p. 1). According to Porter (2010), this goal is what matters most for patients and unites the interests of all actors in the system. If value improves, then everyone (patients, payers, providers, and suppliers) can benefit while the economic sustainability of the health care system is strengthened.

## ◆ Quality Measures for Inpatient Rehabilitation

As Porter (2010) notes in his seminal article, "What Is Value in Healthcare?," value should define the framework for performance improvement in health care. Rigorous, disciplined measurement, and improvement of value is the best way to drive system progress. Yet value in health care remains largely unmeasured and misunderstood. To narrow the scope of this valiant and necessary search, we will focus our discussions on quality measures in inpatient rehabilitation; **Table 8.6** is an example of an outcome hierarchy for knee osteoarthritis. PPACA of 2010 stipulates that "not later than October 1, 2012 . . . the secretary shall publish the measures selected," and further, "for fiscal year 2014 and each subsequent rate year, each rehabilitation facility shall submit . . . data on quality measures . . ." (Patient Protection and Affordable Care Act, 2010, PPACA §3014, Quality Measurement). So we know our timelines for quality measures; now how do we get there? The U.S. offers advanced health care services; however, the care is not always accessible, effective, safe, and efficient. According to Deutsch (2010), health care quality problems include the following:

- Wide variation in health care service utilization

- Underuse of some services

- Overuse of some services

- An unacceptable level of errors

**Table 8.6**   Outcome Hierarchies for Knee Osteoarthritis

| Dimensions | Primary Acute Knee Osteoarthritis Requiring Replacement |
|---|---|
| Survival | Mortality rate (inpatient) |
| Degree of health or recovery | Functional level achieved |
| | Pain level achieved |
| | Extent of return to physical activities |
| | Ability to return to work |
| Time to recovery and time to return to normal activities | Time to treatment |
| | Time to return to physical activities |
| | Time to return to work |
| Disutility of care or treatment process (e.g., diagnostic errors, ineffective care, treatment-related discomfort, complications, adverse effects) | Pain |
| | Length of hospital stay |
| | Infection |
| | Pulmonary embolism |
| | Deep vein thrombosis |
| | Myocardial infarct |
| | Immediate revision |
| | Delirium |
| Sustainability of health or recovery and nature of recurrences | Maintained functional level |
| | Ability to live independently |
| | Need for revision or reoperation |
| Long-term consequences of therapy (e.g., care induced illnesses) | Loss of mobility due to inadequate rehabilitation |
| | Risk of complex fracture |
| | Susceptibility to infection |
| | Stiff knee due to unrecognized complication |
| | Regional pain syndrome |

*Source:* Adapted from Porter, M. E. (2010). What is value in healthcare? New England Journal of Medicine, 363, 2477–2481.

The quality measure that differentiates rehabilitation from all medical specialties is a functional assessment and the consequent functional outcome. We will see in every level of rehabilitation care to be described that each level of care is premised on a "functional assessment." According to Granger et al (2000), "a functional assessment evaluates an individual's abilities and limitations. The essence of it is the measurement of an individual's use of the variety of skills included in performing tasks necessary to daily living, leisure activities, vocational pursuits, social interactions, and other required behaviors" (p. 151). When rehabilitation was refining its outcomes in the early 1980s, acute care was still measuring its health outcomes in a highly binary manner: life or death. Despite rehab's focus on function and quality of life, rehabilitation practitioners are challenged to be definitive and develop some across-the-board accepted tool box of quality measures that will be used to evaluate health care performance in a manner that permits comparisons across facilities and across time. Currently, for example, measurements of aphasia due to stroke vary across the four settings supported by Medicare coverage: home health, SNF, long-term acute care hospital (LTACH), and IRF. So we first need a uniform tool that can compare similar patients across different settings. The CARE tool is the expected final standardized common denominator for all rehabilitation outcomes beginning in 2013, and thus fosters the hope of obtaining condition-specific and multidimensional outcomes for rehab patients.

Health care reform has already established timelines and requirements for quality reporting (IRF and LTACH quality reporting [§3004 in the PPACA]), which will be effective with fiscal year 2014 (which starts October 1, 2013). The measures that will be elaborated on later will be endorsed by National Quality Forum (2011) or other consensus organizations. The Secretary of Health and Human

Services is to publish the consensus measures by October 1, 2012. If a provider fails to report its outcomes on these consensus measures, that failure will result in reduction of annual payment update by 2%.

## Quality Measure Implementation

The quality of health care services has moved from being primarily an issue for regulating, licensing, and accrediting agencies to a concern of clinicians, administrators, researchers, payers, and consumers. The Institute of Medicine (IOM) has defined quality of care as the "the degree to which health services for individuals and populations increase the likelihood of desired health outcomes and are consistent with current professional knowledge" (IOM, 2001, p. 226). The Secretary of Health and Human Services established a national strategy to improve health service delivery, patient outcomes, and population health in section 3011 of PPACA. Secretary Kathleen Sibelius made her first report to congress in January 2011 and is required to produce such an executive summary report annually thereafter. We will discuss the three activities that use quality measures and have been shown to improve health care:

- Public reporting
- Quality improvement
- Pay-for-performance activities

### Public Reporting

Proponents argue that public reporting helps patients, referring physicians, and purchasers of health care make better informed choices about which providers offer the best care. However, public reporting was not associated with higher use of quality information for selecting health providers, but public reporting did stimulate hospitals to engage in quality improvement activities (Fung, Lim, Mattke, Damberg, & Shekelle, 2008). To be even more blunt and critical of public reporting, Kelly, Thompson, Tuttle, Benesch, and Holloway (2008) concluded that publicly reported quality data specifically pertaining to patients with stroke are incomplete, confusing, inaccurate, and distorted. Clearly, transparency must and will continue, because it is hardwired into all federal and most state health care programs. However, the public reports must become more complete, appropriately qualified, and accurate as consumers become more health literate.

### Quality Improvement

Quality improvement has been the bedrock of health care providers' approach to quality for the last quarter of a century. All accrediting bodies now have standards requiring performance improvement (PI) activities as part of their quality and patient safety programs (see Chapter 10). Most PI programs reference Donabedian's model (Donabedian, 1988) that purports to evaluate quality based on structure, process, and outcomes:

- *Structure measures* track whether a particular mechanism or system is in place.
- *Process measures* track performance of a particular action.
- *Outcome measures* consider the end results of care, such as morbidity and mortality resulting.

Tremendous strides have been made in the area of quality in rehabilitation from reducing falls and hospital-acquired pressure ulcers to increasing the percent of patients returning to the community. There are many approaches to quality from the simple Plan–Do–Study/Check–Act cycle of performance improvement to subscribing to manufacturing models like Toyota or Motorola. Weed (2010) features dramatic results when Seattle Children's Hospital embarked on the continuous performance improvement (CPI) journey, which over several years has resulted in tremendous cost savings, improved outcomes, enhanced employee satisfaction, and improved patient experience scores. There is no question that the surviving and thriving providers of health care that are deeply immersed in such dramatic change will need to espouse and embrace CPI or its ilk for the foreseeable future.

### Pay for Performance

In our undergraduate classes on Behavior Management, and in "Parenting 101," we learned that rewards change behavior. So it should come as no surprise to learn that the use of incentives to reward the providers who demonstrate better quality of care based on performance data has been shown to lead to improved care (Deutsch, 2010). The P4P pilot in section 10326 of PPACA (2010) requires that no later than January 1, 2016, a pilot test of value-based purchasing be conducted for:

- IRFs
- LTACHs
- Psychiatric hospitals
- Cancer hospitals
- Hospices

The Secretary of Health and Human Services is legislatively empowered to expand the program anytime after January 1, 2018. It is important to note that payment is linked to *quality*. Thus, DeJong (2010) suggests that providers will be highly motivated to collect quality-related data and will be strongly attuned to quality metrics, their properties, case-mix adjustment, and the like, and finally that they will invest heavily in quality measurement infrastructure, for example, health information technology, an electronic health record, and continuous performance training and programs.

Early in 2008, the Secretary of HHS contracted with the National Quality Forum (NQF) (qualityforum, 2011) to assist in developing and implementing the P4P initiative. The NQF is a nonprofit organization that aims to improve the quality of health care for all Americans through fulfillment of its mission:

- Setting national priorities and goals for performance improvement
- Endorsing national consensus standards for measuring and publicly reporting on performance
- Promoting the attainment of national goals through education and outreach programs

We are most interested in this context of P4P in NQF's formal Consensus Development Process (CDP) (NQF, 2011) to evaluate and endorse consensus standards, including performance measures, best practices, frameworks, and reporting guidelines. The CDP is designed to call for input and carefully consider the interests of stakeholder groups from across the health care industry. The CDP includes nine major steps from a call for intent to submit candidate standards and call for nominations and candidate measures to board ratification and appeals. The CDP is a comprehensive and well-respected approach to the development and vetting of measures. NQF has already made several congressional reports on this issue, and is actively engaged in taking the key steps to finalizing the quality measure including measure development, national selection/endorsement, and measure implementation. The NQF evaluation criteria for these measures are as follows:

- Importance of measure and report
- Scientific acceptability of measure properties
- Usability

- Feasibility
- If competing measures, best-in-class

According to Quality Forum (Qualityforum.com, 2011), scientific acceptability of measure properties requires that the label clearly indicates this criterion applies to measure properties:

- Precise specifications
- Reliability, validity, and discrimination (testing is expected to demonstrate reliability and validity)
- Demonstration of comparability if more than one data source/method is allowed
- Specifications should allow for identification of disparities
- Risk adjustment
- Exclusions

So we are on the verge of finalizing the requisite outcome measures that will get health care in general and more specifically rehabilitation to value-based purchasing, genuine quality, and real patient safety using the best science and practice available.

The challenges to this goal are daunting. Will rehabilitation-focused quality measures arise that meet the litmus test above? We look for rehabilitation to be assigned three types of measures—outcome, process, and efficiency—that will be case-mix adjusted with exclusion criteria/outliers, and finally an agreed-upon threshold or benchmark for a "good" outcome. The considerations that Deutsch (2010) stresses are critical to be considered are the following:

- Medical rehabilitation has primarily measured quality by focusing on outcome measures rather than process or structure measures.
- Patient outcomes are a result of more than just the effectiveness of the rehabilitation treatment provided.
- Patient outcomes also reflect other factors such as the patient's diagnosis, the severity of the patient's illness, comorbidities, and personal characteristics.
- In order for an outcome measure to be a *valid quality measure*, factors other than the treatment effectiveness must be accounted for by case-mix adjustment.

In addition, as we know with any reform, there lurk potential unintended consequences:

- Reduced quality in unmeasured areas (e.g., "teaching to the test")
- Reduced patient access to appropriate care (e.g., providers may limit access to patients who are sicker or for whom care is more challenging)
- Increased disparities in care (by region, race/ethnicity, etc.)
- Gaming of data to obtain incentives

What are the candidates for rehab's quality measures? DeJong's crystal ball (2010) and this author jointly posit the following:

- Functional status/gain
- Discharge destination
- Health status/medical complications
  - —Needs to be condition-specific, e.g., pressure ulcers in spinal cord injury

- Mortality
- Postdischarge emergency room visits
- Rehospitalizations
- Patient satisfaction/experience
- Participation in community

These measures should make conceptual and intuitive sense (content validity), be relatively easy to measure, not be easily gamed, and, of course, reliable and valid. What other considerations might trouble us?

- Potential professional turf battles in selecting process-based quality indicators
  - —Professional associations will sometimes insist that that process variables related to their interventions be included as quality indicators.
  - —Including discipline-specific process quality indicators guarantees the use of the discipline, confers legitimacy, and helps to assure payment.
  - —Not including discipline-specific measures is sometimes seen as threatening.

There are clearly potential positive effects:

- Shift from prestige competition to quality competition; unleash quality competition and dispense with the popularity contest of *Best Hospitals.*
- Stimulate search for best practice and evidence-based practice (EBP).
- Reduce the primacy of randomized-controlled trials in defining EBP.
- Search for best practice replaces prestige competition as the new engine of innovation.
- Transparency makes markets more efficient, and, it is hoped, more accountable.
- Foster research; make the clinical environment more conducive to effectiveness research, and translatable research inquiry, in the search for best practice and EBP.

## Transparency

In the final analysis, health care reform will turn to accreditation's harbinger of value—transparency. As we have learned in purchasing a car or a house, transparency is the critical consumer variable that supersedes all other factors. Transparency, engendered and supported by accreditation in health care, will make markets more efficient and accountable. This prediction is summarized in the following quotation from the Institute of Medicine's *Crossing the Quality Chasm* (IOM, 2001):

> Rule 7: The need for transparency
> The health care system should make information available to patients and their families that allow them to make informed decisions when selecting a health plan, hospital, or clinical practice, or choosing from among alternative treatments. This should include information describing the system's performance on safety, evidence-based practice, and patient satisfaction. (p. 62)

# References

American Association for Accreditation of Ambulatory Surgery Facilities, Inc. (AAAASF), (2011). http://www.aaaasf.org

American Speech-Language-Hearing Association (ASHA). (1992, Sep). Standards for professional service programs in audiology and speech-language pathology. *ASHA, 34*, 63–70

American Speech-Language-Hearing Association (ASHA). (2008). *Incidence and prevalence of speech, voice, and language disorders in adults in the United States: 2008*. Rockville, MD: Author

Annotated Code of Maryland. (2001). COMAR 10.24.01.02(4)(b)

Baldridge National Quality Program. (2011). *Health care criteria for performance excellence*. Gaithersburg, MD: National Institute of Standards and Technology. www.quality.nist.gov/

Berke, J. (2010). Hearing Loss–Demographics–Deafness Statistics: Statistically, How Many Deaf or Hard of Hearing? *About.com Guide.* http://deafness.about.com/cs/earbasics/a/demographics.htm

Blackstone, S. (2011). Personal communication

Boone, B. J. (2011). Accreditation—A quality frame work in the consumer-centric era. In S.R. Flanagan, H. Zaretsky, & A. Moroz (Eds.), *Medical aspects of disability: A handbook for the rehabilitation professional* (4th ed., pp. 687–706). New York: Springer Publishing

Buell, J. M. (2010, Mar-Apr). Lean Six Sigma and patient safety: a recipe for success. *Healthcare Executive, 25*, 26–28, 30, 32 passim

Bush, H. (2008). *Covenant Health's Pledge to Patients*, Hospitals and Health Networks, Fall Supplement, pp. 8–12

Cebul, R. D., Rebitzer, J. B., Taylor, L. J., & Votruba, M. E. (2008, Fall). Organizational fragmentation and care quality in the U.S healthcare system. *Journal of Economic Perspectives, 22*, 93–113

Centers for Medicare and Medicaid Services (CMS). (2004). *Inpatient rehabilitation facility prospective payment system*, August 15, 2005, Final Rule (42 CFR Part 42). gov/InpatientRehabFacPPS/04_IRFPAI.asp; http://www.hhs.cms.gov/irfpai/finalreg.html

Centers for Medicare and Medicaid Services (CMS). (2005). http://cms.gov/deficitreductionsact

Centers for Medicare and Medicaid Services (CMS). (2010a). hhtp://cms.gov/oasis

Centers on Medicare and Medicaid Services (CMS). (2010b). http://cms.gov/EHRIncentivePrograms

Centers for Medicare and Medicaid Services (CMS). (2011). http://cms.hhs.gov

Commission on Accreditation of Rehabilitation Facilities (CARF). (2011). *Medical rehabilitation standards manual*. Tucson, AZ: Author

Community Health Accreditation Program (CHAP). (2011). http://www.chapinc.org

Comprehensive Accreditation Manual for Hospitals (CAMH). (2011). Oakbrook Terrace, IL: The Joint Commission. http://jcrinc.com

Counte, M. A., & Meurer, S. (2001, Jun). Issues in the assessment of continuous quality improvement implementation in health care organizations. *International Journal for Quality in Health Care, 13*, 197–207

DeJong, G. (2010). *Challenges in measuring and reporting quality in rehabilitation programs, a measure for rehab programs*. American Congress of Rehabilitation Medicine-American Society of Neuro Rehabilitation: Joint Educational Conference, Montreal, Quebec, CA

Deutsch, A. (2010). *Quality measures for rehabilitation programs*. American Congress of Rehabilitation Medicine-

American Society of Neuro Rehabilitation: Joint Educational Conference, Montreal, Quebec, CA

Diamond, L. C., Wilson-Stronks, A., & Jacobs, E. A. (2010, Dec). Do hospitals measure up to the national culturally and linguistically appropriate services standards? *Medical Care, 48*, 1080–1087

Disney Institute. (1999). http://www.disneyinstitute.com

Disney Institute. (2009). http://www.disneyinstitute.com

DNV Healthcare. (2011). http://www.dnvaccreditation.com

Donabedian, A. (1988, Sep). The quality of care. How can it be assessed? *Journal of the American Medical Association, 260*, 1743–1748

Eccleston, S. M. (1995). *Managed care and medical cost containment in workers' compensation: A national inventory 1995-1996*. Cambridge, MA: Workers' Compensation Research Institute

Fung, C. H., Lim, Y. W., Mattke, S., Damberg, C., & Shekelle, P. G. (2008, Jan). Systematic review: the evidence that publishing patient care performance data improves quality of care. *Annals of Internal Medicine, 148*, 111–123

Goldberg, A. J., & Young, L. M. (2011, May-Jun). What every CEO should know about Medicare's recovery audit contractor program. *Journal of Healthcare Management, 56*, 157–161

Golper, L., & Brown, J. (Eds.). (2004). *Business matters: a guide for speech-language pathologists*. Rockville, MD: American Speech-Language-Hearing Association

Goonan, K. J. (1994). Using quality assurance systems to change behavior. In T. W. Granneman (Ed.), *Review, regulate or reform? What works to control workers' compensation medical costs* (pp. 247–267). Cambridge, MA: Workers' Compensation Research Institute

Granger, C. V., Kelly-Hayes, M., Johnston, M., Deutsch, A., Braun, S., & Fiedler, R. C. (2000). Quality and outcome measures for medical rehabilitation. In R. L. Braddom (Ed.), *Physical medicine and rehabilitation* (2nd ed., p. 151). Philadelphia: WB Saunders Company

Hasnain-Wynia, R., Yonek, J., Pierce, D., Kang, R., & Greising, C. (2006). *Hospital language services for patients with limited English proficiency: Results from a national survey*. Health Research and Educational Trust. http://www.onlineresources.wnylc.net/pb/orcdocs/LARC_Resources/LEPTopics/HC/2006_HospitalLanguageServicesforLEPPatients.pdf

Hospital Compare. (2011). Hospitalcompare.hhs.gov

Human Rights Campaign Foundation (HRCF). (2011). Healthcare Equality Index 2011. hrfc.org

Institute of Medicine (IOM). (1999). *To err is human*. Washington, DC: National Academy Press

Institute of Medicine (IOM). (2001). *Crossing the quality chasm. A new health system for the 21st century*. Washington, DC: National Academy Press

International Organization for Standardization. (2000). *ISO 9000–2000 (E)*. Geneva, Switzerland: Author

The Joint Commission. (2011). *Comprehensive accreditation manual for hospitals (CAMH)*. Oakbrook Terrace, IL: Author

Joint Commission Perspectives (TJC). (2010). http://www.jointcommission.org

Joint Commission Resources (JCR). (2011). http://www.jcrinc.com

Kelly, A., Thompson, J. P., Tuttle, D., Benesch, C., & Holloway, R. G. (2008, Dec). Public reporting of quality data for stroke: is it measuring quality? *Stroke, 39*, 3367–3371

Leap Frog Group (LFG). (2004). http://www.leapfroggroup.org

Leap Frog Group (LFG). (2011). http://www.leapfroggroup.org

Levey, N. N. (2011). U.S. healthcare spending far outpaces other countries. *Baltimore Sun*, June 30, p. 1

National Business Group on Health (NBGH). (2009). http://www.bussinessgrouphealth.org

National Committee of Quality Assurance. (2003). *Achieving the promise: Transforming mental health care in America. Final Report.* Rockville, MD: Department of Health and Human Services

National Committee of Quality Assurance. (2011). http://www.ncqua.org

National Institute on Deafness and Other Communication Disorders (NIDCD). (2011). *Mission statement.* http://www.nidcd.nih.gov/about/learn/mission.html

National Quality Forum (NQF). (2011). Qualityforum.org

Patient Protection and Affordable Care Act (PPACA). (2010). Public Law 111–148 124 Stat.119. Washington, DC: Government Printing Office

Phillips, S. (2011). *Healthier healthcare with ISO quality standards.* http://www.dnvaccreditation.com

Pleis, J. R., & Lethbridge-Cejku, M. (2006). Summary health statistics for U.S. adults. National Health Interview Survey, 2005. Publication No. (PHS) 2008–1563. National Center for Health Statistics, *Vital Health Statistics, 10.* Hyattsville, MD: U.S. Department of Health and Human Services Center for Health Statistics

Porter, M. E. (2010). What is value in healthcare? *New England Journal of Medicine, 363*, 2477–2481

Porter, M. E., & Teisberg, E. O. (2006). *Redefining healthcare: creating value based competition on results.* Boston: Harvard Business School Press

President's Advisory Commission on Consumer Protection and Quality in the Health Care Industry. (1998). *Quality first: Better care for all Americans.* Washington, DC: Government Printing Office

Rao, P., Ellis, C., & Douglas, S. (2002). *Cultural shift happens: A new value framework.* Invited session presented to CARF's Medical Rehabilitation's International Conference, Tucson, AZ, January

Studer Group. (2011). www.studergroup.com

Tax Equity and Fiscal Responsibility Act (TEFRA). (1982). Public Law 97–248, 96 stat 324. Washington, DC: Government Printing Office

Towers Watson. (2010). *2010 employee survey: National rehabilitation hospital summary of findings.* towerswatson.com

U.S. News and World Repor.t (2011). *Top ranked hospitals.* health.usnews.com/besthospitals/rankings

Walsh, A. (2010). *Dialysis industry prepares for new payment methodology: How might bundling effect providers differently?* http://www.thehealthcareinvestor.com/admin/trackback/189955

Weed, J. (2010). *Factory efficiency comes to the hospital.* Newyorktimes.com./2010/07/11/business/11seattle.html

# Resources

Commission on Accreditation of Rehabilitation Facilities (CARF). (2012). *Standards manual for CARF accreditation.* 4891 East Grant Road, Tucson, AZ 85712. Phone: 800–444–8991. Web site: http://www.carf.org

The Joint Commission. (2011). One Renaissance Blvd., Oakbrook Terrace, IL 60181. Phone: 630-792-5000. Fax: 630-792-5005 Web site: http://www.jointcommission.org

# 9

# Cost-Effectiveness Analysis in Speech-Language Pathology Outcomes

*Richard M. Merson and Michael I. Rolnick*

## ♦ Chapter Focus

This chapter discusses financial data collection, analysis, and reporting, and summarizes the terms and concepts involved in financial outcome analysis as they relate to outcomes data collection and data management in the speech-language pathology environment. Representative examples of financial outcome data are presented and their implications discussed.

## ♦ Introduction

Although an understanding of clinical outcome benefits is critical to the delivery of services to individuals with communication and related disorders (Darley, 1982; Frattali, 1992, 1993; Goldberg, 1993; Trace, 1995; Wertz, 1993), an analysis of the cost-effectiveness data is mandatory for the survival of our profession (Boston, 1994; Keatley, Miller, & Mann, 1995; Rao, 2011; Rolnick & Merson, 1996). National health expenditure costs grew from 5.1% of the gross domestic product (GDP) or $28.65 billion in 1960 to 17.6% of GDP or $2.5 trillion in 2009, and it is projected to reach 19.3% of GDP in 2019 (CMS, 2011). The clinical services delivered to more than 45 million Americans with communication and related disorders will continue to be seriously affected by fiscal health care restraints and evidence-based clinical outcomes (Bello, 1994).

It is with concern that we note from the American Speech-Language-Hearing Association (ASHA) Omnibus Survey that only 42% of reporting speech-language pathologists and 29% of audiologists are collecting and reporting treatment or financial outcome data (Slater, 1995). ASHA now mandates clinicians to engage in evidence-based practice to maintain their clinical competence (Ratner, 2006).

Both clinical and financial outcome data should be collected and integrated using a common tool to answer the financial questions of those who challenge our profession's cost-effectiveness and clinical benefit to our patients. It is not enough to know how much improvement occurred or whether our services made a difference; we must also be cost-efficient and demonstrate the value of our interventions to our patients and our community.

In today's health care environment, we are being asked several important questions. Boston (1994, p. 35) stated that the debate on health care reform can be summed up in a single frustratingly complex question: "Who provides what services, to whom, in what settings, for how long, at what cost, to produce what benefit?" Weintraub (2003), in his widely recognized book, *Cardiovascular Health Care Economics,* made this query simpler, "How do people choose to allocate resources when it is not possible to pay for all desired goods and services?" We must use health care economics to defend the costs to provide a necessary societal benefit in speech-language pathology services. Arthur Rolnick, economist and former senior vice president and director of research at the Federal Reserve in Minneapolis has performed experiments on the return on investment from early childhood development, and found it to be "extraordinary, resulting in better working public schools, more educated workers, and less crime" (Rolnick & Grunewald, 2003, p. 11). He estimates the economic return on investment (ROI) in preschool at up to $17 for every dollar spent. The ROI in early childhood education far exceeds any public expenditures in other areas, for example on billion-dollar sports stadiums (Rolnick, 2011). Our profession should certainly be able to demonstrate the ROI in the treatment and prevention of communication disorders.

Without aggregate data that reflect case-by-case information, we cannot answer the above-mentioned questions in a meaningful way. For instance, it is important to know the average length of treatment for particular client populations. We should be able to determine the average number of treatments needed to achieve optimal benefit from treatment. The average costs to patients and our service institutions for our treatment should also be known in a particular clinical environment. When certain individuals (outliers) exceed the mean values referred to above, we need to have the ability to determine and analyze the reasons for these exceptions.

These pieces of financial information should then be linked to our clients by diagnostic categories. By doing so, we can observe and report the differences that exist in our clinical practice patterns as they affect financial outcomes. It is entirely reasonable to expect that the length of treatment for one communication disorder will be different from that for another. Consequently, the varying costs per case for the treatment of different speech, voice, fluency, language, cognitive-communication, and swallowing disorders will be both identifiable and justified.

## ◆ Differentiating Outcome Data

In general, outcome data can be categorized into *clinical data* and *cost data.* In this way we can separate two very different but related aspects of a clinical program. Clinical outcomes can be considered in relation to the type of client, site of service, type of treatment, different clinicians, or severity of the presenting disorder. *Cost outcomes* can also relate to the above variables but with respect to the actual institutional and community costs (e.g., charges, indirect costs, time expended, cost of being unemployed or underemployed because of a communication disorder, etc.) involved in obtaining specific clinical outcomes.

Clinical outcome is determined, for example, by comparing clients' admission severity status with their discharge severity status using a functional outcome measure. The difference between these two values is a *functional assessment* (Frattali, 1993; Frattali, Thompson, Holland, Wohl, & Ferketic, 1995; Sederer & Dickey, 1996; Seligman, 1995) of improvement, or *clinical outcome.* This aspect of change over time in relation to specific variables should not be confused with *clinical efficacy* (Darley, 1982; McReynolds, 1990; Olswang, Thompson, Warren, & Minghetti, 1990; Pietranton, 1995a; Wertz, 1993), which is a measurement of the effects of a controlled treatment or intervention modality.

Cost outcome data relate to the clinical data that have been obtained for the same client or set of clients. Cost outcome may include information on the length of treatment, number of procedures provided, cost per procedure, or subsequent cost per case. The length of stay (LOS) refers to the amount of time a client remains in the treatment program beginning with the first visit and ending with the final contact for which a charge has been generated. The LOS is usually different for each diagnostic category in the clinical program. The *number of procedures* or treatments provided is the total number of billable contacts generated during the LOS. This number should also differ by diagnosis. *Cost per procedure*, at this point in our discussion, is the actual charge generated for a procedure provided within the LOS time period. Finally, the *cost per case* is determined by multiplying the cost per procedure by the total number of procedures provided during a given length of stay for a particular client.

Assume that Mr. Jones has been referred to your facility for treatment and that you have established an outcome assessment system. Your plan is to collect both clinical and financial outcome data for the period of time that he is under your care. You will first assess his admission status using a selected clinical outcome measure. When Mr. Jones is discharged you will use the same scale for discharge assessment. The difference between the two scores will yield a clinical outcome. The amount of time he actually spends in treatment will be his length of stay. The total number of evaluations and treatments will be added to determine the number of procedures provided. Your total procedures for each case will be multiplied by your institution's cost per procedure, and this amount will then determine the cost per case (the total cost per client). Eventually, Mr. Jones's data will be combined with those of other clients as you develop your database for aggregate outcome analysis.

Both clinical and financial outcome data can be collected and reported as aggregate data to analyze clinical-cost relationships for a comprehensive picture of outcome analysis. In this way, both types of outcome data can serve as invaluable tools in program evaluation and design, and can answer important questions posed by the service delivery industry (Boston, 1994; Eisenberg, 1995; Goldberg, 1993; Ratner, 2006; Rao, 2011; Sederer & Dickey, 1996; Weil, 1995).

## ♦ Cost versus Charges

As changes in the service delivery environment have occurred, financial terms have been redefined. Traditionally, speech-language pathologists have considered the cost of services to be the amount actually billed to the payer. If a clinician treated a client with a diagnosis of stuttering for 10 sessions at $50 per session, then the cost was determined to be $500 for that series of interventions. Actually, the $500 would only be a cost to the *client* or a *payer* who reimbursed the clinician for that amount. More correctly, the $500 is the amount of gross revenue or charges generated, and is not a reflection of the actual costs incurred for providing those services. Furthermore, the revenue charged is very different from the revenue actually collected as many payers only reimburse a portion of the charges (e.g., usual, customary, or reasonable charges).

Actual cost should be considered as the sum total of financial factors for provision of services including salary, supplies, rent, and other direct expenses associated with treatment. This category of direct expenses is different from those indirect expenses incurred when the clinician is working within a business or corporate structure that involves other costs. Administrative and operating expenses that are peripherally related to treatment are examples of *indirect expenses*. These costs are also considered in determining the actual cost per procedure, which can then be used to calculate the cost per case for a particular diagnosis.

With changes in reimbursement methodologies, many speech-language pathology programs have become *cost centers* rather than *revenue centers*. This is especially true under capitation programs and for services reimbursed by Medicare's Prospective Payment Systems associated with diagnosis-related groups (DRGs). Under capitation, an agreed-upon dollar amount is given to the provider per enrollee for any and all services that may be provided to all enrollees. Under a prospective payment arrangement, a predetermined fixed payment is made for all clinical services provided to a client for, in the case of Medicare, a particular diagnosis. Regardless of the reimbursement arrangement, the difference between the payment and the costs of providing the services becomes the profit (or loss). Obviously, if costs exceed the payment structure, no profit is realized. Even in a fee-for-service payment structure, revenue deductions or contractual allowances may be imposed. This occurs when the payers reimburse at a lower rate than the charges being billed. This shortfall reduces the anticipated gross revenue and interacts with the costs affecting the net income. As a cost center, we must be mindful of our direct and indirect costs as they impact our ability to demonstrate a positive "bottom line," or net income, so that we can remain a viable part of the provision of clinical care within the corporate structure.

Increasingly, the charges for treatment become less important than the actual costs of providing that treatment. The program that can track and control direct and indirect costs is better positioned to adjust to a changing case mix as it affects reimbursement. The regular and systematic collection of financial outcome data relating to costs enables a clinical program to determine the average cost per case for all diagnostic categories. It is important to link cost data with clinical data to determine *value* or "effectiveness." This information, when coupled with clinical outcome data, can, for example, be analyzed to show the results of cost-cutting initiatives, re-engineering, or other attempts to modify clinical service delivery. This approach is threatening to many clinicians (Eisenberg, 1995) who fear that clinical outcome and, therefore, quality of care can be compromised by decreasing costs of providing services. However, by collecting defined financial data as well as monitoring quality clinical outcome data carefully, we will obtain the necessary objective information to make appropriate decisions, and to protect the quality of our services to communicatively impaired individuals.

## ◆ Outlier Analysis

If collecting data on the average number of treatments provided, length of stay within the program, and actual cost per case are important, then we must be able to analyze and account for the individual variations that will occur. The concept of *outlier analysis* is employed to look at these variances. Any clients that fall outside the parameters of preestablished financial criteria become outliers.

For example, if the mean length of stay (treatment duration) for 50 clients with vocal fold nodules is 90 days, and seven of those individuals had a length of stay of 150 days, they are considered outliers. The financial component of the outcomes management system should include identifying specific outliers so that the reasons for their outlier status can be analyzed. There may be appropriate clinical reasons for an extended length of stay. There may also be process problems within the program that resulted in the outliers. The system should be capable of conducting this individual client analysis by diagnostic category, treatment site, and individual clinician. All possible factors can then be investigated that could contribute to an individual client's outlier status. If problems are detected, steps can be taken to correct them and thus improve cost-efficiency.

If financial outlier analysis procedures are initiated on an interdisciplinary basis, then speech-language pathologists should link financial data to their clients' clinical outcomes. This linkage may help explain any variances and justify an appropriate intensity of treatment within that interdisciplinary team. Many hospitals are starting to use *service-line management teams* to look at the process of care in specific inpatient populations. These teams of professionals and administrators try to identify duplication and unnecessary work. They will then eliminate the costs associated with redundant processes. For example, rehabilitation for dysphagia and other acute-care speech-language pathology services will be scrutinized along with other hospital services. The program must have the supporting data to justify the service when this type of outlier analysis begins.

## ◆ Value Analysis

*Cost-benefit* and *cost-effectiveness* are two types of economic value analyses used to influence decision making regarding the allocation of resources (American College of Physicians, 2000; Boston,

1994; Granger, Ottenbacher, & Fiedler, 1995; Hoomans, Ament, Evers, & Severens, 2010; Keatley et al, 1995; Weintraub, 2003). These techniques can be employed in speech-language pathology when a provider or payer seeks to maximize the return on those moneys spent for treatment.

When total costs (dollars) are divided by the total benefits (e.g., functional outcome), a *cost-benefit analysis* is being employed. This formula provides a kind of measure of the cost per benefit, or, in economic parlance, the "bang for the buck." Either direct costs, indirect costs, or both can be factored into the formula. You can also perform this analysis with charges. Using charge per procedure, if a client with dysarthria following a stroke received 10 treatments at $120 per treatment, the "cost" would be $1200. If this client was able to return to work 3 weeks earlier than expected as a result of her speech improvement, the cost of treatment would be balanced against the economic benefit of an early return to full employment. This type of benefit analysis might be used on a national scale to demonstrate the value of rehabilitative services to a particular client population such as stroke survivors. In such an example, the total rehabilitation costs would be compared with cost savings involving return to work for the client or his or her spouse. We are exposed to a cost-benefit analysis when we propose payment for a specific treatment regimen to a vocational rehabilitation counselor who then looks at the budget, determines the likelihood of the client's return to work, and either approves or denies our request. When performing a *cost-effectiveness analysis* (CEA), the outcomes and costs of two different interventions are compared. Dr. Robert Nease in his discussion of cost-effectiveness analysis in cardiovascular healthcare economics (Weintraub, 2003) explains this as follows: "CEA is a discipline that seeks to generate insight about the economic efficiency with which various interventions generate health benefit" (Nease, 2003, p. 111).

This is a type of clinical and financial outcome analyses that speech-language pathology administrators and evidenced-practice researchers should be discussing nationally. We should be focused on linking costs with clinical outcomes to demonstrate the value of our interventions in obtaining meaningful and functional results in a cost-effective manner. This, in effect, is the goal of *accountable care organizations* (ACOs) and ASHA's goal of establishing evidenced-based clinical practice guidelines. The challenges and processes for incorporating evidence-based practice guidelines into clinical practice are discussed here and later in Chapter 13.

## ♦ Evidence-Based Practice Guidelines

The concept of a standardized clinical practice guideline is another method of looking at the utility of clinical outcomes, as it provides evidence for cost-effectiveness and patient benefit. In the 1990s we talked about critical pathway analysis as a method of graphing sequence and a roadmap of a multidisciplinary staff's professional treatment activities against a timeline with financial resource constraints for providing the services.

Because the complete interdisciplinary process of treatment is considered in a practice guideline, any variances in that process may affect cost. Indeed, a major motivation for developing clinical guidelines for evidenced-based practice (EBP) is to ensure that the management of the cost of care does not diminish the clinical benefit. Outlier analysis is an important part of this process. Those cases requiring a more intensive level of care over a longer period of time would be looked at carefully during this analysis. The goal is to develop a clinical guideline in which all treatments are appropriate, nonduplicative, timely, and thereby cost-effective. Thus, both length and intensity of care can be controlled and costs can be contained.

The process of EBP development, however, can result in adverse effects on patient care. Any decrease in length of stay or reduction in services should never prevent a positive clinical result. As emphasized by Wilkerson (in Breske, 1995), "Ultimately we're interested in quality outcomes, efficient processes, and reducing costs" (p. 19). Ratner (2006) summarizes the challenges in implementing EBP:

EBP raises questions about defining acceptable forms of evidence for treatment effectiveness and efficacy, the potential roles of nonspecific or common factors, therapist quality in achieving therapy outcomes, and eventual applications of EBP that may overly confine which treatments are considered acceptable and reimbursable. (p. 257)

# ♦ Uses of Cost-Effectiveness Data

To make informed decisions, meaningful data about our program should inform and provide the basis for our actions. Appropriate data constitute a powerful tool when presented to support our professional judgments. CEA or comparative financial outcome data can be used in program evaluation, marketing, answering administrative concerns, and managing third-party reimbursement limits.

As pressures mount in service environments, clinical programs need to look closely at their practice patterns to ensure both quality of care and cost-effectiveness. This process of program evaluation requires the collection, analysis, and reporting of data to take actions that are both appropriate and necessary. Financial outcome data linked to clinical outcome data are the purpose of cost-benefit analysis or CEA. For example, in reviewing the cost per case for various clinicians working within a particular service line, you note that one clinician has consistent outliers. Her clients have longer lengths of stay and a higher average number of treatments when compared with clients of the other clinicians within the group. After discussions with the supervisor, you learn that this clinician has been assigned more complex, severely impaired cases. Furthermore, job dissatisfaction, related to these caseload characteristics, has been expressed by this individual. A solution would be to reassign all cases by distributing levels of complexity and severity on an equitable basis. After further discussions with the supervisor, you discover that this same clinician is unable to discharge clients on a timely basis. A second solution would be to counsel the clinician and ask her to change her practice patterns to coincide with discharge policies. These scenarios are representative of program evaluation and exemplify the benefits of ongoing outcomes data collection and analysis.

Here is a CEA formula for this situation:

$$\text{Cost-Effectiveness} = \frac{\text{Total Costs Clinician 1} - \text{Total Costs Clinician 2}}{\text{Clinical Outcome Gain 1} - \text{Clinical Outcome Gain 2}}$$

Marketing your services to referral sources requires specific data reporting considerations. Consider the case of several physicians who have started a group practice within an ACO. The physicians are *at risk* for the total costs of providing care, including the number of referrals for specialty rehabilitative services. The group is seeking a quality speech-language pathology program that provides cost-efficient treatment. Your program is asked to make a presentation detailing your clinical outcomes and associated length of stay, average number of treatments, and estimated total cost per case. Because the physicians are specialists in neurology and otolaryngology, they are interested only in a specific list of diagnoses. By having cost and clinical effectiveness outcomes available by clinical diagnosis, your presentation can be both credible and quality assuring.

*Administrative concerns* can also be addressed using appropriate data. Assume you need to add a staff member in your acute-care rehabilitation program for dysphagia. The hospital administrators, however, are looking at every staffing request carefully and require full justification. They are especially concerned because a large proportion of patients with dysphagia are covered by Medicare, and any increase in costs may not be covered by its prospective payment structure. Because you have been collecting outcome data and utilizing CEA for this diagnosis you are able to demonstrate a lower number of treatments per case, which is a reduction from the previous year with maintenance in clinical benefit. The clinical outcome remained the same despite the necessary reduced cost of providing the service. You could also demonstrate that your program's intervention strategy hastened discharge because patients were swallowing safely. Finally, and importantly, you could show a lower incidence of rehospitalization for patients with dysphagia who were referred to your service earlier in their hospital stay compared with patients who were referred late as a result of aspiration. This type of information can be documented with CEA outcome analyses that compare both clinical benefit and cost utilizing different staff sizes and intervention strategies.

When *managed care* companies call to question your request for treatment for a specific diagnosis, it would be very effective to support the request with data. A data table that lists the average number of treatments required to obtain a specific clinical outcome for a large number of similar patients with the same communication disorder makes it difficult for the managed care organization to deny the request. In the long term, these types of data tables may facilitate approvals of future requests without the time-consuming and often futile attempts to justify treatment.

## ◆ Benchmarking

Although clinical outcome data can be used for the above-mentioned purposes, advantages are also found by comparing those data with regional and nationally clinical databases. It may be important to know how your program compares with other similar programs to assess your relative effectiveness or position in the marketplace. This comparison process of benchmarking is increasingly evident throughout the health care environment (Rao, 2011; State University of New York at Buffalo, School of Medicine and Biomedical Sciences, The Center for Functional Assessment Research, 1993). The Centers for Medicare and Medicaid Services (CMS) has recognized, certified, and eventually will be mandating the ASHA's National Outcomes Measurement System (NOMS) for establishing EBP guidelines that will reflect benchmarking or outcome data comparisons between national and regional databases to your own clinical program.

Dictionary definitions commonly describe *benchmarking* as a standard by which something can be measured or judged. A working definition of benchmarking is the continuous process of measuring our services or outcomes against those of our toughest competitors or those organizations recognized as leaders. Another term often used interchangeably with benchmarking is *competitive benchmarking.* Competitive benchmarking could be as simple as comparing our department's length of stay by services to that of competing institutions in the same service arena. More advanced competitive benchmarking might include comparing the best patient outcomes for each service site to patient satisfaction measures, social patterns, or levels of economic status within facilities throughout the nation.

In your facility, it would be very helpful to know how your program's length of stay, average number of treatments, or total charges compared with other local providers for particular diagnoses. If you find that your outcome data exceed your regional benchmarks, you may decide to investigate the reasons for this discrepancy. When becoming involved in benchmarking activities, you must be certain that your program is being compared with actual "peer" organizations with comparable attributes (Williams, Baum, & Stein, 1995).

## ◆ Data Collection Mechanisms

Most organizations collect financial data regarding their clinical service programs. Financial officers are responsible for establishing cost accounting systems that meet the needs of a particular corporation, university, school district, or private practice. Although these systems address many of the financial concerns of an organization, it is the clinical program that is usually most concerned with clinical benefit outcome. Because of increased "accountable care" and internal cost containment efforts, each speech-language pathology program will have to decide how to establish an outcome measurement system as a first line of defense for the future.

Advances in computer technology enable the collection of massive amounts of data regionally and nationally (Granger et al, 1995; Mullen, 2004; Pietranton & Baum, 1995b; Ryan, 1995, 1996; Trace, 1995). If there is no active outcome measurement system or data repository process in place within your organization, or if you have no input into what is being measured or if no meaningful cost data are being linked to pertinent clinical information, *it is urgent that your program implement such a system* (Johnson, A.F., 1994; Johnson, D.R., 1995).

# ◆ Available Outcome Measurement Systems

A variety of outcome systems are in use to collect and analyze clinical and financial outcome data in every health care specialty (Eisenberg, 1995; Frattali et al, 1995; Larkins, 1987; Merson, Rolnick, & Weiner, 1995; Sederer & Dickey, 1996; Shelton & Bianchi, 1996; Weintraub, 2003). In nearly all instances, financial data collection is a major component of these systems. The following is a brief description of three clinical outcome systems:

1. Functional Independence Measure–Uniform Data System for Medical Rehabilitation (FIM–UDSmr™) (Granger et al, 1995) is the most widely used rehabilitation system worldwide, with nearly three million patients in their database.

2. Beaumont Outcome Software System© (BOSS) is a small software program (20,000-patient database) developed at William Beaumont Hospital, 1995–2005 (Merson et al, 1995).

3. National Outcomes Measurement System (NOMS) (American Speech-Language-Hearing Association, 2011), developed by ASHA, meets the requirements of the CMS for EBP, Physician Quality Reporting System (PQRS) analyses, and ACOs. NOMS will be increasingly indispensable for all clinical systems in speech-language pathology in the United States.

## Uniform Data System-Medical Rehabilitation

Without question, the most widely used data collection system in rehabilitation in this country and abroad is the UDSmr, which contains FIM and was developed by the State University of New York at Buffalo in 1983. FIM is being used in thousands of facilities in the United States, Canada, and Australia. This is a regional, national, and international database that has been dedicated to inpatient and, to a lesser extent, outpatient rehabilitation programs. It makes use of a standardized set of 18 multidisciplinary functional scales. FIM links its seven-point rating scales to both demographic and financial data. Data are collected locally and conveyed by the Internet to New York for computer analyses. Reports are available online for each participating facility. Each institution's data are benchmarked against nationwide patterns.

In addition to a summary of FIM data, UDSmr uses several integrated financial formulas. For example, *charge efficiency* is defined as the average gain in overall FIM score per dollar (calculated as total FIM gain divided by charges times 1000 to reflect gain per $1000). Further, LOS *efficiency* is the average total FIM gain per day or week (calculated as the total FIM gain divided by the length of stay or by seven to reflect gain per week). Finally, UDSmr provides an analysis system that allows the facility to identify which patients are exceeding the expected length of stay per impairment and severity.

## Beaumont Outcome Software System©

Whereas FIM exemplifies a national and international system, BOSS exemplifies an in-house or facility-specific approach (Merson et al, 1995). Developed at William Beaumont Hospital, Royal Oak,

Michigan, BOSS allows each user to set up specific clinical and outcome data collection parameters and control the collection and analysis functions within the user's facility. Designed as a Microsoft Windows–based program, it was used on personal computers to create tables, charts, and graphs that linked clinical and financial outcomes data, as well as patient satisfaction by different service sites. Analysis by specific clinical diagnoses in speech-language pathology was incorporated. Length of stay, average number of treatments, and cost per case were integrated with clinical outcome. Outlier analysis reports could also be generated, with the user determining the outlier parameters to be analyzed. Although the BOSS database remains for analyses and empirical studies, the Beaumont Health System Speech-Language Pathology Department has completely implemented the ASHA-NOMS system in both its adult and pediatric programs.

### National Outcomes Measurement System

The American Speech-Language Hearing Association developed NOMS through a series of investigations that formed the National Treatment Outcome Data Collection Project (Mullen, 2004; Williams et al, 1995). NOMS uses an Internet-based system of reporting and collecting admission, discharge, treatment, reimbursement source, client satisfaction, and demographic data on each client. NOMS also includes three components: adults, pre-kindergarten, and schools. Comprehensive reports are generated and available on the ASHA NOMS Web site. This system collects information on treatment and evaluation hours per patient that can be used to create local costs per procedure. The ASHA NOMS utilizes a series of seven-point functional communication scales for adults and children. As of 2011, NOMS has an approximate database of 176,000 adults, and 17,000 pre-kindergarten children. It has collected data from 1300 different hospitals, and 270 pre-kindergarten service programs, with 3000 speech-language pathologists certified to report adult data and 1000 certified to report pre-kindergarten (Floyd Roye, Project Administrator, National Center for Evidenced–Based Practice in Communication Disorders of ASHA, personal communication, 2011). Robert Mullen, director of the National Center for Evidence Based Practice in Communication Disorders, provides the founding rationale of NOMS: "Third-party payers, operating in an environment emphasizing return-on-investment, sought data linking expenditures on [speech-language pathology] services with tangible outcomes affecting resource utilization, such as required level of care and ability to discharge" (p. 413). Mullen concludes, "A critical analysis of the evidence supporting clinical practice in speech-language pathology and alignment of the practice with this evidence remains at the core of evidence-based practice" (Mullen, 2004, p. 416).

## ♦ Cost Analysis in Speech-Language Pathology

Assume now, that you have committed your program to the concept of outcomes measurement, advisedly applying the ASHA NOMS, and have selected a system to collect data. As the clinical and financial outcome data becomes available, it is clear that you must be able to link or integrate that data in such a way that critical questions can be both asked and answered. For instance, it is not enough to know the average costs for a large heterogeneous population of individuals with variety of communication disorders. It would be of greater benefit to obtain a more detailed look at cost in the following manner:

• Cost by diagnosis

• Cost by admission severity

• Cost by clinical outcome

• Cost by gender or age

- Cost by clinician

- Cost by clinical site

Although, as a clinical profession, we have been aware of the need to report financial data, we have not had an effective means to do so. By using CEA or examining our costs as a part of the clinical benefit and then comparing intervention strategies, we can begin to respond to payers who ask, "How much?" "How long?" and "What is the beneficial gain?" As well, we can address the questions of corporate financial officers and their comptrollers, such as, "What are the total costs of providing services in different communities with different communication disorder service needs?"

A cost analysis by severity of condition and any comorbidities would be particularly important. Many clients in need of speech-language pathology services in hospitals are referred with more complex medical diagnoses and we are servicing more severe communicative disorders than ever before. Schools are seeing more children who have medical and social histories that include congenital problems, addiction, abuse, severe injury, tracheostomies, dysphagia, and other medical conditions. Clinical benefits as well as cost outcomes are influenced by the severity of disorders being treated. Without the ability to analyze both clinical as well as cost outcome by severity of condition and comorbidities, the outcome data are meaningless. When your outcomes measurement system can analyze data by severity of condition, a more meaningful outcome picture emerges.

Consider also the need to know your costs by clinical site of service. For example, your data may show that the costs of providing rehabilitation within an off-site pediatric program are higher than payer expectations. There may be administrative pressures to reduce costs because of a poor net profit in comparison to other sites staffed by your department. Using an outcomes measurement system, you discover that although costs are high, the clinical benefits exceed those of your other sites. In fact, many families that you serve are actively seeking referrals to your facility's clinics, physicians, and other services because of their satisfaction with the improvement in their child's speech and language. The value of your pediatric program might now be regarded in a different light. This scenario exemplifies how integration of different outcome parameters can support programs and justify variations in costs by clinical site.

The Patient Protection and Affordable Care Act (PPACA), signed into law by President Obama in 2010, attempts to create systems for health care coverage for much larger numbers of Americans than are currently covered. This act will facilitate the formation of ACOs, recognized by the CMS as providing coordinated, monitored, affordable, and beneficial outcomes. ACOs will be formed by health systems (e.g., aggregate hospitals, clinical practices groups in local communities) to closely analyze cost and benefits. The CMS will provide monetary incentives to ACOs. These ACOs must have developed standardized EBP clinical guidelines or practice patterns to control costs and maintain good clinical benefit. By looking at certain practice aspects of an individual practitioner or a group of clinicians' intervention strategies, a *report card* can be generated. That is, practice patterns are analyzed for that individual or group in relation to his or her peers. In many cases, length of stay, intensity of treatments, and subsequent cost generated per case are aspects that are graded on these report cards. Needless to say, many professionals are suspicious of this concept. However, using comparative CEA that is sensitive to individual clinician performance can have an influence on those practice patterns that do not serve the client or the clinical facility in a beneficial manner. If a particular speech-language pathologist demonstrates costs far in excess of others providing the same services, an evaluation of the circumstances can be performed. On balance, these services might deliver such a significant benefit to the community that these extra costs can be justified. A system that allows for this type of analysis will be a valuable tool.

## ♦ Linking Cost and Benefit Outcome Data

**Table 9.1** presents representative outcome data using BOSS for four different clinical sites in our hospital system: voice clinic, outpatient adult rehabilitation, children's clinic, and inpatient adult

**Table 9.1**  Sample Outcomes Data by Clinical Site and Admission Status Discharge Status, Clinical Outcome, Procedures, Length of Stay, and Average Cost Per Case*

| Outcome Variables | Site I<br>N = 253 | Site II<br>N = 293 | Site III<br>N = 136 | Site IV<br>N = 262 |
|---|---|---|---|---|
| **Admission status:**<br>average scale value, where 1 is<br>profound severity and 7 is normal | 2.97 | 2.73 | 3.97 | 4.00 |
| **Discharge status:**<br>average scale value, where 1 is<br>profound severity and 7 is normal | 5.61 | 4.90 | 5.21 | 4.90 |
| **Clinical outcome:**<br>average gain in points on 7-point<br>scale | 2.65 | 2.17 | 1.24 | 0.89 |
| **Length of stay:**<br>average number of days | 50 | 400 | 76 | 19 |
| **Procedures:**<br>average number of evaluations<br>and treatments | 4.5 | 74 | 28 | 18 |
| **Charges:**<br>average cost per case | $463 | $4312 | $3754 | $2179 |

Site I, outpatient voice clinic; Site II, outpatient children's clinic; site III, outpatient adult rehabilitation; site IV, inpatient adult rehabilitation.

*Note: This table does not contain accurate costs. The cost figures are used for illustration purposes only and cannot be interpreted as average charges or costs for speech-language pathology services.

rehabilitation. Both clinical and cost outcomes are presented. This table compares various outcomes by each clinical site and begins the process of comparing the clinical benefit/gain for each site based on cost. It might be interesting to ask, "At what functional level of communication are patients discharged and how do costs differ?" One can see that, although all sites discharged patients at an average severity level of 5 on a seven-point scale, costs were very different. When looking at the number of procedures, length of stay, and case mix, however, these variations can be explained. By viewing this general aggregate display of clinical gain (outcome) and cost (charges per case) data, an explanation of variance of cost at different service sites is possible. Based on specific questions that then arise, a more in-depth analysis can be done to defend the value and sustainability of a program.

**Table 9.2** presents, by specific clinical diagnosis, the same outcome parameters for a single site. Again, discharge seems to occur at about the same level of function, even though different clinical outcome scales are used for each diagnosis in this particular hospital's clinical site. As would be expected, the average number of procedures to attain a comparable clinical gain (outcome) is very different. This number of procedures drives the higher costs for certain diagnoses. One can appreciate how linking cost data to clinical data would enable clinicians to "predict" the average length of stay, average number of visits, or average cost for a particular diagnosis. The use of this type of outcome data to predict both clinical benefit (gain) and cost can be a powerful tool in answering relevant questions from clients, families, administrators, and payers.

Applying cost-benefit-analysis to compare two of the diagnoses in **Table 9.2** (childhood language disorders and vocal nodules), reveals that childhood language disorders was the most costly per benefit (i.e., outcome gain), as illustrated further here, in applying cost-benefit analysis to two diagnoses:

1.  Vocal nodules intervention

$$\text{Cost-Benefit Analysis} = \frac{\text{Cost (\$386)}}{\text{Clinical Outcome Gain (2.6)}} = \$148.46$$

**Table 9.2**    Sample Outcome Data by Communication Diagnosis;[*] Outcome Variables Exhibited for Each Diagnosis

| Outcome Variables | Adult-Aphasia N = 54 | Stuttering N = 17 | Dysphagia N = 41 | Vocal Nodules N = 46 | Childhood Language Disorder N = 43 |
|---|---|---|---|---|---|
| Admission status | 4.0 | 3.8 | 1.9 | 3.1 | 2.7 |
| Discharge status | 5.1 | 5.4 | 5.1 | 5.7 | 4.9 |
| Clinical outcome: gain in points on a 7-point scale | 1.1 | 1.6 | 3.2 | 2.6 | 2.3 |
| Length of stay: average number of days | 78 | 87 | 20 | 40 | 509 |
| Procedures: average number of evaluations and treatments | 32.5 | 6.5 | 4 | 4 | 87 |
| Charges: average cost per case | $4439 | $563 | $799 | $386 | $5221 |

[*]*Note:* This table does not contain accurate costs. The financial figures are used for illustration purposes only and cannot be interpreted as average charges or costs for speech-language pathology services.

2.  Childhood Language Intervention

$$\text{Cost-Benefit Analysis} = \frac{\text{Cost (\$5221)}}{\text{Clinical Outcome Gain (2.3)}} = \$2270$$

A more costly benefit would not necessarily discourage a program from providing this clinical service if other factors were considered, such as a large number of cases referred by physicians and a very substantial amount of funding received from the community. Treating vocal nodules, on the other hand, is far more cost–beneficial, but hiring a full-time clinician to cover a much smaller referral base (for example, spasmodic dysphonia) might discourage a program from offering such a service. A program director could examine several different treatment interventions for childhood language disorders, such as group therapy compared with 100% individual treatment, and examine the CEA.

A similar dilemma is present in comparing the cost-benefit (CB) of stuttering treatment (CB = $563/1.6 gain = $352) and adult aphasia (CB = $4439/1.1 = $4035). The aphasia cost per gain (1.1) is over $4000, but for stuttering is less than $400. CEA would be important for assessing different aphasia intervention strategies to obtain comparable gain and manageable costs.

This information is valuable to program administrators who want to know where their best "bang for the buck" can be found, and marketed. This does not speak to eliminating treatment for aphasia, but rather attempting to make these programs as efficient and standardized in practice guidelines as possible.

**Table 9.3** compares clinical gain and cost outcomes by age, gender, and severity. By using outcomes data in this manner, one can look at the possible effects these variables can have on cost. As can be seen in this hypothetical example, age appears to have some potential effect on both the discharge status and length of stay, but the number of procedures and charges remained essentially the same. Males, on the other hand, although showing more improvement, required more procedures, a longer length of stay, and more dollars expended. As might be expected, the more severe the condition, the greater the charges, length of stay, and number of procedures required; however, more change appeared to occur. These data suggest what is seen in many rehabilitation environments—that more severely involved clients tend to carry a greater cost burden. Although the reasons for these outcomes are not always clear, differences do exist and require additional investigation. Further data

**Table 9.3**   Sample Outcome Data of Adult Clients with Aphasia and Dysarthria Treated in an Outpatient Rehabilitation Program; Outcome Variables Examined Across Age, Gender, and Severity*

| Outcome Variables | Age 56–95 years N = 75 | Age 21–55 years N = 23 | Male N = 49 | Female N = 49 | Mild to Moderate N = 41 | Severe N = 57 |
|---|---|---|---|---|---|---|
| Admission status | 3.9 | 4.1 | 3.9 | 4.1 | 4.8 | 3.5 |
| Discharge status | 5.1 | 5.4 | 5.3 | 5.1 | 5.8 | 5.0 |
| Clinical outcome: gain in points on a 7-point scale | 1.1 | 1.2 | 1.3 | 1.0 | 0.93 | 1.5 |
| Length of stay: average number of days | 80 | 99 | 98 | 68 | 72 | 53 |
| Procedures: average number of evaluations and treatments | 36 | 36 | 43 | 27 | 25 | 111 |
| Charges: average cost per case | $4873 | $4895 | $5871 | $3670 | $3421 | $7095 |

*Note: This table does not contain accurate costs. The cost figures are used for illustration purposes only and cannot be interpreted as average charges or costs for speech-language pathology services.

analysis will begin to explain the differences found and to structure EBP practice guidelines. CEA may shed light on intervention strategies that are more efficient and less costly.

## ♦ Cost-Effectiveness Analysis by Clinician

Cost-effectiveness analysis can be explained as the costs divided by the benefit between interventions. This is calculated by dividing the total costs times the procedures by the average client gain or clinical outcome (i.e., measured in points on a seven-point Functional Communication Scale). CEA can be performed between treatment types as well as between clinicians. Charges for services are not reasonable cost estimates. What programs *charge* for a service and what they are *reimbursed* are highly variable. It is better to utilize your program or corporation's estimate of your *costs per procedure* calculated by including all direct and indirect costs by the number of services you deliver.

$$\text{Cost-Effectiveness} = \frac{\text{Cost per procedure: Clinician 1 – Clinician 2}}{\text{Clinical Outcome: Clinician 1 – Clinician 2}}$$

**Table 9.4** is an example of using *cost-benefit* and *cost-effectiveness* involving two groups of patients with dysphonia secondary to unilateral vocal paralysis treated by two different clinicians. Clinician A achieved a cost-benefit of $82 per clinical outcome, whereas clinician B's costs were higher at $148 per clinical outcome. It would seem that clinician A had a less costly treatment program. However, CEA reveals that the differences in costs divided by gain of the two clinicians were insignificant (CEA = $28, between clinicians A and B). In this hypothetical scenario, the average severity levels of the patients treated by clinician A were higher than those treated by clinician B. Therefore, as in this example, patients who enter treatment with higher severity levels usually demonstrate

**Table 9.4** Cost-Benefit and Cost-Effectiveness Analysis of Treating Clients with Vocal Paralysis Dysphonia by Two Different Clinicians; Outcome Variables Exhibited for Clinician A and Clinician B*

| Outcome Variables | Clinician A | Clinician B |
|---|---|---|
| Admission status | 1.44 (profound) | 2.34 (severe) |
| Discharge status | 5.85 (minimal) | 5.11 (mild) |
| Clinical outcome: gain in points on a 7-point scale | 4.41 | 2.77 |
| Length of stay: average number of days | 22 | 38 |
| Procedures: average number of evaluations and treatments | 3.63 | 4.14 |
| Charges: average cost per case | $363.88 | $411.00 |
| Cost benefit: cost ÷ outcome | $363.88 ÷ 4.41= $82.51 | $411.00 ÷ 2.77 = $148.37 |
| Cost-effectiveness: clinician A versus clinician B | $\dfrac{\$363 - \$411\ (\$48)}{4.41 - 2.77\ (1.7)} = \$28$ | |

*Note: This table does not contain accurate costs. The cost figures are used for illustration purposes only and cannot be interpreted as average charges or costs for speech-language pathology services.

greater gain. It is not unusual, for this diagnosis, that patients with higher admission severity levels attain relatively higher gains because they have more potential gain. CEA, therefore, should be analyzed controlling for different severity levels. Further, it would appear that these severity levels influenced the mean length of stay and average number of procedures, thereby increasing the total charges.

## ♦ Cost Analysis in Benchmarking

Finally, one might consider a formula for cost analyses in *benchmarking* to describe the performance of health systems compared with national and regional data collected on comparable clinical populations. The ASHA NOMS is the only system that makes that possible in speech-language pathology. CMS is expected to require ACOs to benchmark to establish standards of clinical guidelines in regions and throughout the nation. Beaumont Health Systems is completely committed to fully establishing the ASHA NOMS in our outpatient and inpatient programs for children and adults. If your organization has not considered this, it is imperative that you move quickly in this direction.

**Figure 9.1** and **Table 9.5** compare the Beaumont Health System of Michigan with the nation and a Midwest region for the Functional Communication Measure (FCM) for swallowing. The histograms in **Fig. 9.1** illustrate the progress made by a group of adults with dysphagia. The first bar in each pairing illustrates the percent of clients who made no progress, and the second bar illustrates the percent of clients who made progress; 20% of Beaumont clients made no progress and 80% made progress. This compares to regional clients, where 25% made no progress and 74% made progress, and national clients, where 24% made no progress and 75% made progress. To get some insight into cost-effectiveness we need to consider the treatment hours required to obtain these FCM progress data. As you can see in the bottom histogram, Beaumont clients required 10.6 hours to achieve their progress, whereas regional clients required only 6.4 hours and national clients 7.5 hours to achieve their progress. One could reasonably conclude that greater treatment sessions or hours produce more progress. But this

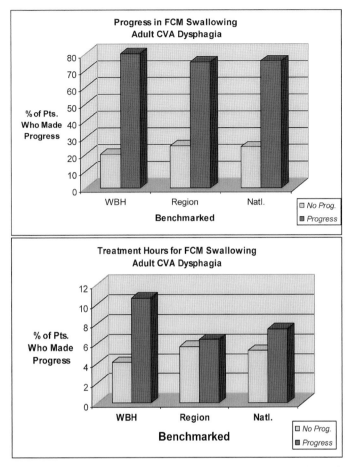

**Fig. 9.1**   Cost-effectiveness parameters-benchmarked: adult dysphagia clients' progress and hours in treatment for William Beaumont Hospital System (WBH), regional Midwest hospitals (Region), and the national outcomes (Natl.). CVA, cerebrovascular accident; FCM, Functional Communication Measure.

**Table 9.5**   Cost Effectiveness Parameters, Benchmarked: Adult Dysphagia Functional Measure; Client's Progress and Hours of Treatment for Beaumont Hospital System Compared with Midwest Regional Hospitals and National Hospitals Using the National Outcome Measure of Swallow

| Functional Measure of Swallow | Beaumont Health System | Midwest Region | Nation |
|---|---|---|---|
| **Progress:** percent of pts. who made progress | 80% | 74% | 75% |
| **No progress:** percent of pts. who did not make progress | 20% | 25% | 24% |
| **Treatment hours:** pts. who made progress | 10.6 | 6.4 | 7.5 |
| **Treatment hours:** pts. who did not make progress | 4.1 | 5.7 | 5.3 |

Cost-Effectiveness Analysis =

$$\frac{(\text{Beaumont Health System Treatment Hours} \times \text{Cost per Hour}) - (\text{Region Treatment Hours} \times \text{Cost per Hour})}{\text{Beaumont Health System Percent Pts. Made Progress} - \text{Region Percent Pts. Made Progress}}$$

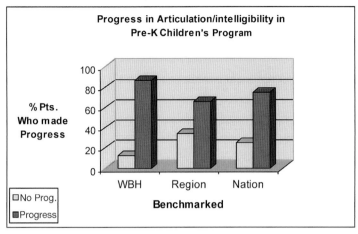

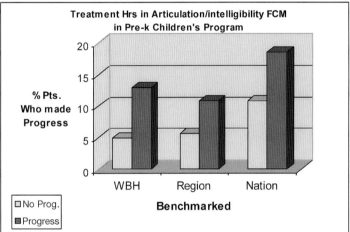

**Fig. 9.2**  Cost-effectiveness parameters, benchmarked: children's progress and treatment hours in Functional Communication Measure of articulation/intelligibility, for William Beaumont Hospital System (WBH), regional Midwest hospitals (Region), and national outcomes (Natl.).

is still incomplete, as we need to know the cost per procedure for the national and regional benchmarks to really examine the cost-effectiveness. What we have is cost-efficiency or progress achieved over time, but we need to include another cost factor to get a more accurate and valid CEA. Note the CEA formula for Beaumont and Region at the bottom of **Table 9.5.**

**Figure 9.2** and **Table 9.6** illustrate the same cost analysis in our Children's Center for Speech-Language Disorders. The NOMS FCM for articulation/intelligibility was used to compare regional and national benchmarks. The Beaumont program had 87% children who progressed on this FCM compared with regional at 66% and national at 75%. The Beaumont program required on average 12.9 hours of treatment to obtain its progress, the regional 10.9 hours, and the national 18.6 hours. The national comparison data indicated many more hours of treatment were required to obtain a level of clinical outcome score that was less than that of Beaumont, so one might conclude that the Beaumont program is more efficient. But we should also look carefully at our corporation's cost per procedure and compare that to the national average to validly identify cost-effectiveness. One might also question if the children seen at Beaumont are comparable in severity, diagnosis, or comorbidities to confidently compare or benchmark these outcomes. Note the CEA formula for Beaumont and Region at the bottom of **Table 9.6**.

**Table 9.6**   Cost-Effectiveness Parameters, Benchmarked: Children's Articulation/Intelligibility, Functional Measure; Progress and Hours of Treatment for Beaumont Hospital System Compared with Midwest Regional Hospitals and National Hospitals Using the National Outcome Measure of Articulation/Intelligibility

| Functional Measure Articulation/Intelligibility | Beaumont Health System | Midwest Region | Nation |
|---|---|---|---|
| **Progress:** percent of pts. who made progress | 87% | 66.2% | 75.1% |
| **No progress:** percent of pts. who did not make progress | 12.9% | 33.8% | 24.8% |
| **Treatment hours:** pts. who made progress | 12.9 | 10.9 | 18.6 |
| **Treatment hours:** pts. who did not make progress | 5 | 5.7 | 10.9 |

Cost-Effectiveness Analysis =

$$\frac{(\text{Beaumont Health System Treatment Hours} \times \text{Cost per Hour}) - (\text{Region Treatment Hours} \times \text{Cost per Hour})}{\text{Beaumont Health System Percent Pts. Made Progress} - \text{Region Percent Pts. Made Progress}}$$

## ♦ Some Caveats

The use of financial outcome formula to reduce complex integrated data into a more manageable concept should be approached with caution. Albert Einstein would often forewarn his colleagues: "Not everything that counts can be counted, and not everything that can be counted counts" (Kevin Harris Website, 1995, Albert Einstein Collected Quotes, 1995). Some of us also recall Wendell Johnson's admonition: "The map is not the territory" (Johnson, 1946). No synthesis or condensation of such data to answer financially related questions can portray the clinical realities that face the patient, family, and clinician in coping with a communication or related disorder. In fact, financial and clinical outcome measures should be understood for what they are *not*. These measures cannot account for all the direct or indirect costs of delivering services, nor can they account for all the costs to the patient to be rehabilitated. Financial outcome measures, when linked to clinical outcome can serve as an innovative shorthand to be used to indicate change over time for purposes of better understanding some of the many variables that might be linked to that change.

## ♦ Conclusion and Future Directions

Teisberg, Porter, and Brown (1994) stated, "Health care reform in the United States is on a collision course with economic reality. . . . In industry after industry, the underlying dynamic is the same: competition compels companies to deliver increasing value to customers. The fundamental driver of this continuous quality improvement and cost reduction is innovation" (p. 131).

Integrating cost and clinical outcome data, although indispensable to clinic managers in developing and evaluating treatment programs, will demand careful inferences about the value of our services. This activity, however, is critical if we are to sustain our programs in the presence of rapid and unpredictable change. Databased clinical outcome systems must be embraced and implemented across the country, so that data can be collected, accessed, and examined from multiple perspectives. This should prompt our profession to think differently about how we approach our interventions, and to adopt new terminology and data analysis so that we might achieve the highest possible clinical outcomes, within responsible evidenced-based practice guidelines, at an appropriate and supportable cost.

# References

American College of Physicians. (2000). *Effective clinical practice primer on cost-effectiveness analysis, 3,* 5, 253–255. http://www.acponline.org

American Speech-Language-Hearing Association. (2011). *National Outcomes Measurement System (NOMS).* National Center for Evidence-Based Practice in Communication Disorders. Rockville, MD: Author. http://www.asha.org

Bello, J. (1994). *Communication Facts.* American Speech-Language Hearing Association, Research Information Section. Rockville, MD: ASHA

Boston, B. O. (1994, Nov). Destiny is in the data. A wake-up call for outcome measures. *ASHA, 36,* 35–38

Breske, S. (1995). Forging critical paths for outcomes management. *ADVANCE for Speech-Language Pathologists & Audiologists, November* 5, p. 19

Centers for Medicare and Medicaid Services (CMS). (2011). *NHE fact sheet.* http://www.hhs.gov

Darley, F. L. (1982). The effect of treatment. In F.L. Darley. *Aphasia* (pp. 144–184). Philadelphia: WB Saunders

Eisenberg, L. (1995, Jul). Medicine—molecular, monetary, or more than both? *Journal of the American Medical Association, 274,* 331–334

Frattali, C. M. (1992). Functional assessment of communication: Merging public policy with clinical views. *Aphasiology, 6,* 63–83

Frattali, C. M. (1993, Jan–Mar). Perspectives on functional assessment: its use for policy making. *Disability and Rehabilitation, 15,* 1–9

Frattali, C. M., Thompson, C. K., Holland, A. L., Wohl, C. B., & Ferketic, M. M. (1995). *Functional Assessment of Communication Skills for Adults (ASHA FACS).* Rockville, MD: ASHA

Goldberg, B. (1993, Jan). Translating data into practice. *ASHA, 35,* 45–47

Granger, C. V., Ottenbacher, K. J., & Fiedler, R. C. (1995, Jan–Feb). The Uniform Data System for Medical Rehabilitation. Report of first admissions for 1993. *American Journal of Physical Medicine & Rehabilitation, 74,* 62–66

Harris, K. (1965). Albert Einstein Collected Quotes. Retrieved from: http://www.alangil.org/quotations/einstein.html

Hoomans, T., Ament, A. J., Evers, S. M., & Severens, J. (2010). Implementing guidelines into clinical practice: what is the value? *Journal of Evaluation in Clinical Practice, ISSN 1356–1294,* Blackwell Publishing, October 4, pp. 1–9

Johnson, A. F. (1994). *Creating and applying data base technology for outcome measurement.* Presented at the Outcomes, Reform and Efficacy Conference, Department of Speech-Language Sciences and Disorders, Henry Ford Hospital Medical Center, Detroit, MI

Johnson, D. R. (1995). Integrated computer software helps manage information: A better way to prove outcomes and track costs. *Rehabilitation Outcomes Review in Hospital Rehab,* Atlanta, GA, pp. 119–122

Johnson, W. (1946). *People in quandaries: The semantics of personal adjustment.* New York: Harper & Row

Keatley, M. A., Miller, T. I., & Mann, A. (1995). Treatment planning using outcome data. *ASHA, 37,* 49–52

Larkins, P. G. (1987). Program Evaluation System (PES): Determining quality of speech-language and hearing services. *ASHA, 24,* 21–25

McReynolds, L. (1990). Historical perspective of treatment efficacy research. In L. B. Olswang, C. K. Thompson, S. F. Warren, & N. J. Minghetti (Eds.), *Treatment efficacy research in communication disorders* (pp. 5–14). Rockville, MD: American Speech-Language-Hearing Association

Merson, R. M., Rolnick, M. R., & Weiner, F. (1995). *The Beaumont Outcome Software System© (BOSS).* West Bloomfield, MI: Parrot Software

Mullen, R. (2004, Sep–Oct). Evidence for whom?: ASHA's National Outcomes Measurement System. *Journal of Communication Disorders, 37,* 413–417

Nease, R. F. (2003). Introduction to cost-effectiveness analysis. In W. S. Weintraub (Ed.), *Cardiovascular health care economics* (pp. 111–121). Totowa, NJ: Humana Press

Olswang, L. B., Thompson, C. K., Warren, S. F., & Minghetti, N. J. (1990). *Treatment efficacy research in communication disorders.* Rockville, MD: American Speech-Language-Hearing Foundation

Pietranton, A. (1995a). *Treatment efficacy bibliography.* Rockville, MD: American Speech-Language Hearing Association, Health Services Division

Pietranton, A. A., & Baum, H. M. (1995b, Nov–Dec). Collecting outcome data. Existing tools, preliminary data, future directions. Task Force on Treatment Outcome and Cost Effectiveness. *ASHA, 37,* 36–38

Rao, P. (2011). Evidence-based practice: The coin of the realm in CSD. *The ASHA Leader,* June 7

Ratner, N. B. (2006, Oct). Evidence-based practice: an examination of its ramifications for the practice of speech-language pathology. *Language, Speech, and Hearing Services in Schools, 37,* 257–267

Rolnick, A. (2011). *Getting the Most Bang for the Buck: Quality Early Education and Care,* U.S. Senate, Subcommittee Hearing

Rolnick, A., & Grunewald, R. (2003). Early childhood development: Economic development with a high public return. *FedGazette,* December, pp. 6–12

Rolnick, M. I., & Merson, R. M.(1996). User Friendly Computer System tracks speech outcomes. *Rehabilitation Outcomes Review in Hospital Rehab,* Atlanta, GA, March, pp. 35–38

Ryan, C. R. (1995). Creating specialized information systems. *Transitions, 2,* 18–21

Ryan, C. R. (1996). *R/Com plus resource management and program evaluation modules.* Seattle, WA: R/Com

Sederer, L. I., & Dickey, B. (1996). *Outcomes assessment in clinical practice.* Baltimore, MD: Williams & Wilkins Press

Seligman, M. E. P. (1995, Dec). The effectiveness of psychotherapy. The Consumer Reports study. *The American Psychologist, 50,* 965–974

Shelton, R., & Bianchi, B. (1996). Patient tracking system helps manage outcomes, *costs. Rehabilitation Outcomes Review in Hospital Rehab,* Atlanta, GA, pp. 7–10

Slater, S. (1995). *Omnibus survey results.* Rockville, MD: American Speech-Language-Hearing Association, Science and Research Department

State University of New York at Buffalo, School of Medicine and Biomedical Sciences, The Center for Functional Assessment Research. (1993). *Guide for the uniform data set for medical rehabilitation,* Version 4.0. Buffalo, NY: UB Foundations

Teisberg, E. O., Porter, M. E., & Brown, G. B. (1994, Jul–Aug). Making competition in health care work. *Harvard Business Review, 72,* 131–141

Trace, R. (1995). Outcomes measures lead to increased accountability. *Advance for Speech-Language Pathologists and Audiologists,* 6–7

Weil, T. P. (1995, Winter). How do Canadian hospitals do it? A comparison of utilization and costs in the United States and Canada. *Hospital Topics, 73,* 10–22

Weintraub, W. S. (2003) *Cardiovascular health care economics.* Totowa, NJ: Humana Press

Wertz, R. T. (1993, Jan). Adult-onset disorders. *ASHA, 35,* 38–39

Williams, P. S., Baum, H. M., & Stein, M. E. (1995). *ASHA data collection instruments for measurement of treatment outcomes.* Presented at the American Speech-Language Hearing Association Annual Convention, Orlando, FL

# 10

# Defining Quality Through Patient Safety and Satisfaction Outcomes

*Nancy B. Swigert*

## ♦ Chapter Focus

This chapter suggests that quality is a *construct*, an aspiration, that is difficult to describe or define objectively without referencing the outcome measurements associated with it. Quality, as a whole, seems to be best understood by looking at the shape and size of its parts. The performance expectations defining quality in health care services have been drawn from a variety of sources and commentary over the past decade, but two broad areas seem to dominate the outcome expectations associated with quality in health care today: patient *safety* and patient *satisfaction*. This chapter discusses why and how patient safety and patient satisfaction are so prominent and integral to quality, and describes some of the safety and satisfaction initiatives that are evident in health care policies and practices.

## ♦ Introduction

The trio of topics covered in this chapter—quality, patient safety, and patient satisfaction—are presented in this order by design. Many consider quality as the overarching principle and patient safety as one of the most important outcomes, if not the most important outcome, of quality services. The two are inextricably linked in research, in quality measures, and in many definitions. The Institute of Medicine (IOM) states that patient safety is "indistinguishable from the delivery of quality health care" (Aspden, Corrigan, Wolcott, & Erickson, 2004, p. 4). In fact, the IOM's report, *To Err is Human: Building a Safer Health System*, first published in 1999, (Kohn, Corrigan, & Donaldson, 2009) is often considered the impetus for the quality initiatives we are experiencing today, even though quality initiatives have been present since the early 1990s.

Of course, maintaining patient safety is not the only desired outcome of quality services. There is also the hoped for impact on the *health* of the patient (e.g., cure, remission, improved health, extended life expectancy, etc.). A patient might have a safe experience with the health care system but a poor health outcome, and thus might feel that quality services had not been rendered. For example, a patient with cancer might undergo a course of chemotherapy administered in a safe fashion, only to have a recurrence of the disease because the current standard of care (e.g., concomitant chemoradiation treatment) was not followed. Safe? Yes. Quality? No.

To differentiate patient satisfaction from its relationship to quality and patient safety would be an artificial distinction. Patient satisfaction undoubtedly makes a significant contribution to patients' perceptions that they received quality care. But a separate body of literature focuses on patient satisfaction and thus it is addressed as the third topic in this chapter, allowing the discussion of quality and patient safety to be intertwined.

## ♦ Quality

To discuss quality, we must first define it. But the definition of quality has evolved over the past 25 years. In 1990, the Committee to Design a Strategy for Quality Review and Assurance in Medicare issued a report, *Medicare: A Strategy for Quality Assurance* (Lohr, 1990), that defined quality as "the degree to which health services for individuals and populations increase the likelihood of desired health outcomes and are consistent with current professional knowledge." Quality is an abstract concept. Therefore, most current definitions are linked to measures or indicators of quality. It is difficult to find a definition of quality that does not merely determine how it will be measured. The reliance on measurement may be necessary, but it does not totally define quality. David Loxtercamp, a self-described "country doctor," said in an interview that "quality is more than metrics" (Loxtercamp, 2011). As consumers of health care, each of us would agree we know quality when we experience it. We know the outcome we expect.

Although the 1990 definition in the Medicare report focused on achieving a positive health outcome, the report included quality indicators that were also designed to avoid unfavorable consequences: death, disease, disability, discomfort, and dissatisfaction. Since those initial attempts to define quality, the emphasis has shifted to include a focus on positive outcomes rather than simply avoiding these negative outcomes.

### Initiatives for Quality Improvement

In the late 1990s, President Clinton formed the President's Advisory Commission on Consumer Protection and Quality in the Health Care Industry. The commission was charged to "advise the president on changes occurring in the health care system and recommend such measures as may be necessary to promote and assure health care quality and value, and protect consumers and workers in the health care system" (President's Advisory Commission on Consumer Protection and Quality in Health Care, 1998, p. 1). The commission did not define quality, but identified the following national aims for improvement of health care quality:

- "reducing the underlying causes of illness, injury, and disability;

- expanding research on new treatments and evidence on effectiveness;

- assuring the appropriate use of health care services;

- reducing health care errors;

- addressing oversupply and undersupply of health care resources; and,

- increasing patients' participation in their care" (President's Advisory Commission on Consumer Protection and Quality in the Health Care Industry, 1998, p. 3).

The commission also indicated that a key element of improving quality was the ability to measure specific indicators or objectives and report these to the public. In addition, the measures should be standardized and developed in such a way as to ensure their validity, utility, and meaningfulness. It was the stated desire of the commission that the comparative information on health care quality would be widely available in the public domain. The commission cited the need for public–private partnerships for leadership in the quality initiative. It also promoted a strategy to engage consumers in their own health care management by educating them and providing the information they need to make informed decisions about care.

In 2001, the Committee on Quality of Health Care in America released the report, *Crossing the Quality Chasm: A New Health System for the 21st Century* (Committee on Quality of Health Care in America, 2001). This report followed an earlier report (Kohn et al, 2001) that focused on patient safety. The 2001 report broadened the scope to assess all aspects of quality and listed six aims that health care should be:

- "Safe—avoiding injuries to patients from the care that is intended to help them.

- Effective—providing services based on scientific knowledge to all who could benefit, and refraining from providing services to those not likely to benefit (avoiding underuse and overuse, respectively).

- Patient-centered—providing care that is respectful of and responsive to individual patient preferences, needs, and values, and ensuring that patient values guide all clinical decisions.

- Timely—reducing waits and sometimes harmful delays for both those who receive and those who give care.

- Efficient—avoiding waste, including waste of equipment, supplies, ideas, and energy.

- Equitable—providing care that does not vary in quality because of personal characteristics such as gender, ethnicity, geographic location, and socioeconomic status" (Committee on Quality of Health Care in America, 2001, pp. 5–6).

These six aims have guided most quality efforts in the public (e.g., Medicare) and private arenas and perhaps provide the best definition of quality in health care. Health care should be safe, effective, patient-centered, timely, efficient, and equitable. The committee recommended continued funding by Congress to establish monitoring and tracking processes and cited the need for transparency:

> The health care system should make information available to patients and their families that allows them to make informed decisions when selecting a health plan, hospital, or clinical practice, or choosing among alternative treatments. This should include information describing the system's performance on safety, evidence-based practice, and patient satisfaction. (Committee on Quality of Health Care in America, 2001, p. 8)

The report also suggested aligning financial performance with outcomes, what is commonly called *pay for performance* (P4P), in its recommendation: "Private and public purchasers should examine their current payment methods to remove barriers that currently impede quality improvement, and to build in stronger incentives for quality enhancement" (Committee on Quality of Health Care in America, 2001, p. 18).

Thus two fundamental components of health care reform, public reporting and pay for performance, were suggested. Pay for performance was subsequently mandated by the Benefits Improvement and Protection Act of 2000 and the Medicare Prescription Drug, Improvement, and Modernization Act (MMA) of 2003. P4P, "depending on the context, refers to financial incentives that reward providers for the achievement of a range of payer objectives, including delivery efficiencies, submission of data and measures to payer, and improved quality and patient safety" (McNamara, 2006, p. 6S).

## Private Insurers and Pay for Performance

Reimbursement by private third-party payers is often heavily influenced by Medicare policies, but the relationship is symbiotic. Policies and trends in the private insurance arena have had an impact on Medicare policies. Private payers experimented with P4P for physician services, which increased policy makers' interest in the concept. Not surprisingly, some of the pioneering work in P4P was done in California under the oversight of a voluntary organization, Integrated Healthcare Association. Physician organizations and insurers developed a series of measures of quality, and higher payments are made to practices that score higher. Some insurers in Boston use a P4P format based on quality data already available in standard claims data. A large part was based on cost measures, such as the percent of generic prescriptions (Ginsburg, 2007).

## Who Defines Quality?

With the advent of public reporting, the definitions of quality that matter are prescribed by policy making, accrediting, regulatory, and funding agencies. These definitions, and the indicators by which they are measured, matter most because they drive reimbursement in the P4P model. Individual facilities must not only abide by these external definitions of quality but also have data to back up their claims. More and more quality indicators are being publicly reported, and increasingly consumers are relying on these public reporting sites for information that shapes their health care buying decisions.

The agencies defining quality do so based on evidence and best practice. Typically they complete a review of the literature when defining quality. They may also rate or grade the quality of the research that is reviewed, giving more weight to a randomized-controlled trial (RCT), for example, than to a consensus report. They define all aspects of the indicator: the population or disorder being measured; the goal or target; how measurement will be done; over what period of time the measurement takes place; the sample size needed for reporting, including the numerator and denominator; and what constitutes an outlier. All parameters are clearly defined so that comparisons can be made among facilities.

## National Quality Forum

The National Quality Forum (NQF) originated in 1999 by a coalition of public- and private-sector leaders in response to the recommendations made in the report of the Advisory Commission on Consumer Protection and Quality in the Health Care Industry (National Quality Forum, 2011a–d). The commission recommended that an organization like NQF was needed to focus on patient protection and quality in health care. The recommendation was that this would be accomplished through measurement and public reporting. It receives both public and private funding.

As part of the Medicare Improvements for Patients and Providers Act of 2008 (MIPPA), the U.S. Department of Health and Human Services (DHHS) awarded a contract to NQF to "help establish a portfolio of quality and efficiency measures that will allow the federal government to more clearly see how and whether health care spending is achieving the best results for patients and taxpayers" (National Quality Forum, 2011c).

"NQF evaluates and endorses tools for standardized performance measurement, including: performance measures that assess structure, process, outcomes, and patient perceptions of care; preferred practices that suggest a specific process that, when executed effectively, lead to improved patient outcomes; and frameworks that provide a conceptual approach to organizing practices. These performance standards can be used by institutions, providers, and health care consumers to:

- Create reliable, comparative performance information on which consumers can rely to make informed decisions about their care;

- Ensure practitioners and provider organizations are held accountable for the quality and efficiency of their performance; and

- Support quality improvement activities" (National Quality Forum, 2011a–d).

The NQF states that the data it gathers improves health care through:

- Public reporting to external agencies, which then share the information with the public.

- Reimbursement methodologies like pay for performance, in which institutions are rewarded financially for meeting quality standards and penalized if they don't.

- Institutional use of the data for internal quality improvement.

**Table 10.1**    Examples of the Functional Communication Measure (FCM) of Swallowing, Endorsed by the National Quality Forum (NQF)

Project Name: NVCS (National Voluntary Consensus Standards) for the Prevention and Management of Stroke Across the Continuum of Care

Status: Time-limited endorsed

Original endorsement date: July 31, 2008

Steward(s): American Speech-Language-Hearing Association

Description:
This measure describes the change in functional communication status subsequent to speech-language pathology treatment of patients who exhibit difficulty in swallowing

**Details**

Numerator:
Level of functioning on a seven-point scale at the conclusion of the first speech-language pathology treatment session

Denominator:
Level of functioning on the same seven-point scale at the time of discharge from speech-language pathology services

*Source:* From National Quality Forum. (2011b). Functional communication measure—swallowing. http://www
.qualityforum.org/MeasureDetails.aspx?SubmissionId=682#k=speech&e=1&st=&sd=&mt=&cs=&s=n&so=a&p=1
Exclusion: patients discharged from speech-language pathology services after only one treatment session.

The NQF uses a consensus development process to evaluate and endorse consensus standards. Its Web site currently includes a list of over 600 performance measures it has endorsed, with plans to add lists of other types of consensus standards, including preferred practices and measurement frameworks (National Quality Forum, 2011a).

A search of these performance measures using the term *speech* reveals ten measures listed, including eight Functional Communication Measures (FCMs) from the American Speech-Language-Hearing Association's (ASHA) National Outcomes Measurement System (NOMS): spoken language comprehension, spoken language expression, reading, writing, motor speech, memory, attention, and swallowing. Having these measures endorsed by the NQF means they can be used by speech-language pathologists (SLPs) in P4P reimbursement (**Table 10.1**).

The two other endorsed measures are the percentage of patients aged 18 years and older with the diagnosis of ischemic stroke or intracranial hemorrhage who receive any food, fluids, or medication by mouth and who underwent a dysphagia screening process before taking any foods, fluids, or medication by mouth; and the tympanostomy tube hearing test.

## Agency for Healthcare Research and Quality: National Quality Measures Clearinghouse

Another important entity in quality measurement is the Agency for Healthcare Research and Quality (AHRQ), a part of the U.S. Department of Health and Human Services. The AHQR administers the National Quality Measures Clearinghouse™ (NQMC), which is described as a "public resource for evidence-based quality measures and measure sets." It provides information on how to select, apply, and interpret measures. Unlike the NQF, the NQMC "does not develop, produce, approve, or endorse the measures represented" on its site. It is merely a repository for measures, in seven domains, that meet its inclusion criteria (Agency for Healthcare Research and Quality, 2011c):

- "A *process of care* is a health care service provided to, on behalf of, or by a patient appropriately based on scientific evidence of efficacy or effectiveness.

- An *outcome of care* is a health state of a patient resulting from health care.

- *Access to care* is a patient's or enrollee's attainment of timely and appropriate health care.

- *Experience of care* is a patient's or enrollee's report concerning observations of and participation in health care.

- *Structure of care* is a feature of a health care organization or clinician relevant to its capacity to provide health care.

- A *use of service* is the provision of a service to, on behalf of, or by a group of persons defined by geographic location, organizational or non-clinical characteristics without determination of the appropriateness of the service for the specified individuals. Use of service measures can assess encounters, tests, interventions as well as the efficiency of the delivery of these services.

- *Population health* is the state of health of a group of persons defined by geographic location, organizational affiliation or non-clinical characteristics. (Eligibility for measures of population health is not restricted to recipients of clinical care.)" (Agency for Healthcare Research and Quality, 2011b, p. 1).

The National Quality Measures also include 15 of ASHA's Functional Communication Measures. In addition to those endorsed by NQF, the NQMC also lists alaryngeal communication, augmentative-alternative communication, fluency, pragmatics, problem solving, voice following tracheostomy, and voice (Agency for Healthcare Research and Quality, 2011c).

## Centers for Medicare and Medicaid Services

The Centers for Medicare and Medicaid Services (CMS) do not typically have a role in developing or endorsing quality measures. However, because CMS policies have a significant impact on the entire health care delivery system, what it says about quality is important to all providers in all settings. CMS developed its Roadmap for Quality Measurement in the Traditional Medicare Fee-for-Service Program (CMS, 2009), and it states that its goal is to "guide future CMS decisions in selecting and strategically implementing quality measures in the health care system" (p. 3). This report encourages attention to conditions that are prevalent in the Medicare population (e.g., heart disease, diabetes, pneumonia, chronic obstructive pulmonary disease [COPD]) and indicates that the measures should focus on health outcomes for the patient, transitioning the patient across settings, and resources used to treat the patient. Although the report spotlights these high utilization conditions, it states that CMS should continue to take interest in measures regarding topics such as patient safety, patient experience, end of life and palliative care, and efficient use of health information technology.

The CMS Roadmap for Quality Measurement indicates that the measures should provide information that will enable outcomes-driven, evidence-based care for all patients. The measures should also make the information transparent and easily accessible to consumers, payers, and providers. And, highlighting perhaps the most significant change in quality in the last decade, connecting quality outcomes to reimbursement, the report states that the quality measures should "align financial incentives to reward providers that work together to deliver high quality care" (p. 2). Currently, as illustrated by the 2008 trustees' report, the findings of which are summarized in **Fig. 10.1**, CMS has over 375 quality measures in place that cover all settings except laboratories, durable medical equipment, and hospices.

Similar to the NQMC, the CMS quality measures fall into different domains:

- "Efficiency measures or measures of resource use (e.g., is an MRI used to diagnose pneumonia vs. the more standard chest x-ray?)

- Structure measures to track if a mechanism or system is in place (e.g., IT tools)

- Process measures to track the performance of a particular action, such as use of a particular medication administered to treat a specific disorder

- Intermediate outcome measures to target a test result (e.g., did the treatment lower the blood pressure to the desired level?)

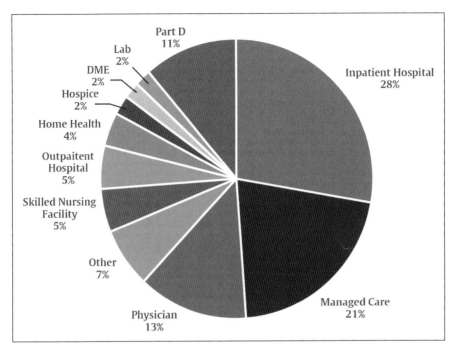

**Fig. 10.1**  Settings that are covered by quality measures: percentage of 2008 total expenditures by setting ($450.5 billion), including Medicare Advantage. Note: The percentages are calculated based on total Medicare spending, including Medicare Advantage.

• Outcome measures to track morbidity and mortality resulting from a specific disease

• Patient centeredness measures that reflect the experience of the patient with the systems and providers" (p. 3).

Of particular interest to SLPs in private practice providing services to patients with Medicare is the provider category of physician and other professionals. In this category, providers can participate in P4P through the Physician Quality Reporting Initiative (PQRI). Established in 2006, the PQRI, for which there are 153 quality measures, is a voluntary incentive payment program for eligible health care professionals. PQRI is intended to support improvements in quality of care to Medicare beneficiaries through the tracking of practice patterns. Private practice SLPs who provide services to adult patients with stroke covered under Medicare Part B are eligible to receive an incentive payment at the end of the year for reporting on the approved quality measures. Eight of ASHA's NOMS Functional Communication Measures have been identified as PQRI quality measures (American Speech-Language-Hearing Association, 2011).

In a section of the Roadmap for Quality Measurement report describing the future of quality measurement, measures that focus on transitioning of care are discussed. Such measures would help move the health care system from a silo approach to a more integrated approach to care. CMS states that when these measures are paired with appropriate financial incentives, they could foster improved coordination of care. The measure could assess care provided in more than one setting by more than one provider type, and measure the care over a longer time frame, for example, the care provided to a patient at the hospital for a specific disease, and the follow-up care provided at the physician's office after discharge.

Speech-language pathology services can play an integral role in these initiatives for quality. As the quality movement in Medicare focuses on high utilization conditions (heart disease, diabetes, cancer, renal disease, joint disease, pneumonia and influenza, COPD) speech-language pathology services for both communication and swallowing disorders will have an impact. If the goal is to focus coordination of care across settings, speech-language pathology services are already provided in each setting in which these patients may receive care for the disorder. CMS also wants the focus to be on quality and value. Treatment of communication and swallowing disorders inarguably improves quality of life, and these services have been shown to be a good value.

## Institute for Healthcare Improvement

It is not just government agencies that focus on quality measures and initiatives to improve quality. The Institute for Healthcare Improvement (IHI) is an independent not-for-profit organization focused on

- "Building the *will* for change
- Cultivating promising improvement *ideas*
- Putting those ideas into action through effective *execution*" (Institute for Healthcare Improvement, 2011, p. 5).

The IHI sponsors an annual conference, National Forum on Quality Improvement in Health Care; collaborates with health care facilities; and disseminates information on best practices. One of its goals is to facilitate the dissemination of research into practice. One of the best known examples is the *ventilator bundle,* a collection of effective processes designed to eliminate ventilator-associated pneumonia. Most hospitals across the country have instituted the ventilator bundle. Other well-known initiatives of the IHI are the use of *rapid response teams* in hospitals, which are designed to intervene when a patient's status first begins to decline, and *medication reconciliation,* in which health care facilities reconcile medications prescribed by different providers. The IHI publishes improvement reports from facilities that have implemented evidence-based projects resulting in improved quality outcomes. These reports cover a wide range of topics including critical care, chronic conditions, palliative care, system improvement, reducing mortality, and health care–associated infections.

## Will Consumers Use the Data?

In a survey completed by the Kaiser Family Foundation in 2008, 30% of Americans said they had seen information comparing the quality of different insurance plans, hospitals, or doctors, whereas only 14% had used such information (Kaiser Family Foundation, 2008). That was slightly higher than what was reported in previous years. For example, a 2007 survey by Harris Interactive revealed that 23% of respondents had seen hospital comparative quality (Harris Interactive, 2008).

A systematic review of research assessing consumer use of publicly reported quality data confirmed that consumers are not regularly utilizing such data in their health care decision making (Faber, 2009). Some of the findings include the following: if consumers do not understand the information, they consider it irrelevant and then it is not used in decision making (Hibbard & Jewett, 1997); quality information was used to select a provider only when it confirmed the patients' expectations; even when quality scores of the patient's own physician were low, the patient would not change physicians (Marshall, Hiscock, & Sibbald, 2002); the sensitivity to quality information increases if consumers are dissatisfied with their current provider (McCormack, Garfinkel, Hibbard, Norton, & Bayen, 2001).

Multiple new applications ("apps") for various media appear on an almost weekly basis. Free "apps" for phones and tablets cover topics as wide ranging as weight loss, migraines, and heart disease. There are 8000 health-related applications available through iTunes alone. Unfortunately, only a small percentage of those users who download these applications actually use them (iHealth Beat, 2011). These applications are for management of health. The U.S. Department of Health and Human

Services sponsored a competition in 2010 for the development of "apps" that would make health quality data more accessible to consumers (Consumer Apps to Visualize Health Care Quality, 2010).

Most private health care in this country is purchased through employers. Therefore, it may be more important that employers who purchase health care plans utilize the quality data when making purchasing decisions. In fact, the first systematic approach for public reporting of health plans was the Health Plan Employer Data and Information Set (HEDIS) (National Committee of Quality Assurance, 2011). As part of the Patient Protection and Affordable Care Act (PPACA), a proposed rule would allow organizations that meet certain qualifications to have access to patient-protected Medicare data to produce public reports on physicians, hospitals, and other health care providers. This would offer employers an advantage in making health care decisions. Currently they rely on data from within their own plant to determine if quality and affordable care is being provided (The Voyager: Helping Physicians Navigate the Health Care Industry, 2011).

### Is Quality Improving?

Given the multitude of measures and the agencies monitoring them, one wonders if health care quality is improving. The Joint Commission (formerly known as the Joint Commission on Accreditation of Healthcare Organizations [JCAHO]) issues an annual report on quality and safety, and the 2010 report focuses, for the first time, on accountability measures. There are 19 measures that have been followed since 2002, including heart attack care, heart failure care, pneumonia care, surgical care, and children's asthma care. Each has associated metrics to measure improvement. Data were reported from 3000 accredited hospitals. The report indicates that all but one measure showed improvement over the reporting range. The Joint Commission cites these improvements as evidence of gains in hospital quality performance. The National Healthcare Quality Report (Agency for Healthcare Research and Quality, 2011c,e) indicates that quality improvement is progressing at a slow rate of 2.3% a year. These data are based on more than 200 health care measures, many of which have been described in this chapter. The best gains were seen in the treatment of acute illnesses or injuries (e.g., patients suffering a heart attack getting the right medication in a timely way). There were modest gains in rate of screening for preventive services and immunizations. Measures of lifestyle modifications (e.g., smoking cessation, reducing obesity) saw no improvement. An accompanying report showed that disparities in quality of care and access to care for minorities did not improve (Agency for Healthcare Research and Quality, 2011c).

## ◆ Patient Safety

Quality in health care, as stated earlier, can encompass many aspects of the care provided. Patient safety, however, is a critical component of quality. Awareness of problems with patient safety generated the movement for improved quality. Safety is considered the "first domain of quality" and refers to "freedom from injury" (Kohn et al, 2009, p. 18).

Reports of adverse events have long appeared in the news: wrong limb amputated; child dies from administration of wrong medication; serious complication caused when patient acquires infection in the health care facility. Data extrapolated from the Harvard Medical Practice Study indicate adverse events occurred in 2.9% of hospitalizations in Colorado and Utah and 3.7% of hospitalizations in New York (Brennan, Leape, Laird, Hebert, Localio, et al, 1991). Between 6.6% and 13.6% of those adverse events led to death. Adverse events are injuries caused by medical management rather than the underlying condition of the patient. If the adverse event can be attributed to an error, it is considered *preventable* (Brennan et al, 1991). When data from the Harvard study were extrapolated, the implication was that at least 44,000 Americans die each year as a result of medical errors, with the number possibly being as high as 98,000. And other data indicate the number may be much higher than that. The Agency for Health Care Quality and Research indicates that over 770,000 people die or are injured annually just from adverse drug events. These events cost millions of dollars each year *per hospital* (U.S. Department of Health and Human Services, 2001).

## Medical Errors and Adverse Events

An error is a failure of a planned action to be completed as intended, or the use of a wrong plan to achieve the action. These can be considered errors in execution, when the correct action does not achieve the intended result, or errors of planning, when the intended action is not correct (Reason, 1990). Although the terms *error* and *adverse event* are sometimes used interchangeably, there is generally a distinction made between medical errors and adverse events. Medical errors are "failures in the process of care and, while they have the potential to be harmful, numerous reports have shown that they are often not linked to the injury of patients. Instead they are often 'caught' by the system before they can lead to injury" (Resar, Rozich, & Classen, 2003, p. ii39). Often when errors reach the patient they do not result in any harm. Adverse events are "directly linked to actual harm resulting from medical care" (Resar et al, 2003, p. ii39). Of course, adverse events can occur even when the correct care is given (e.g., complications), but in that case there was no error.

Cognizant of the difference in an error and an adverse event, consider the types of errors as characterized by the Harvard study:

- Diagnostic
  - Error or delay in diagnosis
  - Failure to employ indicated tests
  - Use of outmoded tests or therapy
  - Failure to act on results of monitoring or testing
- Treatment
  - Error in the performance of an operation, procedure, or test
  - Error in administering the treatment
  - Error in the dose or method of using a drug
  - Avoidable delay in treatment or in responding to an abnormal test
  - Inappropriate (not indicated) care
- Preventive
  - Failure to provide prophylactic treatment
  - Inadequate monitoring or follow-up of treatment
- Other
  - Failure of communication
  - Equipment failure
  - Other system failure (Leape, 1993)

When considering these types of errors, one logically thinks of medication errors or surgical errors. However, in the context of providing dysphagia services, it is easy to imagine examples of each of these types of errors, shown in **Table 10.2**. They may or may not lead to an adverse event.

It is likely that the numbers of adverse events reported are an underestimation of the occurrence of preventable adverse events for the following reasons: only patients with a specified level of injury were included in the studies cited; there was a high threshold to determine if the event was preventable; and only errors documented in the patient records were included (Andrews et al, 1997).

**Table 10.2**   Types of Errors Applied to Dysphagia Management

*Diagnostic*
- Error or delay in diagnosing dysphagia
- Failing to proceed to instrumental assessment of swallowing when indicated, relying solely on bedside exam results to plan treatment
- Determining on the instrumental assessment that the patient is aspirating but doing nothing to change the patient's diet or how he or she eats

*Treatment*
- Teaching swallowing exercises incorrectly
- Selecting the wrong treatment techniques

*Preventive*
- Failing to instruct all caregivers on the feeding precautions
- Failing to check that the patient is following precautions

*Other*
- Failing to communicate the results of the swallowing study to the nurse or physician

## Center for Patient Safety

Many consider the IOM's report, *To Err Is Human*, first published in late 1999, to be the most influential document that spurred action regarding patient safety (Kohn et al, 2009). It was the first report generated by the Quality of Health Care in America project. Initiated in 1998, the project was charged with developing a strategy to result in "threshold improvement" in quality over the next 10 years (p. xi). The IOM report concluded that the way to prevent medical errors was to build a safer system. It acknowledged that other industries had become safer (e.g., aviation) and looked to those industries for ways to make health care delivery safer. The IOM recommended that Congress create the Center for Patient Safety in the AHRQ, which would set annual goals, track progress, and issue an annual report. The center was also to develop a research agenda, fund centers for excellence, and disseminate information about patient safety.

The IOM also recommended a nationwide mandatory reporting system that would collect standardized information about adverse events. This mandatory reporting system has not been implemented.

The site on the AHRQ page Patient Safety Net (Agency for Healthcare Research and Quality, 2011d) contains a weekly update of citations of patient safety reports, journal articles, newspaper or magazine articles, grants, press releases, and even audiovisual resources such as webinars. It also includes contains a searchable collection organized by approaches to improving safety, clinical areas, error types, setting of care, and so on.

The site also provides primers on the key concepts of patient safety. These address processes used in providing health care services. Some focus on standardizing processes to reduce or prevent errors (e.g., rapid response systems, use of checklists), and others highlight processes that can be used to analyze problems (e.g., root cause). A few of these key concepts with which SLPs are involved are summarized in the following subsections.

### Adverse Events After Hospital Discharge

Many patients experience an adverse event within 3 weeks after discharge from a hospital (Forster, Murff, Peterson, Gandhi, & Bates, 2003). Because the focus is on preventing readmissions to the hospital, eliminating these adverse events could reduce readmissions. Most of these errors involve medications, but hospital-acquired infections also contribute. Although many patients who have received speech-language pathology services will be referred to another level of care (e.g., skilled nursing facility, inpatient rehabilitation facility), those being discharged to home could be at risk if appropriate discharge instructions are not provided about managing the patient's dysphagia.

*Checklists*

A checklist is an algorithm used by health care workers to ensure that no step in a process is omitted. They have long been used in other industries (e.g., aviation safety) and are credited with many significant successes in patient safety. Checklists are used in many procedural areas and in control of infection. With the rise in multidrug resistant organisms, particularly those that can live on surfaces for long periods of time (e.g., *Acinetobacter baumannii*), speech-language pathology departments should design checklists for cleaning of their endoscopic swallowing (FEES®) cart and equipment when used in any isolation room.

*Computerized Physician Order Entry*

Most medication errors occur at the ordering or transcribing stage (Bates et al, 1995). Any clinician working in health care has struggled to read what a physician or physician-extender has written in the chart, so it is easy to see how such medication errors might occur. Computerized Physician Order Entry (CPOE) refers to any system in which the clinician directly enters the order into the system.

*Handoffs and Signouts*

Errors in communication between caregivers pose a significant safety risk. It is the nature of health care that patients will be cared for by multiple providers during their stay. Even if it is an outpatient procedure, the patient will likely encounter multiple professionals providing a different aspect of care. If the SLP takes the patient to another area of the facility for a procedure or treatment, a handoff has occurred.

*Health Care–Associated Infections*

Health care–associated infections (HAIs) are the most common complication of hospital care (Thomas et al, 2000). The Centers for Disease Control and Prevention (CDC, 2011) report that nearly 1.7 million HAIs occur each year, with approximately 99,000 deaths each year (Klevens, 2007). The four most common infections are surgical site infections, catheter-associated urinary tract infections, central venous catheter-related bloodstream infections, and ventilator-associated pneumonia. These account for more than 80% of HAIs (Warren & Kollef, 2005). Although SLPs are not involved in some of the actions to prevent these specific infections (e.g., performing readiness-to-wean assessments of patients on ventilators; prompt removal of urinary catheters), they and all other health care providers must be involved in the one action that can serve to reduce all of these infections: proper *hand hygiene* before and after patient contact (see additional discussion in Chapter 8).

*Medication Reconciliation*

When patients transition from one level of care to another, there is a heightened risk for medication errors. A medication prescribed in one setting may not be carried over to the next. A change in the patient's condition may warrant the addition of a new medication or a change in dosage. Patients or their caregivers may not be aware of all medications that were being administered at the other facility. Improving the process of reconciling these differences reduces potential errors. If patients' communication deficits interfere with their participation in the medication reconciliation process, the SLP may be involved.

*Voluntary Patient Safety Event Reporting*

Often called incident reports, voluntary patient safety event reporting relies on frontline personnel to complete a form (paper or electronic) to report an incident or event. It is considered a passive form of surveillance to capture near-misses or unsafe conditions. SLPs may fill out incident reports when they observe unsafe conditions. For example, if the patient is on a dysphagia diet and the SLP observes that the tray delivered to the patient's room contains foods the patient cannot safely swallow, the patient has been placed at risk. Of course, SLPs may observe events unrelated to their management of the patient that should still be reported by them. For example, if a confused patient is left unattended in a wheelchair in the hall, this could place the patient at risk and would be reportable.

### Trigger Tools to Measure Errors

Other methods for measuring errors or adverse events, also considered passive methods, include retrospective or concurrent chart reviews and observations. Each method has inherent weaknesses. Staff members often perceive incident reports to be punitive and thus may fail to complete them. Chart reviews are time-consuming and may be inaccurate. There are advantages to quantify harm (adverse events) rather than errors (Kilbridge, 2002). Errors are process related and typically evaluate an individual's role in the event. Focusing on harm tends to place the emphasis on the system rather than on the individual and also analyzes methodology to improve the clinical outcome. This approach reduces the staff's concern that these investigations are punitive in nature (Kilbridge, 2002).

In contrast to these passive methodologies, the use of a trigger tool is considered a more accurate and more active way to identify adverse events (Resar et al, 2003). The trigger method uses specific events (e.g., ordering certain drugs, certain abnormal laboratory values) as the "triggers" to initiate a more detailed concurrent chart review. For example, each time a patient is prescribed a medication that is considered a trigger (potential for adverse event), the pharmacy is notified and performs an in-depth concurrent review. The methodology is based on the hypothesis that surveillance of events closely linked to harm will help develop an effective strategy to reduce injury (Kilbridge, 2002).

Resar and colleagues (2003) have refined this methodology and developed functional trigger tools. Each of the triggers on a tool has a rationale for use. For example, on the intensive care unit (ICU) trigger tool, a positive blood culture is a trigger because bloodstream infections are frequently iatrogenic and associated with poor outcomes in the ICU. Pneumonia onset in the ICU is a trigger because all nosocomial pneumonias are considered an adverse event (Resar et al, 2003). This methodology produces consistent and reliable data at a low cost (Rozich, Haraden, & Resar, 2003).

### The Joint Commission's National Patient Safety Goals

In 2002, the Joint Commission established its National Patient Safety Goals (NPSG) program that went into effect in January 2003 (Joint Commission, 2011a,b). The goals are updated annually, and many continue from year to year, though the emphasis or specific requirements may change. The goals apply to any health care setting the Joint Commission accredits (e.g., ambulatory health care, critical access, behavioral health, laboratory, long term care, home care, hospitals). The goals, also discussed in Chapter 8, include such items as the following:

• Using two patient identifiers

• Using hand hygiene to prevent infections

• Getting important test results to the right patient at the right time (Joint Commission, 2011a,b)

The NPSG program is not the only safety initiative of the Joint Commission. The accrediting agency also places significant focus on patient safety through other current safety initiatives, including the following:

• Do-not-use abbreviation list

• Advancing effective communication, cultural competence, and patient- and family-centered care

- Speak-up: the Joint Commission's award-winning patient safety program
- Infection control

Speech-language pathologists should familiarize themselves with all of these, but of particular importance is the emphasis on advancing effective communication. The Joint Commission defines effective communication in this way:

> The successful joint establishment of meaning wherein patients and health care providers exchange information, enabling patients to participate actively in their care from admission through discharge, and ensuring that the responsibilities of both patients and providers are understood. To be truly effective, communication requires a two-way process (expressive and receptive) in which messages are negotiated until the information is correctly understood by both parties. Successful communication takes place only when providers understand and integrate the information gleaned from patients, and when patients comprehend accurate, timely, complete, and unambiguous messages from providers in a way that enables them to participate responsibly in their care. (The Joint Commission, 2010, p. 1)

Who better to be involved in implementing this standard than SLPs? The report even states, "Contact the Speech Language Pathology Department, if possible, to provide the appropriate augmentative and alternative communication (AAC) resources needed to help a patient who has a communication impairment due to a current medical condition" (Joint Commission, 2010, p. 9).

## Patient Protection and Affordable Care Act and Safety

Patient safety remains at the forefront in the United States. The Patient Protection and Affordable Care Act (PPACA) requires the secretary of the Department of Health and Human Services to establish a national strategy for quality improvement in health care, the National Quality Strategy. Its three broad aims are better care, healthier people and communities, and affordable quality care for all. The first initiative listed in the report is "making care safer."

The report summarizes examples of two federal initiatives. One of them is the Michigan Keystone Intensive Care Unit Project. Noting that nearly one in every 20 hospitalized patients in the U.S. each year acquires an HAI, an AHRQ-funded project was aimed at reducing central intravenous line-associated bloodstream infections, as they are one of the most deadly types of HAI, with a mortality rate of 12 to 25%. Implementation of CDC recommendations to reduce central-line bloodstream infections in 100 intensive care units throughout Michigan reduced the rate of these central-line bloodstream infections by two thirds within 3 months. Over 18 months, the program saved more than 1500 lives and nearly $200 million. These significant improvements have been sustained for 5 years, and the approach used is now being spread to all 50 states and the District of Columbia (President's Report to Congress: National Strategy for Quality Improvement in Health Care, 2011).

## International Focus on Safety

Improving patient safety is an international concern. In October 2004, the World Health Organization (WHO) launched its patient safety initiative in response to a World Health Assembly resolution (WHO, 2002) urging the WHO and its member states to attend to the problem of patient safety. Its establishment highlighted the importance of patient safety as a global health care issue (WHO, 2011). Their focus is on many of the same areas already discussed, such as encouraging hand hygiene, using technology to improve safety, using standardized processes (e.g., checklists), researching adverse effects, and empowering patients to champion patient safety.

Recognizing that the risk of patient harm may be greater in developing countries, the WHO indicated the risk is made greater by limitations in the capacity to carry out research regarding patient safety. The WHO has developed Core Competencies for Patient Safety Researchers. This tool is designed to strengthen research methods and science regarding patient safety. The WHO has also developed a standard classification for key safety concepts, the International Classification for Patient

Safety. The goal is to standardize how the concepts are discussed so that information sharing across borders will lead to improved patient safety (WHO, 2011).

### Safety from the Patient's Perspective

Consumers Advancing Patient Safety (CAPS) was formed in 2003 as a result of a workshop sponsored by AHQR that brought together consumers, health care providers, accrediting agencies, educators, and legal system stakeholders with the aim of achieving patient-focused safety goals. CAPS's mission is to

- be a champion for patient safety in a new health care culture;
- be a voice for individuals, families, and healers who wish to prevent harm in health care encounters through partnership and collaboration; and
- teach the health care community what consumers and providers need to know whenever they interact within health care systems (Consumers Advancing Patient Safety, 2011).

CAPS works with agencies like the WHO to achieve its goals. CAPS also provides patient education resources to help patients play a more active role in ensuring their safety in the health care environment.

In 2008, CAPS sponsored the Chicago Patient Safety Workshop (CPSW). The participants discussed and developed action plans for each of these important areas:

- Patient reporting of medical errors
- Engaging patients and families in quality improvement (QI) and patient safety
- Patient and family involvement in their own care
- Effective patient/clinician communication
- Preventing error through patient/provider partnership
- Disclosure, root cause analysis, learning, and emotional support (Chicago Patient Safety Workshop, 2008)

Although the recommendations were designed specifically for the Chicago community, the areas of focus for improved patient safety inform everyone in the medical community. For example, AHRQ is currently investigating the establishment of a mechanism for consumers to report patient safety events (Agency for Healthcare Research and Quality, 2009). In addition, most facilities participate in root cause analysis of patient safety events, and many have established a mechanism for partnership with consumers regarding patient safety.

## ♦ Patient Satisfaction

Given that most errors do not reach the patient, or if they do, there is no harm done, then patients are largely unaware of many of the safety issues that exist in health care. So when rating quality of care, patients consider many things besides safety. Obviously the patient expects a quality outcome. Was the procedure successful? Was the patient's health status improved? But patients' satisfaction often centers on the quality of the service provided.

Health care facilities have long measured patient satisfaction. However, as a result of PPACA, getting good results on patient satisfaction in hospitals has taken on a new level of importance. PPACA mandates implementation of a *value-based purchasing* (VBP) program, which will reward hospitals for the quality of care they provide as demonstrated by their performance on measures of quality of care. A part of the Medicare reimbursement for a hospital is at risk if the hospital does not reach performance goals. Outcomes measures are slated to be introduced into the VBP, including AHQR patient safety indicators, nursing sensitive care, and specific disease-related measures. The weighting of the total score that determines how much of the at-risk payment a hospital may retain will be based 70% on how closely hospitals follow the best clinical processes and 30% on patient experience of care. Thus, patient satisfaction scores will no longer be just a target for improvement. They will have a direct impact on revenues (Newsroom, 2011).

## National Benchmarking

The survey tool to be used by hospitals is the Hospital Consumer Assessment of Healthcare Providers Survey (HCAHPS). It is part of a group of tools included in the National CAHPS® Benchmarking Database, established in 1998. In addition to the hospital tool, the database includes a clinician and group survey component and a health plan survey database (Agency for Healthcare Research and Quality, 2011a). The hospital tool (HCAHPS) comprises 22 items that, in general, assess the following areas:

- Communication with nurses
- Communication with doctors
- Clean and quiet environment
- Responsiveness of hospital staff
- New medications explained
- Management of pain
- Information provided on discharge
- Overall hospital rating (Consumer Assessment of Healthcare Providers Survey, 2011).

As part of the National CAHPS Benchmarking Database, there is also a measure of consumer satisfaction with health plans, the Consumer Assessment of Health Plans Study (CAHPS). It includes information on commercial plans, Medicaid, and Medicare. It measures many of the same items as the physician measures, but related to these services being covered by the health plan: getting the care the patient needs, getting care quickly, and how well the doctor communicates (U.S. Department of Health and Human Services, 2011a,b).

## Satisfaction with Physician Services

Patient satisfaction is measured in most settings, not just hospitals. As part of the National CAHPS Benchmarking Database, the component for clinician and group survey is a measure specifically of physician services. Physicians can compare their services to others in the database. Over 1000 practice sites are represented in the database with more than 330,000 surveys. This measure has been endorsed by the National Quality Forum (U.S. Department of Health and Human Services, 2011b).

The NQMC includes two related categories of measure for patients' overall rating of their physician and for patients' overall rating of their physician's office (National Quality Measures Clearinghouse, 2011). The patient's overall rating of their physician contains a 10-point scale for rating patient satisfaction with the physician (Camacho, Feldman, Balkrishnan, Kong, & Anderson, 2009). Items include attitude, time spent, how well questions were answered, and treatment success. The overall rating of the physician's office measures items such as friendliness of staff, convenience of location, ability to get all the care needed at the same clinic, and ability to see the same physician each visit.

Private organizations, such as Healthgrades, also provide the consumer with information to compare physicians on items such as trust, communication, time spent with the patient, office friendliness, wait time, and so on. Consumers can enter scores to rate the physician (Healthgrades, 2011).

## Typical Patient Satisfaction Measurements

As demonstrated by the questions on some of the survey instruments mentioned above, consumers do not rate a service solely on the outcome, but also on their perceptions of the entire process of service delivery. For example, the communication disorder for which they sought treatment is improved through therapy, but the office staff was rude and there was frequently a long wait at each appointment. The outcome was good, but parts of the process were not. In addition, it is only the patient who can determine the criteria that matter when measuring satisfaction (Shelton, 2000). Shelton summarizes areas of patient satisfaction typically measured. Most of these are easily applicable to an outpatient setting in which speech-language pathology services are rendered. In addition to the patient's perception of the quality of the service received, these include the following:

- Access
  - How easy is it to schedule appointments by phone?
  - How easy is it to schedule the next appointment at the front desk?
  - Is there a long wait between when the patient wants to be seen and when the appointment is set?
  - Is there a long wait in the waiting room?
  - How easy is it to see the provider the patient chooses?
- Convenience
  - Is the office located in an area easy to reach?
  - Are the hours of operation convenient?
  - Is parking available and easy to access?
- Communication
  - What is the patient's first impression of the provider?
  - How well does the provider explain the problem?
  - How well does the provider explain any procedures?
  - Is the communication good between the provider and other members of the staff?
  - Does the provider listen?
  - Does the provider give necessary information for management of the problem?
- Personal caring
  - Were all staff in the office friendly?
  - Was the provider friendly?
  - Was the patient shown respect by all individuals?
- Facilities and equipment
  - What is the overall appearance of the office?
  - Is signage effective and easy to read?
  - Is the office clean?

## Speech-Language Pathology Specific Patient Satisfaction Tools

When ASHA first developed NOMS in the 1990s, it included a consumer satisfaction measure. The items were developed based on input from a consumer focus group and included items such as time-liness of appointments, friendliness of support staff, clean and quiet environment, amount of time spent, as well as the perception that services were effective (American Speech-Language-Hearing Association, 1989). After several years of data collection revealed consistently high scores on all items in all settings, this component was discontinued (see Chapter 5 for further discussion).

Related to satisfaction measurements are quality-of-life measurements that focus more on the outcomes than on the process of the service provided. There are tools measuring quality-of-life aspects related to communication and swallowing disorders. The Washington Quality of Life (University of Washington, 1999) contains a speech domain. The Voice Handicap Index (VHI) (Jacobson, et al, 1997) and the Voice Related Quality of Life (VRQOL) (Hogikyan & Sethuraman, 1999) are specific to quality of life related to voice disorders. The SWAL-QOL is a measure of quality of life with a swallowing disorder (McHorney et al, 2000). Further discussion of quality of life outcomes measurement is found in Chapter 2.

## Using Patient Satisfaction Data

Anyone working in a health care organization that gathers patient satisfaction data realizes that gathering the data is only the first, and least important, step in the process. What really matters is what the organization does with the data to improve the patient satisfaction scores. And even harder than improving the scores is maintaining those improvements.

Numerous authors have written about approaches to establishing service excellence as the culture of the organization. It is essential to establish and maintain a culture of service excellence, because virtually every factor that contributes to the patient's perception of satisfaction depends on the behavior of staff. Shelton (2000) describes it as building and sustaining a service-oriented organizational culture. He summarizes the work of other authors (Deal, 1982; Peters & Waterman, 1982; Wall, 1999; Wellington, 1995) in describing essential elements in establishing a patient-focused, service-oriented health care organization. Common themes emerge:

- The organization builds service excellence into the mission/values.
- Systems are put in place to maintain a customer focus:
  - Continuous communication about these values
  - Celebrations/rewards for success
- Staff members are hired who demonstrate a belief in the tenets of a service culture and held accountable for demonstrating good service.
- Staff members are involved in the process.
  - For example, they are empowered to address problems immediately.
- Teamwork is encouraged.

## Building Service Excellence

Three recommended resources on the topic of service excellence are summarized briefly here:

*Hardwiring Excellence:* Quint Studer (2003) describes a Healthcare Flywheel™ that shows "how organizations can create a momentum for change by engaging the passion of their employees to apply prescriptive actions guided by Nine Principles of service and operational excellence to achieve bottom-line results" (p. 26). Studer bases the approach on nine principles, including measuring what is important, creating and developing leaders, building individual accountability, and communicating at all levels (Studer, 2003).

*Baptist Health Care Journey to Excellence: Creating a Culture that WOWs!:* Al Stubblefield (2005) describes the changes implemented at his health care organization to gain a competitive advantage in the mid-1990s. He did this by focusing on patient satisfaction. His book provides a description of his five keys to service and operational excellence: creating and maintaining a great culture; selecting and retaining great employees; committing to service excellence; continuously developing great leaders; and hardwiring success through systems of accountability.

*If Disney Ran Your Hospital: 9½ Things You Would Do Differently:* Fred Lee (2004) summarizes the approach he helped develop, the Disney approach to quality service for the health care industry. One of the most interesting aspects is his contention that the concept of work should be changed to the concept of theater. He posits that if employees acted as if they were on stage while interacting with patients, they could more easily demonstrate the behaviors needed for a culture of service.

The experience of the National Rehabilitation Hospital with the Disney approach to culture coaching is discussed in Chapter 8. There are numerous other resources on utilizing patient satisfaction information to change the culture across the organization and improve the quality of services provided. Many facilities and health care systems have embraced this concept and endorse a specific approach or methodology.

## ◆ Conclusion and Future Directions

It is clear that the health care arena will continue to focus on improving quality and safety of services, as they are integral to improving patient satisfaction. With the increasing importance placed on involving the consumer in the health care process, the outcome data obtained through patient satisfaction surveys will help shape how the services are provided. Financial incentives by CMS and third-party payers increase the urgency with which health care organizations will implement needed systems and culture changes to achieve these results.

The ultimate goal of collecting and making available to the public performance data on quality, safety, and satisfaction is for consumers to use this information to make wise choices for their health care. However, as noted in a provocative commentary, "Health Care Quality Transparency: If You Build It, Will Patients Come?" Ginsburg and Kemper state (2009), "turning passive patients into active consumers who factor cost and quality into decisions about which doctors or hospitals to choose or which treatment options to pursue is an elusive goal in the U.S. health care system" (p. 1).

In Chapter 8, Rao argues that the evidence points toward a more consumer-centric future in health care, but much still remains to be done to move consumers from passive to active participant in the management of their own health. "Until consumers are motivated to use quality information to choose providers, the main value of public quality reporting will likely be to motivate providers to improve their performance" (Ginsburg & Kemper, 2009, p. 4). That alone is not an unworthy result.

## References

Agency for Healthcare Research and Quality. (2009, May). Designing Consumer Reporting Systems for Patient Safety Events. No. 09-M023. http://www.ahrq.gov/qual/consrep flyer.htm

Agency for Healthcare Research and Quality. (2011a). *Consumer assessment of healthcare providers survey.* U.S. Department of Health and Human Services. https://www.cahps.ahrq.gov/content/NCBD/NCBD_Intro.asp?p=105&s=5

Agency for Healthcare Research and Quality. (2011b). *Frequently asked questions.* U.S. Department of Health and Human Services. http://www.qualitymeasures.ahrq.gov/faq.aspx

Agency for Healthcare Research and Quality. (2011c). *National quality measures.* U.S. Department of Health and Human Services. http://www.qualitymeasures.ahrq.gov/browse/by-organization-indiv.aspx?orgid=2086

Agency for Healthcare Research and Quality. (2011d). *Patient safety net (PSnet).* http://www.psnet.ahrq.gov/

Agency for Healthcare Research and Quality. (2011e). *Research activities.* Silver Spring, MD: U.S. Department of Health and Human Services

American Speech-Language-Hearing Association. (1989). *Consumer satisfaction measure.* Rockville, MD: Author

American Speech-Language-Hearing Association. (2011). *Speech-language pathology and the Physician Quality Reporting Initiative (PQRI).* http://www.asha.org/Members/research/NOMS/PQRI/

Andrews, L. B., Stocking, C., Krizek, T., Gottlieb, L., Krizek, C., Vargish, T., et al. (1997, Feb). An alternative strategy for studying adverse events in medical care. *Lancet, 349,* 309–313

Aspden, P., Corrigan, J. M., Wolcott, J., & Erickson, S. M. (2004). *Patient Safety: achieving a new standard for care.* Washington, DC: National Academies Press

Bates, D. W., Cullen, D. J., Laird, N., Petersen, L. A., Small, S. D., Servi, D., et al.; ADE Prevention Study Group (1995, Jul). Incidence of adverse drug events and potential adverse drug events. Implications for prevention. *Journal of the American Medical Association, 274,* 29–34

Brennan, T. A., Leape, L. L., Laird, N. M., Hebert, L., Localio, A. R., Lawthers, A. G., et al. (1991). Incidence of adverse events and negligence in hospitalized patients: Results of the Harvard Medical Practice Study I. *The New England Journal of Medicine, 324,* 370–376

Camacho, F. T., Feldman, S. R., Balkrishnan, R., Kong, M. C., & Anderson, R. T. (2009, Jan-Feb). Validation and reliability of 2 specialty care satisfaction scales. *American Journal of Medical Quality, 24,* 12–18

Centers for Disease Control and Prevention. (2011, March 17). Health-related quality of life. http://www.cdc.gov/hrqol/concept.htm#six

Centers for Medicare and Medicaid Services (CMS). (2009). *Roadmap for quality measurement in the traditional medicare fee-for-service program.* http://www.cms.gov/Medicare/Quality-Initiatives-Patient-Assessment-Instruments/QualityInitiativesGenInfo/downloads/QualityMeasurementRoadmap_OEA1-16_508.pdf

Chicago Patient Safety Workshop. (2008, March). http://patientsafety.org/file_depot/0-10000000/20000-30000/24986/folder/58345/The+Chicago+Patient+Safety+Workshop+Proceedings+Report+Final+102808.pdf

Committee on Quality of Health Care in America. (2001). *Crossing the quality chasm: A new health system for the 21st century.* Washington, DC: National Academies Press

Consumer Apps to Visualize Health Care Quality. (2010). Challenge.gov: http://challenge.gov/HHS/57-consumer-apps-to-visualize-health-care-quality?sso=c808f37f38b448582e02f4e74336f834996f0329e4403011b1d4df6e59789ce516f5229aad7951f24cc8c74ecfce68fb75b5#detailed_description

Consumer Assessment of Healthcare Providers Survey. (2011, March). *Hospital survey. Hospital care quality information from the consumer perspective.* http://www.hcahpsonline.org/surveyinstrument.aspx

Consumers Advancing Patient Safety. (2011, March 8). Patient safety.org: http://www.patientsafety.org/file_depot/0-10000000/20000-30000/24986/folder/58345/capsfactsheet.pdf

Deal, T. (1982). *Corporate cultures: The rites and rituals of corporate life.* Menlo Park, CA: Addison-Wesley

Faber, M. B. (2009). Public reporting in health care: How do consumers use quality-of-care information? Medical Care, 1–8.

Forster, A. J., Murff, H. J., Peterson, J. F., Gandhi, T. K., & Bates, D. W. (2003, Feb). The incidence and severity of adverse events affecting patients after discharge from the hospital. *Annals of Internal Medicine, 138,* 161–167

Ginsburg, P. (2007). Private payer roles in moving to more efficient health spending. In A. A. Antos (Ed.), *Restoring fiscal sanity 2007: The health spending challenge* (pp. 153–171). Washington, DC: Brookings Institution Press

Ginsburg, P., & Kemper, N. M. (2009). Health care quality transparency: If you build it, will patients come? *Commentary: Insights into the Health Care Marketplace,* 1–4

Harris Interactive. (2008). *Just looking: Consumer use of the Internet to manage care.* Oakland, CA: California Health-Care Foundation

Healthgrades. (2011). *Find a doctor.* http://www.healthgrades.com/find-a-doctor?yaid=hg

Hibbard, J. H., & Jewett, J. J. (1997, May-Jun). Will quality report cards help consumers? *Health Affairs (Project Hope), 16,* 218–228

Hogikyan, N. D., & Sethuraman, G. (1999). Validation of an instrument to measure voice-related quality of life (V-RQOL). *Journal of Voice, 13,* 557–569

iHealth Beat. (2011, March 22). *Mobile health.* http://www.ihealthbeat.org/articles/2011/3/22/mobile-health-apps-popular-but-efficacy-in-question-experts-say.aspx

Institute for Healthcare Improvement. (2011). *Closing the quality gap.* http://www.ihi.org/about/Documents/IntroductiontoIHIBrochureDec10.pdf

Institute of Medicine, Lohr, K. N. (Ed.). (1990). *Medicare: A strategy for quality assurance.* Washington, DC: National Academy Press

Jacobson, B., Johnson, A., Grywalski, C., Silbergleit, A., Jacobson, G., Benninger, M. S., et al. (1997). The Voice Handicap Index (VHI). *American Journal of Speech-Language Pathology, 6,* 66–70

Joint Commission. (2010). *Advancing effective communication, cultural competence, and patient- and family-centered care: A.* Oakbrook Terrace, IL: Author

Joint Commission. (2011a). *Facts about the national patient safety goals.* http://www.jointcommission.org/facts_about_the_national_patient_safety_goals/

Joint Commission. (2011b). *2011 national patient safety goals.* http://www.jointcommission.org/assets/1/6/2011_NPSG_Hospital_3_17_11.pdf

Kaiser Family Foundation. (2008). *Update on consumers' view of patient safety and quality information.* Menlo Park, CA: Author. www.kff.org/kaiserpolls/posr101508pkg.cfm

Kilbridge, P. (2002). Surveillance for adverse drug events: history, methods and current issues. *VHA Research Series,* 1–48

Klevens, R. E. (2007). *Estimating health care-associated infections and deaths in U.S. hospitals, 2002.* Atlanta: Public Health Reports

Kohn, L. T., Corrigan, J. M., & Donaldson, M. O. (2001). *To err is human: Building a safer health system.* Washington, DC: National Academies Press

Leape, L. L. (1993). Preventing medical injury. *Quality Review Bulletin,* pp. 144–149

Lee, F. (2004). *If Disney ran your hospital: 9 1/2 things you would do differently.* Bozeman, MT: Second River Healthcare Press

Lohr, K. C. (1990). *Medicare: A strategy for quality assurance.* Vol. 1. Washington, DC: National Academy Press

Loxtercamp, D. (2011, May 29). A follow-up visit with a country doctor. (L. Hansen, interviewer.) http://www.npr.org/2011/05/29/136765593/a-follow-up-visit-with-a-country-doctor

Marshall, M. N., Hiscock, J., & Sibbald, B. (2002, Nov). Attitudes to the public release of comparative information on the quality of general practice care: qualitative study. *BMJ (Clinical Research Ed.), 325,* 1278

McCormack, L. A., Garfinkel, S. A., Hibbard, J. H., Norton, E. C., & Bayen, U. J. (2001, Jul). Health plan decision making with new medicare information materials. *Health Services Research, 36,* 531–554

McHorney, C. A., Bricker, D. E., Robbins, J., Kramer, A. E., Rosenbek, J. C., & Chignell, K. A. (2000, Summer). The SWAL-QOL outcomes tool for oropharyngeal dysphagia in adults: II. Item reduction and preliminary scaling. *Dysphagia, 15,* 122–133

McNamara, P. (2006, Feb). Foreword: payment matters? The next chapter. *Medical Care Research and Review, 63*(1, Suppl), 5S–10S

National Committee of Quality Assurance. (2011). *HEDIS and quality measurements. Measuring quality, improving health care.* http://www.ncqa.org/tabid/59/default.aspx

National Quality Forum. (2011a). *Endorsed standards.* http://www.qualityforum.org/Measures_List.aspx

National Quality Forum. (2011b). *Functional communication measure—swallowing.* http://www.qualityforum.org/MeasureDetails.aspx?SubmissionId=682#k=speech&e=1&st=&sd=&mt=&cs=&s=n&so=a&p=1

National Quality Forum. (2011c, May). *Funding.* http://www.qualityforum.org/About_NQF/Funding.aspx

National Quality Forum. (2011d). *Improving healthcare quality.* http://www.qualityforum.org/Setting_Priorities/Improving_Healthcare_Quality.aspx

National Quality Measures Clearinghouse. (2011). *Measure summary.* http://www.qualitymeasures.ahrq.gov/content.aspx?id=14865

Newsroom. (2011, April 29). http://www.healthcare.gov/news/factsheets/valuebasedpurchasing04292011a.html

Peters, T., & Waterman, R. N. (1982). *In search of excellence.* Glasgow, UK: HarperCollins

President's Advisory Commission on Consumer Protection and Quality in Health Care. (1998, June 19). *Preamble.* http://www.hcqualitycommission.gov/charter.html

President's Advisory Commission on Consumer Protection and Quality in the Health Care Industry. (1998). *Executive summary.* http://www.hcqualitycommission.gov/prepub/recommen.htm

President's Report to Congress: National Strategy for Quality Improvement in Health Care. (2011, March). http://www.healthcare.gov/center/reports/nationalqualitystrategy032011.pdf

Reason, J. T. (1990). *Human error.* Cambridge: Cambridge University Press

Resar, R. K., Rozich, J. D., & Classen, D. (2003, Dec). Methodology and rationale for the measurement of harm with trigger tools. *Quality & Safety in Health Care, 12*(Suppl 2), ii39–ii45

Rozich, J. D., Haraden, C. R., & Resar, R. K. (2003, Jun). Adverse drug event trigger tool: a practical methodology for measuring medication related harm. *Quality & Safety in Health Care, 12,* 194–200

Shelton, P. (2000). *Measuring and improving patient satisfaction.* Gaithersburg, MD: Aspen

Stubblefield, A. (2005). *The Baptist health care journey to excellence: creating a culture that WOWs!* Hoboken, NJ: John Wiley & Sons

Studer, Q. (2003). *Hardwiring excellence.* Gulf Breeze, FL: Firs Starter Publishing

Thomas, E. J., Studdert, D. M., Burstin, H. R., Orav, E. J., Zeena, T., Williams, E. J., et al. (2000, Mar). Incidence and types of adverse events and negligent care in Utah and Colorado. *Medical Care, 38,* 261–271

U.S. Department of Health and Human Services. (2001, March). http://www.ahrq.gov/qual/aderia/aderia.htm

U.S. Department of Health and Human Services. (2011a). *The CAHPS benchmarking database: health plans.* https://www.cahps.ahrq.gov/CAHPSIDB/Public/Trending.aspx

U.S. Department of Health and Human Services. (2011b). *The CAHPS benchmarking database: clinician and group.* http://www.qualitymeasures.ahrq.gov/content.aspx?id=14866

University of Washington. (1999). *Quality of life questionnaire (UWQOL).* http://depts.washington.edu/otoweb/research/head_neck_cancer/uw_qol_r_v4.pdf

The Voyager: Helping Physicians Navigate the Health Care Industry. (2011, June 6). *Major new effort to give consumers and employers better information about quality of care.* http://atlanticfinancial.wordpress.com/2011/06/06/major-new-effort-to-give-consumers-and-employers-better-information-about-quality-of-care/

Wall, B. S. (1999). *The mission-driven organization.* Rocklin, CA: Prima

Warren, D. K., & Kollef, M. H. (2005, Feb). Prevention of hospital infection. *Microbes and Infection, 7,* 268–274

Wellington, P. (1995). *Kaisen strategies for customer care: How to create a powerful customer care program—and make it work.* London: Pitman

World Health Organization (WHO). (2002) *Fifty-fifth World Health Assembly WHA55.18; agenda item 13.9: quality of care: patient safety*

World Health Organization (WHO). (2011). *Patient safety.* http://www.who.int/patientsafety/research/strengthening_capacity/training_leaders/en/index.html; or http://www.who.int/patientsafety/about/en/index.html

# 11

# Outcome Assessment for Improving Organizational Efficiencies

*Tamala S. Bradham*

## ◆ Chapter Focus

This chapter provides an example of a quality management problem as a means of illustrating how the quality models and tools and quality improvement processes discussed in the chapter can assist managers and providers in improving efficiencies and the quality of services within organizations.

---

**A Quality Fable**

**Part One: We Have a Problem**

Abel, the manager of 15 speech-language pathologists, just left a meeting with his boss. He was given some negative news about his department's performance. How is he going to share this with his staff? How is he going to address these issues? Everyone felt they were working hard, did not get paid enough, and, well, management just does not understand! What is he going to do?

---

## ◆ Introduction

In 2009, over the course of just one year, the national health care cost in the United States grew 4% to about $2.5 trillion (or $2486 billion to be exact). This accounts for 17.6% of the gross domestic product. Medicare spending grew 7.9% to $502.3 billion, and Medicaid grew 9% to $373.9 billion (CMS, 2011). Although the U.S. has the highest per capita health care costs of any industrialized nation, many other developed countries are also experiencing the same cost increases (Kowdley & Ashbaker, 2011). Increasing costs are reducing access to care, and constitute an ever heavier burden on employers and consumers. Yet as much as 20 to 30% of these costs may be unnecessary, or even counterproductive, to improved health (Wennberg, Brownless, Fisher, Skinner, & Weinstein, 2008).

The impact is not exclusive to health care. Educational settings are also challenged to serve more children who have been identified with communication disorders. To ensure quality services, the

American Speech-Language-Hearing Association (ASHA) recommended several years ago that the caseloads of school speech-language pathologists (SLPs) not exceed 40 students under any circumstances, and for special populations, ASHA recommended a maximum caseload of 25 students (ASHA, 1984, 1993). The actual average number of students within the SLPs' caseloads, however, has remained significantly higher than these recommendations. Based on the 2010 ASHA survey, the median school-based SLP caseloads is 50 students, with some SLPs' caseloads being as large as 80 students (ASHA, 2010).

Addressing these unwanted costs and unrealistic caseloads is essential if we are to continue providing quality clinical services. One avenue to reducing unwanted costs while maintaining quality of services has been termed *quality management*. Some argue that implementing quality management programs is costly. But others would argue that poor quality is even more costly. The Centers for Medicare and Medicaid Services (CMS) defines quality as "how well the health plan keeps its members healthy or treats them when they are sick. Good quality health care means doing the right thing at the right time, in the right way, for the right person—and getting the best possible results" (CMS, 2008). The Institute of Medicine (IOM) states, "Quality of care is the degree to which health services for individuals and populations increase the likelihood of desired health outcomes and are consistent with current professional knowledge" (IOM, 1990, p. 21).

To improve our organizational effectiveness and efficiencies, both leaders and service providers in all settings need to make changes in current practices. Hence, this chapter discusses introducing changes, developing teams, and setting goals. It also discusses program evaluations, selecting items to change, and suggesting models and tools used for measuring performance improvement to obtain the best outcomes.

---

### Part Two: The Team

Abel scheduled a meeting with his staff and presented the results of the department's performance outcomes over the past year. It was stone quiet.

Then, Ann said, "So, what do we need to do?"

Abel replied, "We are going to work together, form teams, and address these issues. At the end of today's meeting, you will all be given your team assignments with your specific goals. Each team will first meet with a facilitator to review ground rules, timelines, and expectations."

---

## Change: How to Begin?

To make any system improvement requires change. The change may be simple or complex, minor or significant. *Change* is simply a state that is different from the status quo. This change may be positive or negative, better or worse than the status quo, so deciding what needs to be changed, and how it will be changed, is important. This is particularly important when considering changes in service delivery, because such changes usually require an across-the-board change in a *process*, and thus engagement of multiple providers.

The manner in which the changes are introduced will impact the manner in which employees embrace new service delivery paradigms. Although one individual can make changes, the most effective and efficient way to make and maintain these changes is through engagement of all appropriate "stakeholders" in the process. Traditionally, the work model employed in organizations has been a top-down style of management: "Do as I say and respect my decisions no matter what." Today, however, employees bring their own ideas about how the workplace should run, and express a desire to be a part of the process. Professionals respect outcomes and results more than positions of authority, prefer to share in the decision-making and hold the position that people can manage themselves as long as everyone understands on the job responsibilities and expectations.

Understanding that employees tend to embrace change at their own pace is important. How quickly an organization embraces change depends on the following five factors:

1. Recognizing and accepting the need for change.

2. Setting the course for the future through direction and planning.

3. Moving forward and carrying out the action plan.

4. Managing negativity.

5. Integrating the changes through the system.

Acknowledging that change takes time, commitment, consistency, and ongoing communication is essential in creating the necessary culture of change. Creating a culture of change in any organization is an ongoing journey. Although some may find this frustrating, there are always things that can be improved. That is the essential engine behind *continuous quality improvement* (CQI) programs, the implementation of which requires that a team of individuals work together to improve the organization's performance. Improvement is ongoing; it is not a fixed end point for the provider teams. A team is a group of individuals working toward a common purpose. Stamatis (2011) states the following three criteria are essential for an effective team:

- Team members share the same goals and view themselves as part of the team working together on a specific project for a specified time period.

- The teams are appropriately sized to allow for effective (and preferably face-to-face) communication (i.e., five to nine people). Also, the chair of the group should not be the supervisor or manager of the members on the team.

- The team should consist of both multidisciplinary (e.g., physicians, audiologists, speech-language pathologists, administrators, etc.) and cross-functional (e.g., schedulers, billing, records, compliance officers, etc.) members.

In addition to these criteria, the individuals on the team must be willing to share expertise and data, and look for opportunities to succeed. They must also all be open to learning and be actively engaged throughout the process. Negativity, hidden agendas, and or personal grudges should be left outside the workplace.

---

### Part Three: The Goals

The meeting was over and Abel was preparing to hand out the team assignments and goals. His unit had been through a lot during the past couple of years. He had been receiving coaching from an outside consultant in managing his group. His unit had been on retreats; read some management motivational books such as *The Five Dysfunctions of a Team* by Patrick Lencioni (2002), *Who Moved My Cheese?* by Spencer Johnson (2000), and *Crucial Conversation: Tools for Talking When Stakes Are High* by Patterson, Grenny, McMillan, and Switzler (2011); and had been having effective staff meetings. He was now reading *Hardwiring Excellence* by Quint Studer (2003) and had asked the staff to read it as their next team-building homework assignment. They were poised for change, but what changes did they need to make? They decided to focus on patient satisfaction outcomes and time management efficiencies.

Their patient satisfaction scores were slightly below the expected benchmarks. The four areas that affected their overall score were (1) time spent with the patient, (2) explanation of test results, (3) delays in scheduling, and (4) wait times in the clinic. Based on these scores, Abel and his team developed the following goal:

*Goal 1:* To improve patient satisfaction regarding the services delivered, the staff will evaluate the current patients' perspectives on services in these four areas, utilize performance improvement tools and processes to better understand the nature of the problems, and implement action plans within the next 3 months.

Abel also had to address the budget concerns. His unit was almost 5% over their budgeted expenses, and their revenue was 20% below what they had projected. He had to address this problem without the staff members feeling they were not supported and preferably without having to let someone go. After evaluating the expenses and staff relative value units (RVUs), he developed the following goal:

*Goal 2:* To meet budget requirements, the staff members will evaluate current inventories, how they spend their day (billable versus nonbillable time), and review how long it takes a patient to receive services from the time of the referral to the first visit. This first part should be completed within 2 months.

Although these goals were just the first step, Abel felt that they would give the staff some direction as well as freedom to explore how to best address these areas of concerns.

## Identifying Areas of Improvement and Writing Goals

Once the team agrees that change is needed to provide safe, high-quality, efficient, and cost-effective care, deciding where to begin can be a daunting task. Obtaining employee suggestions; reviewing practice data such as patient satisfaction questionnaires, adverse events reports, or financial information; and evaluating both national and local trends will assist the organization in identifying targeted areas. The Joint Commission also has some suggested targeted areas (Brown, 2009; Stamatis, 2011):

- *Appropriateness:* The degree to which the care and services provided are relevant to an individual's clinical needs, given the current state of knowledge (i.e., doing the right thing based on the need).

  —Are there areas within your service program that do not add any value to the services you provide?

- *Availability*: The degree to which appropriate care and services are accessible and obtainable to meet an individual's needs (i.e., access to care).

  —Can your students/patients/clients obtain the care they need in a timely manner? Do you have an access issue (i.e., access to medical records, access to individualized education program (IEP) goals, opportunity to ask questions and get a response quickly, access to other providers providing care)?

- *Competency:* The degree to which the practitioner adheres to professional and organizational standards of care and practice.

  —Are you practicing within your scope of care? Do you have a system to document competency within your business/institution/organization?

- *Effectiveness:* The degree to which care is provided in the correct manner, given the current state of knowledge, to achieve the desired or projected outcomes for the individual.

  —Is it written down? Is there consistency in delivery?

- *Efficacy/work flow improvement/continuity:* The power of a procedure, treatment, or intervention to improve the overall health status of the individual or population and the coordination of needed health care services for an individual or population among all practitioners and across all organizations over time.

  —Are there processes in the work flow that could improve?

- *Efficiency/eliminating or reducing waste:* The relationship between the outcomes and the resources used to deliver the care.

  —Are there better ways of providing that service?

- *Respect and caring:* The degree to which those providing services do so with sensitivity for the individual needs, expectations, and differences as well as for the individual and family members are involved in their own care and service decisions.

  —Are there avenues that allow customers/patients/clients to share their views about services received?

- *Safety:* The degree to which the health care intervention minimizes risks of adverse outcome for both the individual and the practitioner.

  —Is there a "blameless" reporting system for staff to use to report less than standard of care incidents?

- *Appropriate inventory:* The degree to which the minimum inventory is available to address the needs of the population served.

  —What inventory is absolutely necessary to have on hands? Where is it stored?

- *Timeliness:* The degree to which care is provided to the individual at the most beneficial or necessary time.

  —Is wait time for services a problem? What is the lead time for delivery of products (i.e., hearing aids, Frequency Modulation (FM) systems, augmentative communication devices, therapy supplies)?

With these target areas in mind, asking the questions "What can we do better?" and "Is there a better way to accomplish this task?" will help both the leaders and employees select what areas should be targeted for change.

After the target area is selected, goals should be developed for the quality improvement project. To quote the American philanthropist Elbert Hubbard, "Many people fail in life, not for lack of ability or brains or even courage, but simply because they have never organized their energies around a goal." Goal writing comes naturally to specialists in communication disorders. Our clinical training has taught us to conceptualize clinical change by establishing long- and short-term goals. We engage in goal writing almost every day treating the populations we serve. Goal writing is equally important for the quality improvement projects we undertake. To maximize communication between the organization and the project teams, consider using *SMART goals* as a starting point. SMART in a mnemonic for specific, measureable, attainable, realistic, and timely:

- *Specific:* The goals must be clear and unambiguous. The specific part of the goal answers the what, why, and how of the goal.

- *Measurable:* The goal needs to have a concrete criterion to measure the progress toward attainment of the goal. Furthermore, measuring the outcome will help employees stay motivated to complete their goals.

- *Attainable:* Goals must be reasonably attainable by the employees. The goals should encourage the employees to push themselves within reason to achieve the desired outcome. That is, the goals are neither out of reach nor below standard performance.

- *Realistic/relevant:* The goals must be meaningful and reflect your organization's mission and vision. The goal should be worthwhile to complete.

- *Timely:* The goals must provide a time line, specifically starting and ending points and fixed durations.

The task of identifying areas in which improvements can be made is relatively easy. Writing the goals, however, takes time. It is essential that the goals truly communicate to the team the essence and expectations for the project.

---

**Part Four: The Model**

Abel knew the staff members had questions after they received their goals. He knew that he needed to give them some time to process and discuss these objectives. The facilitator, whom he had selected, would be able to guide his staff on the process of implementing these goals. They would first set the ground rules, such as listen actively, be committed to the purpose, do your fair share and help others, be nonjudgmental, leave negativity at the door, and tolerate disagreement. The first step in the process was to evaluate the problem; then they would generate ideas, try them out, and finally evaluate the outcome. He knew his staff would take on the challenges.

---

# ♦ Quality Improvement Models and Tools

## Models

Over the years many models have been proposed to evaluate processes that we employ in our work environment. One of the original and most widely known is called the Plan, Do, Check, Act (PDCA) cycle. PDCA was originally developed by Walter Shewhart, a statistician at Bell Laboratories in the U.S. during the 1930s, and is referred to as the Shewhart cycle. In the 1950s, a quality expert, W. Edwards Demining, started to use this concept, now also known as the Deming wheel. This model reiterates that programs must start with careful planning and execution and improvement is a continuous cycle.

### Plan-Do-Check-Act

• *Plan:* Determine what is not working and develop ideas to solve the problems.

• *Do:* Implement the plan. The plan should be on a small or experimental scale at first to minimize disruption to the day-to-day activities.

• *Check:* Study your data and determine if you received the desired outcome or not. Check often during the implementation stage to identify any new problems that may arise.

• *Act:* If you received the desired outcome, implement this change across your program. Share your findings with others and if needed, update your policy and procedure manual to reflect these current findings.

   After you have completed one cycle, return to the plan stage and work on the next problem that was discovered. If the experiment did not achieve the desired outcome, skip Act and return to Plan to develop some new ideas, and go through the cycle again.
   There are many variations on PDCA, of which several are worth mentioning. The one that most resembles PDCA is Plan, Do, Study, Act (PDSA). The *Lean method* (Stamatis, 2011) for quality improvement, which will be discussed later in this chapter, often refers to PDCA as being synonymous with PDSA. Although everything is essentially the same, instead of *check* they use the term *study*. It is, however, important to do both: study your data to measure the effectiveness of your project, and check your data during the project to make sure that you are going in the right direction.
   The Standardize, Do, Check, Act (SDCA) variation is another model that is used in the Lean method. The word *kaizen,* in Japanese, which means improvement or change for the better, requires that you standardize your process, specifications, systems, procedures, etc. Your work should be measured and perform to a specific standard. After implementation, standardization is important to achieve consistency.

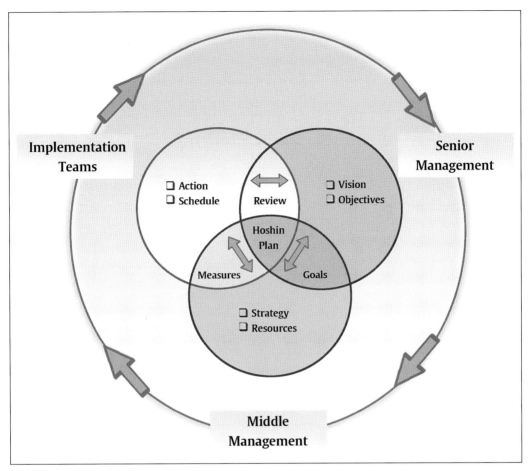

**Fig. 11.1**   The Hoshin plan. [From Akao, Y. (1991). *Hoshin Kanri policy deployment for successful TQM.* New York: Productivity Press. Reprinted by permission.]

### Hoshin

The Check, Act, Plan, Do (CAPD) process, also called the *Hoshin Kanri* methodology, is also used in both Lean and *Six Sigma,* to be discussed later in this chapter. *Hoshin* means pointing the direction or compass and *Kanri* means control or management. This methodology began in Japan in the early 1960s and later was called total quality control (TQC). The importance of this methodology or model is that it involves both planning and deployment of policies starting with the management level. Using strategic plans, the management sets the goals for the entire organization. When implementing this model, the organization begins with "check" so that the current process or system is fully understood prior to moving to the traditional PDCA cycle. Consider the model provided in **Fig. 11.1**.

### Pareto Principle

Another renowned quality expert often discussed in quality management is Joseph Juran, who is known in this area for many things, including the application of the *Pareto principle* to quality. The Pareto principle essentially separates the "vital few" from the "useful many" by suggesting that 80% of the problem is due to 20% of the causes. Adding the human dimension to quality is Juran's trilogy, the cross-functional management approach to quality (quality planning, quality control, and quality improvement). The Juran's model for quality improvement includes the following:

1. Identify the problem—something that went wrong that negatively impacted your service delivery.

2. Establish a project.

3. Prior to any intervention, measure and analyze the current process/problem to establish the baseline performance.

4. Generate and test theories as to the causes of the problem.

5. Prove the "root causes" of the problem.

6. Develop remedial improvements/changes to the process that remove or manage the causes of problem.

7. Establish new controls to prevent recurrence and to sustain the new standards.

8. Deal with resistance to change.

9. Replicate the result and start a new project (Juran Institute, 2009).

Juran's model of quality improvement complements the traditional PDCA by reminding us of the details that truly effect change.

### FOCUS-PDCA

A leading health care organization, Hospital Corporation of America (HCA), originated the FOCUS-PDCA model, which assumes that processes are already in place for quality improvement. The components of the FOCUS-PDCA acronym are as follows:

- *Find a process for improvement:* Define the process, identify the population that will most benefit, and understand how this process fits within the organization and strategic plans.

- *Organize the appropriate team:* Select an appropriate team, keeping in mind the size, and develop a method to document the team's progress toward the goals.

- *Clarify the current knowledge about the process:* Review the current process and analyze the difference between what is expected and what is truly happening.

- *Understand the variables and causes:* Begin data collection, measure the outcomes, and learn the causes of the problems or variations in the process.

- *Select the process involvement:* Identify the plan that will improve the process, and support your recommendations with data.

- *PDCA:* Use after the plan/strategy is selected for implementation across the organization (Brown, 2009).

### Ten-Step Benchmarking

The Xerox Ten-Step Benchmarking model serves as a tool for industries, including health care, by finding and implementing best practices using benchmarks as a guide. Camp and Tweet (1994) from Xerox developed the ten-step benchmarking model, which has been modified by others through the years. The model is as follows:

- *Planning*

  —Step 1. Identify what is to be benchmarked.

—Step 2. Identify comparative companies/providers/schools.

—Step 3. Determine the data collection methods and collect the data.

- *Analysis*

—Step 4. Determine current performance levels and gaps.

—Step 5. Project future performance levels.

—Step 6. Communicate benchmark findings and gain acceptance.

- *Integration*

—Step 7. Establish functional goals.

—Step 8. Develop action plans.

- *Action*

—Step 9. Implement specific actions and monitor progress.

—Step 10. Recalibrate benchmarks.

### Accelerated/Rapid-Cycle Change Approach

The Accelerated/Rapid-Cycle Change Approach model may be considered when time is of the essence. For many managers and employees, the thought of committing 6 months or longer to a quality improvement project can be overwhelming. Furthermore, managers already feel that they do not have the time or staff to spare as everyone is fully committed. With the accelerated approach, the projects can take as little as a week to complete. This is due to good planning, participation by key stakeholders and leadership, and commitment to the change and process. The "pre-work" is the key to the success of this model. Prior to the first meeting, the following should be completed:

- State the problem.
- Gather data that depict the problem, including root cause analysis if needed.
- Prepare flowcharts of the process problems.
- Review the literature regarding the problem, if available.
- Identify team members and establish agreements about resource allocations (i.e., staff time and financial resources).
- Prepare meeting schedules.

The work flow then may look something like the following:

- Meeting 1/Day 1/Week 1: Select the team (if needed), discuss the process and issues, present the current flowchart or processes, prepare data collection plan and tools that will be used, and develop and agree upon the action plan.
- Meeting 2/Day 2/Week 2: Use creativity tools (i.e., brainstorming), collect additional data, identify and validate lower level causes of variation, revise process/flowcharts, complete cost benefit analysis, and identify potential solutions.
- Meeting 3/Day 3/Week 3: Complete solution design and pilot the solution(s) with dates and decide who is responsible.
- Meeting 4/Day 4/Week 4: Analyze data, fine tune, and plan for full implementation.
- Meeting 5/Day 5/Week 5: Execute plan (Brown, 2009).

   The meeting/day/week for each item can vary based on the agreed-upon resource allocation and the scope of the project. Furthermore, the success of this model is contingent on the quality of data, management involvement, and the appropriate tools selected to implement the change.

### Lean

Another widely known and frequently referenced model for quality management, called Lean, was first mentioned in a master's thesis by John Krafcik in 1988 at the Massachusetts Institute of Technology (MIT). This thesis was based on behavioral observations made at the Toyota Motor Company. As written in the thesis, the notion behind the term Lean was that a company

- could accomplish more with less;
- be customer service driven;
- adopt a culture of change through continuous, incremental improvement;
- keep things moving in a "value-added, effective manner;" and
- maintain the respect of its employees.

   When an organization embraces Lean, there will be evidence of the following:

- Activities are viewed as processes while considering the customer/patient and eliminating the wasteful, non–value-added steps.
- *Kaizen* events are held to brainstorm on how to eliminate the waste and to implement PDCS or other models.
- Communication occurs through *value-stream maps*, team meetings, process flow diagrams, or other instruments to communicate the message.
- Everyone is involved and makes suggestions.
- Activities are deliberate and decisive. The workplace is standardized. Meetings are short and effective.
- The staff and leadership embrace learning and sharing knowledge, and are open to changes and new ways of doing things.
- Long-lasting relationships are formed with employees, patients/customers, vendors and suppliers, and the community.

   A basic principle of Lean includes understanding "customer value" (willingness of the person to give you payment for the product or service when he/she feel that it is a fair exchange of value), identifying and analyzing the stream of activities that create that customer value, evaluating and maintaining your system flow, scheduling practices of the work flow that should keep a steady and achievable pace based on the actions of the customer, and continuing the journey of striving for perfection. There are many tools used in Lean that will be described in the next section.

### Six Sigma

A close cousin to Lean is Six Sigma, which emerged in the mid-1990s at Motorola and General Electric. The implementation of Six Sigma principles is credited with helping companies eliminate significant waste and saving money. Many of the Fortune 500 companies practice Six Sigma, with an estimated combined savings exceeding $427 billion over a 20-year period, with the average savings being approximately 2% of total revenue each year (Marx, 2007). Due to this demand and ensuring that qualified people implement this model, this approach provides four different levels (expressed as "belts") of "certification." An individual with a *Yellow Belt* has a solid basic knowledge of Six Sigma methodologies with an understanding of quality versus profit. A *Green Belt* does much of the legwork of the project by gathering the information and executing experiments. *Black Belts* are directly responsible for executing the Six Sigma project within the organization. They help the team achieve the overall goals of the project while saving the organization significant money in the process. The *Master Black Belts* are full-time experts in Six Sigma who help integrate Six Sigma across the entire organization. The scope of the project will determine how many Yellow, Green, and Black Belt facilitators you need to help execute the project. Six Sigma is a way to identify and control variations that affect performance and profit. Six Sigma deploys five phases, referred to as DMAIC:

- *Define* the problems, the customer's concerns, project goals, and cost-benefit analysis.

- *Measure* the current process and collect relevant data.

- *Analyze* the data and verify cause and effect relationships. Seek out root causes of the problems.

- *Improve* the situation by offering solutions, and implement the pilot projects to address the problems.

- *Control* the process to ensure that improvements are maintained and can be performed by anyone in the organization.

Six Sigma has been embraced by various industries as it offers a structured, analytical, and logistical approach to problem solving with a strong organizational framework for implementation (Stamatis, 2011).

All the above models have very similar characteristics. They all embody continuous improvement concepts around planning your project; systematically addressing the concerns; involving the entire organization; collaborating to ensure interdisciplinary, cross-functional involvement; utilizing tools for data collection and measuring performance; assessing the outcomes; and fully integrating successful projects across the organization before starting the process over again.

**Part Five: Let the Fun Begin**

The teams took to the challenge and over the next couple of months they used a variety of tools to gather data and study the problems, employed several graphical tools introduced by the facilitator to assist them with system improvements, and then analyzed their data to target effective outcomes.

To address customer satisfaction, the team with goal 1 decided to have simple conversations with their patients using a "rounding" technique they recently learned from Abel to collect their data. Based on the information they gathered, they employed the AIDET technique (Studer, 2003) to help with overall communication and satisfaction:

- *Acknowledge:* "You are important." Make eye contact, shake hands, acknowledge everyone in the room, get down to the child's level, ask or make a relationship-building question or statement (e.g., "Your shirt says 'Isle of Palms'; my family vacations there every summer. My children love to eat at the . . .").

- *Introduce:* "Welcome to our team. You are in good hands." Give your name, specialty, years of experience, and mention a referring physician to position yourself as a colleague. For example, "I'm Jane Smith, your speech-language pathologist. I want you to know that I've worked with more than 500 children with feeding issues and their families during the 10 years I've been in practice in this specialty area. I also see that Dr. Johnson referred you to me. We've worked together as a team for many years. You're fortunate to have such an excellent doctor."

- *Duration:* "I anticipate your concerns." Tell patients what to expect (e.g., how long will the test take, what will happen, can they bring a special toy, when will they know the test results, how long is the average length of therapy, if we go twice a week versus once a week, does insurance cover this, etc.).

- *Explanation:* "I want you to be informed and comfortable." Carefully listen to your patient's story and use language the patient can understand when describing the treatment plan.

- *Thank You:* "I appreciate the opportunity to care for you." Thank the patient for choosing your practice or school, for coming in today, and for waiting to see you, if necessary.

In closing, ask "What other questions do you have?" Not only did the team's scores improve, the team members received an award for exceeding their required benchmarks that were set by the organization.

While managers typically develop and oversee the day-to-day operations and budgets, wise use of financial resources is the responsibility of everyone. Staff members recognized that they did play a part in the overall finances. They employed *value stream maps*, *5 Whys*, *flow charts*, and *cause-and-effect diagrams*. The data indicated that they were spending on average 2.5 hours a week on nonbillable tasks, such as tracking down patient bills, handling mail, answering the phone when the assistant was out, cleaning toys used in the sessions, and finding a computer to complete their documentation. For 15 staff members, this added up to 37.5 hours of work a week, or almost $150,000 in lost gross billings a year, which justified adding another support staff member and purchasing a computer to handle these nonbillable tasks. Even with these added costs, the department still wound up saving money because the clinical staff members were then able to use their newly freed-up time to schedule an additional 30 office visits a week.

## Tools and Resources for Improving Organizational Efficiencies

A quality improvement program is an ongoing and dynamic process that should be sufficiently nimble to respond whenever an inefficient process/system is discovered, as well as in response to changes in the organizational priorities. When evaluating targeted areas for improvement, there are many strategies that can be employed, from simply brainstorming solutions with colleagues to a full-fledged formal, facilitated, structured process. There is a continuum of tools available to meet your specific needs. When selecting an approach to address the issue(s), bear in mind that it needs to make sense to the employees, leaders, and the teams who will be involved with the quality improvements. One approach, process, or tool, does not meet all needs or situations, so being familiar with a variety of tools and data collection techniques is helpful.

### Data Collection and Monitoring

Data can be both qualitative and quantitative. Having systems in place to collect both types of data is essential in any quality improvement program. Qualitative data can be collected through simple conversations or using Internet data capture tools such as *Survey Monkey* (www.surveymonkey.com) or *REDCap* (Harris et al, 2009), discussed in Chapter 2. Quantitative data capture is also important for any project because you need baseline data or benchmark references prior to implementing your project to measure the effectiveness of the project after completion against the starting point or an outside standard. Using easily accessible spreadsheets, such as *Microsoft Excel* (http://office.microsoft .com/en-us/excel/), or a database designed for large-scale research and organizational data capture, such as *REDCap* (Harris et al, 2009), is helpful when collecting quantitative data. For example, in the Department of Hearing and Speech Sciences at Vanderbilt University, we use a variety of automated, electronic data collection tools, such as *Audbase* (www.audbase.com), *MediLinks* (www.mediserve .com), and *REDCap* (www.redcap.vanderbilt.edu). *Audbase* enables the automatic capture of quantitative and qualitative clinical data such as audiometric thresholds, speech perception scores, immittance thresholds, and demographic data. Within the *MediLinks* clinical documentation system, in addition to offering a method for efficient clinical documentation linked to billing codes and automatic charge entries, efficiency measurements also can be obtained, such as timeliness of completion of documentation, the duration of time required to meet short-term and long-term goals, attendance and "no-show" rates across populations/diagnoses, and demographic data (such as zip codes). The Research Electronic Data Capture, or REDCap system, is a secure, Web-based meta-data capture application principally designed to facilitate and support data capture for research studies. REDCap is now used worldwide by its university network partners and provides support for organizational quality improvement projects and surveys. REDCap provides (1) an intuitive interface for validated data entry, (2) audit trails for tracking data manipulation and export procedures, (3) automated export procedures for seamless data downloads to common statistical packages, and (4) procedures for importing data from external sources (Harris et al, 2009). The Department of Hearing and Speech Sciences at the Vanderbilt Bill Wilkerson Center has used REDCap in several projects and processes, including tracking all the quality improvement projects, developing a database for speech-language-auditory outcomes on children who are deaf or hard of hearing, and conducting employee performance evaluations and targeted satisfaction surveys. Having access to computerized data capture, reporting, and monitoring systems can assist in the early identification of problems and trends that are less than favorable to patient care, educational outcomes, or risk management issues, as well as for research data capture support.

### Anecdotal and Qualitative Data

**Conversation**   A simple conversation about a problem area can provide essential anecdotal, qualitative data that allow us to consider individual perspectives. These conversations can occur between employees, between supervisors and staff, with the individuals and their families for whom we provide care, with community partners, and with other stakeholders, such as contracting agencies and organizations. Studer (2003) advocates for organizations to use a structured conversation, called *Rounding* (Studer, 2003), to collect on-site information from employees and to allow for "eyes-on" observations of the provision of services.

### Rounding for Outcomes with Employees (Studer, 2003)

- Rounding can be performed individually or in small groups. The following questions are samples of what staff could be asked by managers during rounding:

  —What do you think is working well?

  —Is there anyone I should recognize for doing great work?

  —Are there any systems that need improvement?

  —Do you have the basic tools and equipment to do your job?

  —Do you have any tough questions?

  —Is there anything I can help you with right now?

- Then, when finished, close with something like, "Thank you for making a difference to our organization!"

### Leaders Rounding with Patients/Families (Studer, 2003)

- Prior to meeting with the patient/family, ask the person who provides direct services if there is anything you need to know before talking with the patient/family?

- Ask the family in a conversational way, the following questions:

  —Is there anyone on staff who has done a good job caring for you?

  —Is there anything I can do for you right now?

- Then, close with something like, "Thank you for choosing our facility for your care!"

**5 Whys**    Another tool that is used for elucidating and determining the underlying cause of a problem is called the *5 Whys* (Miller, 2007). With this conversation, you ask questions starting with the word why to learn about the presented problem. To demonstrate this principle, let's use a scenario in which speech-language test manuals are not being returned to the test file in a timely manner.

- First why: *Why does this happen?* Answer: The test manual remains on the clinician's desk after the evaluation.
- Second why: *Why?* Answer: The clinician is seeing students back to back.
- Third why: *Why?* Answer: The clinician had to take the student who was tested back to the classroom and pick up the other student for a scheduled therapy session.
- Fourth why: *Why?* Answer: The current schedule does not allow time for the clinician to return materials to their proper place between sessions.

With this example, it took only four "whys" to identify the root of the problem. The issue is the clinician's schedule. The five main steps used with this conversational technique are as follows:

- Describe the problem.
- Ask why the problem has occurred.
- Continue to ask why until a clear answer is reached.
- Take steps to correct the problem and document what you did. If the problem is resolved, then no further action is needed.
- If the problem continues, then repeat the process or use another technique to eliminate the problem.

When using this technique, you need to probe deeply but carefully. You may need to go to different people and get different perspectives to truly examine the problem.

**Questionnaires**    The use of questionnaires is also helpful in data collection. Questionnaires can collect both qualitative and quantitative data. The most common questionnaire used in our field is the patient/client satisfaction questionnaire.

**Graphical Tools**    There are a variety of tools that can be used to sketch the relationship of variables and visually study and manage the projects to address the problems. Graphical representations can communicate an overall message and relationships better than the raw data or a narrative report. Using graphical tools often makes it easier to see the problem, steps in a process, and to demonstrate improvement after a solution has been implemented.

## Graphic Analysis

### Cause and Effect: Fishbone Diagrams

This diagram is also known as an *Ishikawa diagram* named after Kaoru Ishikawa, who first applied this method to the shipyards of Kobe, Japan, in the 1940s. With this diagram, you identify the major categories of the influence on the problem. Within each category you identify the causes and their connections. **Figure 11.2** illustrates the Fishbone diagram that was used by Abel's team.

### Pareto Chart

This is a special chart that uses both a bar graph and a line graph with the absolute number and the percentage of contribution. As you recall earlier, the Pareto principle, discussed earlier, is based on the notion that 20% of the causes are responsible for 80% of the outcomes. The line depicts the

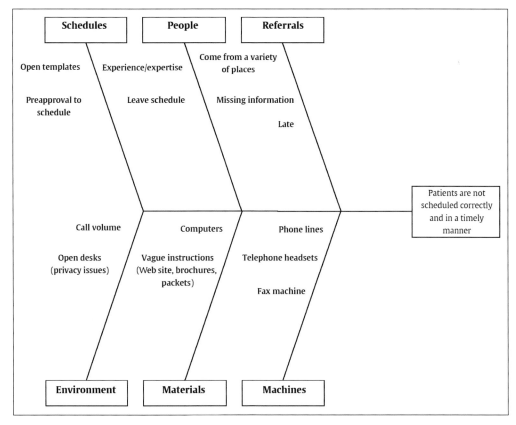

**Fig. 11.2**    A Fishbone diagram used to examine sources for delays in scheduling.

cumulative percentage total up to 100%. As **Fig. 11.3** illustrates, 80% of the delays in scheduling the intake visit were attributable to the insurance authorization process, as compared to other causes (missing information, the need for an interpreter, difficulties with the family's schedule, or the need for a special team or provider).

*Check Sheets*

In real time, your team may want to gather data using a check sheet to see what is happening as the activity is occurring. For example, you may have a check sheet for tallying how many referrals you receive each day by email, phone, and fax. Another example would be a work sample where you would indicate how time is spent in each category identified for tracking. See **Table 11.1** for an example from Abel's team.

*Scatter Plots: Looking for Relationships*

Although this is the simplest of all plots, the scatter plot often provides some valuable insight on relationships and trends. When Abel's team members looked at their revenue over time, they noticed changes in their referrals sources that led them to implement a quality improvement project to make access to care easier. Based on the data in the chart (**Fig. 11.4**), they found essentially little change in school referrals, an increase in audiology referrals, and a decrease in physician referrals (i.e., pediatricians and otolaryngologists).

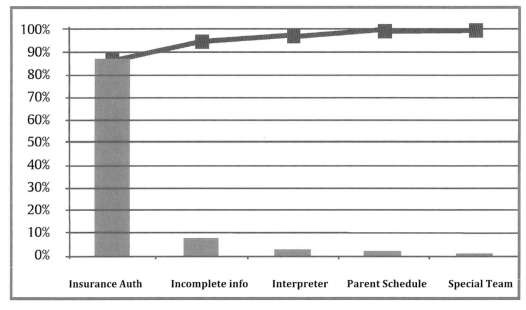

**Fig. 11.3**    Example of a Pareto chart.

### Bar Charts and Histograms

Bar charts provide a great way to illustrate the data, understand the ranges, compare conditions, and identify trends. A histogram is a type of bar chart that is organized with equal widths and displays the distribution of data. The histogram helps the analyzer to see how processes relate and the degree of variations that can influence performance. As shown in **Fig. 11.5**, the team learned that the clinic wait times varied by specialty areas, which may have been due to the distance between the treatment rooms and the waiting area, or a provider factor.

### Value Stream Map

Used in Lean and Six Sigma, the value stream map (VSM) is a graphical representation of all the steps in the process and the flow of information that starts the process. It is essentially a flow chart of every step in the process from start to finish. VSMs are often hand-drawn, but there are some soft-

**Table 11.1**    Check Sheet: Work Sample

| Clinician's name: Ben Courage<br>Date: August 1, 2011 | |
|---|---|
| | **Count** |
| Direct patient contacts | ЦН ЦН
 ЦН ЦН
 || |
| Nondirect patient time | ЦН†
 ЦН†
 |

Direct patient contacts: ЦНТ ЦНТ ЦНТ ЦНТ ||
Nondirect patient time: ЦНТ ЦНТ

*Key:* Each hash mark represents 15 minutes.

*Notes:* Spent 30 minutes with mailing letters, 30 minutes answering the phone for secretary, 1 hour cleaning toys, 30 minutes on Facebook (waiting for late patient).

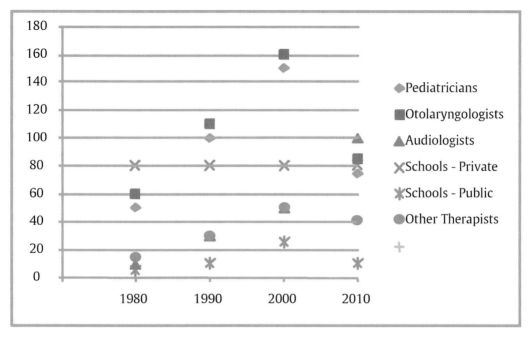

**Fig. 11.4**   A scatter plot of tracking referral sources over time.

ware tools available to make more elaborate maps. Lean and Six Sigma have special icons and ways to depict the flow of the process. The VSMs can include who is responsible, the time it takes, and the equipment, space, and resources used in the process. Once you have the process down, then you search for *muda* (the Japanese term for waste or inefficiencies in the system). To identify *muda*, the team evaluates each step in the VSM and designates it as "value-added" (VA) or "non–value-added" (NVA)

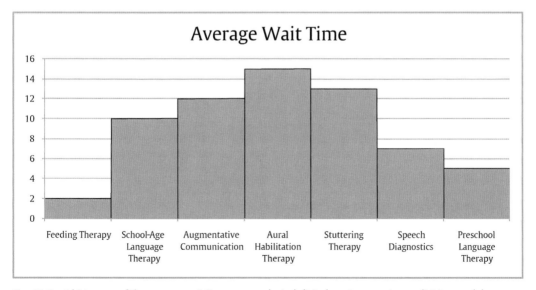

**Fig. 11.5**   A histogram of the average wait time across selected clinical service areas in a pediatric speech-language pathology department.

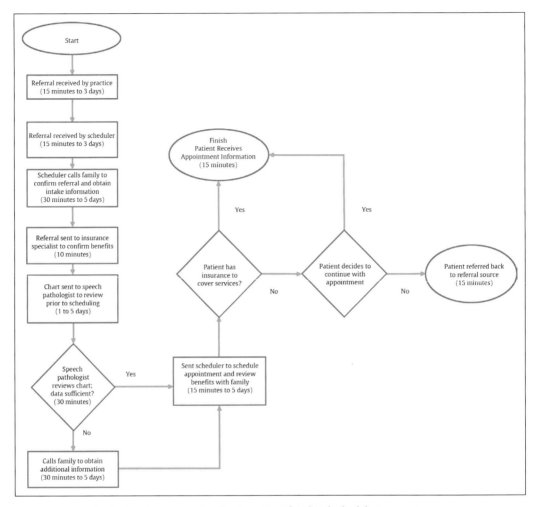

**Fig. 11.6** Example of value stream mapping the steps in a referral and scheduling process.

items. In Abel's example, the team created a simple VSM on the process of scheduling a patient to identify *muda* (**Fig. 11.6**). By examining their VSM, the team was able to identify both VA and NVA properties in each step. The team could then could apply *5 Whys* to explore the issues in each NVA step and develop quality improvement plans to address those issues using the PDCA model to achieve a positive outcome!

**Part Six: The Tiger Examines Its Stripes**

As Abel was reviewing the outcomes from the team projects with his boss, he shared with her some of the lessons they learned. He outlined each of them:

1. The support from the leadership was truly valued. Giving the staff the release time from their clinic schedules, financial support for the facilitators, and room space, and, most importantly, the leadership's involvement and participation in the team truly made the difference.

2. The team members' engagement and readiness were also a key to their success. They left the negativity at home and truly engaged in the process. They also felt empowered and appreciated.

3. The institution creating a culture of change, encouraging it at all levels. The staff members did not feel alone in the process because they knew their colleagues in other services areas at the institution were doing the same thing.

At the end of the day and only targeting two areas, the boss told Abel that his team saved the institution over $450,000 after all the costs were deducted, patient satisfaction scores improved significantly, and quality of patient care had improved. The boss's closing words to Abel were, "I truly value all that you do for the population you serve and the employees you represent. Thank you!"

## ◆ Conclusion and Future Directions

Choosing specific, well-defined areas to target for implementing an integrative quality management program can potentially reduce deficiency, improve customer satisfaction, and reduce expenditures. As we know, there is great waste (unnecessary steps, paper processes that could be automated, hand-off communications that could be more efficient) in every system. These inefficiencies affect both patient and employee satisfaction with the organization and the quality of care.

Given the ever-pressing push to "do more with less" while maintaining quality of services in the schools and in the clinic, the following recommendations are offered:

1. Although some argue that it takes money to operate an effective program, the reality is we truly cannot "buy" what we need most: *great leaders* who can help the system to improve, and *motivated employees* ready to embrace these changes. Those are qualities and attitudes individuals bring to the job with them. Leaders need to have the curiosity and tenacity to look critically at what they are doing, reflect on what works and what does not, and find better, more efficient ways to deliver safe, high-quality care as well as be supportive of the people in the trenches delivering these changes (Wellman, Hagan, & Jeffries, 2011).

2. Once your organization enters into a commitment to create a culture of caring that defines their quality improvement program, openness to change will be integrated into all aspects of your system. New perspectives and new processes will not be considered an extra responsibility or burden. Always looks for better ways of delivering care, be a team player, and leave negativity at the doorstep.

3. Once you learn a new process, share it with your colleagues in your community and nationally. The first rule of efficiency is "don't reinvent the wheel!" Work collaboratively and share your knowledge and experience to make service provision across the discipline available to those who need it. Ultimately, our goal is to help our patients/clients/students reach their fullest communication abilities with the least amount of time and resources.

4. Finally, after implementing your quality improvement project, it is important to codify your new process or procedure. By writing down what steps you took to improve a system, you ultimately will help others to address similar situations going forward, and assist in sustaining the new standard, practice, or process to achieve consistency.

Although it takes time and effort to implement a quality improvement program to improve organizational performance, the costs are too high not to do this for ourselves and our patients. As the American Speech-Language-Hearing Association's Special Interest Group 11 Steering Committee stated in 1996, "Improving quality requires a scientific and systematic way of thinking, discipline, and unwavering commitment from the top. Thus it is not for all organizations. But in this age of accountability . . . it would seem irresponsible to choose a lesser alternative" (Steering Committee of the Quality Improvement Study Section, 1996, p. 3).

# References

Akao, Y. (1991). *Hoshin Kanri policy deployment for successful TQM*. New York: Productivity Press

American Speech-Language-Hearing Association (ASHA). (1984). *Guidelines for caseload size and speech-language services in the schools* (pp. 53–58). Rockville, MD: Author

American Speech-Language-Hearing Association (ASHA). (1993, Mar). Guidelines for caseload size and speech-language service delivery in the schools. Ad Hoc Committee on Service Delivery in the Schools. *ASHA Supplement, 35*(3, Suppl 10), 33–39

American Speech-Language-Hearing Association (ASHA). (2010). *2010 schools survey report: SLP caseload characteristics.* www.asha.org/research/memberdata/SchoolsSurvey.htm

Brown, J. A. (2009). *The healthcare quality handbook: A professional resource and study guide* (24th ed.). Pasadena, CA: JB Quality Solutions

Camp, R. C., & Tweet, A. G. (1994, May). Benchmarking applied to health care. *The Joint Commission Journal on Quality Improvement, 20,* 229–238

Centers for Medicare and Medicaid Services (CMS). (2008). *Glossary.* http://www.medicare.gov/Glossary/search.asp?SelectAlphabet=Q&Language=English

Centers for Medicare and Medicaid Services, Office of the Actuary, National Health Statistics Group (CMS). (2011). *National health care expenditures data.* http://www.cms.gov/NationalHealthExpendData/25_NHE_Fact_Sheet.asp#TopOfPage

Harris, P. A., Taylor, R., Thielke, R., Payne, J., Gonzalez, N., & Conde, J. G. (2009, Apr). Research electronic data capture (REDCap)—a metadata-driven methodology and workflow process for providing translational research informatics support. *Journal of Biomedical Informatics, 42,* 377–381

Institute Of Medicine, Lohr, K. N. (Ed.). (1990). *Medicare: A strategy for quality assurance* (p. 21). Washington, DC: National Academy Press

Johnson, S. (2000). *Who moved my cheese?* New York: Putnam Adult

Juran Institute, Inc. (2009). *Quality improvement.* http://www.juran.com/solutions_improve_quality_of_products_and_services_quality_improvement.html

Kowdley, G., & Ashbaker, D. (2011, May-Jun). Health care costs in America—technology as a major driver. *Journal of Surgical Education, 68,* 231–238

Lencioni, P. (2002). *The five dysfunctions of a team.* San Francisco, CA: Jossey-Bass

Marx, M. (2007). Six Sigma saves a fortune. *Six Sigma Magazine, 3.* http://www.i360institute.com/files/pdf/fortune500sixsigma.pdf

Miller, J. (Ed.). (2007). *Taiichi Ohno's work place management.* Mukilteo, WA: Gemba Press

Patterson, K., Grenny, J., McMillan, R., & Switzler, A. (2011). *Crucial conversation: Tools for talking when stakes are high.* New York: McGraw-Hill

Stamatis, D. H. (2011). *Essentials for the improvement of healthcare using Lean & Six Sigma.* New York: Productivity Press

Steering Committee of the Quality Improvement Study Section. (1996). Quality improvement: The basics. In *Special Interest Division 11: Administration and supervision* (pp. 1–3). Rockville, MD: ASHA

Studer, Q. (2003). *Hardwiring excellence* (pp. 94, 142–153). Gulf Breeze, FL: Fire Starter Publishing

Wellman, J., Hagan, P., & Jeffries, H. (2011). *Leading the Lean healthcare journey: Driving culture change to increase value.* New York: Productivity Press

Wennberg, J. E., Brownless, S., Fisher, E. S., Skinner, J. S., & Weinstein, J. N. (2008). An agenda for change: Improving quality and curbing health care spending: opportunities for the Congress and the Obama Administration. *A Dartmouth Atlas White Paper* (pp. ii). http://www.dartmouthatlas.org/downloads/reports/agenda_for_change.pdf

# IV

# Research

# 12

# Treatment Research

## *Lesley B. Olswang and Barbara A. Bain*

## ♦ Chapter Focus

This chapter expands upon questions that were posed by Olswang in the 1998 edition of this text in her discussion of treatment efficacy research. Here treatment research is examined by highlighting the differences between efficacy and effectiveness research. The chapter focuses on the types of research questions each addresses, and provides an overview of the research structure for each with regard to designs, independent and dependent variables, and forms of data analysis. The relative contributions of different types of treatment research studies are considered, and the argument is made for expanding clinically applicable treatment research of all forms.

## ♦ Introduction

Over the past 20 years, treatment research in communication disorders has grown impressively. This trend no doubt reflects the interest in and commitment to evidence-based practice (EBP) as embraced by individual researchers and national organizations, including the American Speech-Language-Hearing Association (ASHA), the American Speech-Language-Hearing Foundation (ASHF), and the Academy of Neurologic Communication Disorders and Sciences (ANCDS). The priority of EBP for our profession has become apparent; university programs are incorporating major concepts of EBP into their curricula, and clinicians are urged to do the same in their practices (ASHA, 2011c). Some urgency has accompanied this emphasis on EBP, based not only on ethical considerations but also on economic factors as well. In the current climate of health care and education reform, and a growing population of diverse clientele, speech-language pathologists are faced with new challenges in the delivery of services. Limited resources are exacerbating these challenges, thus creating an urgent need to address the efficacious delivery of services to those individuals, pediatric to geriatric, in need of treatment for speech and language disorders. Treatment research is more in demand now than ever before.

The primary trend in treatment research in communication sciences and disorders (CSD) has been to examine the *efficacy* of treatments designed to change behaviors in individuals with communication disorders under controlled conditions. Less common has been *effectiveness* research designed to explore the benefits of treatment in everyday practice under everyday conditions. As our competence in EBP continues to grow, both efficacy and effectiveness research need to keep pace.


# ◆ Treatment Research Structure


Dollaghan (2007) has provided a practical definition of EBP for our discipline that identifies three critical components: *external evidence* from systematic research, *internal clinical practice evidence,* and evidence concerning *client preference*. Treatment research, as discussed in this chapter, refers to the external evidence component, which complements clinician expertise, including collected data (internal evidence) and client perspective (client preference). Treatment research entails using valid, systematic scientific methodology to investigate intervention protocols and document trends in clinical outcomes via data collection. Robey (2004) argues that the organizing structure for treatment research is anchored by two major terms/concepts: treatment efficacy and treatment effectiveness. *Treatment efficacy* refers to the extent to which an intervention produces favorable outcomes under ideally controlled conditions. Robey (2004) notes that "the ideal conditions of efficacy testing result directly from an imperative for preserving internal validity. The researcher's task is to assure that only the effect of the independent variable (i.e., the treatment protocol) on the dependent variable (i.e., the clinical-outcome) plausibly accounts for observed changed in the outcome measure" (p. 402). Treatment efficacy relies upon rigorous, reliable, and systematic control in the research methodology under ideal conditions with participants similar in characteristics. As such, efficacy research examines treatment protocols that may well be driven and utilized by conventional wisdom, but whose benefits are yet to be reliably documented. Efficacy research examines such treatments under rigorously controlled and reliable conditions in an attempt to prove the relationship between treatment implementation and positive change. Because of the tightly controlled methodology under ideal conditions, the results of efficacy research are limited in population generalization. The Institute of Education Sciences (IES) states, "The goal of efficacy trials is to determine if an intervention can work to improve student outcomes with a limited and specified sample as opposed to if an intervention will work when implemented under conditions of routine practice" (Institute of Education Sciences, 2011, p. 45).

*Treatment effectiveness* refers to the extent to which intervention produces favorable outcomes under usual or everyday conditions. Effectiveness research evaluates treatment in the complex and variable context of applied settings. As Robey (2004) states, "Treatment efficacy warrants the expectation of reasonable benefits. . . . Treatment effectiveness puts that expectation to test in clinical practice" (p. 403). One dimension of treatment effectiveness research addresses issues of service delivery in regard to efficacious treatment strategies, particularly examining the value and usefulness of standard care procedures. Of significance in this type of research is the exploration of treatments from the perspectives of a variety of stakeholders, including patients, caregivers, and providers. In education, for example, effectiveness research of this type might include the creation and testing of demonstration projects. This dimension of treatment effectiveness is widely observed in health disciplines under health service research (AcademyHealth, 2011). Another dimension of treatment effectiveness research takes the next step in examining well-tested treatments in a broader context of practice. The IES refers to these studies as "scale-up evaluations," where effectiveness of fully developed and proven interventions are examined in authentic educational delivery settings as part of routine practice with diverse samples (IES, 2011, p. 57). Ultimately, effectiveness research must address the implementation of programs and practices in everyday practice, to improve the delivery of services in all social, health care, and educational services. This dimension of effectiveness research, termed *implementation science,* has the widest generalizability, which can then impact policy development (Fixsen, Naoom, Blase, Friedman, & Wallace, 2005). As such, effectiveness research has more extensive population generalization than efficacy research.

The terms *efficacy* and *effectiveness* are used exclusively in this chapter, but as should be apparent from the introduction above, terminology varies across disciplines, reflecting distinctions in conceptual emphases. For example, efficacy might be referred to as "effects" and "efficiency" research. Some disciplines refer to "laboratory research" or possibly even "bench science" to refer to research delivered under ideal conditions with well-defined samples yielding causal conclusions. Even more varied is the terminology applied to effectiveness research. As mentioned above, a term commonly used in the health care world is *health services research,* which refers to research examining factors impacting *access, quality,* and *cost* of health care (AcademyHealth, 2011). This type of research has also been called "health systems research" and "operations research." *Scale-up evaluations* are considered a form of effectiveness research, where proven programs are tested in routine practice settings. This terminology comes from the broader concept of "scaling up" as used in health care to describe the science of implementing proven innovations "to benefit more people and to foster policy and programme development on a lasting, sustainable basis" (Simmons, Fajans, & Ghiron, 2007, p. i). Another related term, *implementation science,* refers to the "scientific study of methods to promote the systematic uptake of clinical research findings and other evidence-based practices into routine practice" to improve the quality of education and health care on a large scale (Implementation Science, 2011, p. 1).

*Scaling up* and *implementation science* embody the effort to translate evidence-based findings into common practice—*translational research.* Because large-scale implementation is the focus of this research, unique approaches to methodology are required. Even the term *outcome research* has been used in discussions of effectiveness. The nuances surrounding the terminological differences will not be explored in this chapter; so often, terminology differences are an artifact of different disciplines speaking about shared concepts. Regardless of the terms mentioned above, one can appreciate that they describe a continuum of clinical research with the following three anchor points: (1) examining treatment strategies under tightly controlled, ideal conditions; (2) investigating these strategies under typical, "real-world" conditions; and (3) investigating the implementation of these strategies as they become part of large-scale social service, education, and health care programs. In this chapter, we will consistently use the terms *efficacy* and *effectiveness*, and focus our discussion on the first two anchor points on the continuum. We will certainly draw from other disciplines and conceptual models to elaborate our themes. Our attempt in this chapter is to introduce the concepts behind treatment efficacy and effectiveness to begin describing the breadth of treatment research in CSD. This orientation, in turn, will provide a framework for suggesting directions for where the discipline of CSD, particularly in the profession of speech-language pathology, should be moving in its EBP efforts, always mindful that ultimately our goal is to have our research evidence be implemented in practice on the broadest scale possible.

Both treatment efficacy and treatment effectiveness are designed to examine and provide evidence for the benefits of intervention, but each with a slightly different perspective. The differences in evidence between the two are probably most clearly understood by appreciating the structure of research. The major elements of the research create that structure; they are research questions, designs, independent variables, dependent variables, and data analysis and interpretation. The sections that follow will briefly discuss the basic contours of each element with regard to treatment research, with an emphasis on efficacy research and highlighting notable differences between efficacy and effectiveness. The reader is referred to Hegde (2003), Hulley, Cummings, Browner, Grady, and Newman (2007), and Schiavetti, Metz, and Orlikoff (2011) for elaborated descriptions of the elements that define the structure of clinical research.

## ◆ Research Questions

Research questions lie at the heart of the structure; they serve as the objective of the study. Research questions define the uncertainty about a particular problem that the investigator wishes to resolve

(Hulley et al, 2007). The questions define and determine the nature of the research and the methodology. Efficacy research questions are, by definition, clinical, and they attempt to establish a direct, causal relationship between the implementation of treatment and a change in client behavior. Effectiveness research questions are also clinical, but investigate treatment in the context of natural environment and issues concerning service delivery. Robey (2004) helps us appreciate the difference between efficacy and effectiveness research by describing them in terms of a five-phase model of research. The five phases correspond to a proposed sequence: from early studies of feasibility through testing the worth of a treatment. Briefly, the five phases are as follows (see Robey, 2004, for details):

- Phase I—documenting a treatment's therapeutic effect, which corresponds to change that is associated with treatment implementation

- Phase II—documenting the dimensions of the therapeutic effect, for example, exploring variations in client characteristics, examining magnitude of change, and refining treatment protocols

- Phase III—conducting a clinical trial to test and documenting efficacy; in behavioral research, this is the gold standard for controlling external threats to validity

- Phase IV—exploring efficacious treatment protocols in the field, by examining treatment benefits under average conditions, which includes different service delivery approaches

- Phase V—examining the cost-effectiveness of treatment as it is delivered in clinical practice

The discussion that follows further defines efficacy and effectiveness research by highlighting the variety of questions that each addresses in speech-language pathology. Efficacy questions, which correspond to Robey's (2004) phases I to III, examine the nature of the relationship between a treatment and the change that is observed in the client. Appreciating the complexity of the relationship is critical to understanding how treatment influences client change. First, efficacy questions can examine and attempt to confirm the benefits of treatment. This means linking treatment manipulations to client behavioral change. Questions verifying the benefits of treatment must address issues of validity and reliability, specifically addressing whether a particular treatment (or treatment strategy/technique) is directly responsible for client change and whether the change is trustworthy under varying controlled conditions. These questions document validity issues, that is, that the treatment, and not some other cause, is responsible for behavior change (Schiavetti et al, 2011). These are basic questions of an evidence-based practice discipline. For example, Fey et al (2006) investigated if *responsivity education/prelinguistic milieu teaching* (RE/PMT) significantly increased children's rate of imperative acts, declarative acts, and overall communicative acts compared with the use of these same acts by children who did not receive RE/PMT. Cream et al (2010) investigated the efficacy of video self-monitoring following speech restructuring treatment to improve the maintenance of treatment effects. Petersen, Gillam, Spencer, and Gillam (2010) investigated the effects of narrative language intervention on the macrostructure and microstructure of oral narratives of school-age children. And Ingersoll and Lalonde (2010) investigated whether object and gestural imitation training increase the language use in children with autism spectrum disorders.

Efficacy research can also include questions that explore the phenomenon of change in communication, examining which aspects of treatment differentially influence which behavior, that is, the *effects* of treatment. These questions focus on generalization issues, exploring ways in which behaviors change in relationship to each other as a product of treatment. For example, Ballard, Robin, McCabe, and McDonald (2010) investigated whether treatment targeting whether treatment for children with apraxia of speech that targets improved control of relative syllable durations in three-syllable nonwords that represent strong-weak and weak-strong stress patterns generalize to other nonword and real word stimuli. Finally, efficacy research can address the rate and magnitude of change over time, that is, *efficiency*. These questions explore the relative benefits of two or more treatments. They also examine rate and degree of change by dissecting the components of a treatment package. Examples of these questions include the following: Is there a difference in the efficacy of *responsive education and prelinguistic milieu teaching* and the *Picture Exchange Communication System* on spoken communication of preschoolers with autism spectrum disorders (Yoder & Stone, 2006)? And is there a difference in generalization to treated and not treated sounds when children with phonological disorders are treated with nonwords versus real words as treatment stimuli (Gierut, Morrisette, & Ziemer (2010)? The essence of efficacy questions is that they address the direct link between what the clinician implements as part of treatment and the client behaviors that change in response. The questions are framed so that they can be answered in controlled situations, with external and internal variables constrained as much as possible.

Effectiveness questions, in contrast, define investigations that explore confirmation of treatment effects in a broader context; these correspond to Robey's (2004) phases IV and V. Effectiveness questions explore the delivery of research-verified treatment packages and techniques (as answered via efficacy research) in natural contexts, where control of external and internal variables is neither feasible nor desired. Robey (2004) defines treatment effectiveness as research that examines "the potency of a treatment protocol for bringing about change in the real world" (p. 402). Therefore, effectiveness questions can also be viewed as investigating service delivery, including questions that explore setting and clinician variations and dosage or cost effectiveness issues. To illustrate the examination of an evidence-based treatment in applied settings, Miller and Guitar (2009) conducted a study that asked would the Lidcombe program for early stuttering treatment have a similar outcome with inexperienced speech-language pathologists as compared with outcomes when implemented by the developers? Different agents of change (e.g., clinicians, family members, professional assistants or aides) are considered in this set of questions as they inform clinician variations in the delivery of services. In additional examples, Binger, Kent-Walsh, Ewing, and Taylor (2010) investigated whether trained educational assistants could facilitate message productions of students who require augmentative and alternative communication (AAC), and Kent-Walsh, Binger, and Hasham (2010) investigated if instructed parents could use the least-to-most prompting strategy on the turn-taking skills of their children who use AAC. Correspondingly, patient-oriented care questions form a category of effectiveness questions. These questions also tackle issues concerning patient/client and family expectations and satisfaction. For example, Mullen and Schooling (2010) examined parent satisfaction as part of their study of the *National Outcomes Measurement System* (NOMS) regarding speech-language pathology intervention for the pediatric population.

Also under the umbrella of effectiveness research are questions addressing the broad category of *cost-effectiveness.* These include investigating issues of treatment dosage, feasibility, and accountability in regard to delivery of specific treatment protocols, treatment packages and coordination among providers. Barriers to service delivery are also areas that are researched, such as questions that address caseload size and ethical versus legal mandates for service. Certainly questions addressing *informatics* and data management as they apply to the cost-effective service delivery come under the broad category of effectiveness questions. Often effectiveness questions of this type are driven by health care decision makers versus research scientists, although ideally these stakeholders should come together to generate questions for investigation (Ginsburg, Lewis, Zackheim, & Casebeer, 2007). As an example of this type of effectiveness question in our discipline, Katz, Maag, Fallon, Blenkarn, and Smith (2010) conducted a study examining school-based speech-language pathologists' mean caseload size, asking whether there is a threshold at which caseload size begins to be perceived as unmanageable, and what are the variables that seem to predict the likelihood that a speech-language pathologist makes this judgment?

As should be apparent, the range of questions from efficacy to effectiveness is tremendous, reflecting how much we need to learn about treatment for communication disorders. In treatment research, correctly identifying the question is critical. For example, Schlosser, Koul, and Costello (2007) provide a thoughtful discussion regarding *clinical questions* in the area of AAC. The question that is asked serves to provide the framework for guiding the structure of the methodology, including selection of the research designs and the independent and dependent variables.

## Designs

Treatment research should employ many types of designs. The variety reflects the range of questions for investigating efficacy and effectiveness. The research question will drive the design choice, but because the emphasis is on ***unassailable*** evidence, the designs must provide that capability. This section briefly discusses basic design strategies and, in doing so, suggests how they might apply to efficacy versus effectiveness questions, and how they could be incorporated into Robey's (2004) five-phase model. The purpose of this section is to introduce broad design types and suggest their most typical application to treatment research. The emphasis is on experimental (versus descriptive) designs, as we are focusing our interests on treatment research that corroborates therapeutic change. Hegde (2003), Schiavetti et al (2011), and Hulley et al (2007) provide clear, elaborated descriptions of designs used in treatment research in communicative disorders.

Questions that first explore the feasibility of therapeutic benefits often use within-subject or time-series designs. These questions ask how a particular manipulation (i.e., treatment) alters behavior over time and thus are often associated with Robey's (2004) phase I research. This approach to research attempts to explore treatment efficacy by systematically introducing treatment to an individual and carefully measuring the corresponding performance over time. At the heart of within-subject methodologies is _applied behavioral analysis_. The environment is manipulated by the experimenter in methodical, predetermined ways (i.e., treatment), and critical behaviors are measured repeatedly over time. Of significance is the focus on individual performance over time. An intervention outcome is demonstrated by systematic change in a subject's performance as treatment is introduced, altered, or withdrawn. This is accomplished by separating conditions into phases: _baseline, treatment,_ and _withdrawal_ (see the discussion in Chapter 14, by Kearns and de Riesthal, on single-subject research designs and case reports). _Replication_, either within subjects across phases or across subjects, is essential to establishing a relationship between the treatment and the outcome. The more replications, the more powerful will be the evidence. Replications across subjects, particularly when yoked in time, provide increased experimental control and allow for greater generalization of results. Case studies are ones in which a single subject is observed independently from other subjects; however, a case study by itself will have limited experimental control and thus provides weaker evidence for generalization to a larger sample. The beauty of time-series single-subject research is the opportunity to examine the unfolding nature of change. The approach allows the researcher to document how treatment changes an individual over time. The power of this observation is that it yields extraordinary insight into the therapeutic process, by revealing how treatment interfaces with particular disorders and subject/client characteristics.

Questions that ask whether a group of individuals, on average, changed more often than not with the implementation of treatment, lend themselves to between-group strategies. Examples include the case-control study, the randomized trial, the cross-sectional study, and the cohort study. These designs cut across efficacy and effectiveness research, and phases II to V in Robey's (2004) model. One of the major challenges in group design is identifying homogeneous groups of individuals, treating some and not others, or providing one treatment to one group and a different treatment to another, similar group. The minimum number of groups is always two, and groups are formed on the basis of either randomization or matching. Group differences are examined to determine the benefits of treatment, or the benefits and efficiency of one treatment versus another. Between-group designs are important for determining whether individuals with similar characteristics will respond to treatment and to what degree. Confirmation of a treatment effect is demonstrated by differences in group performances on pre- and posttest measures as tested by statistical procedures or other analyses. The results yielded by these designs become more powerful with larger groups of individuals, but they often become difficult to implement because homogeneity among subjects is frequently difficult to achieve. Efficacy studies attempt to control these group differences, whereas effectiveness studies might embrace the differences across groups as part of the exploration of a treatment into a less controlled, natural context. Between-group designs are important when generalization of findings is a goal—that is, if the intent is to suggest that the findings apply to a large proportion of a population. The application to efficacy and effectiveness questions is obvious; however, the trade-off is that these designs are not meant to provide information about individual variation in performance. Thus, their application to some efficacy questions will be limited.

Questions asking how particular contextual variables influence behaviors can also be addressed by _qualitative_ designs. This research strategy, employing a variety of design types, explores the natural relationship between client performance and contextual/environmental influences, such as setting, persons, activities, and so on (see Damico & Simmons-Mackie, 2003, for a tutorial). Although this type of research is considered a descriptive rather than experimental study, it still has a valuable place in treatment research. Qualitative, observational research examines behaviors in natural contexts. The investigator observes events in a natural context without influencing or altering them. The evidentiary support for the findings is substantiated via tools for documenting credibility and plausibility (Lincoln & Guba, 1985), a point to be discussed later in this chapter. Because qualitative designs are essentially descriptive (rather than experimental), they might be considered as more appropriately contributing to effectiveness research—Robey's (2004) phase IV. However, if phase I is viewed as including feasibility studies, then qualitative designs might be considered applicable. The essence of this type of research is acknowledging that performance cannot be separated from context; as such, performance must be studied within the variability of context (Bogdan & Biklen, 1992).

Questions that address the occurrence of a disease or health-related disorder and environmental influences utilize _epidemiological_ designs. This research strategy explores treatment from the perspective of the population at large, and thus can address issues concerning incidence and prevalence of disease or disorders. Large samples reflecting the population are used to show trends in treatment benefits. The designs include both descriptive/observational and experimental methodological studies and are illustrated by the four major epidemiologic prototypes: the case-control study, the randomized trial, the cross-sectional study, and the cohort study. As such, epidemiologic designs overlap with group designs. Because of the necessity for large sample sizes to reflect populations, sophisticated statistical analyses are used. Robey (2004) indicates that these questions and designs are primarily used for examining treatment effectiveness, specifically phases IV and V.

As efficacy and effectiveness research accrues regarding a given treatment, a desire to synthesize the findings builds. Variations among the studies will naturally exist, but researchers and clinicians will hope to bring together the results in a cohesive manner. This research strategy encompasses _systematic reviews_. "A systematic review is a comprehensive overview of the research literature that addresses a specific clinical question" (Schiavetti et al, 2011, p. 400). Well-designed studies can also be grouped and analyzed statistically as a whole using a _meta-analysis_ statistical methodology, discussed in Chapter 15 by Ntourou and Lipsey. Robey (2004) states, "The integration and synthesis is accomplished through a set of mathematical procedures collectively termed 'meta-analysis'" (p. 406). Note that meta-analyses can apply to both efficacy and effectiveness research, but as Robey (2004) notes, a systematic review will not mix efficacy and effectiveness studies, as each type of research addresses different questions. Meta-analyses play a major role in the creation of evidence-based practice guidelines. For additional discussion regarding systematic reviews and practice guidelines, see Dijkers (2009), and Moher, Liberati, Tetzlaff, and Altman (2009).

All of the design strategies discussed above allow an opportunity to observe human behavior under different conditions of treatment and/or no treatment. All of the designs can provide powerful information to our knowledge base about communication and related disorders, the role of treatment, and service delivery. And all begin with a question; thus, the research question will drive the design choice, and, in turn, the design will shape the methodology.

## Independent Variables

The independent variables of a study refer to the conditions that are manipulated to produce change, or more generally, differences among conditions that are likely to influence subject performance. As such, independent variables include subject/participant characteristics and the treatment attributes. Treatment research demands that researchers know and clearly delineate which variables they wish to manipulate and which they wish to control. This applies to both subject characteristics and treatment attributes. Because efficacy research is conducted under controlled conditions, the subject characteristics and treatment attributes will be systematically proscribed. In effectiveness research, the independent variables are defined by clinical practice in the setting(s) being examined. Our discussion of independent variable starts from the perspective of efficacy research.

Subject characteristics need to accurately and completely describe the participants in all respects that might be critical to the outcome of a study. The researcher must specify which characteristics subjects must share to be included in the study, the *inclusionary criteria,* and which characteristics are not desirous, the *exclusionary criteria.* Typically, certain characteristics are critical and will need to be controlled across subjects, whereas others are less important and can vary. In efficacy research the subject characteristics are very often systematically manipulated to determine how subject characteristics might interact with a treatment. For example, subjects' language level, age, educational background, or site of lesion may be manipulated while the treatment is held constant to determine how efficacy might change with different subject characteristics. Differences in performance across individuals with varying characteristics provide insights into how the treatment might be working.

The independent variable is most often defined by the treatment itself and the manipulation of it. Treatments can be manipulated in many ways, including in their strength and integrity (Yeaton & Sechrest, 1981). *Strength* refers to the intensity of a treatment (length of session, number of exposures to teaching items, etc.). *Integrity* refers to identifying and manipulating the various components of the treatment, including the steps/phases, the instructions (prompts, cues, consequences, reinforcements), and the person implementing the treatment, the setting, the activities, and the materials. In efficacy research these aspects of treatment implementation are specified (controlled) and systematically implemented or varied. Because the focus of efficacy research is on manipulating subjects or the treatment protocol to explore concomitant changes in performance, subject assessments and treatment implementation must be conducted reliably. This form of reliability is known as *procedural reliability* or *fidelity.* It demonstrates that the procedures for including subjects and implementing treatment can be trusted and replicated (Billingsley, White, & Munson, 1980; Kearns, 1990; LeLaurin & Wolery, 1992; also see Chapter 14 by Kearns and de Riesthal).

Effectiveness research manages independent variables somewhat differently. In effectiveness research, these are exactly the variables that define clinical practice. Whereas efficacy research will control and manipulate these variables, effectiveness research will describe the variables as they occur in the day-to-day practice. Recall that effectiveness questions primarily ask whether the outcomes documented in efficacy research are *translatable* and will hold up within the natural settings of clinical practice. Clinical practice serves heterogeneous subjects, and treatment implementation must respond to less controlled conditions. Variations in clientele, particularly with regard to socioeconomic status and cultural background, often become important aspects of investigation for effectiveness research. Service delivery models also may vary due to setting constraints, thus effectiveness research is required to determine how different models might alter the outcomes of treatment protocols found to be efficacious in controlled settings. Consider, for example, the independent variables of dosage as it includes session length and frequency of treatment delivery. Treatment efficacy research may substantiate the benefits of a given treatment protocol when it is provided three times a week, 50 minutes per session in a controlled clinical laboratory; however, when the same treatment is implemented two times a week, 20 minutes per session in a community center, the results might not be shown to be as effective. Recently, Schmitt and Justice (2011) have discussed the importance of examining three particular independent variables in school settings that might impact on intervention benefits: *classroom quality, teacher self-efficacy*, and *school climate*. The constraints of real-life practice will likely alter the fidelity of treatment procedures that have been deemed successful in the laboratory. Investigating the influence of these variations is an important aspect of effectiveness research.

## Dependent Variables

The *dependent variables* of a study refer to what to measure and how to measure. In treatment research, the dependent variables are the measurable performance areas that are predicted to change (are dependent upon) the intervention. These measurement decisions are driven by the research questions. Dependent measures are selected because they reflect the construct of interest for the research, and they are sensitive to the type and magnitude of change that is expected with treatment. Because communication is complex, the researcher should always consider "multiple measures." The measures are most often *behavioral*; these include overt, observable behaviors, which can be collected in controlled, structured elicitation tasks or through more naturalistic observation. Measures may also be of nonobservable phenomenon, such as attitudes, beliefs, or opinions, which can be assessed by _self-reports, inventories, questionnaires_, or _scales_. Finally, measures may be _psycho-physiological_. These are measures that allow for the examination of biological events as they reflect psychological and physiological states, and that are measured through appropriate instrumentation (e.g., cardiovascular measures through heart rate, breath flow measures through spirometry, or neurological measures through MRI/fMRI or biofeedback measures in fluency). The challenge in identifying measures is determining data that will reflect change that is associated with the therapeutic manipulation.

At first glance, measuring "change" in behavior seems like a relatively simple concept. We want to know if treatment alters communication in some way. The simplicity vanishes quickly when entering the clinical world. Change can take many forms: it occurs at different times during the therapeutic process and at different levels of communication. Therefore, examining change must be _multidimensional_. Both quantitative and qualitative data are important to collect to yield full views of change (see Bogdan & Biklen, 1992; Hegde, 2003). Treatment, probe, and control data (Olswang & Bain, 1994) are used to measure different types of behaviors, including specific behaviors that are targeted in treatment (target behaviors) versus behaviors that might change as a result of treatment (generalization behaviors), or behaviors that are not expected to change as a result of treatment (control behaviors). These behaviors and the corresponding measures allow for different views of change and are critical in determining whether treatment is efficacious. In this chapter, two dimensions will be suggested for viewing and measuring change: levels of change and temporal aspects of change. These two dimensions will serve to show the breadth of dependent variables that might be considered in both efficacy and effectiveness research.

Levels of change are appropriately examined using the framework provided by the World Health Organization's International Classification of Functioning, Disability, and Health (ICF) (WHO, 2011). Accordingly, the three levels correspond to structures/functions, activities/participation, and environmental factors associated with disease and/or related health issues, including communication disorders. Measures of structures/functions will describe psychological, physiological, anatomical behaviors, including linguistic forms, phonological features, airflow, and so on. These are typically overt behaviors that describe the symptoms or topology of communication impairment, and the processes of language comprehension and production. Activities correspond to behaviors of communication used functionally in everyday situations. These include behaviors that reflect how individuals are participating in their life's events. Measures addressing environmental factors include the family's support, societal attitudes, physical and technologic factors, setting-specific factors (e.g., living situation), and educational and health policies. In addition, the ICF considers personal factors, which include the client's attitude, temperament, and emotional status as facilitators or barriers to communication, and other personal factors that impact quality of life and well-being (see Chapter 3 by Threats, this text).

Efficacy research has its origins in examining the relationship between treatment and the nature of disorders (Rosenbek, 1995). As our understanding of communication disorders has increased, we have altered our treatments to better address the nature of the disorders by targeting change in not only structures and functions, but also increasingly in activities and environmental factors (Rogers, Alarcon, & Olswang, 1999). Very often, the primary measure for efficacy research is structures/functions, with secondary or generalization measures of activities and environmental factors. Such studies help to clarify the effects of treatment and to further enlighten our understanding about the nature of disorders. Effectiveness research most commonly turns the perspective around, measuring activities and environmental factors as primary outcomes; this reflects the emphasis of therapeutic change in a "real-world" context. Both quantitative and qualitative data serve these measures quite well, acknowledging that quality-of-life and well-being variables are often best measured by rating scales and questionnaires (quantitative) or interviews (qualitative). For example, Angell, Bailey, and Stoner (2008) conducted semistructured interviews of family members of children with dysphagia to identify factors that facilitate or inhibit effective school-based management of dysphagia. Mullen and Schooling (2010) reported the results of the _Parent Satisfaction Form and the Teacher Survey_, both rating scales, in their study of outcomes using the NOMS for pediatric speech-language pathology.

Change can also be examined along a time dimension. Temporal aspects of change refer to how and when the treatment shows its effect. A framework that has proven useful in examining temporal aspects of change is borrowed from Rosen and Proctor (1978, 1981); it differentiates intermediate, instrumental, and ultimate change. _Intermediate change_ is the change that occurs session to session, as an immediate consequence of the treatment process—that is, the acquisition of skills, knowledge, and beliefs that move the client forward in the therapeutic process. An aspect of efficacy is documenting intermediate change as necessary evidence for continued intervention with the prescribed treatment strategies and techniques. Treatment data, typically quantitative, are used to explore outcomes concerning intermediate change. _Instrumental change_ is the change that occurs with treatment, which leads to other change without further treatment. That is, once attained, these changes serve as the instruments for the attainment of other change. Instrumental change, if linked to the desired target of treatment, can become a criterion for treatment success. These changes have often been thought of as the triggers for automaticity and generalization of the desired target. Using quantitative probe data of untrained words, Olswang and Bain (1985) demonstrated that preschoolers' success in the production of phonemes at the single-word level using untrained pictures could be used as the criterion for withdrawing treatment, with the target objective being productions in conversation. Finally, _ultimate change_ is the final product, the long-term goal and final objective of treatment. Ultimate change describes the behavior that is desired to result from the therapeutic process. It either reflects normalized performance or socially appropriate performance. Measures of social validity typically are used to measure ultimate change; they employ probe quantitative or qualitative data to measure activities and environmental factors related to performance. They reference change in a subject compared with relevant peers (social comparison) (Beilinson & Olswang, 2003) or as measured by subjective evaluation by the subject him- or herself or by significant others. For example, Pollard, Ellis, Finan, and Ramig (2009) obtained qualitative data from participants through weekly written logs and exit questionnaires to assess some of the effects of a _SpeechEasy_ device in therapy for stuttering. The researcher may be interested in one type of change more than another, or perhaps the relationship between the different temporal aspects of change. The research questions will guide the selection of the dependent measures.

Consider the following example as a reflection of multiple measures that would be valuable in an efficacy study. If a researcher were investigating a treatment for dysarthria of speech, where the focus was on breathing and spacing that would ultimately transfer to conversational speech, the following measures might be selected: (1) measures of coordination of breathing with speech during treatment using "Respitrace," respiratory inductive plethysmography, yielding size changes to the rib cage and abdomen (estimating respiratory shape and lung volume levels with speech and providing quantitative treatment data to reveal immediate change); (2) measures of intelligibility (percent intelligible) of items on a single-word list, structured sentences, or reading of the Rainbow Passage (quantitative probe data to reveal instrumental and/or ultimate change); and (3) ratings of intelligibility and naturalness of conversational speech, and client satisfaction revealed by an interview (quantitative and qualitative probe data to reveal ultimate change). A control behavior for the dysarthric client might be vital capacity, because this is related to the problem but is not a part of the treatment. Multiple target measures allow for an investigation of treatment effects, and provide important information regarding the breadth of change that has resulted from the treatment (Spencer, 2011).

With all of this discussion about types of data and measures, a key element is the researcher's (and consumer's) confidence in the _truthfulness_ and _trustworthiness_ of the data. Truthfulness refers to the _validity_ of the data, or how accurately the data measure the construct or phenomenon of interest. To ensure valid data, the researcher must observe behaviors that will representatively reflect change. Using multiple measures, considering temporal aspects and levels of change, data will appropriately address questions regarding the benefits of treatment. The researcher must maintain a broad perspective in attempting to document change due to treatment and not to other external or internal forces. Both qualitative and quantitative data must be valid. To ensure validity, we must have adequate amounts of data, an adequate variety of data, and adequate confirming and disconfirming evidence to demonstrate plausibility. The bottom line is that the data must reflect what we know and believe to be true about the communication development and disorders.

*Reliability* refers to the trustworthiness of our data. This means that the data must be "repeatable" across examiners and settings, and amenable to collection over time without concern for variability in performance other than what is "true" for the client, rather than being in the "mind of the beholder." The researcher must be able to trust the data to be credible over time, truly fluctuating as a result of the subject's changing abilities. For quantitative data, reliability is ensured in part by having independent observers sample the collection of the same data. For qualitative data, credibility is ensured by having different sources of data yield the same conclusions (Lincoln & Guba, 1985). The bottom line for reliability and credibility is that the data do not purely reflect what is in the researcher's mind, but rather that others can have trust in the data as they have been collected.

## Data Analysis and Interpretation

Persuasive evidence for documenting the efficacy of treatment will come in many forms, depending on the research question, the research design, and data. The evidence may be statistical or clinical, but in either case the goal is to document significant change—change that is neither random nor unimportant (Bain & Dollaghan, 1991; Kazdin, 1980; Schiavetti et al, 2011). Recently, Bothe and Richardson (2011) offered a framework for examining treatment outcomes using four different constructs of significance: statistical, practical, clinical, and personal. Their tutorial defines each form of significance and explores how each contributes to our understanding of the magnitude and meaning of our clinical efforts to change and help our clients. For this discussion, we will focus generally on statistical and clinical evidence of change, but the reader is encouraged to read Bothe and Richardson (2011) for a more complete discussion of the constructs supporting the different forms of significance. Statistical procedures examine *significance of change* ($p$ values) and *degree of change* (effect size). Significance addresses to some degree whether change is due to "chance." Typically a confidence level ($p <.05$ or $p <.01$) is preselected by the researcher as the criterion for determining statistical significance. Changes in performance are examined with a statistical test that yields a probability *(p)* value. Statistical significance is judged by whether the probability level is equal to or below the level of confidence selected. To find that a relationship in an experiment (i.e., a relationship between the introduction of treatment and behavior change) is statistically significant does not necessarily mean a genuine *cause-and-effect* relationship exists between the two. The statistical analysis only indicates the probability that the result was or was not due to chance, but chance is never completely eliminated. Other causes, such as sampling error, could have yielded the results; however, convention and logic argue that when a probability level is as low as .05 or .01, one can safely assume that the relationship between the independent and dependent variables of interest has been demonstrated.

*Effect size* is another valuable statistical tool in treatment research. Effect sizes include a variety of quantitative indices that examine the strength of relationships between variables, including measures of *standardized mean difference, standardized regression coefficient,* and the *odds ratio* (Hedges, 2008). They have value in efficacy studies by comparing performance under one set of conditions to performance under another, including within-subject/time-series data, for example, when comparing performance across baseline, treatment, and withdrawal phases. One of the advantages of using effect size is that results of a particular research can be summarized in a way that is not only clinically understandable and useful but also in a form that can be compared across studies. As described earlier, research questions will determine outcome measures, and as such, variability will exist across studies regarding the presentation of results. Effect size using similar quantitative indices serve to allow for comparison of therapeutic change. According to Hedges (2008), "Effect sizes are intended to communicate a research study's findings about strength of relations between variables in a manner that captures the essential features of results but that can be broadly understood and compared with findings from other studies" (p. 167). Utilizing effect size analyses is particularly valuable for effectiveness research, as the relative importance of change can be captured in terms of strength of relationships.

Statistical analyses require careful selection of procedures. This is not a simple task. Although the goal and underlying assumption of statistical forms of evaluation is to conduct a relatively bias-free and consistent method of data analysis and interpretation, bias can slip into the picture. Selection of tests, criteria for significance, and, even more basic, a flaw in the design (e.g., sample size, heterogeneity of subjects, variations in procedures) may yield suspect or invalid results. The use of statistics to analyze data are not the end-all in efficacy and effectiveness research, particularly if interest lies in determining how subjects change and whether change is important in real life.

Clinical forms of data analysis also attempt to document that change is significant and not due to chance or other threats to validity. In the current discussion, we are viewing this form of data analysis as nonstatistical but not necessarily nonnumerical. A valuable nonstatistical yet numerical procedure for evaluating quantitative data is visual inspection. Visual inspection is commonly used in within-subject/time-series designs (single-subject research designs), where repeated, continuous data are available for individual subjects. The examiner views the data for each subject separately and then in comparison to other subjects or behaviors to determine trends in the rate and degree/magnitude of change with the introduction and withdrawal of different types of manipulations. The researcher looks for trends during the initial phase in which no treatment is provided (baseline probes), changes in the trends when treatment is introduced, how the trends change as the treatment unfolds or other manipulations are introduced, and changes and trends in the data when treatment is withdrawn. In addition, control measures (measures of behaviors that are not related to the treatment target but related to the problem, and that are not expected to change) can be a part of the design and an important part of data analysis and visual inspection. The assumption is that if target behaviors change and control behaviors do not, then the change is more likely to be attributable to the treatment than to some other cause (e.g., maturation, spontaneous recovery). The validity of visual inspection is increased by having naïve observers view the data and report trends.

Replication of trends within subjects (across behaviors and conditions) and across subjects lends further credence to the validity of the findings. The availability of repeated, continuous data makes examination of data through visual inspection less arbitrary than one might expect. The unfolding nature of treatment benefits can be observed and analyzed with these data, where pre- and posttest data make such an analysis difficult, if not impossible. As with statistical procedures, nonstatistical visual inspection requires criteria for suggesting significance. Changes in performance need to be robust and immediately apparent, making statistical procedures often seem redundant. Well-constructed designs and clear trends in the data increase the validity of interpretation. On top of this, replication across subjects powerfully increases the generalization of results. This latter point can best be appreciated by clinical researchers (and practitioners) who know only too well about individual variation among even the most homogeneous subjects. When robust, clear trends in change are replicated over and over across subjects, and observed by independent inspectors, the validity of the phenomenon is enhanced and the ability to generalize the findings increases. Visual inspection speaks directly to quantitative data.

Other nonstatistical means of analyzing qualitative data also exist. For a complete discussion of this topic, the reader is referred to Lincoln and Guba (1985), Bogdan and Biklen, (2007), Glesne and Peshkin (1992), and Bothe and Richardson (2011) as beginning references. Data analysis of qualitative data is the process of systematically searching and arranging the data that have been collected to better understand the phenomenon of interest. This entails working closely with the data, "organizing them, breaking them into manageable units, synthesizing them, searching for patterns, discovering what is important and what is to be learned" (Bogdan & Biklen, 1992, p. 153). Patterns and trends in the data lead to conclusions. Conclusions become more credible and plausible in several ways. First, the researcher must have adequate amounts of data. Prolonged engagement in a setting, yielding numerous examples of patterns and trends, contribute importantly to the strength of the interpretation. Second, the researcher must have adequate variety of evidence; this is known as "triangulation." Credibility increases when data come from different sources, methods, and investigators. _Different sources_ can mean multiple versions of one type of source (e.g., interview respondents—parent, siblings, teacher), or different sources of the same information (e.g., verifying an interview with field notes). _Different methods_ means different data collection modes or types of data (e.g., interview, questionnaire, observation, behavioral measurement). *Different investigators* means using data from another study or working on a team with different questions but overlapping data. Third, the researcher must recognize and utilize concordance and discrepancy in the data. Disconfirming or negative evidence often sheds light on a particular trend or helps reach a particular conclusion. The researcher needs to look for such evidence, and if found, it needs to be analyzed in light of the patterns. Fourth, credibility and plausibility are enhanced with dramatic data that are so noteworthy as to be difficult to ignore. However, a caution must be made: "whiz bang" effects must never stand alone. Recall that several years ago the success of *facilitated communication* as a treatment for children with autism was documented by reports of startling effects. Observations of extraordinary communication breakthroughs in communication via computers were used as proof of treatment efficacy. These claims, unfortunately, were bold and misleading. Extraordinary, "whiz bang" effects must always be viewed in light of other confirming and disconfirming evidence, and must be accompanied by triangulation. Qualitative data have a place in efficacy research. These types of data afford researchers a unique look at how treatment alters subjects' behaviors in context. As with quantitative data, analysis must proceed in line with the assumptions of the data. No doubt, someday clinical researchers will become better equipped to utilize quantitative and qualitative data as complementary sources of valid information.

Clinically, significant change also addresses whether or not changes in performance are important, and whether or not the results are real to the subject (or relevant others). Many years ago Wolf (1978) introduced the notion of social validity or social acceptability of treatment. Bothe and Richardson (2011) have referred to this perspective as "personal significance." "The acceptability of treatment includes several areas, such as whether the focus of treatment, the procedures used, and the results of treatment are acceptable to the client or those in contact with the client. Essentially, social validation of clinical importance of behavior change can be determined in two ways, which have been referred to as the social comparison and subjective evaluation methods" (Kazdin, 1980, pp. 365–366). *Social comparison* compares behavior of the subject before and after treatment with the behavior of "nondeviant peers." The question asks whether the subject's behavior following treatment is distinguishable from that of relevant peers. The emphasis here must be on relevant peers. For example, subjects with developmental disabilities would be compared with others with this diagnosis, but for whom the "treatment target" is *not* of concern. *Subjective evaluation* examines the importance of behavior change by assessing the opinions of the client and individuals who are likely to have contact with the client about the benefits of treatment. This type of evaluation has been termed *consumer satisfaction* (Baer, 1988; Schwartz & Baer, 1991). Subjective evaluations most appropriately examine whether changes are important in terms of communication function and quality of life. Social validity has become increasingly important in clinical research, and, appropriately, the science and technology for examining social validity has improved (Schwartz & Baer, 1991). Clinical significance is no longer the pale sidekick of statistical analysis. Its place in research, and the advancement of science, has been proven and adopted. Whereas efficacy research will often address social validity, effectiveness research, arguably, has at its core the examination of socially valid responses to the therapeutic process.

## ♦ Impact of Treatment Research on the Profession

In the first edition of this book (Frattali, 1998), this chapter ended with a call for efficacy research to address not only practice issues but also theoretical issues (Olswang, 1998). We continue that call now, emphasizing that the process of conducting treatment research, and the results obtained, can and will contribute to the discipline of CSD in critical ways. By examining how manipulations of the environment (i.e., treatment) alter communication behaviors in individuals with disorders, we have much to gain in our understanding of communication itself and of the nature of disorders. The beauty of treatment research truly is that it naturally addresses both clinical and theoretical questions simultaneously (see Olswang, 1993). Gains in theory ultimately advance our efforts to demonstrate accountable clinical practice; similarly, our gains in practice ultimately advance our knowledge in theory.

As early as 1989, ASHF sponsored a landmark conference on treatment efficacy in communication disorders (Olswang, Thompson, Warren, & Minghetti, 1990). This set the stage for the subsequent attention to and enthusiasm for investigating the efficacy of our treatments. Since that time, EBP driven by treatment research has become a common phrase across our discipline. The momentum has continued to grow over the last two decades, culminating in the arrival of the 21st century and a priority to adopt EBP as the norm. To illustrate, in 2003 ASHA sponsored the 13th Annual Research Symposium on Outcomes Research and Evidence-Based Practice, co-sponsored by a grant from the National Institute on Deafness and Other Communication Disorders (NIDCD). This symposium was designed to update researchers on advances in outcomes research, including exposure to designs, scales for examining levels of evidence, and principles of EBP related to health care. In 2004, the Research and Scientific Affairs Committee of ASHA (2004) produced a technical report entitled "Evidence-Based Practice in Communication Disorders," which had four purposes:

> (a) to provide an overview of some of the principles and procedures of EBP; (b) to describe the relevance of EBP to current clinical issues in speech-language pathology and audiology; (c) to raise awareness of the importance of EBP research as one component of the research mission of the American Speech-Language-Hearing Association; and (d) to recommend potential steps toward increasing the quantity of credible evidence to support clinical activities in the professions (American Speech-Language-Hearing Association, 2004, p. 1).

This report highlighted the value of clinical research alongside basic science research, stating that EBP research is a key component of the research mission of ASHA. Finally, this report outlined steps to increase the quantity of credible evidence to support the practice of professionals, which included, among other recommendations, making evidence more readily available to practitioners, encouraging universities to include information on EBP in their curricula, and promoting the publication of well-crafted and implemented clinical research in the ASHA journals.

In 2005, ASHA created a Joint Coordinating Committee on Evidence-Based Practice, which produced a position statement stating "audiologists and speech-language pathologists incorporate the principles of evidence-based practice in clinical decision making to provide high quality clinical care" (ASHA, 2005). Practitioners are called upon to continually evaluate evidence and appropriately apply their knowledge to the needs, abilities, and preferences of their clients. Currently, ASHA's Web site offers a large section dedicated to EBP, which includes terminology and definitions, links to valuable resources such as systematic reviews addressing treatment for a growing number of disorders, and five EBP Web-based tutorials: basic principles, question framing, evidence searches, evidence evaluation, and decision making using evidence (ASHA, 2011a). The Academy of Neurologic Communication Disorders and Sciences (ANCDS) initiated its commitment to conduct systematic reviews and publish EBP guidelines in 1998 (Golper et al, 2001a,b), and has also been providing high-quality and easily accessible practice guidelines based on systematic reviews since 2001 (see Chapter 13 by Yorkston and Baylor). This compilation of information is valuable to both researchers and practitioners, and clearly reflects a commitment by our professional societies to EBP.

## Treatment Research Within the Profession: What Is the Evidence?

Certainly, in the last decade, clinical evidence concerning efficacious treatments for communication disorders has increased. To take the pulse on how our discipline has moved forward in its commitment to expanding treatment research, a journal review was conducted to examine the extent of treatment studies that were published during a 5-year period in the three primary ASHA journals of interest to speech-language pathology: *Journal of Speech, Language, and Hearing Research (JSLHR)*; *Language, Speech and Hearing Services in the Schools (LSHSS)*; and the *American Journal of Speech-Language Pathology (AJSLP)*. The following data were collected for each journal and each issue from

2006 to 2010: (1) total number of articles per issue, (2) number of treatment articles per issue, and (3) type of each treatment article. Treatment articles were defined as *data-based* research that investigated treatment of individuals with speech or language impairments. In keeping with the focus of this chapter and the perspective that treatment research should be designed to examine and provide evidence for the benefits of intervention, we elected to include only data-based articles. On that basis, articles were categorized as either efficacy or effectiveness studies. Efficacy research had to utilize methodology that demonstrated *experimental control*, that is, employing either group or single-subject designs, or be conducted under carefully controlled conditions. We also included systematic reviews and meta-analyses in this category. Effectiveness research included data-based studies employing a variety of methodologies, but that were conducted in naturalistic contexts under "every day/average" conditions, and were studies addressing questions pertinent to application of treatment in clinical contexts or settings. For completeness, we included data-based case studies without experimental control but categorized them separately. The specific review procedures, including the inter-rater reliability can be found in the appendix, below.

*Findings*

The review found that a total of 763 articles were published in the three journals over the 5-year period. Seventy-four (10%) were classified as treatment studies. Of the total number of treatment studies published, 73% were judged to be efficacy studies, 19% effectiveness studies, and 8% case studies. The data show that treatment research represented only a small proportion of published studies in our discipline (10%), with efficacy studies being the majority. Thus, not surprisingly, effectiveness studies were quite limited in our journals. Further, the research categorized as effectiveness focused primarily on questions examining implementation of treatments in natural environments. Three of the effectiveness studies were extensions of efficacy research, and only one addressed issues related to cost-effectiveness of standard care. This review of the literature indicates a need for increased treatment studies of all types. Certainly, the percentage of treatment articles published (10%) does not likely reflect the proportion of time that clinicians spend providing treatment. In short, the data from this literature review indicate that the discipline continues to provide relatively little evidence to influence clinicians' treatment decisions and activities. Further, the absence of research exploring treatment implementation in clinical settings (i.e., effectiveness research) is even more apparent and of concern—a topic we will return to in the concluding section of this chapter.

Convention programs also reflect the increased awareness of and interest in evidence to guide practitioners' decision making. The enthusiasm for increasing awareness of EBP in university programs is apparent in ASHA's Quality Indicators for Integration of Clinical Practice and Research: Program Self-Assessment, which was created in 2005 as a way to help faculty assess their curricula in regard to EBP content (ASHA, 2011b). Whether or not practitioners are utilizing EBP principles and appropriately considering external evidence, internal evidence, and client perspective in their decision making is difficult to determine. Although recent graduates and committed professionals certainly are exposed routinely to the principles, vocabulary, and ethics of conducting research-guided, evidence-based services, it is not clear how well EBP has really penetrated clinical services across the country. The difficulty with bringing EBP into clinical service generally and suggestions to make research more accessible are discussed in Chapter 13 by Yorkston and Baylor.

## ♦ Conclusion and Future Directions

Without a doubt, the full-throttle emphasis on treatment efficacy research must continue bringing the discipline and profession closer to the standard of knowledge and practice that is expected and required for the future. Efficacy research must continue to identify treatment protocols that successfully achieve the outcomes for which they are designed. We need to better understand the nature of communication disorders and how they respond to treatment strategies that are grounded in theory. Researchers in our discipline are skilled in planning and implementing controlled experiments to document treatment efficacy. As we continue our paths of programmatic research, more and more clinical trials will emerge, as will systematic reviews, providing stronger evidence on which practitioners can base their clinical decisions. As efficacy research continues to mature and amass, effectiveness research must, correspondingly, keep pace. The need for an increased effort in effectiveness research cannot be minimized, particularly in this climate of health care and education reform and increasing diversity in clientele.

The first decade of the 21st century ushered in an expansion in service delivery expectations for practitioners. Populations in need of our services have grown, including infants through geriatrics. Further, as we become a more global society, multicultural caseloads are becoming the norm. As the diversity in our clientele expands, either through age or cultural identity, so too do the disorder types. More children are being referred for assessments in the public schools, and the incidence of some diagnoses is increasing (e.g., autism spectrum disorders, fetal alcohol spectrum disorders). Further, with advances in medicine, many of our adult patients are living longer with chronic or degenerative conditions. These expansions have also resulted in the extension of service delivery settings, with the prime example being the federal mandate to provide services to children from birth to age 3 in the least restrictive environment, which in many states has been translated to mean the families' homes. The next generation of service delivery providers is facing challenges never encountered before in the context of expanding populations creating an urgent need to address the efficacious delivery of services to individuals in need. Compounding these challenges is the current environment of limited resources and the need to conduct our practices differently.

The most significant reflection of the need to do business differently is the passage of the Patient Protection and Affordable Care Act (PPACA, or ACA), the health care reform bill, in 2010. The discussion about this congressional act has increased awareness and need for cost-effective and efficient service delivery for more people. Although treatment efficacy research is expanding in communication disorders, a disparity exists between service delivery and science. To improve services to individuals with communication disorders, scientific discoveries must be translated into practical applications. As noted by the Division of Program Coordination, Planning, and Strategic Initiatives at the National Institutes of Health, translational research is a *two-way street*. Scientists provide clinicians with new tools for patient care, and clinicians provide scientists with novel observations that lead to new investigations (National Institutes of Health, Division of Program Coordination, Planning, and Strategic Initiatives, 2011). The need to bring together efficacy and effectiveness research is paramount. Investigations of the implementation of service in natural settings are a critical aspect of EBP (i.e., effectiveness research). This current and future state of health care and education is requiring an expanded scientific approach to the delivery of services. Research must keep pace with the prevailing level of knowledge and real-world needs, enabling quality, cost-effectiveness services and access for all persons with communication disorders. As such, treatment research needs to be planned with an eye toward implementation of innovative, evidence-based strategies in practice, and as such, needs to include a variety of stakeholders in the research process.

Effectiveness research not only must examine proven treatment protocols under less controlled situations in real-world settings, but also effectiveness must include targeted research on service delivery models. This requires employing state-of-the-art methodologies for investigating systems and organizational structure as their impact on cost-effective service delivery. This focus on effectiveness research suggests following the model of EBP in medicine, where new approaches to delivery of health care are utilizing principles from a variety of disciplines. Health service research reflects this perspective, defined as "the multidisciplinary field of scientific investigation that studies how social factors, financing systems, organizational structures and processes, health technologies, and personal behaviors affect access to health care, the quality and cost of health care, and ultimately our health and well-being. Its research domains are individuals, families, organizations, institutions, communities, and populations" (AcademyHealth, 2011, p. 1). The emphasis is on examining not only what services are efficacious, but also how they are provided, by whom, and under what conditions. This includes research exploring service delivery models for individual patients/clients, groups of patients/clients, *coordination* among providers, and patient satisfaction. Research is needed to examine barriers to quality care and methods for overcoming barriers across a variety of settings, disorders, ages, and delivery models (acute versus chronic care) in communication sciences and disorders. Of course, such research is not limited to speech-language pathology services in health care settings, as was so clearly illustrated by Schmitt and Justice (2011) in their discussion of classroom variables that impact treatment fidelity and benefits. If the goal is implementing best practices in everyday practice, then primary stakeholders need to assist in planning the direction of future research. This focus is essential in creating a better quality of care and more client-centered care through cost-effective service delivery. Areas such as health care informatics, which attempts to manage patient data to allow for the most cost-effective and efficient service delivery, might become an important component of our treatment effectiveness research. Further research directly addressing efficiency of service delivery as it relates to patient/client satisfaction might become an arm of this body of effectiveness research. Such innovative directions in our treatment research effort will require an influx of new support along three major dimensions: education of researchers (awareness and training in methods), interdisciplinary research collaboration (epidemiology, health care engineering, management science, public health, health service research), and financial support in the form of grant commitments.

The future holds the promise for more treatment research. The climate is ripe for continued investigation of the efficacy of our treatment approaches, with a solid push toward more systematic investigations that result in clinical trials. So too are we ready for documenting the effectiveness of our services as they are implemented within contexts of real-world societal demands and constraints. As our body of treatment research accumulates, we must be actively considering how science and practice can blend. Implementation of scientific innovations into practice requires that practitioners and other stakeholders become part of the research conversation, including participation in the entire research process. The motivation to provide services to individuals with communication disorders with the most current evidence-based treatments exists. The challenges are huge, but so too are the stakes.

## ◆ Appendix: Journal Review of Treatment Articles

To verify and amplify some of comments in this chapter, a literature review was conducted to examine the number and type of treatment studies that were published during a 5-year period in the three primary professional journals published by the American Speech-Language Hearing Association: *Journal of Speech, Language, and Hearing Research (JSLHR); Language, Speech and Hearing Services in the Schools (LSHSS);* and the *American Journal of Speech-Language Pathology (AJSLP).* The following data were collected for each journal and each issue from 2006 to 2010: total number of articles per issue, number of treatment articles per issue, and type of each treatment article. Procedures for the review of each issue began by examining the tables of content to identify the total number of articles and treatment studies. Audiology and hearing-related or hearing science articles were excluded from the total number of articles for *JSLHR* and *LSHSS.* In addition, notes or reports from editors, letters to the editors, commentary/second opinion, and errata were also excluded from the total. Supplemental articles, clinical forums, and clinically focused articles were included in the total count if they pertained to speech-language pathology.

To identify treatment studies, the titles, the abstracts, and, when necessary, the full text of the articles were reviewed. Studies were categorized as "treatment studies" if they were data-based, examined some aspect of treatment for speech or language or dysphagia/swallowing, and described complete methodology. Treatment research could employ any of the following: systematic reviews of the literature, meta-analyses, or data-based studies that employed group designs with experimental control, single-subject designs with experimental control, or case studies without experimental control. Studies involving participants "at risk" but not identified as having disorders or for

**Table 12.1** Comparison of Total and Type of Treatment Studies, 2006–2010

|  | 2006 | 2007 | 2008 | 2009 | 2010 | Total |
|---|---|---|---|---|---|---|
| Total No. of articles | 136 | 142 | 155 | 161 | 169 | 763 |
| Total No. (%) of treatment articles | 12 (9%) | 8 (6%) | 25 (16%) | 11 (7%) | 18 (11%) | 74 (10%) |
| No. (%) of treatment efficacy articles | 8 (67%) | 7 (88%) | 18 (72%) | 7 (64%) | 14 (78%) | 54 (73%) |
| No. of articles employing group or single-subject experimental designs | 6 | 7 | 13 | 3 | 10 | 39 |
| No. of treatment systematic review and meta-analysis articles | 2 | 0 | 5 | 4 | 4 | 15 |
| No. (%) of treatment effectiveness articles | 3 (25%) | 1 (13%) | 3 (12%) | 3 (27%) | 4 (22%) | 14 (19%) |
| No. (%) of treatment case studies articles | 1 (8%) | 0 | 4 (16%) | 1 (9%) | 0 | 6 (8%) |

*Note:* The percentage of treatment articles is based on the percentage from the total number of articles published in a given year, whereas the percentage of the different types of treatment articles is based on the total number of treatment articles for a given year.

whom English was a second language were excluded. Also excluded were those studies that involved treatment not administered by speech-language pathologists, such as cochlear implants and pharmacological agents. Studies were also excluded if they only presented an historical perspective of treatment for a disorder or a summary, and not a systematic review of a treatment. Studies involving speech-language pathologists' perceptions of particular treatments were also excluded.

After treatment articles were identified, they were classified into the following categories: efficacy studies that demonstrated experimental control employing either group or single-subject designs and administered under "ideal" conditions, effectiveness studies that were conducted in natural settings and represented typical clinical conditions, systematic reviews, meta-analysis studies, and case studies that included pretreatment information and a careful description of the treatment but did not control extraneous variables for experimental control (McReynolds & Kearns, 1983). Reference information was recorded for all treatment articles.

Point-by-point reliability for identifying the total number of articles and the number and types of treatment articles was obtained for 28% of the issues analyzed during the time period of 2006 to 2010. A second reviewer randomly selected four issues from each year, one each from *LSHSS, AJSLP,* and *JSLHR,* plus one extra also selected randomly. This resulted in a total of 20 issues reviewed for purposes of reliability assessment. Of a total of 205 articles, only one reviewer disagreement occurred. **Table 12.1** and **Table 12.2** present the results of this review.

**Table 12.2** Comparison of Treatment Studies by Journals

|  | JSLHR | LSHSS | AJSLP | Total |
|---|---|---|---|---|
| No. of articles in 5-year period | 431 | 183 | 149 | 763 |
| No. (%) of treatment articles in 5-year period | 30 (7%) | 16 (9%) | 28 (19%) | 74 (10%) |

# References

AcademyHealth. (2011, June 9). *What is HSR section, paragraph 1?* http://www.academyhealth.org/About/content.cfm?ItemNumber=831&navItemNumber=514

American Speech-Language-Hearing Association (ASHA). (2004). *Evidence-based practice in communication disorders: An introduction* [technical report]. www.asha.org/policy

American Speech-Language-Hearing Association (ASHA). (2005). *Evidence-based practice in communication disorders* [position statement]. www.asha.org/policy

American Speech-Language-Hearing Association (ASHA). (2011a, June). *Evidence-based practice.* http://www.asha.org/members/ebp/

American Speech-Language-Hearing Association (ASHA). (June 2011b). Quality indicators for integrating research and clinical practice into communication sciences and disorders (CSD) programs: Program self-assessment. http://www.asha.org/uploadedFiles/academic/teach-tools/QualityIndicators.pdf

American Speech-Language-Hearing Association (ASHA). (2011c, Jan). *Standards for accreditation of graduate education programs in audiology and speech-language pathology.* www.asha.org/Academic/accreditation/accredmanual/section3.htm

Angell, M. E., Bailey, R. L., & Stoner, J. B. (2008, Apr). Family perceptions of facilitators and inhibitors of effective school-based dysphagia management. *Language, Speech, and Hearing Services in Schools, 39,* 214–226

Baer, D. (1988). If you know why you're changing a behavior, you'll know when you've changed it enough. *Behavioral Assessment, 10,* 219–223

Bain, B., & Dollaghan, C. (1991). Treatment efficacy: the notion of clinically significant change. *Language, Speech, and Hearing Services in Schools, 22,* 264–270

Ballard, K. J., Robin, D. A., McCabe, P., & McDonald, J. (2010, Oct). A treatment for dysprosody in childhood apraxia of speech. *Journal of Speech, Language, and Hearing Research: JSLHR, 53,* 1227–1245

Beilinson, J., & Olswang, L. (2003). Facilitating peer group entry in kindergarteners with deficits in social communication. *Language, Speech, and Hearing Services in Schools, 34,* 154–166

Billingsley, F., White, O., & Munson, R. (1980). Procedural reliability: a rationale and an example. *Behavioral Assessment, 2,* 229–241

Binger, C., Kent-Walsh, J., Ewing, C., & Taylor, S. (2010, May). Teaching educational assistants to facilitate the multisymbol message productions of young students who require augmentative and alternative communication. *American Journal of Speech-Language Pathology, 19,* 108–120

Bogdan, R., & Biklen, S. (1992). *Qualitative research for education: An introduction to theory and methods.* Boston: Allyn & Bacon

Bogdan, R., & Biklen, S. (2007). *Qualitative research for education: An introduction to theories and methods* (5th ed.). Boston: Allyn & Bacon

Bothe, A. K., & Richardson, J. D. (2011, Aug). Statistical, practical, clinical, and personal significance: definitions and applications in speech-language pathology. *American Journal of Speech-Language Pathology, 20,* 233–242

Cream, A., O'Brian, S., Jones, M., Block, S., Harrison, E., Lincoln, M., et al. (2010, Aug). Randomized controlled trial of video self-modeling following speech restructuring treatment for stuttering. *Journal of Speech, Language, and Hearing Research: JSLHR, 53,* 887–897

Damico, J. S., & Simmons-Mackie, N. N. (2003, May). Qualitative research and speech-language pathology: a tutorial for the clinical realm. *American Journal of Speech-Language Pathology, 12,* 131–143

Dijkers, M. (2009). *When the best is the enemy of the good: The nature of research evidence used in systematic reviews and guidelines.* Austin, TX: SEDL: National Center for the Dissemination of Disability Research

Dollaghan, C. (2007). *The handbook for evidence-based practice in communication disorders.* Baltimore, MD: Paul H. Brookes Publishing

Fey, M. E., Warren, S. F., Brady, N., Finestack, L. H., Bredin-Oja, S. L., Fairchild, M., et al. (2006, Jun). Early effects of responsivity education/prelinguistic milieu teaching for children with developmental delays and their parents. *Journal of Speech, Language, and Hearing Research: JSLHR, 49,* 526–547

Fixsen, D. L., Naoom, S. F., Blase, K. A., Friedman, R. M., & Wallace, F. (2005). *Implementation research: A synthesis of the literature* (FMHI Publication No. 231). Tampa, FL: University of South Florida, Louis de la Parte Florida Mental Health Institute, The National Implementation Research Network

Frattali, C. (1998). *Outcomes measurement in speech-language pathology.* New York: Thieme Medical Publishers

Gierut, J. A., Morrisette, M. L., & Ziemer, S. M. (2010, May). Nonwords and generalization in children with phonological disorders. *American Journal of Speech-Language Pathology, 19,* 167–177

Ginsburg, L. R., Lewis, S., Zackheim, L., & Casebeer, A. (2007). Revisiting interaction in knowledge translation. *Implementation Science: IS, 2,* 34. 10.1186/1748-5908-2-34

Glesne, C., & Peshkin, A. (1992). *Becoming qualitative researchers: An introduction.* White Plains, NY: Longman

Golper, L., Katz, R., Myers, P., Wertz, R. T., Yorkston, K., Beeson, P., et al. (2001b). Practice guidelines: Project report. Proceedings of the Academy of Neurologic Communication Disorders and Sciences. *Journal of Medical Speech-Language Pathology, 9,* ix–x

Golper, L., Wertz, R. T., Frattali, C. M., Yorkston, K., Myers, P., Katz, R., et al. (2001a). *Evidence-based practice guidelines for the management of neurogenic communication disorders: An introduction.* http://www.ancds.org

Hedges, L. (2008). What are effect sizes and why do we need them? *Child Development Perspectives, 2,* 167–171

Hegde, M. (2003). *Clinical research in communicative disorders: Principles and strategies.* Austin, TX: Pro-Ed

Hulley, S., Cummings, S., Browner, W., Grady, D., & Newman, T. (2007). *Designing clinical research* (3rd ed.). Philadelphia, PA: Lippincott Williams & Wilkins

Implementation Science. (2011, June 14). *About implementation science.* http://www.implementationscience.com/about

Ingersoll, B., & Lalonde, K. (2010, Aug). The impact of object and gesture imitation training on language use in children with autism spectrum disorder. *Journal of Speech, Language, and Hearing Research: JSLHR, 53,* 1040–1051

Institute of Education Sciences (IES). (2011). *Special education research grants, request for applications.* CFDA number 84.324A

Katz, L., Maag, A., Fallon, K., Blenkarn, K., & Smith, K. (2010). What makes a case-load (un)manageable: School-based speech-pathologists speak. *Language, Speech, and Hearing Services in Schools, 31,* 139–152

Kazdin, A. (1980). *Research design in clinical psychology.* New York: Harper & Row

Kearns, K. (1990). Reliability of procedures and measures. In L. Olswang, C. Thompson, S. Warren, & N. Minghetti (Eds.), *Treatment efficacy research in communication disorders* (pp. 79–90). Rockville, MD: American Speech-Language-Hearing Foundation

Kent-Walsh, J., Binger, C., & Hasham, Z. (2010, May). Effects of parent instruction on the symbolic communication of children using augmentative and alternative communication during storybook reading. *American Journal of Speech-Language Pathology, 19,* 97–107

LeLaurin, K., & Wolery, M. (1992). Research standards in early intervention: defining, describing, and measuring the independent variable. *Journal of Early Intervention, 16,* 275–287

Lincoln, Y., & Guba, E. (1985). *Naturalistic inquiry.* Beverly Hills, CA: Sage Publications

McReynolds, L., & Kearns, K. (1983). *Single-subject experimental designs in communication disorders.* Baltimore, MD: University Park Press

Miller, B., & Guitar, B. (2009, Feb). Long-term outcome of the Lidcombe Program for early stuttering intervention. *American Journal of Speech-Language Pathology, 18,* 42–49

Moher, D., Liberati, A., Tetzlaff, J., & Altman, D. G.; PRISMA Group (2009, Oct). Preferred reporting items for systematic reviews and meta-analyses: the PRISMA statement. *Journal of Clinical Epidemiology, 62,* 1006–1012

Mullen, R., & Schooling, T. (2010, Jan). The National Outcomes Measurement System for pediatric speech-language pathology. *Language, Speech, and Hearing Services in Schools, 41,* 44–60

National Institutes of Health, Division of Program Coordination, Planning, and Strategic Initiatives. (2011, Feb). *Translational research.* http://commonfund.nih.gov/clinical research/overview-translational.aspx

Olswang, L. (1993). Treatment efficacy research: A paradigm for investigating clinical practice and theory. *Journal of Fluency Disorders, 18,* 125–131

Olswang, L. (1998). Treatment efficacy research. In C. Frattali (Ed.), *Outcomes measurement in speech-language pathology* (pp. 134–150). New York: Thieme Medical Publishers

Olswang, L., & Bain, B. (1985). Monitoring phoneme acquisition for making treatment withdrawal decisions. *Applied Psycholinguistics, 6,* 17–37

Olswang, L., & Bain, B. (1994). Data collection: Monitoring children's treatment progress. *American Journal of Speech-Language Pathology, 3,* 55–66

Olswang, L., Thompson, C., Warren, S., & Minghetti, N. (1990). *Treatment efficacy research in communication disorders.* Rockville, MD: American Speech-Language-Hearing Foundation

Petersen, D. B., Gillam, S. L., Spencer, T., & Gillam, R. B. (2010, Aug). The effects of literate narrative intervention on children with neurologically based language impairments: an early stage study. *Journal of Speech, Language, and Hearing Research: JSLHR, 53,* 961–981

Pollard, R., Ellis, J. B., Finan, D., & Ramig, P. R. (2009, Apr). Effects of the SpeechEasy on objective and perceived aspects of stuttering: a 6-month, phase I clinical trial in naturalistic environments. *Journal of Speech, Language, and Hearing Research: JSLHR, 52,* 516–533

Robey, R. R. (2004, Sep-Oct). A five-phase model for clinical-outcome research. *Journal of Communication Disorders, 37,* 401–411

Rogers, M. A., Alarcon, N. B., & Olswang, L. B. (1999, Nov). Aphasia management considered in the context of the World Health Organization model of disablements. *Physical Medicine and Rehabilitation Clinics of North America, 10,* 907–923, ix

Rosen, A., & Proctor, E. (1978). Specifying the treatment process: the basis for effectiveness research. *Journal of Social Service Research, 2,* 25–43

Rosen, A., & Proctor, E. K. (1981, Jun). Distinctions between treatment outcomes and their implications for treatment evaluation. *Journal of Consulting and Clinical Psychology, 49,* 418–425

Rosenbek, J. C. (1995, Fall). Efficacy in dysphagia. *Dysphagia, 10,* 263–267

Schiavetti, N., Metz, D., & Orlikoff, R. (2011). *Evaluating research in communicative disorders.* Upper Saddle River, NJ: Pearson Education

Schlosser, R. W., Koul, R., & Costello, J. (2007, May-Jun). Asking well-built questions for evidence-based practice in augmentative and alternative communication. *Journal of Communication Disorders, 40,* 225–238

Schmitt, M. B., & Justice, L. (2011). Schools as complex host environments: aspects that may influence clinical practice and research. *The Asha Leader, 16,* 8–11

Schwartz, I. S., & Baer, D. M. (1991, Summer). Social validity assessments: is current practice state of the art? *Journal of Applied Behavior Analysis, 24,* 189–204

Simmons, R., Fajans, P., & Ghiron, L. (2007). *Scaling up health service delivery: From pilot innovations to policies and programmes.* Geneva, Switzerland: WHO Press

Spencer, K. (2011). Personal communication

Wolf, M. M. (1978, Summer). Social validity: the case for subjective measurement or how applied behavior analysis is finding its heart. *Journal of Applied Behavior Analysis, 11,* 203–214

World Health Organization. (2011, June 20). *International Classification of Functioning, Disability and Health (ICF).* http://www.who.int/classifications/icf/en/

Yeaton, W. H., & Sechrest, L. (1981, Apr). Critical dimensions in the choice and maintenance of successful treatments: strength, integrity, and effectiveness. *Journal of Consulting and Clinical Psychology, 49,* 156–167

Yoder, P., & Stone, W. L. (2006, Aug). A randomized comparison of the effect of two prelinguistic communication interventions on the acquisition of spoken communication in preschoolers with ASD. *Journal of Speech, Language, and Hearing Research: JSLHR, 49,* 698–711

# 13

# Evidence-Based Practice: Applying Research Outcomes to Inform Clinical Practice

*Kathryn M. Yorkston and Carolyn R. Baylor*

## ♦ Chapter Focus

This chapter summarizes the benefits and challenges of adopting an evidence-based practice approach to clinical decision making in the field of speech-language pathology, and offers suggestions for clinicians who wish to integrate evidence-based practice strategies into their practice. Three elements—clinician expertise, client preferences, and research—are considered equally important in weighing treatment decisions, but particular emphasis is placed on the research component of EBP and on strategies for strengthening the traditionally weaker presence of research evidence in clinical decision making.

## ♦ Introduction

One widely accepted source describes evidence-based practice (EBP) as "the conscientious, explicit, and judicious use of current best evidence in making decisions about the care of an individual patient" (Sackett, Rosenberg, Gray, Haynes, & Richardson, 1996, p. 71). The three key sources of evidence used in making evidence-based decisions are clinician expertise, client values and preferences, and research evidence from studies of treatment outcomes. EBP was endorsed by the American Speech-Language-Hearing Association (ASHA) in a 2004 position paper (ASHA, 2004). Clinician opinion about EBP varies considerably from those who are "excited" or "intrigued" to those who believe it is "alien," "scary" or "trendy" (Le May, Mulhall, & Alexander, 1998). There are several reasons for this range of reactions to EBP. First, EBP is relatively new to the field of speech-language pathology, and experience with its clinical application has only recently begun. Second, we are facing the challenge of taking a process that has been developed in different fields of medicine, particularly those that rely on drug interventions, and applying it to our work, which relies largely on behavioral interventions. Another reason for the differences of opinion is that EBP is both beneficial and challenging. One of the challenges, and the element of EBP that might be most "alien" to many clinicians, is the application of research outcomes to treatment decision making. Speech-language pathologists (SLPs) have a long tradition of fostering clinician excellence through our training programs, and with recent trends in health care toward shared decision making (Edwards, Davies, & Edwards, 2009) and participation-focused treatment goals (Kagan & Simmons-Mackie, 2007), client values and preferences are incorporated into treatment decisions with greater regularity. However, digesting and integrating research evidence into clinical practice is one area in which clinicians often struggle.

## ◆ Benefits of Evidence-Based Practice

The broad goals of EBP are consistent with the goals of clinical practice, that is, to improve treatment outcomes by evaluating the quality and consistency of treatment. When it is working as intended, EBP forms a link among stakeholders: clients, clinicians, researchers, educators, and policy makers. EBP can benefit all of these stakeholders. For clients, EBP provides a mechanism to understand what treatment options are available and why certain options may or may not be feasible or appropriate when weighing the variables of research evidence, clinician capabilities, and the clients' own preferences. If clients are made privy to the EBP decision-making process, they might better understand why clinicians make the recommendations they do. For clinicians, EBP provides a method to filter and evaluate information to make it readily accessible. EBP can help clinicians identify candidates for a particular treatment or best practices for treatment. For researchers, EBP helps to identify gaps in our knowledge and thus spurs future research directions. EBP can also help researchers to disseminate the outcomes of their investigations to a broad audience of researchers, clinicians, educators, policy makers, and patients by helping these audiences understand the purpose and role of different studies in clinical decision making. For educators, EBP can provide a method for teaching students how to make systematic and transparent clinician decisions. Finally, for policy makers, EBP provides information about treatments strongly supported by evidence.

## ◆ Challenges of Evidence-Based Practice

Despite the positive features of EBP, a number challenges limit its widespread implementation. A general discussion of concerns about EBP across different fields of clinical practice is followed by a discussion of the particular challenges faced by rehabilitation fields such as speech-language pathology.

### General Challenges Across Clinical Fields

Many fields of clinical practice face a similar set of challenges in applying the principles of EBP. Perhaps the most obvious challenge is the lack of high-quality research to support EBP decisions. Because clinical trials, which are the foundation of the research component of EBP, are expensive and time-consuming and require enormous resources, such trials are not available for every topic of interest. Much of the research evidence, therefore, consists of studies that have lower levels of research control than the ideal randomized-controlled clinical trials, and therefore the causal link between treatments and outcomes is weaker. Beyond questions of research design, other issues may limit the ability of research to yield convincing evidence. These issues include the overall quality of the research as well as the scope of the research. For example, some studies may be so narrowly focused that the population of interest to a clinician is not included, whereas others may be so broad that the results are impossible to apply directly to an individual patient (Caplan, 2001).

Another challenge in utilizing research outcomes in EBP relates to interpreting the results of clinical trials. Many researchers focus on reporting the statistical significance of the findings, for example, reporting that there is a small likelihood (<5%) that the results have occurred by chance alone.

However, small changes that may be statistically significant may be of no important to the patient. Recently, clinical researchers have called for a broader perspective that requires not only statistical significance but also meaningful change (Make, 2007). The term *minimal important difference* (MID), or minimal clinically important difference, has been applied to these meaningful differences. Specifically, these differences have been described as the smallest difference in a measure that *patients perceive* as beneficial (Jaeschke, Singer, & Guyatt, 1989). Bothe and Richardson (2011) have proposed the term *personal significance* to serve a similar purpose. Currently, information about minimal clinically important differences or personal significance is not available for many treatment outcomes measures, and determining the change needed for a clinically or personally significant result may be difficult because individual patients may have different perceptions of what is meaningful change for them.

The final challenge faced by practitioners of EBP is consumer skepticism. In a recent study including focus groups, interviews, and an online survey, few consumers understood the terms *medical evidence* and *quality guidelines* (Carman et al, 2010). Consumers believed that medical guidelines are inflexible and limit the physician's ability to provide the needed care. These beliefs seriously limit consumer engagement in evidence-based decision making.

## Challenges for the Profession of Speech-Language Pathology

In addition to the challenges faced by all fields of clinical practice, speech-language pathology and other fields of rehabilitation face additional problems. Many of these challenges arise as a result of the nature of our interventions. Our treatments are typically multidimensional and individualized to the patient because many patients have different patterns of impairment from one person to the next even within a single diagnosis. For example, when managing dysarthria associated with a traumatic brain injury (TBI), different speech production components such as the respiratory, phonatory, velopharyngeal, and oral articulatory systems may be affected. Some speakers may have more difficulty with articulation precision, whereas others may have problems affecting other speech parameters such as rate and stress patterning. In a complex diagnosis such as TBI, the patients' constellations of dysarthria symptoms may exist in the context of other unique TBI manifestations such as the extent and nature of cognitive-communication impairments. The patients' treatment plans will also be heavily influenced by their communication needs in their daily environments as well as by the supports and barriers in their environments, such as environmental noise or communication partners. Finally, speech pathology intervention must also be considered within the context of personal factors that are not under the control of the rehabilitation team (Dijkers, 2009).

## Randomized-Controlled Trials

Randomized-controlled trials (RCTs) are considered among the highest levels of research evidence in EBP frameworks. Yet, RCTs are challenging in the field of speech-language pathology for several reasons. First, for all the reasons presented in the previous paragraph, interventions provided by SLPs are often highly individualized. Clinicians make decisions about specific, unique, and complex cases, whereas RCTs provide information about the "average case" (Tate, Kalpakjian, & Kwon, 2008). Ylvisaker and colleagues offered another challenge of RCTs by suggesting an inverse relationship between the heterogeneity of the clinical population and usefulness of large-*n* studies (Ylvisaker et al, 2002). The more diverse the clinical population, the greater the likelihood that a particular patient will *not* resemble those enrolled in an RCT. RCTs do not adequately handle complex behavioral interventions (Johnston, Sherer, & Whyte, 2006). Finally, RCTs require control groups receiving placebo treatment or no treatment at all. Placebos are not available for many interventions, and many researchers are uncomfortable with the ethics of withholding treatment particularly if there are critical windows for intervention, such as soon after an injury, or if withholding intervention renders people unable to communicate optimally. Because RCTs are considered the "gold standard" study design in many fields of medicine, speech-language pathology is often viewed as have low levels of research evidence because of the lack of RCTs.

Another significant challenge in implementing principles of EBP by SLPs involves the concept of _information literacy_—the extent to which SLPs are comfortable accessing and interpreting research about treatment outcomes. In a survey completed by 208 SLPs, the results indicated that clinicians were more likely to consult colleagues, take part in continuing education activities, or search the open Internet than read scholarly journal articles as an aid in clinical decision making (Nail-Chiwetalu & Bernstein Ratner, 2007). By far the most commonly cited barrier in obtaining quality research information was lack of time, followed by difficulty searching for and locating appropriate research and having access to that research. Thus, if EBP practices are to be implemented clinically, information literacy education should be incorporated in training curricula, and clinical summaries of research evidence should be made available to the field.

## ♦ How to Make Evidence-Based Practice Work for You

Evidence-based practice is a method of helping clinicians make decisions about which treatments are appropriate for particular patients. Because no single source of information is sufficient for clinical decision making, several sources must be combined. The traditional EBP framework incorporates three key sources of evidence: _clinician expertise,_ the _values and preferences_ of the individual client, and _research evidence_. Other frameworks are available. For example, Tonelli (2006) (Tonelli, 2006) suggests five important sources. The first, _empirical evidence_, is derived from clinical research. This evidence must be supplemented by _experiential evidence_ derived from personal clinical experience or the clinical experience of others (expert opinion). The third source of information is the _pathophysiologic rationale_ or justification based on what the field knows about speech or language production and guidelines such as principles of motor learning or language processing. Added to these sources of information are _patient preferences,_ derived from interaction with each patient, and _system features,_ including available resources and legal and cultural concerns. All of these sources contribute to clinical decisions. Sources of information are combined and tested in what has been called patient-specific hypothesis testing (Ylvisaker et al, 2002). This often takes the form of treatment trials or diagnostic teaching.

The following subsections offer suggestions for clinicians who are seeking current evidence from clinical research to help guide treatment decisions. Applying research findings to clinical decision making is well within the capabilities, and certainly within the responsibilities, of individual clinicians, and these suggestions are intended to help SLPs navigate treatment outcomes research and to locate additional resources to help with the process. Key steps in the process of integrating research into clinician decision making include (1) asking good questions of the research, (2) finding the most helpful research, (3) extracting the useful information from the research, and (4) integrating the research findings with other sources of information for treatment planning.

### Asking Good Questions of the Research

A literature search is somewhat like a research study. You must start with a question that is meaningful and answerable. Start by thinking about the specific question you would like to have answered to guide you in treatment planning. If your question is too general, you may be overwhelmed with too many studies to digest, or you may have trouble finding information specific enough for your situation. For example, the question "Is speech treatment for dysarthria effective?" is a very broad question and precise answers may not be possible. On the other hand, if your questions are too specific you may not find any studies on that very narrow topic. For example, the following question is very specific and it may be difficult to generalize the findings beyond these specific conditions: "Do respiratory exercises performed daily increase the sustained phonation time for children between 3 and 5 years of age with spastic cerebral palsy?"

Templates are available to assist clinicians in building answerable questions (Schlosser, Koul, & Costello, 2007). The PICO template suggests that the question should include information about the patient, intervention, comparison, and outcome. For example, does alphabet supplement (the intervention) improve speech intelligibility (the outcome) more than does clear speech (the comparison) for people with moderate to severe dysarthria (the patient)? Be prepared to reformulate your question if initial searches yield either too much or too little research evidence.

## Finding the Most Helpful Research

Literature searches are becoming increasingly easier with the wide range of online resources available. We can offer suggestions to keep in mind to ensure that the search yields the needed information to answer the questions in the most efficient way possible. Most people start by searching a research database. Choosing the database and the specific search terms to use can impact the research studies located, and searches should cover multiple databases and use several search terms to be most effective. Information about search techniques is available through consultation with a librarian at your practice site, through general literature search guides (Garrard, 2007), or through articles particularly focusing on searches related to topics of communication disorders (Schlosser, Wendt, Angermeier, & Shetty, 2005). It is generally a good idea to use more than one source of information because not all databases cover all speech/language related journals. Medline (accessed through PubMed) is a free resource that is developed and maintained by the National Center for Biotechnology Information (NCBI) at the U.S. National Library of Medicine (NLM), located at the National Institutes of Health (NIH). The Cumulative Index of Nursing and Allied Health Literature (CINAHL) covers over 1600 journals from allied health professions. Web of Science is a multidisciplinary database covering journals in the sciences, social sciences, and arts and humanities, with searchable cited references. Google Scholar (http://scholar.google.com/) is also helpful because in addition to traditional journals it provides quick access to books, book chapters, dissertations, professional societies' publications, and other online sources.

Other search strategies may help you locate key manuscripts. For example, finding a classic article that is central to your topic may help to refine the search terms. Use of search terms from this central article will help in identifying other similar articles. Once you have located one or two manuscripts that seem central to your topic, further targeted searches can occur through ancestral and cited reference searches. Ancestral searches involve looking at the reference lists in key articles to locate articles that were cited in these manuscripts that might be useful for your topic. Cited reference searches are searches to look for articles published more recently that cite the key article you have located. Cited reference searches are facilitated in many databases that provide links to manuscripts citing the one you are reading. The Web of Science has a database dedicated to cited reference searches as well. Cited reference searches are particularly important to ensure that you are retrieving the most up-to-date research evidence available.

When conducting a literature search, the logical concern arises regarding the extent to which the articles located represent the body of work being done, and published, in any particular field of study. In statistical terms, this question is asking about sampling bias. Were the studies selected in such a way that all of the relevant studies were found? **Figure 13.1** illustrates several possible sources of sampling bias in a literature search. The largest oval represents the universe of all studies that have been conducted, both those that are published and those that should have been published but were not. The next largest oval represents published studies. Because not all published studies are indexed in research databases, the next largest oval represents indexed studies. A still smaller oval represents those indexed studies that were retrieved using a specific search strategy. The smallest oval represents those studies judged to be relevant from the larger group of studies retrieved from the search. The ideal situation is illustrated by the shaded oval, in which all relevant studies are found across all these conditions. The figure suggests that sampling bias can occur as part of the publication process. This is known as publication bias, where studies reporting statistically significant results are more likely to be published than those that do not. Sampling bias can also occur during the process

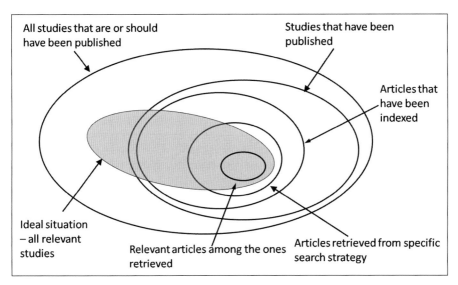

**Fig. 13.1**   Sampling bias is illustrated with a series of nested ovals ranging from the largest, indicating all studies that are or should have been published, to the smallest, indicating relevant articles among the ones retrieved. The shaded oval represents the ideal situation, indicating all relevant studies. (M. Ciol, personal communication, 2011.)

of searching the databases. Use of inappropriate or incomplete search strategies will result in missing relevant articles.

In the likely situation that a search yields many possible relevant articles, the next question is which articles should busy clinicians choose to focus on in their reading to obtain the best possible research evidence to guide them. Most EBP guidelines suggest focusing on the studies with the highest "levels of evidence." *Levels of evidence* refers to the amount and quality of experimental control in research studies. *Experimental control* is the extent to which the outcomes of the study can be attributed to the treatment condition as opposed to possible extraneous or confounding variables. Studies that have higher levels of experimental control can make stronger cause-effect conclusions between treatments and outcomes and are regarded as having the strongest levels of research evidence. These studies are generally given more weight when gleaning evidence from the research literature. EBP guidelines typically draw attention to RCTs as the research design regarded as having the highest level of evidence for experimental control.

There are dozens of schemes available to guide readers in rating the quality of evidence in research studies. Some simply rely on the study design (experimental control). For example, the American Academy of Neurology (AAN) (http://www.aan.com/professionals/practice/) ratings range from class I (prospective, randomized-controlled clinical trials with a masked outcome assessment in a representative population) to class IV (uncontrolled studies, case series, case reports, and expert opinion). Other schemes include more factors. For example, the Grading of Recommendations Assessments, Development, and Evaluation (GRADE) system (http://www.gradeworkinggroup.org/) (GRADE Working Group, 2004) includes not only study design but also study quality, consistency across studies, and the directness (the people, interventions, and outcomes are similar to those of interest). These components are combined into four levels or grades of evidence, from high (further research is very unlikely to change the confidence in the effect size) to very low (any estimate of effect is very uncertain). Thus the GRADE rating defines the quality of evidence in terms of the extent to which there is confidence that the effect size is correct.

Studies may also be rated according to the quality of the reporting in the article. The Consolidated Standards of Reporting Trial (CONSORT) (Moher, Schulz, & Altman, 2001) contains a checklist of 22 items that specify in detail what should be included in the article. These checklists have been applied as a scheme for rating the quality of research studies (J. Law & Plunkett, 2006). Generally, there is a trend to move away from rating systems that depend on a single criterion such as study design. More complex and flexible rating systems may more adequately reflect the quality of research.

Clinicians and researchers searching the speech-language pathology literature from an EBP viewpoint will often be frustrated by the lack of published studies with the highest levels of evidence. RCTs are sparse in many topics in our field. The paucity of RCTs often leads clinicians and researchers to bemoan the absence of evidence in our profession. However, experienced researchers recognize that there is a continuum of increasing evidence that starts not with RCTs but rather with earlier phases of research. Campbell and colleagues (2000) suggest a five-phase continuum of treatment outcomes research that begins with a preclinical phase in which the relevant theories are explored, (Campbell et al, 2000) and moves up through developing the elements of treatment feasibility, treatment protocols, and outcomes measures that are required preparation for well-designed RCTs. Robey (1998) provide a similar research hierarchy adapted to the field of speech-language pathology. Of course, it is possible to conduct a well-designed RCT in the area of communication disorders. However, to obtain adequate sample sizes and robust control, these studies run the risk of addressing a narrow subset of speakers with similar communication disorder symptoms and associated characteristics, and narrowing the focus might limit the usefulness of the study to answer more general clinical questions about the range of *typical* patients.

When considering the range of research evidence available (or not available as the case may be), it is important to recognize the distinction between best "available" evidence and best "possible" evidence. The authoritative definition of EBP cited at the beginning of this chapter proposes that EBP involves using "current best evidence" in addition to clinical expertise and client preferences to make decisions (Sackett et al, 1996). Dijkers (2009) suggests that many in the field interpret "best" as "best possible" rather than "best available." Frequently, the best possible evidence or studies of the highest quality are not always available. When "best" is defined as the best available evidence, a more inclusive evidence review is encouraged including observational studies, single-case design research, or case series. Such inclusive searches are typically more useful in fields related to rehabilitation. Therefore, clinicians are encouraged to recognize that there can be much useful information in research studies at many different levels of evidence. As long as readers do not overstep the research and attribute definitive cause-and-effect relationships to treatment outcomes that lower-level studies are not intended to support, even studies at lower levels of experimental control can provide highly useful information about relationships and associations among variables, likely outcomes of interventions under development, and additional information to guide treatment decisions.

## Systematic Reviews and Meta-Analyses

Fortunately, two types of research studies that are regarded most highly in EBP are also highly useful to research consumers because they provide summaries of existing research evidence. These two products are systematic reviews and meta-analyses. Review articles are common in the literature, but there is a difference between *narrative reviews* and *systematic reviews.* Narrative reviews are conducted by experts using informal, subjective methods to collect and interpret information. These reviews frequently reflect the opinion of a single author or a small group of collaborators and do not provide enough detail to allow replication or updating of the review. *Systematic reviews* are rapidly replacing these narratives. A systematic review is an attempt to collate all empirical evidence that fits pre-specified eligibility criteria to answer a specific research question (Institute of Medicine, 2011). Professional organizations often sponsor these reviews to ensure a board prospective. For example, the Academy of Neurologic Communication Disorders and Sciences (ANCDS) has developed a series of systematic reviews on topics including aphasia, acquired apraxia of speech, dysarthria, dementia, and traumatic brain injury that are available on their Web site (http://www.ancds.org/). See **Table 13.1** for a list of the topics, year of publication, and number of articles examined in these reviews. Components of systematic reviews include a clear set of objectives and research questions, reproducible search techniques and criteria for study inclusion, well-defined methods for rating the quality and validity of research, and a systematic synthesis of the research findings (Liberati et al, 2009). *Meta-analyses* are similar to systematic reviews in that they are a systematic compilation of

**Table 13.1**    Systematic Reviews Available from the Academy of Neurologic Communication Disorders and Sciences (http://www.ancds.org/)

| Topic | Year of Publication | Number of Articles | Topic | Year of Publication | Number of Articles |
|---|---|---|---|---|---|
| Acquired apraxia of speech | 2006 | 59 | Dementia: caregiver education | 2007 | 7 |
| Aphasia: overall language performance | 2007 | 73 | Dementia: computer-assisted cognitive interventions | 2005 | 3 |
| Aphasia: lexical retrieval | 2008 | 123 | Dementia: Montessori-based intervention | 2006 | 5 |
| Aphasia: syntax | 2006 | 63 | Dysarthria: loudness, rate or prosody | 2007 | 51 |
| Aphasia: speech production/fluency | 2009 | 28 | Dysarthria: spasmodic dysphonia and related disorders | 2003 | 103 |
| Aphasia: written language—reading | 2008 | 56 | Dysarthria: behavioral management of respiratory/phonatory dysfunction | 2003 | 35 |
| Aphasia: written language—writing | 2007 | 52 | Dysarthria: velopharyngeal function | 2001 | 33 |
| Aphasia: alternative communication | 2005 | 75 | TBI: behavioral intervention | 2007 | 65 |
| Dementia: simulated presence therapy | 2006 | 5 | TBI: external aids for memory | 2007 | 54 |
| Dementia: group reminiscence therapy | 2006 | 7 | TBI: behavioral and social interventions | 2005 | 59 |
| Dementia: spaced-retrieval training | 2005 | 18 | TBI: direct attention training | 2003 | 6 |
| Dementia: caregiver active cognitive stimulation | 2007 | 14 | TBI: intervention for executive functions | 2008 | 15 |
| | | | Unilateral vocal fold Paralysis | 2006 | 92 |

TBI—traumatic brain injury

studies collected to answer a specific research question. However, meta-analyses go beyond the qualitative summaries of systematic reviews. Meta-analyses involve compiling the data from all included studies and reanalyzing them as a single data set to provide a statistical summary of the treatment effects of the intervention under consideration. Meta-analyses are a statistical means of synthesizing results of related but independent studies (Normand, 1999). Meta-analyses are used to increase the statistical power to detect an effect and to estimate an average effect, which can be particularly useful when results of individual studies are conflicting. A discussion of meta-analysis is provided in Chapter 15 by Ntourou and Lipsey. Examples of meta-analyses are available in the speech-language pathology literature (Robey, 1998; Robey, McCallum, & Francois, 1999).

Research consumers may want to start their literature searches with systematic reviews and meta-analyses because these studies provide efficient and traceable summaries of the research on a topic. However, as with all studies, readers should be aware that systematic reviews and meta-analyses will not necessarily include all studies on a topic; they include only those studies that directly apply to the research question chosen by the authors of the systematic reviews/meta-analyses, and include only those studies that met specific selection criteria. Furthermore, as with all published research, readers need to be alert for additional studies published since the systematic review or meta-analysis that might provide more up-to-date information. These updates can be completed quite efficiently with systematic reviews because the methods of these papers should include the search strategies used to locate studies for these projects (databases and search terms), and those searches can be repeated and updated by the interested reader at any time.

## Other Types of Research Designs

In addition to the types of research described above, research consumers should also be alert to studies that, by their design, are not included in most traditional EBP evidence hierarchies. Two examples highly relevant to the field of speech-language pathology are single-subject designs and qualitative research designs. Single-subject designs can address many of the challenges of large group studies relevant to the field of speech-language pathology such as the inherent heterogeneity in our patient populations. Single-subject designs get around the sometimes insurmountable task of finding enough subjects with similar characteristics to form experimental and control groups. Single-subject designs also address ethically uncomfortable control group issues by allowing each subject to serve as his or her own control through multiple baselines, withdrawal periods, and other design elements. Because single-subject designs cannot be accurately evaluated by the same levels of evidence hierarchies used for group designs, other systems for rating the quality of these studies are available (Logan, Roberts, Pretto, & Morey, 2002; Tate et al, 2008). For example, the Single-Case Experimental Design (SCED) Scale (Tate et al, 2008) rates whether or not the report meets criteria in 11 areas: history, target behavior, design, baseline, behavior during treatment, raw data, inter-rater reliability, independent assessor, statistical analysis, replication, and generalization. Although single-subject designs do not have the power of well-controlled group designs, they can bring high-quality control to investigate treatment outcomes when group designs are not feasible. Single-subject research designs and case reports are described in greater detail in Chapter 14 by Kearns and de Riesthal.

_Qualitative research_ can also provide highly informative data for treatment planning. Qualitative research is a diverse field of research with many different traditions, methods, and theoretical approaches available to use for different research questions. Much qualitative research focuses on describing phenomena not easily captured through quantification, and much of it focuses on documenting the "lived experiences" of people with, in our field, communication disorders. Qualitative research can provide valuable insight into the experiences and manifestations of treatment approaches beyond the cut-and-dried question of whether or not significant change was observed after treatment. Data from qualitative research may supplement other research data to provide a more well-rounded picture of the experiences associated with interventions and their outcomes, and this additional information may be very useful to clinicians and clients in the decision-making process (M. Law et al, 1998).

Other information should be taken into account when choosing the most relevant articles. Although research design and quality of the research evidence are important, readers should also consider whether or not the patient populations, clinic settings, resources, or other features of the study are relevant enough to the situation at hand to make the study directly useful. If a study provides very strong research evidence about a novel treatment technique, but that technique is not feasible in your clinic due to the need for specialty equipment or training that is not readily available, the clinician may need to pursue additional reading of other studies that address treatment approaches that are feasible in that clinician's particular setting at that time.

## Extracting the Useful Information from the Research

Once the clinician has chosen the articles from the literature that appear to be most relevant to the question at hand, the next step in utilizing the research evidence in EBP is to extract the information from the articles and to understand how that information can be applied to clinical practice. Readers are wise to remember that research studies are rarely conducted in a "perfect world" in which all resources are readily available to conduct the ideal study. Like clinical practice, research takes place in the "real world" where there are constraints on time, resources, access to patient populations, and other constraints that may shape the size, nature, and quality of research studies. Readers therefore need to be prepared to make their own judgments about the quality of the research, how relevant the studies are to their own particular situations, and to what extent they can apply information from the studies to their clinical needs.

Tools are available to help readers summarize and organize information from manuscripts in a way that will lead them to decisions about the extent to which the research is applicable to their own clinical situations. For example, Dollaghan (2007) provides a series of checklists and guidelines for digesting and applying research evidence to clinical situations. These include guidelines for the *Critical Appraisal of Treatment Evidence* (CATE), *Critical Appraisal of Systematic Reviews and Meta-analyses* (CASM), and a *Checklist for Appraising Patient/Practice Evidence* (CAPE), among others (see appendices in the Dollaghan text). These guidelines direct the reader through elements of the study such as clarifying the specific research question addressed by the study, examining the strength of the research design, examining the quality of the methods including the reliability and validity of measures and methods, interpreting the meaningfulness of outcomes, and considering practical issues such as cost-benefit comparisons.

Because of their appeal to readers as summaries of research evidence, specific criteria that might be used to judge the quality and relevance of systematic reviews will be presented in further detail here. General schemes for rating the quality of systematic reviews are available (ASHA, 2004; Moher, Liberati, Tetzlaff, & Altman, 2009). **Table 13.2** lists 27 items to include in systematic reviews. Although such a checklist is valuable, it is also useful to ask several simple questions when evaluating the quality of the review. Some of these questions are similar to those asked of other research studies, whereas some are unique to systematic reviews.

### Who Conducted the Review?

Because systematic reviews are commonly a combination of research or empirical evidence and expert opinion when no evidence is available, the authors should be recognized authorities on the topic. Frequently, professional organization, such as ANCDS, will sponsor systematic reviews that are authored by a group of experts who represent a range of opinions on the topic. The authors also typically represent a variety of practice sites and academic locations. A broad range of expertise helps to minimize the bias of a single researcher or research group. Information about sponsorship, funding, or potential conflict of interest is available either in the introduction or in the acknowledgment section. Authorship by an authoritative, unbiased group is preferred over that by a single researcher or research group with a potential conflict of interest.

### Was the Question Both Answerable and Important?

A specific question or set of questions should be provided. Readers should pay close attention to the research question, because if the question addressed in the review differs notably from the question the reader has, it is possible the systematic review will not cover the research literature that might be most relevant to that particular reader.

### What Search Strategies Were Used to Locate Studies for the Review?

It is important to know the information source (databases used and dates of inclusion), eligibility requirements (study design, publication characteristics), and search terms used. Knowing this information allows for replication and updating of reviews. It is also gives the reader information about what sources of information were *ignored*. For example, does the review include only randomized clinical trials when heterogeneity of the population suggests that single-case design research is both

**Table 13.2**   List of Items Typically Contained in a Systematic Review

| | |
|---|---|
| Title | Results |
| Structure abstract | Study selection |
| Introduction | Study characteristics |
| Rationale | Risk of bias with studies |
| Objectives | Results of individual studies |
| Methods | Synthesis of results |
| Protocol or registration | Risk of bias across studies |
| Eligibility criteria for study inclusion | Additional analysis |
| Information sources | Discussion |
| Search strategies | Summary of evidence |
| Study selection | Limitations |
| Data collection process | Conclusions |
| Data items | Funding |
| Risk of bias in individual studies | |
| Summary measures | |
| Synthesis of results | |
| Risk of bias across studies | |
| Additional analysis | |

common and perhaps more appropriate? Knowing the eligibility requirements also allows the reader to evaluate whether the studies are similar enough to be pooled for a summary.

### How Is "Best" Evidence Being Defined and How Is the Evidence Rated?

The quality of the evidence in systematic reviews is constrained by the quality of the research evidence in the studies that are included in the review. Even though systematic reviews are generally placed high on the tier of evidence in EBP protocols, if the reviews contain only studies with low levels of experimental control, the overall evidence presented by the review remains similarly low. On the other hand, some EBP practitioners suggest that *only* RCTs be included in systematic reviews to ensure that such reviews do indeed occupy the highest tiers of EBP evidence rating systems. Rating systems that penalize all but RCTs, or reviews that include only RCTs, often result in what are known as "empty reviews" (Schlosser & Sigafoos, 2009). These are reviews that may be of high technical quality, with the standard review protocol clearly described, a variety of relevant sources searched, an extensive list of search terms employed, and the characteristics of excluded studies provided. However, if all studies but RCTs are excluded, there may be no studies located at all to include in the review. Abstracts of these empty reviews will contain phrases such as there is "no evidence of the quality required to support or refute the effectiveness" of treatment (Sellars, Hughes, & Langhorne, 2005). Such restrictions may limit the usefulness of these reviews for both clinicians and researchers because they exclude many important sources of evidence (Yorkston & Baylor, 2009). This is one point at which the question regarding best *possible* evidence versus best *available* evidence is of interest in terms of determining what evidence to consider. Regardless of your philosophy on the issue of RCTs, a systematic review should clearly identify the level of evidence and other key elements of research quality for the search strategies and for each included study so that the reader can make an informed judgment of the strength of research evidence in the review.

### Are the Conclusions Useful?

Typically, systematic reviews provide some synthesis of the findings in narrative form. The analysis of the results will depend on the topic and the objectives of the review. For example, several approaches to data analysis have been taken by the ANCDS dysarthria writing committees. When examining evidence for the management of the velopharyngeal system, results were reported as a list of factors related to candidacy for palatal lift fitting (Yorkston et al, 2001). Factors including the muscular tone of the soft palate, adequacy of oral articulation, rate of change, and cognitive function contributed to judgments of candidacy. When reviewing the effect of Botox on adductor spasmodic dysphonia, conclusions were in the form of statement of trends (Duffy & Yorkston, 2003). This review suggested that Botox injection, "results in a substantial degree of improvement for a substantial percentage of patients, with benefits generally lasting for three to four months" (p. l). When reviewing the evidence related to speech supplementation (Hanson, Beukelman, Heidemann, & Shutts-Johnson, 2010; Hanson, Yorkston, & Beukelman, 2004), raw data indicating speech intelligibility with and without supplementation were provided. Thus, the clinician could use this information to estimate the degree of expected change.

Although many of the guidelines for evaluating systematic reviews also apply to meta-analyses, there are a few additional points about the latter studies to consider. Just as with systematic reviews, readers should be cautious in interpreting meta-analyses because combining poorly designed studies in a meta-analysis does not overcome the quality of the original studies. Statistical analysis of treatment outcomes is also dependent on adequate outcome measures. If the outcome measures are inappropriate or imprecise, the combination of studies will not improve the strength of the evidence. Bias may also arise from the fact that studies showing no significant results may not be published and so cannot be included in the statistical analysis.

### Integrating Research with Other Sources of Information for Treatment Planning

For all research evidence, the final critical decision for clinicians is *how does the research evidence contribute to clinical decision making*? When answering this question caution is warranted. It is unlikely that any single research study, including systematic reviews or meta-analyses will have all the answers for a specific patient. The evidence provided as part of the research component of the EBP process must be combined with the other two components of EBP: clinician expertise and client preferences and values. These three combined elements facilitate the process of shared decision making in which the clinician and patient both contribute to the decision, which maximizes patient autonomy and the use of medical expertise (Makoul & Clayman, 2006). The clinician is responsible for knowing about the best available research evidence for a particular intervention and for placing that evidence in the context of expert opinion and the particular clinical situation at hand. In short, it is the clinician's responsibility to provide the patient with all of the evidence upon which to make an informed decision. This process can sometimes be challenging. Although well-recognized procedures have been developed to review the research literature (Liberati et al, 2009), methods for incorporating expert opinion and client perspectives are less well established. However, including clients in the decision-making process utilizing the principles of shared decision making (Edwards et al, 2009) can be a productive start to integration of research evidence, clinician expertise, and client preferences.

## ◆ Conclusion and Future Directions

With both its benefits and its challenges, EBP has become a part of clinical practice. Montgomery and Turkstra (2003) provide a fitting analogy when they suggest that EBP is "like 'smelling salts,' an antidote to the fuzzy-headedness of the past, and noxious but welcome relief" (Montgomery & Turkstra, 2003) (p. xii). EBP is designed to wake us up and to raise our consciousness about the practices of the past, and it is beneficial in that it forces us to examine previous assumptions that have frequently been made on expert opinion alone. It is noxious because it is not always a pleasure to reflect on the shortcomings of our past and current practice. Finally, it is a welcome relief because it clearly identifies in what direction our field needs to go in the future. There are several urgent needs for the future. Most importantly, as Olswang and Bain argued in Chapter 12, we need the primary research to investigate *efficacy* and the *effectiveness* of our interventions beginning at the appropriate phase of research and leading to clinical trials. Next, systematic reviews and meta-analyses are needed to assess and interpret the outcomes of the primary research. These reviews should pose clinically important yet answerable questions, and we need to follow up these reviews with the research called for in their conclusions to clarify outcomes when they are not clear. Finally, we need to address the critical issue of research literacy for clinicians. Clinicians are essential to the EBP process by bringing the research findings to their clinical practices, and in turn informing researchers about areas in which research can serve their clinical work in meaningful and practical ways. If we are able to accomplish the agenda outlined by the process of EBP, our field and our ability to care for people with communication disorders will advance.

# References

American Speech-Language-Hearing Association (ASHA). (2004). *Evidence-based practice in communication disorders: An introduction* [technical report]. http://www.asha.org/members/deskref-journals/deskref/default

Bothe, A. K., & Richardson, J. D. (2011). Statistical, practical, clinical, and personal significance: Definitions and applications in speech-language pathology. *American Journal of Speech-Language Pathology, 20,* 233–242

Campbell, M., Fitzpatrick, R., Haines, A., Kinmonth, A. L., Sandercock, P., Spiegelhalter, D., et al. (2000, Sep). Framework for design and evaluation of complex interventions to improve health. *British Medical Journal, 321,* 694–696

Caplan, L. R. (2001, Nov). Evidence based medicine: concerns of a clinical neurologist. *Journal of Neurology, Neurosurgery, and Psychiatry, 71,* 569–574

Carman, K. L., Maurer, M., Yegian, J. M., Dardess, P., McGee, J., Evers, M., et al. (2010, Jul). Evidence that consumers are skeptical about evidence-based health care. *Health Affairs, 29,* 1400–1406

Dijkers, M. (2009). *When the best is the enemy of the good: The nature of research evidence used in systematic reviews and guidelines.* Austin, TX: SEDL, National Center for the Dissemination of Disability Research

Dollaghan, C. A. (2007). *The handbook of evidence-based practice in communication disorders.* Baltimore, MD: Paul H. Brookes Publishing

Duffy, J. R., & Yorkston, K. M. (2003). Medical interventions for spasmodic dysphonia and some related conditions: A systematic review. *Journal of Medical Speech-Language Pathology, 11,* ix–lviii

Edwards, M., Davies, M., & Edwards, A. (2009, Apr). What are the external influences on information exchange and shared decision-making in healthcare consultations: a meta-synthesis of the literature. *Patient Education and Counseling, 75,* 37–52. 10.1016/j.pec.2008.09.025

Garrard, J. (2007). *Health sciences literature review made easy: The matrix method* (2nd ed.). Sudbury, MA: Jones & Bartlett Publishers

GRADE Working Group. (2004, Jun). Grading quality of evidence and strength of recommendations. *British Medical Journal, 328,* 1490–1494

Hanson, E. K., Beukelman, D., Heidemann, J. K., & Shutts-Johnson, E. (2010). The impact of alphabet supplementation and word prediction on sentence intelligibility of electronically distorted speech. *Speech Communication, 52,* 99–105

Hanson, E. K., Yorkston, K., & Beukelman, D. (2004). Speech supplementation techniques for dysarthria: A systematic review. *Journal of Medical Speech-Language Pathology, 12,* ix–xxix

Institute of Medicine. (2011). *Finding what works in health care: Standards for systematic reviews: Consensus Report.* http://www.iom.edu/Reports/2011

Jaeschke, R., Singer, J., & Guyatt, G. H. (1989, Dec). Measurement of health status. Ascertaining the minimal clinically important difference. *Controlled Clinical Trials, 10,* 407–415

Johnston, M. V., Sherer, M., & Whyte, J. (2006, Apr). Applying evidence standards to rehabilitation research. *American Journal of Physical Medicine & Rehabilitation, 85,* 292–309

Kagan, A., & Simmons-Mackie, N. (2007). Beginning with the end: outcome-driven assessment and intervention with life participation in mind. *Topics in Language Disorders, 27,* 309–317

Law, J., & Plunkett, C. (2006). Grading study quality in systematic reviews. *Contemporary Issues in Communication Science and Disorders, 33,* 28–36

Law, M., Stewart, D., Lette, L., Pollock, N., Bosch, J., & Westmorland, M. (1998). *Guidelines for critical review form— Qualitative studies.* http://www-fhs.mcmaster.ca/rehab/ebp/pdf/qualguidelines.pdf

Le May, A., Mulhall, A., & Alexander, C. (1998, Aug). Bridging the research-practice gap: exploring the research cultures of practitioners and managers. *Journal of Advanced Nursing, 28,* 428–437

Liberati, A., Altman, D. G., Tetzlaff, J., Mulrow, C., Gøtzsche, P. C., Ioannidis, J. P., et al. (2009, Oct). The PRISMA statement for reporting systematic reviews and meta-analyses of studies that evaluate health care interventions: explanation and elaboration. *Journal of Clinical Epidemiology, 62,* e1–e34

Logan, K. J., Roberts, R. R., Pretto, A. P., & Morey, M. J. (2002). Speaking slowly: Effects of four self-guided training approaches on adults' speech rate and naturalness. *American Journal of Speech-Language Pathology, 11,* 163–174

Make, B. (2007, Sep). How can we assess outcomes of clinical trials: the MCID approach. *Journal of Chronic Obstructive Pulmonary Disease, 4,* 191–194

Makoul, G., & Clayman, M. L. (2006, Mar). An integrative model of shared decision making in medical encounters. *Patient Education and Counseling, 60,* 301–312

Moher, D., Liberati, A., Tetzlaff, J., & Altman, D. G.; PRISMA Group (2009, Oct). Preferred reporting items for systematic reviews and meta-analyses: the PRISMA statement. *Journal of Clinical Epidemiology, 62,* 1006–1012

Moher, D., Schulz, K. F., & Altman, D.; CONSORT Group (Consolidated Standards of Reporting Trials) (2001, Apr). The CONSORT statement: revised recommendations for improving the quality of reports of parallel-group randomized trials. *Journal of the American Medical Association, 285*, 1987–1991

Montgomery, E. B., & Turkstra, L. (2003). Evidence-Based Medicine: Let's be reasonable. *Journal of Medical Speech-Language Pathology, 11*, ix–xii

Nail-Chiwetalu, B., & Bernstein Ratner, N. (2007, Apr). An assessment of the information-seeking abilities and needs of practicing speech-language pathologists. *Journal of the Medical Library Association, 95*, 182–188, e56–e57

Normand, S. L. (1999, Feb). Meta-analysis: formulating, evaluating, combining, and reporting. *Statistics in Medicine, 18*, 321–359

Robey, R. R. (1998, Feb). A meta-analysis of clinical outcomes in the treatment of aphasia. *Journal of Speech, Language, and Hearing Research: JSLHR, 41*, 172–187

Robey, R. R., McCallum, A. F., & Francois, L. K. (1999, June). *A meta-analysis of single-subject research on treatments for aphasia.* Paper presented at the Clinical Aphasiology Conference, Key West, Florida

Sackett, D. L., Rosenberg, W. M., Gray, J. A. M., Haynes, R. B., & Richardson, W. S. (1996, Jan). Evidence based medicine: what it is and what it isn't. *British Medical Journal, 312*, 71–72

Schlosser, R. W., Koul, R., & Costello, J. (2007, May–Jun). Asking well-built questions for evidence-based practice in augmentative and alternative communication. *Journal of Communication Disorders, 40*, 225–238

Schlosser, R. W., & Sigafoos, J. (2009). 'Empty' reviews and evidence-based practice. *Evidence-Based Communication Assessment and Intervention, 3*, 1–3

Schlosser, R. W., Wendt, O., Angermeier, K. L., & Shetty, M. (2005). Searching for evidence in augmentative and alternative communication: Navigating a scattered literature. *Augmentative and Alternative Communication, 21*, 233–255

Sellars, C., Hughes, T., & Langhorne, P. (2005). Speech and language therapy for dysarthria due to non-progressive brain damage. *Cochrane Database of Systematic Reviews, 3*, CD002088

Tate, D., Kalpakjian, C., & Kwon, C. (2008). The use of randomized clinical trials in rehabilitation psychology. *Rehabilitation Psychology, 53*, 268–278. DOI 10.1037/A0012974

Tate, R. L., McDonald, S., Perdices, M., Togher, L., Schultz, R., & Savage, S. (2008, Aug). Rating the methodological quality of single-subject designs and n-of-1 trials: introducing the Single-Case Experimental Design (SCED) Scale. *Neuropsychological Rehabilitation, 18*, 385–401

Tonelli, M. R. (2006, Jun). Integrating evidence into clinical practice: an alternative to evidence-based approaches. *Journal of Evaluation in Clinical Practice, 12*, 248–256

Ylvisaker, M., Coehlo, C., Kennedy, M. R. T., Sohlberg, M. M., Turkstra, L., Avery, J., et al. (2002). Reflections on evidence-based practice and rational clinical decision making. *Journal of Medical Speech-Language Pathology, 10*, ix–xxxviii

Yorkston, K., & Baylor, C. (2009). The lack of RCTs on dysarthria intervention does not necessarily indicate there is no evidence to guide practice. *Evidence-Based Communication Assessment and Intervention, 3*, 79–82

Yorkston, K., Spencer, K., Duffy, J. R., Beukelman, D., Golper, L. A., Miller, R. M., et al. (2001). Evidence-Based Practice Guidelines for Dysarthria: Management of Velopharyngeal Function. *Journal of Medical Speech-Language Pathology, 9*, 257–274

## Resources

Academy of Neurologic Communication Disorders and Sciences. (n.d.). *Practice guidelines.* http://www.ancds.org/

Center for Reviews and Dissemination. (n.d.). *Undertaking systematic reviews of research on effectiveness.* http://www.york.ac.uk/inst/crd/report4.htm

Edlund, W., Gronseth, G., So, Y., Franklin, G., & American Academy of Neurology. (2004). *Clinical practice guideline process manual.* http://www.aan.com/professionals/practice/pdfs/2004_Guideline_Process.pdf

Guyatt, G., Rennie, D., Meade, M., & Cook, D. (2008). *Users' guides to the medical literature: Essentials of evidence-based clinical practice.* New York: McGraw-Hill Professional

Institute of Medicine. (2011). *Finding what works in health care: Standards for systematic reviews: Consensus report.* http://www.iom.edu/Reports/2011

Liberati, A., Altman, D. G., Tetzlaff, J., Mulrow, C., Gøtzsche, P. C., Ioannidis, J. P., et al. (2009, Oct). The PRISMA statement for reporting systematic reviews and meta-analyses of studies that evaluate health care interventions: explanation and elaboration. *Journal of Clinical Epidemiology, 62*, e1–e34

National Center for the Dissemination of Disability Research. (n.d.). http://www.ncddr.org/sqr/standreport.htm

# 14

# Applying Single-Subject Experimental Research to Inform Clinical Practice

*Kevin P. Kearns and Michael R. de Riesthal*

## ♦ Chapter Focus

This chapter considers the unique contributions made by studies using a single-subject experimental design (SSED) to the body of intervention research evidence in communication disorders. Single-subject research and case study methods incorporating SSEDs are described as a way to monitor and report patient outcomes in clinical care and to build the practice-based evidence literature. Drawing from examples in the aphasia literature, the authors review the key principles and methods of SSED to emphasize how an understanding of these methods will enable clinicians to become better consumers of the treatment literature and clinician-scientists. The authors identify the essential strategies for determining the quality and validity of single-subject research findings so that clinicians are better able to decide whether interventions may prove valuable for helping to improve the communication abilities of their clients. Examples of published studies and an example case study incorporating an SSED protocol are provided to demonstrate the power and elegance of this approach to intervention research and the utility in clinical practice.

## ♦ Introduction

Single-subject designs are arguably one of the most useful research design methods for answering the types of clinical questions that interest clinicians (Barlow, Hayes, & Nelson, 1984; Barlow & Hersen; 1984; Kazdin, 1982; Kearns, 1986, 2000). This approach to intervention research is most often used to answer practical clinical questions, such as: Does a given treatment work better than no intervention at all? What components of a treatment package contribute most to improvement? Does adding a component to treatment improve it? How does the treatment of interest compare with other treatments? The direct parallel between important clinical questions and a methodology that is used to investigate the answers to such questions facilitates the translation of research findings into clinical practice (Kearns, 2000). Rosenbek, LaPointe, and Wertz (1989) further argue that the use of single-subject research designs in clinical practice is essential, because it "provides a means for testing theory and principles, for comparing what we think we are doing with what we are doing" (p. 129). The application of single-subject ($N = 1$) designs differs from a group research paradigm. In group designs, a large number of participants and control subjects usually need to be recruited to provide sufficient power to test the hypothesis of the study. Research methods in SSED studies are just as rigorous as group experimental methods in the planning, execution, and subject selection, and are most appropriate for intervention questions involving a single individual serving as his or her own control. Single-subject experimental methods, thus, provide a fundamental link between intervention research and clinical practice. Knowledge about the methods of single-subject designs not only allows the clinician to evaluate the merits of $N = 1$ research reports, and become a better clinician-scientist as a consumer of these published studies, but also provides a basic clinical tool for empirical evaluation of an intervention with individual patients.

# ♦ The Clinical-Scientist as a Consumer of Single-Subject Research

Well in advance of the outcomes and evidence-based practice (EBP) movements, Hayes, Barlow, and Nelson-Gray (1999) argued that "scientist practitioners" should be consumers of research, accountable for measuring the outcomes of their interventions, and when opportunities present themselves, they should be active research collaborators. The term *clinician-scientist*, an appropriate synonym for *scientist practitioner,* captures the centrality of clinical roles of speech-language pathologists who care for individuals with communication disorders. As research consumers, clinician-scientists must become knowledgeable about basic research principles and methodologies so that that can critically analyze published research to determine the relevance of findings to clinical practice. This notion can be extended in the age of EBP to the ability to evaluate and compare individual studies and levels of evidence in support of a particular treatment approach. The second role of the clinician-scientist, accountability, is a moral imperative as much as it is an expected skill set. That is, this role assumes that knowledge of clinical outcome measures and the ability to use data to drive intervention decisions are ethical requirements for clinical practice. The final core principle, active involvement in clinical research through collaboration, is often an aspiration that may or may not be fulfilled depending on one's employment setting and opportunities for collaboration. Clearly, busy case loads, productivity expectations, and funding models often limit opportunities for clinician-scientists to actively participate in research. Increasingly, however, research funding from the National Institutes of Health (NIH) and other agencies is pushing researchers toward more immediate application of their discoveries. Research programs that examine how well an intervention works in controlled, experimental conditions are being expanded to ascertain how well an intervention works under typical clinical conditions. There is, in essence, movement away from an EBP model in which research steers the direction of clinical practice and toward a practice-based evidence model wherein researchers are collaborating with clinicians to develop and test experimental treatments in the "real world."

## Clinician-Scientist Collaboration

*Examples from the Aphasia Literature*

The evolution of clinical research toward a model of true collaboration between researchers and clinicians may provide additional opportunities for clinician-scientists in the future. Consider, for example, the opportunities for clinician-scientist collaborations in aphasia intervention. Over 900 treatment studies of aphasia interventions in the published literature and meta-analyses of the literature support the conclusion that language intervention for aphasia is efficacious (Robey, 1994, 1998). Treatments have been guided by a variety of rationales and theories including psycholinguistic, cognitive neuropsychological, pragmatic, and models of oral/written naming, sentence comprehension and production, minor hemisphere mediation, and so on. Pharmacological and neurological interventions have also been explored. The depth and breadth of the efficacy literature provides a rich resource for clinicians who are committed to using evidence-based treatments and documenting their efforts with appropriate outcome measures. The fact that the literature has been carefully reviewed and summarized in a fashion that allows clinicians to evaluate the quality of the clinical research base and draw preliminary conclusions regarding the strength of evidence supporting the variety of interventions for aphasia is enormously helpful in this regard. The Academy of Neurologic Communication Disorders and Sciences (ANCDS) Practice Guidelines Project (http://aphasiatx .arizona.edu/) and the American Speech-Language-Hearing Association (ASHA) National Center for Evidence-Based Practice in Communication Disorders (N-CEP) evidence-based summaries and practice guidelines (www.asha.org/members/ebp/compendium) provide invaluable resources for clinicians and researchers alike.

Despite obvious progress in our efforts to develop, summarize, and provide evidence-based treatments for individuals with aphasia, clinicians face increasing pressure to document the outcomes of treatment. They are routinely asked to critically evaluate research, use data to make clinical decisions, and to sift through a large, rapidly growing and increasingly sophisticated literature with limited training or experience to guide them. Importantly, the challenge for clinicians is exacerbated by the inherent limitations of the evidence base that they are being asked to evaluate. As Kazdin (2004) points out, a major problem that is often overlooked is the fact that evidence from well-controlled studies may not generalize to clinical settings. Attempts to generalize findings from research to practice is made difficult because intervention research and clinical practice are conducted in dramatically different settings, with different patients/participants, contrasting recruitment and selection methods, divergent outcome assessments, and vastly different training and experience of the treating clinicians. Unfortunately, we have very limited data to inform us about the effectiveness of published treatment research in typical clinical conditions. Criteria for demonstrating evidence are very different and often contradictory across research versus clinical environments. Whereas clinical significance is the coin of the realm in practice settings, this standard is often eschewed and replaced with statistical significance by researchers.

The National Academies Roundtable on Evidence-Based Practice (Olsen, Aisner, & McGinnis, 2007) amplifies this concern and concludes that prevailing approaches to obtaining clinical evidence are currently inadequate and maybe irrelevant in the future. The expert panel notes there is an overdependence on randomized-controlled trials (RCTs) as the gold standard for treatment research. This is particularly problematic in aphasiology, where single-subject experimental designs and nonstatistical criteria have been the predominant method used to evaluate treatment efficacy (Thompson, 2006; Thompson & Kearns, 1991). Furthermore, perspectives of stakeholders, researchers, clinicians, patients, and payers vary significantly and may influence the formulation and clinical implementation of evidence-based clinical guidelines. It is safe to conclude that, despite significant progress in recent years, approaches to interpreting and summarizing research evidence are inconsistent and sometimes confusing for clinicians attempting to incorporate the best evidence into their practice. It is clear that clinicians cannot rely solely on others to analyze and interpret the aphasia intervention literature. As research consumers, clinician-scientists must develop the knowledge base and analytical skills necessary to critically evaluate the evidence that drives their clinical practice.

Over the past 30 years SSEDs have been the most prevalent methodology used for conducting aphasia treatment research (Thompson, 2006). For this reason alone it is important for clinicians to understand the essential components of this approach to intervention research. Although this chapter provides a tutorial introduction to this approach, more comprehensive summaries of single-subject research are available for those interested in furthering their knowledge of the topic (Bailey & Burch, 2002; Connell & Thompson, 1986; Hayes et al, 1999; Kazdin, 1982; Kearns, 1986, 2000; Kennedy, 2005; McReynolds & Kearns, 1983; McReynolds & Thompson, 1986; Thompson, 2006).

## Single-Subject Experimental Designs

Single-subject experimental research designs have been known by several labels including single-case research, single-subject research, single-case designs, and single-participant research. Although all of these labels are acceptable, the term *single-subject experimental design* is preferred because it makes clear that these designs are *experimental* and not descriptive, as compared with case reports lacking experimental methods. One could argue further that the generic term *single-subject* is a misnomer in the sense that across-subject replication is a key to establishing the believability of single-subject research results, and published studies that report findings for a single individual must be replicated with additional subjects before the results can be considered reliable. That is, although the emphasis in this approach is on the intense study of individuals over time, single-subject researchers typically publish the results of an intervention on three or more individuals at a time.

Although there are obvious and important differences between single-subject designs and group experimental approaches to intervention research, they share many common characteristics, including the requirement for demonstrating that the coding or scoring of target communication behaviors are *reliable* (consistent and replicable), and that care has been taken to demonstrate *experimental control* (i.e., internal validity). Given the nature of single-subject designs there are stringent requirements for clear and precise definitions of all aspects of a study including definitions of the *independent* (treatment) variable(s) and the *dependent* (outcome) variable(s) for single-subject research. This emphasis on providing detailed descriptions of treatment protocols and research participants provides obvious advantages for clinicians who are evaluating research in the hopes of gleaning intervention ideas that may be used in clinical practice. We provide a real-life example of that application later in this chapter. The application of single-subject findings to the clinical settings is facilitated by the fact that, similar to clinical practice, the single-subject researcher conducting an intervention study tracks the pattern of change in treated behaviors before, during, and after intervention to determine the success of treatment.

### Single-Subject Versus Group Experiment Methods

An important difference between single-subject and group treatment research methods is that whereas group researchers use statistical methods to determine the significance of findings, single-subject researchers emphasize clinical significance (Meline & Wang, 2004) as the gold standard for evaluating the results of intervention research. This aspect of single-case studies facilitates clinical understanding and logical generalization of findings from the clinical research literature to the clinic. This is not to imply that statistical analyses are not critical judgment aids for both forms of research. Appropriate statistical methods are now available for single-subject research (Borckardt et al, 2008; Fisher, Kelley, & Lomas, 2003) and should be considered a *required* and fundamental element of high-quality single-case research.

### Single-Subject Experimental Designs in Efficacy Research

Single-subject experimental designs are ideally suited for conducting efficacy research that explores the cause-effect relationships between interventions and outcomes through experimental manipulations. These designs provide an experimental means of developing, testing, and extending treatments. Initial findings with a handful of participants are extended through a process of direct and systematic replication (Kearns, 1992). The programmatic use of single-subject research to replicate initial positive findings and explore the power and limits of interventions provide a powerful means of developing and testing treatment approaches, particularly in aphasia intervention (see Thompson & Shapiro, 2007).

### Design Considerations

As noted earlier, single-subject designs are experimental, not observational. Subjects serve as their own control by receiving both nontreatment (baseline) and treatment conditions. As the examples that follow demonstrate, juxtaposition of baseline (A) and treatment (B) phases provides mechanism for experimental control. Similar to the logic used to assess findings from group research studies, single-subject investigators carefully compare the results of individuals with aphasia's performance during baseline (control) conditions and treatment (experimental) conditions to judge whether or not the intervention being examined is responsible for positive changes observed in the participants' performance. Baseline and treatment conditions are carefully arranged to determine if intervention effects are apparent when (and only when) treatment is applied. Observable change in performance across pretreatment (baseline) and treatment phases that directly correlate with the application or removal of intervention provide evidence that the intervention is efficacious.

Experimental control in single-subject research is based on within- and across-subject comparisons of treatment versus no-treatment conditions, and within- and across-subject replication increases the believability of the findings. Single-subject research has a rich tradition of using visual–graphic analysis as a primary means of judging the efficacy of treatment. That is, each individual participant's data are graphed to display performance over time during treatment and no-treatment phases of a single-subject intervention study. The graphed data are then carefully analyzed for temporal patterns of change through visual inspection of level, slope, trend, and variability within and across treatment and no-treatment conditions. Thus, visual-graphic analysis is used as a primary means of judging the clinical significance of findings. Appropriate statistical analyses should also be used to confirm visual observations and rule out sources of interpretative bias (Borckardt et al, 2008; Fisher et al, 2003).

### Experimental Phases

**Baseline Phase**   The baseline, or A phase, of a single-subject experiment is the pretreatment period of testing used to establish level of performance before intervention takes place. Multiple assessments over time are necessary to determine the level and stability of responding before treatment occurs. A minimum of three and, ideally, five or more baseline test sessions are required to assess any trends in baseline data (Kratochwill et al, 2010). It is particularly important to demonstrate that pretreatment performance is stable during baseline. Obviously, a trend toward improvement in performance during baseline would provide evidence that the targeted behavior was already improving before treatment occurred, and this would make it difficult to demonstrate that the intervention was responsible for the observed change in performance. An important assumption in single-subject research is that performance during baseline is the best predictor of future performance if treatment did not occur. Thus, a long and stable rate of baseline performance serves as a standard against which subsequent treatment effects can be evaluated.

**Treatment Phase**   Similar to the baseline phase, intervention sessions occur during the treatment, or B phase, at regular intervals, generally several times per week. This helps ensure that there are sufficient data to examine patterns of change over time and to monitor the possible influence of extraneous factors that may be influencing performance. Investigators also take care to ensure that the same tasks and stimuli used to examine baseline performance are also administered as the outcome variable during the treatment phase of single-subject studies. This allows a direct comparison of performance during the pretreatment baseline testing and the treatment phase. Given the high value placed on analysis of graphed data by single-subject researchers, it is important to be explicit about the criteria to determine the length of baseline and treatment phases.

A priori decisions about when to begin or end treatment help to avoid inadvertent bias that may occur when researchers terminate phases (Kearns, 1992, 2000). Similar to clinical practice, the length of a treatment phase is often based on how long it takes to reach a preestablished performance criterion rather than being based on an arbitrary number of treatment sessions.

### Design Options

Although case studies continue to proliferate in the aphasia literature, it is worth reiterating that even the most careful case studies cannot be used to determine if a treatment is efficacious. Despite superficial similarities to single-subject research designs, case studies do not include the experimental controls necessary to rule out the influence of extraneous variables, such as pharmacology or other concurrent interventions, on an individual. Consequently, case studies cannot reveal whether or not a treatment being observed is responsible for any improvements seen in a patient's performance.

This is not to denigrate the value of case study observations for describing rare disorders, noting apparent correlations between brain behavior relationships, and identifying areas for future experimental study, as we discuss later in this chapter. It is important to note, however, that case studies alone do not inform us about whether a treatment "works" (i.e., is efficacious or effective). Clinicians cannot, therefore, use observations from case studies as support for evidence-based interventions.

The emphasis in this chapter is on presenting basic principles of single-subject designs and analysis techniques to serve as a foundation for clinician-scientists who wish to improve their skills as consumers of research. Although a comprehensive review of single-subject experimental research is beyond the scope of this chapter, excellent sources are available for a more in-depth coverage of this topic (Hayes et al, 1999; Kazdin, 1982, 2010; Kennedy, 2005; McReynolds & Kearns, 1983).

The type of single-subject design chosen for a treatment study depends on the nature of the research question posed by the investigators (Kearns, 2000; Kratochwill et al, 2010). Relating general evaluations strategies to clinical research questions and single-subject designs helps organize the variety of experimental designs available. Kearns (1986, 2000) identifies four evaluation strategies:

1.  Treatment–no treatment comparisons

2.  Component assessment

3.  Successive level analysis

4.  Between-treatments comparisons

These strategies represent the range of issues that are evaluated using single-subject designs. The strategy names are self-explanatory. Design options are available for comparing the efficacy of treatment versus no-treatment (control) conditions, for evaluating the relative contribution of treatment components, for examining successive levels of treatment, and for comparing the power of two or more treatments. Although a variety of single-subject design options are available for examining these types of issues for communicatively impaired individuals, most are permutations of one of two prototypical designs: the *withdrawal* (or reversal designs) and *multiple baseline designs*. Understanding these designs provides a basis for understanding the more sophisticated designs as well as the use of combined designs to answer complex clinical questions.

Again, referencing the aphasia literature as an example, it should be noted that relatively few *reversal* or *withdrawal* studies have been published (Kearns & Salmon, 1984; Renvall, Laine, & Martin, 2005). Multiple baseline designs are by far the most prevalent single-subject designs used to investigate aphasia treatments. A clear understanding of these designs will provide clinician-scientists with a strong foundation for analyzing and interpreting the aphasia treatment research and developing evidence-based clinical interventions. Given the paucity of withdrawal designs in the aphasia literature, we will only briefly describe these options. An example is provided for the more common multiple baseline designs, and it will serve as the basis for discussing the steps used to analyze single-subject research (Raymer et al, 2001; Renvall et al, 2005).

**Withdrawal and Reversal Designs**   Although they are the prototypical single-subject designs, relatively few reversal or withdrawal designs have been published in the aphasiology literature (Kearns & Salmon, 1984; Raymer et al, 2001; Renvall et al, 2005). The primary reason for this is that experimental control with these designs requires that treatment effects be reversed (returned to baseline) following a successful intervention. This reversal is often examined by simply withdrawing treatment and returning to baseline phase to determine if treatment effects are transient once the active intervention phase is terminated. Reversal designs are a more complicated variant of this approach in which the experimenter actively manipulates the target of treatment to "force" a reversal of the treatment effect (Kearns & Salmon, 1984).

Obviously many behaviors of interest to clinical aphasiologists, such as language and cognition, are not readily reversible once improvement has occurred as a result of treatment. Thus, a primary consideration in using or evaluating these designs is whether or not the therapeutic effect can be reversed. Despite the obvious limitations of withdrawal and reversal designs for our clinical science, a basic understanding of these options is essential for comprehending the nature of achieving experimental control with single–subject designs.

The basic format for withdrawal is the straightforward "A-B-A" design, in which a period of baseline testing (A) is followed by an intervention phase (B), and, once the treatment criteria are met, a final baseline testing (A) phase. Renvall and colleagues (2005) used an A–B–A design to study the effects of contextual priming in a patient with anomia. They speculated that contextual priming treatment would be effective but that, when treatment was withdrawn in the second baseline phase, the effects of treatment would not be maintained. Their results supported this hypothesis.

The classic format for a withdrawal design is the A-B-A-B design, in which the experiment ends on following a second treatment phase. In the A-B-A-B withdrawal design, a treatment is alternately applied and withdrawn across successive experimental phases, to determine if changes in the target behavior are clearly associated with the presence or absence of treatment. The advantages of adding a second treatment phase to the basic A-B-A design sequence is that this enhances the opportunity to demonstrate experimental control by replicating the treatment effect for the individuals under study. In addition, it could be argued that terminating a study following an active treatment phase gives participants the best opportunity to benefit from the intervention.

A convincing demonstration of treatment efficacy is apparent when the target of treatment is stable during baseline pretesting (A), there is an immediate and obvious effect of treatment (improvement) during the intervention phase (B), followed by a clear decrease in performance to near pretreatment levels when treatment is withdrawn (A), and a replication of the treatment effect following the reintroduction of intervention during the final (B) phase of an A-B-A-B study.

Raymer and her colleagues (2001) used an A-B-A-B withdrawal design to study the effects of the drug bromocriptine on the verbal fluency of a patient with crossed nonfluent aphasia. The design involved five sessions of baseline testing of the person with aphasia's verbal fluency prior to intervention (A), followed by a 3-week treatment phase (B) in which the drug bromocriptine was administered in doses increasing to 20 mg per day, followed by a second, 2-month baseline (A) phase in which the drug was withdrawn, and then a second treatment (B) phase in which the drug was readministered to the patient. The researchers also monitored the patient's verbal fluency for a period of time after the study and after the drug was again withdrawn. Although the effects of the drug on verbal fluency did not reverse during the withdrawal phases, the authors had incorporated other experimental controls that allowed them to conclude that long-lasting verbal fluency improvements were a result of the drug treatment for their patient.

As the previous examples demonstrate, withdrawal designs provide a powerful means of examining the efficacy of a single treatment for individuals. Visual–graphic analysis of individual performance over time during baseline and treatment conditions can be used to establish the efficacy of an intervention. An idealized graph of hypothetical data from a single-subject A-B-A-B study is presented in **Fig. 14.1** to demonstrate this process.

For the clinician–scientist examining these hypothetical data, there are several factors that would indicate that the treatment was primarily responsible for improvements in the subject's target behavior. First, prior to intervention, during the initial baseline (A phase, sessions 1 to 7), the individual with aphasia produced a consistently low and fairly stable (5 to 15% correct) rate of the target behavior. One would assume that if no treatment is introduced, the same low level of performance would continue. With the introduction of the treatment phase (B phase, sessions 8 to 14), there was an obvious and immediate increase (improvement) until a preestablished criterion was met (90% correct; session 14). Looking at the data across the first two phases, it is obvious that there is a dramatic difference in the level, slope, and trend of the data before (A) and after the introduction of treatment (first arrow). With the withdrawal of active treatment (A phase, sessions 15 to 21), it is apparent that the individual's performance deteriorated until it approximates the original baseline level of responding. Comparing the treatment (B1) and withdrawal phases (A2), it is again apparent that there is a fairly obvious and dramatic difference in the level, slope, and trend of the data. Finally, reintroduction of treatment in the final phase (B2 phase, sessions 22 to 28) of the study replicated the initial finding that improvement was immediate and continued throughout the second treatment

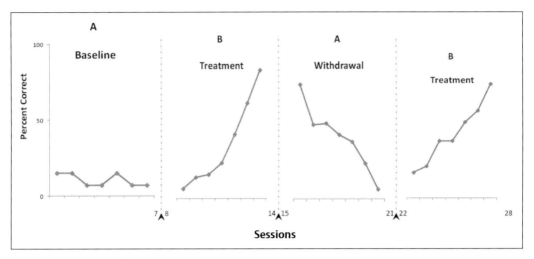

**Fig. 14.1**   Hypothetical illustration of A-B-A-B withdrawal data.

phase. Thus, following a stable, pretreatment baseline, it is clear that there is a close correlation between the introduction or removal of treatment, shown in the arrow in **Fig. 14.1**, and change in the communication behavior being treated.

One could conclude that a visual inspection of the graph of this subject's performance during this hypothetical study supports the conclusion that treatment was efficacious for this individual. Replication of this data pattern with other individuals with aphasia would further strengthen the believability of this conclusion. A similar process of visual analysis is used to analyze and interpret data from other types of SSEDs including multiple baseline designs, the most prevalent design used to examine aphasia treatment efficacy. This flexible and common design strategy is discussed below.

**Multiple Baseline Designs**   Single-subject withdrawal designs are used to determine treatment efficacy by applying treatment to a single behavior, such as verbal fluency, and then withdrawing treatment. By contrast, experimental control is established for multiple baseline designs by staggering treatment across behaviors (different treatment targets), subjects, or settings. Variants of multiple baseline designs, including the multiple-probe and changing-criterion design, are also available to examine questions relating to steps in a treatment sequence and the acquisition of gradually acquired behaviors (Kazdin, 1982, 2010; Kennedy, 2005; McReynolds & Kearns, 1983; Simmons-Mackie, Kearns, & Potechin, 2005; Thompson, 2006). For both withdrawal and multiple baseline designs, within- and across-phase analysis of data patterns and observations of change in the dependent (treatment) variable associated with the presence or absence of active treatment are used to judge experimental control and determine if treatment is effective.

Like their withdrawal counterparts, multiple baselines are ideally suited for examining treatment efficacy questions. These designs have also been widely used to examine generalization issues and important theoretical questions in aphasiology (Kiran & Thompson, 2003; Kiran, Sandberg, & Sebastian, 2011; Thompson & Shapiro, 2007). The most common type of multiple baseline is the across-behaviors design. With this design a single form of treatment is examined by applying it to two functionally related target behaviors within the same individual. Multiple-baseline across-behaviors designs require an assumption that treatment of one behavior could conceivably affect others in the sequence. That is, all behaviors being studied should have equal susceptibility to extraneous influences and have a reasonable probability of being affected by the treatment under study.

With the multiple-baseline across-behaviors design, baselines are obtained for two or more similar but independent behaviors, and a single treatment is subsequently staggered across both. That is, a series of baseline probes is obtained for each of the target behaviors to establish baseline stability.

Following baseline testing, treatment is individually and sequentially applied to one target behavior at a time while baseline testing continues for the remaining untreated behaviors. After the criterion is met for the first target behavior, treatment is sequentially applied to the remaining behaviors. Baseline testing continues for target behaviors not undergoing treatment. This type of design was applied in the case example we discuss later in this chapter.

Experimental control is established when it can be shown that untreated behaviors remain relatively stable and unchanging until treatment is directly applied to that target behavior. When treatment does occur, there should be a visually obvious improvement in the behavior being treated as evidenced by a change in the level, slope, and trend of the graphed data. As with the withdrawal designs, there should be a marked difference between performance data graphed for baseline and treatment conditions; a contrasting pattern must be replicated for each behavior treated in the study. Thus, data from the baseline assessment phase should be stable and relatively unchanging, whereas data from the treatment phase should document immediate and obvious improvement in the targeted behaviors. Within-subject replication of the treatment effect is crucial for establishing treatment efficacy in a multiple-baseline across-behaviors design, and across-subject replication further establishes the believability of the findings. One obvious advantage of multiple-baseline designs is that a reversal of the treatment effect is not required to establish control and demonstrate efficacy. These designs, therefore, are much more practical for examining the efficacy of treatments for non-reversible target behaviors having to do with language and cognition.

Thompson, Kearns, and Edmonds (2006) examined the effectiveness of a cuing hierarchy for facilitating improvements in word retrieval for an individual with anomic aphasia. They employed a multiple-baseline across-behaviors design to examine the efficacy, generalization, and maintenance of their intervention. In this study the design called for baseline assessment of four lists of nouns that were matched according to spoken and written frequency of occurrence. The subject's pretreatment ability to name the four sets of words was assessed on four separate occasions during the initial baseline period. Following baseline testing, a word retrieval intervention was sequentially applied to the word lists (the "behaviors" in the multiple-baseline design) and generalization of improved naming ability was examined to the untrained word lists. The data from this study are displayed in **Fig. 14.2**.

The important points for our current discussion pertain to the graphic display of the data and how a visual inspection of **Fig. 14.2** supports the authors' conclusion that the cuing hierarchy used in this study was primarily responsible for improvement in the subject's word retrieval ability on the treated word lists. The four word lists that served as the "behaviors" in this multiple-baseline across-behaviors design are labeled A1 through B2 on the graph. The number of sessions conducted during the study is displayed across the bottom of the graph, and the percent correct naming on the word lists is displayed along the left side of the graph. The graph displays time series data for each of the phases of the study: baseline (A), treatment (B), and maintenance (A)—the final data panel on the right.

Visual inspection of the baseline data for each of the word lists reveals that this individual with anomic aphasia consistently produced approximately 20% of the words correctly from each list prior to treatment; see **Fig. 14.2** (baseline, A phase). In addition, the variability in the percent correct responding was fairly minimal across the baseline session. Based on these observations, one could conclude that the baseline was stable. In other words, prior to treatment this individual with aphasia demonstrated significant difficulty retrieving and producing the words on the lists, and there was no indication that his ability to do so was improving over time. Examination of the treatment phase shows that each time intervention was sequentially applied to the four word lists, there was a visually obvious treatment effect for training (B phase). Importantly, the treatment effect was specific to the list being trained, and there was minimal improvement evident for the untrained lists that remained at baseline. Thus, when treatment was applied to the first list, there was no discernable improvement in the individual's performance on the remaining lists for which baseline testing continued (i.e., lists A2, B1, and B2). Similarly, each time treatment was conducted for the subsequent word lists, there was essentially no discernible improvement in the subject's ability to produce the remaining untreated word lists. The finding that treatment effects are specific to the word list being

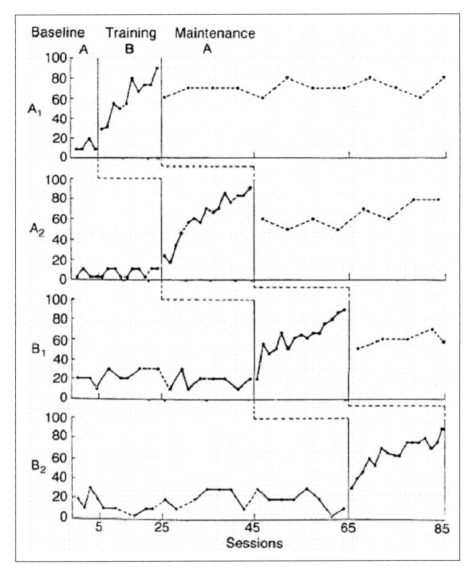

**Fig. 14.2**    Percent correct naming for a patient with anomic aphasia on word lists A1, A2, B1, and B2. [From Thompson, C. K., Kearns, K. P., & Edmonds, L.A. (2006). An experimental analysis of acquisition, generalization, and maintenance of naming behavior in a patient with anomia. *Aphasiology, 20,* 1226–1244. Reprinted by permission of Psychology Press.]

trained while untrained control items (the remaining untrained word lists) remain stable is the basis for demonstrating experimental control with a multiple-baseline across-behaviors designs. Notably, a treatment effect was replicated four times within this individual with aphasia. Thus, there were obvious improvements in the percentage of accurately named words associated with treatment as compared with baseline for each of the four word lists.

It should be apparent that the process of visual inspection of single-subject research findings can be enormously helpful for clinician-scientists who want to improve their ability to critically analyze and adopt new treatments into their EBP. Moreover, the visual inspection process is similar regardless of the type of single-subject design being reviewed. Within- and across-phase visual-graphic

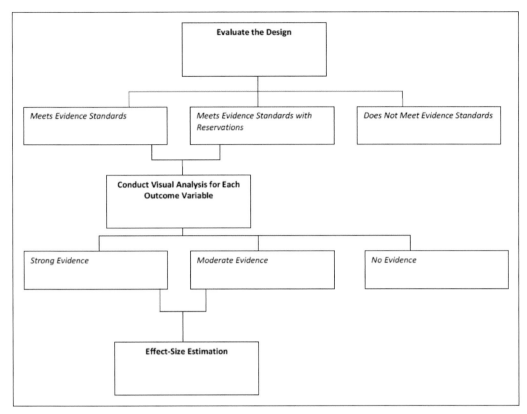

**Fig. 14.3**    Process for evaluating single-subject designs and assessing strength of evidence. [From U.S. Department of Education, Institute of Education Sciences, What Works Clearinghouse. (2010, June). *Single-Case Design Technical Documentation (Version 1.0).* http://www.whatworks.ed.gov.]

analysis is based on a careful inspection of the level of performance (e.g., percent correct), the trend in data over time (stable, increasing, or decreasing performance), the range and variability in the data, overlap across phases, and the consistency of the data pattern across adjacent and similar phases.

The process of visual–graphic inspection has recently been disused and codified by an expert panel for the What Works Clearinghouse (Kratochwill et al, 2010). This expert panel provides a step-by-step approach to the visual–graphic approach to evaluating single-subject treatment research. In addition, Kratochwill et al (2010) discuss standards for evaluating evidence from single-subject research, shown in **Fig. 14.3**. Design standards are proposed to assess the internal validity of single-subject designs. Studies evaluated using these criteria are classified as follows:

1. Meets the standards

2. Meets the standards with reservations

3. Does not meet the standards

To fully meet the standards for a quality single-subject research design, the expert panel suggests that, at a minimum, the following criteria must be evident. First, the treatment (independent variable) must be actively manipulated by the investigator across three points in time or three different phases of the study (baseline, treatment). Thus, the label "experimental" in the term *single-subject experimental design.* Second, each dependent (outcome) variable must be measured over time, and reliability must be demonstrated for both the independent (treatment) and dependent (outcomes) variables. Third, in terms of the time series nature of these designs, the panel requires that a minimum of three or more data points be reported during each phase of an A-B-A-B reversal/withdrawal design, and five or more data points per phase for multiple baseline designs. This requirement is important for demonstrating that there are sufficient data to judge the reliability of apparent trends. In general, it is important to provide a sufficient sample of data for visual inspection of the results of an intervention study.

A related criterion used to assess the internal validly is that there must be a clear demonstration of inter-rater reliability by two or more individuals for a sample of 20% or more of the sessions conducted during each phase of a study. This standard is essential for ensuring that appropriately trained observers arrive at the same scores and conclusions while independently viewing a subject's performance. This requirement helps to ensure that the experimenter objectively applies the criteria for determining how to score a subject's response. Careful operational definitions of how to score a subject's response are crucial for demonstrating interobserver reliability. Of course, minimal acceptable levels of inter-rater agreement must be met to be convincing.

It is also crucial that experimenters fully and accurately follow all steps in a treatment program, and that all subjects in a treatment study receive the intervention as intended. Thus, an evaluation of treatment integrity, or the degree to which interventions are performed as specified, is another standard that must be demonstrated for single-subject research studies that fully meet the standards proposed by Kratochwill et al (2010). Unfortunately, very few published single-subject aphasia treatment studies meet this standard.

In addition to *design standards* that assess the internal validity of single-subject research, Kratochwill et al (2010) also discuss *evidence standards* to assess the overall strength of evidence for a treatment effect that has met the design standards. They categorize studies as providing strong evidence, moderate evidence, or no evidence of a treatment effect. To be classified as strong evidence, there need to be three or more "points of proof" of treatment effectiveness across three periods of time. In other words, convincing demonstrations of an effect through visual-graphic analysis of level, trend, variability, immediacy of the effect, across-phases differences, data overlap, and consistency of patterns of across similar phases. As noted in our discussion of single-subject withdrawal and multiple baseline designs, there should be clear and repeated evidence that there is a distinction in performance between baseline and intervention phases, and there should also be a visually obvious effect on performance each time treatment is applied or withdrawn during a study. Again, within- and across-subject replication of a treatment effect is the key to establishing the believability of single-subject research findings. Further confidence in the strength of the evidence is proved when effect size estimates are provided (Beeson & Robey, 2006) or appropriate statistical procedures are used to confirm the conclusions from a visual inspection of the data (Borckardt et al, 2008; Fisher et al, 2003).

Tate and colleagues (2008) developed and evaluated the Single-Case Experimental Design (SCED) Scale to help assess methodological quality and assist with critical appraisal of the literature. This rating scale also formalizes the process for evaluating single-subject research and provides a useful tool for clinicians interested in becoming better consumers of the single-subject treatment literature.

## ♦ Clinician-Scientist Collaboration

The principles of data collection and knowledge of SSEDs can be used not only to inform research consumers but also to assist with clinical accountability. Clinicians are seldom in a position to carefully design a single-subject experiment to evaluate treatment efficacy, as a truly experimental study requires time, design sophistication, and resources that are not typically available in the clinical setting. Without core SSED elements, including operational definitions, reliability, and experimental control, clinical studies inevitably are observational case studies. However, clinicians can adopt SSED principles, including the use of time series data and graphic analysis of treatment results, for clinical accountability purposes. The following discussion and example of a case study demonstrates how clinical accountability may be enhanced by adopting components of SSEDs.

## Case Reports and Case Studies

Case reports and case studies with descriptive observations and empirical data have been used in the behavioral and medical sciences for centuries to describe the clinical characteristics and novel treatment approaches for interesting or rare diseases and disorders (Petrusa & Weiss, 1982). Returning to examples from the aphasia literature, a classic example of the influence a case report can have on a field of study is Paul Broca's (1861) description of two patients with the disorder *aphemia* (later termed aphasia) and its association with damage to the third left frontal convolution, now known as Broca's area. A few years later, Carl Wernicke (1874), a German neurologist, produced detailed case reports of patients with language comprehension deficits following damage to the left posterior temporal gyrus, now known as Wernicke's area. Since the publication of Broca's and Wernicke's case reports, countless studies across a century and a half of neurology and aphasiology literature, using increasingly rigorous scientific methods, have tested the observations of aphasia localization that stem from these early case reports.

Case reports continue to have an elemental place in the study of neurogenic communication disorders. For example, case reports can be found in the contemporary literature to describe the cognitive, communicative, and anatomical changes that occur in progressive speech and language disorders (Gorno-Tempini, Murray, Rankin, Weiner, & Miller, 2004), the use of new technologies in treating individuals with chronic aphasia (Naeser et al, 2010), and the use of experience sampling method to measure psycho-emotional variables in an individual with aphasia (Fitzgerald-DeJean, Rubin, & Carson, 2012). Although case studies are not "experimental," in these examples, the authors identify key findings that warrant further consideration in research studies. There is a well-demonstrated utility of case reports and case studies in spurring further scientific discovery; however, critics caution that these reporting methods are of limited utility in clinical decision making because the findings are only relevant to the case being reported and cannot be generalized to the population (Hoffman, 1999); thus, the data from case reports should be interpreted with caution.

Although the results of case reports cannot be generalized to the population, they are an integral step in scientific discovery and in the development of novel treatments for speech and language disorders. Robey and Schultz (1998) describe an adaptation of the five-phase, universal model for treatment outcomes research. References to the five-phase model are discussed elsewhere in this text (see Chapters 1, 2, and 12). In this model, each phase of research targets specific objectives, which build upon observations and data from the previous phase and guides the design and development of studies in the subsequent phases. These phase-related objectives may be accomplished using a variety of research designs. In phase I, the objectives are to determine the potential therapeutic effect of a treatment, develop the treatment protocol, and determine the safety of the procedure (Robey & Schultz, 1998). Among the various research methods employed in this phase, case studies play an important role, because they identify a potential therapeutic effect of a novel treatment or a modification of an existing treatment that might warrant further study and refinement. In phase II, the protocol and independent variables that need to be controlled are defined, and then the intervention is administered to selected subjects or a targeted clinical population. The selection of the appropriate subjects for this intervention may be based on clinical expertise or a theoretical construct. The empirical data from the case study may be used to inform the development or refinement of the treatment protocol and the outcome measures that are then applied in subsequent phases. As authors have stated in other chapters, the five-phase model for treatment outcomes research is a useful roadmap for systematic analysis of the efficacy, effectiveness, and efficiency of interventions. Case studies may make an important contribution to this process.

In addition to the development of treatment data, case studies play a role in EBP. EBP is generally referenced in the context of clinical decision making based on an integration of the best (least biased) research evidence from the treatment outcomes literature, clinical expertise, and the values of the patient (Sackett, Richardson, Rosenberg, & Haynes, 2000). As discussed above, case studies can contribute to the research evidence by identifying a promising intervention procedure. The process for engaging in EBP has been described as follows:

1. Develop the clinical question.

2. Search for related research evidence.

3. Appraise the validity, strength, and relevance of the evidence.

4. Apply evidence to clinical practice.

5. Evaluate the outcome of the intervention in a population or individual.

The last two steps in this process require that the clinician carefully plan the implementation of the treatment and employ a mechanism for evaluating the patient's success. Data on the patient's ability to perform the behaviors targeted in treatment at baseline, during treatment probes, and after treatment tasks are completed may be collected by borrowing methods found in single-subject research designs described above (e.g., multiple-baseline design, changing-criterion design, etc.). The resulting *clinical* data can provide a validation of the clinical decision making, or the lack of a validation can inform the clinician-scientist of the need to alter the course of treatment.

## Case Report Methods

There are two main types of case study reports: retrospective and prospective. In a *retrospective* case report, the clinician abstracts existing data of interest from the patient's medical record to report on the assessment, diagnosis, treatment outcome, or full management of the patient (Green & Johnson, 2006). In a *prospective* case report, the clinician identifies the opportunity to develop a case report, such as a rarely occurring condition, and carefully selects the tools that will be needed to collect the necessary data for the report (Green & Johnson, 2006). In both scenarios, a case is appropriate for reporting only if it adds new information or insight to the literature. That is, it describes a new or unique feature of a disorder or disease; it describes a new assessment, treatment, or management plan for the disorder or disease; or it provides negative evidence of a prevailing theory.

To accomplish these purposes, case reports follow a structure that includes a clear introduction, a description of methods and results, and a discussion. In the introduction, pertinent background information related to the case should be provided that highlights the unique nature of the case and its contribution to the literature. In the methods section, the specific details of the case, including patient history, assessment, treatment protocol, and outcome measures, should be described so that other providers or researchers can evaluate the clinical decision making. This will permit the reader to judge the overall validity of the results and discussion (Green & Johnson, 2006). If the case study report is intended to evaluate the outcome of a novel intervention, or test the effectiveness of an intervention that has been reported, then single-subject research methods are advantageous.

### Integrating Single-Subject Experimental Designs into Clinical Practice: An Example

The following case report was presented at an ASHA convention (de Riesthal, 2007). It describes a treatment that was implemented for an individual with aphasia who was seen in an outpatient clinical setting under typical clinical conditions. The data used in the report were drawn from clinical records examined retrospectively after the patient was discharged from treatment. The intervention employed in the clinic was a modification of a published treatment protocol. The protocol was amenable to a type of single-subject multiple baseline.

The patient, H.R., was a 61-year-old, right-handed man, with a severe nonfluent aphasia (Western Aphasia Battery AQ = 15.6) subsequent to an infarction of the majority of the left middle cerebral artery (MCA) distribution. At the time he was referred for outpatient treatment, he was 12-months post–onset of aphasia. His spontaneous speech consisted primarily of variations on the recurring stereotypy "yes, yes, yes, no, no." He was stimulable for some single-word utterances with sentence completion or repetition. He had a moderate-severe coexisting apraxia of speech (AOS). His auditory comprehension was significantly impaired, but a relative strength compared with verbal expression. He was able to hold a pen/pencil in his left hand and copy letters and words.

Due to transportation issues, H.R. was able to attend only one therapy session each week. This limited treatment options to those whose intensity could be maximized by home practice or caregiver training. One such option, Copy and Recall Treatment (CART), was a writing treatment designed to improve single-word writing in individuals with severe aphasia by strengthening and improving access to the graphemic representations of treated words (Beeson, Rising, & Volk, 2003). The treatment program consists of individual sessions and homework assignments that include repetitive copying tasks targeting selected words.

The therapeutic effect of CART on single-word writing performance in individuals with severe aphasia has been demonstrated in the intervention literature (Beeson, Hirsch, & Rewega, 2002). Beeson and colleagues (2003) further refined the treatment protocol and provided data for the selection of potential ideal candidates for the treatment. All participants had a severe aphasia and were 2 to 7 years post-onset. Four of the eight participants with aphasia reached criterion (80% accuracy) for each of the targeted five-word sets. Post-hoc analyses indicated these participants demonstrated a relatively preserved semantic system, adequate processing of visual information, and the ability and willingness to complete the daily homework. Moreover, these participants demonstrated the ability to recall the target words in the first two treatment sessions. The authors suggest that these factors, including assessment of performance in a trial of CART, are good predictors of a participant's success in developing a corpus of meaningful written words with the treatment.

In addition to written naming performance, Beeson et al (2003) reported that several participants demonstrated improvement on verbal repetition tasks, spoken naming of treatment picture stimuli, and spontaneous use of spoken words in communicative interactions. These unexpected changes were attributed to the participants' exposure to the spoken name of each item during treatment and the vocal rehearsal of the target words during the writing task.

Based on H.R.'s demographic information and aphasia assessment, his clinician concluded he possessed several characteristics similar to the successful participants in the Beeson et al (2003) study of CART. In particular, H.R. demonstrated adequate processing of visual information and the ability and willingness to complete homework, and he was able to learn to write several of the words after a trial of the CART program. It was felt that successful performance in the CART program would provide H.R. with a corpus of functional words for communication with his family. Moreover, it was hypothesized that modifying the CART protocol by introducing vocal rehearsal of the target words into the treatment would improve the patient's ability to write and speak each word.

### Intervention

H.R. participated in weekly treatment sessions and completed homework 6 days per week. The CART and spoken repetition protocol during the weekly treatment session was designed in an 8-step protocol, as follows:

1. A picture card was presented and the clinician said the target word.

2. H.R. repeated the word. The word was provided up to three times for repetition.

3. If H.R. was not successful, he was provided with a sentence completion cue.

4. H.R. wrote the word on lined paper.

5. If the word was spelled correctly, the next picture card and corresponding word was presented.

6. If the word was spelled incorrectly, the printed word was provided and H.R. copied it three times.

7. H.R. then attempted to write the word without the printed cue.

8. If incorrect, steps 6 and 7 were repeated.

As part of this treatment protocol, H.R. was provided with daily homework sheets to practice writing. The homework sheets contained a picture of each target word and the printed target word. Six lines were provided beside each picture to copy the word. H.R. was also provided with a dedicated alternative and augmentative communication device, MessageMate 40™ (http://www.words-plus .com/website/products/hand/mm.htm) to practice saying the target words. The buttons on the MessageMate 40 contained pictures of the five target words. H.R.'s correct production of each word was recorded on each button. The homework protocol was as follows:

1. H.R. pressed the button for the target item and attempted to repeat the word.

2. H.R. copied the target word six times.

3. After practicing the set of words, H.R. completed a self-assessment for each word without the printed word.

H.R. maintained a stable baseline for each of the four sets of five words in both spoken and written naming, shown in **Fig. 14.4**. In written naming, he reached criterion (80% accuracy over two sessions) for the written productions of the target words in two to five treatment sessions. He was able to maintain 60 to 100% accuracy after treatment for each of the four sets. In spoken naming, he was unable to say the target label for more than two items in any of the four sets of five words. His wife reported that he was not consistent in performing the repetition task during homework trials, but there was an increase in his use of writing to communicate at home and the production of spoken words.

The data from the case report suggest that CART is successful in improving single-word writing for individuals with severe aphasia even with fewer copying attempts during homework. The number of copying attempts needed may vary among individuals with aphasia. The data did not demonstrate improvement in the ability to say the target words with the added repetition component. This is likely related to the participant's inconsistent practice and the presence of AOS. However, the inclusion of a repetition component in CART using auditory and visual stimuli to elicit a correct production warrants further investigation.

The results of the case study report led to the development of a prospective study of CART and spoken repetition in individuals with severe aphasia and a coexisting AOS. In this subsequent study, Ball, de Riesthal, Breeding, and Mendoza (2011) included audio-video clips of a clinician saying the target words to improve the likelihood of successful repetition during home practice. All of the participants improved in their ability to write the words targeted in treatment. However, although the audio-video clips improved the participants' ability to engage in the home practice repetition program, none made significant progress in spoken word production of the target stimuli.

## ♦ Conclusion and Future Directions

This chapter discussed the important contributions that are made by SSED and the case-based perspective. Key SSED principles and research designs were outlined, and an example of a case report integrating SSED methods to evaluate the effect of an intervention program was provided. It was argued that knowledge of these designs will allow clinicians to become better consumers of the treatment literature, and judicious adaptation of SSED principles may also improve clinical accountability. Essential strategies for determining the quality and validity of single-subject research findings were presented so that clinicians are better able to decide whether published interventions are truly evidenced based. Given the prevalence of SSED for studying novel interventions, particularly in disorder populations that are highly variable, such as aphasia, practitioners who become knowledgeable about them will be positioned to become clinician-scientists. Trends in the application of EBP are increasingly embracing the "clinician experience" perspective, and systematic reviews and

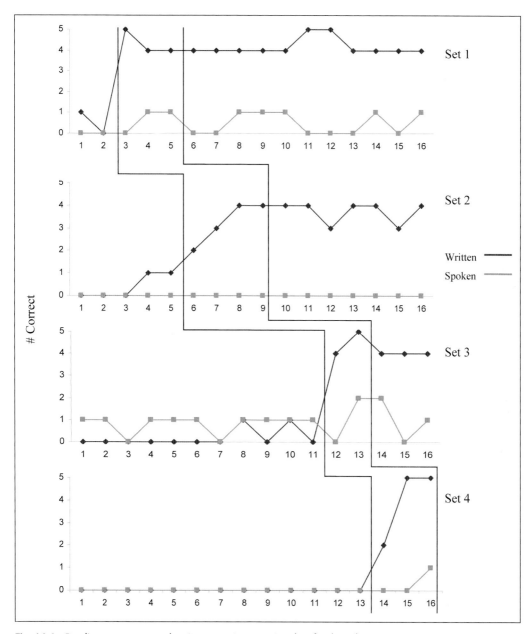

**Fig. 14.4**  Baseline, treatment, and maintenance intervention data for the aphasic patient H.R.

meta-analyses are increasingly including studies using single-subject experimentation as legitimate forms of efficacy research. With the drift toward practice-based evidence in studies of clinical outcomes in health care, there is a growing interest in the sort of real-world, applied evidence that SSED provides. Thus, improving one's ability to evaluate treatment SSED research and applying these methods to clinical data collection will contribute to reducing uncertainty in our clinical decision making (Dollaghan, 2007; Kamhi, 2011) and, ultimately, allow us to provide the best possible care for the patients we serve.

# References

Bailey, J. S., & Burch, M. R. (2002). *Research methods in applied behavior analysis*. Thousand Oaks, CA: Sage

Ball, A., de Riesthal, M., Breeding, C., & Mendoza, D. (2011). Modified ACT and CART for severe aphasia. *Aphasiology, 25,* 836–848

Barlow, D. H., Hayes, S. C., & Nelson, R. O. (1984). *The scientist practitioner: Research and accountability in clinical and educational settings*. New York: Pergamon Press

Barlow, D. H., & Hersen, M. (1984). *Single-case experimental designs: Strategies for studying behavioral change* (2nd ed.). Boston: Allyn & Bacon

Beeson, P. M., Hirsch, F. M., & Rewega, M. A. (2002). Successful single-word writing treatment: Experimental analysis of four cases. *Aphasiology, 16,* 473–491

Beeson, P. M., Rising, K., & Volk, J. (2003, Oct). Writing treatment for severe aphasia: who benefits? *Journal of Speech, Language, and Hearing Research: JSLHR, 46,* 1038–1060

Beeson, P. M., & Robey, R. R. (2006, Dec). Evaluating single-subject treatment research: lessons learned from the aphasia literature. *Neuropsychology Review, 16,* 161–169

Borckardt, J. J., Nash, M. R., Murphy, M. D., Moore, M., Shaw, D., & O'Neil, P. (2008, Feb-Mar). Clinical practice as natural laboratory for psychotherapy research: a guide to case-based time-series analysis. *The American Psychologist, 63,* 77–95

Broca, P. (1861). Remarques sur le siege de la faculté du langage articulé; suivies d'une observation d'aphemie. *Bulletin des Societés Anatomiques de Paris, 6,* 330–357

Connell, P. J., & Thompson, C. K. (1986, Aug). Flexibility of single-subject experimental designs. Part III: Using flexibility to design or modify experiments. *Journal of Speech and Hearing Disorders, 51,* 214–225

De Riesthal, M. (2007). *Changes in written and spoken naming with a modified CART program*. Poster presented at the 2007 American Speech-Language-Hearing Association Convention, Boston

Dollaghan, C. (2007). *The handbook for evidence-based practice in communication disorders*. Baltimore, MD: Brookes

Fisher, W. W., Kelley, M. E., & Lomas, J. E. (2003, Fall). Visual aids and structured criteria for improving visual inspection and interpretation of single-case designs. *Journal of Applied Behavior Analysis, 36,* 387–406

Fitzgerald-DeJean, D. M., Rubin, S. S., & Carson, R. L. (2012). An application of the experience sampling method to the study of aphasia: A case report. *Aphasiology, 26,* 234–251

Gorno-Tempini, M. L., Murray, R. C., Rankin, K. P., Weiner, M. W., & Miller, B. L. (2004). Clinical, cognitive and anatomical evolution from nonfluent progressive aphasia to corticobasal syndrome: A case report. *Neurocase, 10,* 426–436

Green, B. N., & Johnson, C. D. (2006, Summer). How to write a case report for publication. *Journal of Chiropractic Medicine, 5,* 72–82

Hayes, S. C., Barlow, D. H., & Nelson-Gray, R. O. (1999). *The scientist practitioner: Research and accountability in the age of managed care* (2nd ed.). Needham Heights, MA: Allyn & Bacon

Hoffman, J. R. (1999, May). Rethinking case reports. *The Western Journal of Medicine, 170,* 253–254 [Editorial]

Kamhi, A. G. (2011). Balancing certainty and uncertainty in clinical practice. *Language, Speech, and Hearing Services in Schools, 4,* 59–64

Kazdin, A. E. (1982). *Single-case research designs: Methods for clinical and applied settings*. New York: Oxford University Press

Kazdin, A. E. (2004). Evidence-based treatments: Challenges and priorities for practice and research. In B. J. Burns & K. E. Hoagwood (Eds.), *Child and Adolescent Psychiatric Clinics of North America, 13,* 923–940

Kazdin, A. E. (2010). *Single-case research designs: Methods for clinical and applied settings* (2nd ed.). New York: Oxford University Press

Kearns, K. P. (1986). Within-subject experimental designs: II. Design selection and arrangement of experimental phases. *Journal of Speech and Hearing Disorders, 51,* 204–214

Kearns, K. P. (1992). Methodological issues in aphasia treatment research: A single-subject perspective. In J. A. Cooper (Ed.), *Aphasia treatment: Current approaches and opportunities* (Monograph 93–3424, pp. 7–16). Bethesda, MD: NIH-NIDCD

Kearns, K. P. (2000). Single-subject experimental designs and treatment research. In L. J. Gonzalez-Rothi, B. Crosson, & S. E. Nadeau (Eds.), *Aphasia and Language: Theory to Practice* (pp. 421–441). New York: Guilford Publications

Kearns, K. P., & Salmon, S. J. (1984, May). An experimental analysis of auxiliary and copula verb generalization in aphasia. *Journal of Speech and Hearing Disorders, 49,* 152–163

Kennedy, C. H. (2005). *Single-case designs for educational research*. Boston: Allyn & Bacon

Kiran, S., Sandberg, C., & Sebastian, R. (2011, Aug). Treatment of category generation and retrieval in aphasia: effect of typicality of category items. *Journal of Speech, Language, and Hearing Research: JSLHR, 54,* 1101–1117

Kiran, S., & Thompson, C. K. (2003, Aug). The role of semantic complexity in treatment of naming deficits: training semantic categories in fluent aphasia by controlling exemplar typicality. *Journal of Speech, Language, and Hearing Research: JSLHR, 46,* 773–787

Kratochwill, T. R., Hitchcock, J., Horner, R. H., Levin, J. R., Odom, S. L., Rindskopf, D. M., et al. (2010). *Single-case designs technical documentation*. What Works Clearinghouse Web site: http://ies.ed.gov/ncee/wwc/pdf/wwc_scd.pdf

McReynolds, L. V., & Kearns, K. P. (1983). *Single-subject experimental designs in communicative disorders*. Austin, TX: Pro-Ed

McReynolds, L. V., & Thompson, C. K. (1986, Aug). Flexibility of single-subject experimental designs. Part I: Review of the basics of single-subject designs. *Journal of Speech and Hearing Disorders, 51,* 194–203

Meline, T., & Wang, B. (2004, Aug). Effect-size reporting practices in AJSLP and other ASHA journals, 1999-2003. *American Journal of Speech-Language Pathology, 13,* 202–207

Naeser, M. A., Martin, P. I., Lundgren, K., Klein, R., Kaplan, J., Treglia, E., et al. (2010, Mar). Improved language in a chronic nonfluent aphasia patient after treatment with CPAP and TMS. *Cognitive and Behavioral Neurology, 23,* 29–38

Olsen, L. O., Aisner, D., & McGinnis, J. M., (Eds.). (2007). *IOM roundtable on evidence-based medicine*. National Academies Press. http://www.nap.edu/catalog/11903.html

Petrusa, E. R., & Weiss, G. B. (1982, May). Writing case reports: an educationally valuable experience for house officers. *Journal of Medical Education, 57,* 415–417

Raymer, A. M., Bandy, D., Adair, J. C., Schwartz, R. L., Williamson, D. J., Gonzalez Rothi, L. J., et al. (2001, Jan). Effects of bromocriptine in a patient with crossed nonfluent aphasia: a case report. *Archives of Physical Medicine and Rehabilitation, 82,* 139–144

Renvall, K., Laine, M., & Martin, N. (2005, Nov). Contextual priming in semantic anomia: a case study. *Brain and Language, 95,* 327–341

Robey, R. R. (1994, Nov). The efficacy of treatment for aphasic persons: a meta-analysis. *Brain and Language, 47,* 582–608

Robey, R. R. (1998, Feb). A meta-analysis of clinical outcomes in the treatment of aphasia. *Journal of Speech and Hearing Research, 41,* 172–187

Robey, R. R., & Schultz, M. C. (1998). A model for conducting clinical-outcome research: an adaptation of the standard protocol for use in aphasiology. *Aphasiology, 12,* 787–810

Rosenbek, J. C., LaPointe, L. L., & Wertz, R. T. (1989). *Aphasia: A clinical approach.* Austin, TX: Pro-Ed

Sackett, D. L., Richardson, W. S., Rosenberg, W., & Haynes, R. B. (2000). *Evidence-based medicine: How to practise and teach EBM.* London: Churchill-Livingstone

Simmons-Mackie, N. N., Kearns, K. P., & Potechin, G. (2005). Treatment of aphasia through family member training. *Aphasiology, 19,* 583–593

Tate, R. L., McDonald, S., Perdices, M., Togher, L., Schultz, R., & Savage, S. (2008, Aug). Rating the methodological quality of single-subject designs and n-of-1 trials: introducing the Single-Case Experimental Design (SCED) Scale. *Neuropsychological Rehabilitation, 18,* 385–401

Thompson, C. K. (2006, Jul-Aug). Single subject controlled experiments in aphasia: the science and the state of the science. *Journal of Communication Disorders, 39,* 266–291

Thompson, C. K., & Kearns, K. P. (1991). Analytical and technical directions in applied aphasia analysis: The Midas touch. In T. E. Prescott (Ed.), *Clinical Aphasiology* (Vol. 19, pp. 41–54). Minneapolis, MN: BRK Publishers

Thompson, C. K., Kearns, K. P., & Edmonds, L. A. (2006). An experimental analysis of acquisition, generalization, and maintenance of naming behavior in a patient with anomia. *Aphasiology, 20,* 1226–1244

Thompson, C. K., & Shapiro, L. P. (2007, Feb). Complexity in treatment of syntactic deficits. *American Journal of Speech-Language Pathology, 16,* 30–42

Wernicke, C. (1874). *Der aphasische Symptomenkomplex.* Breslau, Poland: Cohn, Weigert

# 15

# Meta-Analysis in Outcomes Research

*Katerina Ntourou and Mark W. Lipsey*

## ♦ Chapter Focus

This chapter describes the principles and methods of meta-analysis to provide the reader with a framework that will promote basic understanding of the logic of meta-analysis and facilitate critical appraisal of published meta-analyses. The authors discuss the role of meta-analysis in speech-language pathology. Though many different kinds of empirical research findings can be addressed with meta-analysis, the application of meta-analysis is of particular importance to the evaluation of outcomes research in speech and language.

## ♦ Introduction

> Science is cumulative, and scientists must cumulate scientifically!
>
> —Sir Iain Chalmers

Unlike their long history in disciplines such as psychology and educational research, systematic reviews and meta-analyses were relatively sparse in the field of communication sciences and disorders until the late 1990s (Robey & Dalebout, 1998). Typically, the task of combining and summarizing existing scientific evidence to derive conclusions regarding a specific topic had been undertaken in narrative reviews. However, over the last decade, with a steady transformation to a field that is evidence-based (Justice, 2008) and the fast accumulation of new scientific knowledge, the use of systematic reviews and meta-analyses has increased considerably.

A systematic review is "a review of a clearly formulated question that uses systematic and explicit methods to identify, select, and critically appraise relevant research, and to collect and analyze data from the studies that are included in the review" (Cochrane Collaboration, 2011). The statistical methods of meta-analysis may or may not be used to analyze and summarize the results of the included studies. Thus, *meta-analysis* is not synonymous with *systematic review,* but rather is a form of systematic review that can be used when summary data from included studies are available, sufficient, and amenable to statistical analysis. Our focus in this chapter is meta-analysis, also referred to as *quantitative research synthesis*.

# ♦ Overview of Meta-Analysis

### What Is Meta-Analysis?

According to Gene V. Glass, one of pioneers in the field of quantitative research synthesis,

> Meta-analysis refers to the analysis of analyses. . . . The statistical analysis of a large collection of analysis results from individual studies for the purpose of integrating the findings. It connotes a rigorous alternative to the casual, narrative discussions of research studies which typify our attempts to make sense of the rapidly expanding research literature. (Glass, 1976, p. 3)

Thus, meta-analysis refers to the statistical synthesis of quantitative findings from a set of empirical studies to provide answers to research questions. Meta-analysis involves techniques that may also be able to reconcile and explain inconsistencies in the findings across studies by identifying "moderator" variables that can account for different results from different studies.

In meta-analysis the units of observation are individual *studies* rather than participants. To allow meaningful numerical combination and comparison of findings from the studies, these findings are converted to a common standardized metric, generally referred to as *effect size*. For intervention studies, an effect size represents the difference between the treatment and control groups on a particular outcome variable in a form that allows comparison across studies even when the outcome was measured in different ways. In the simplest form of meta-analysis, an effect size estimate is computed for each study and then an overall mean is calculated for the set of effect sizes from all the studies. Not all effect sizes have equal influence on that overall mean, however. The effect sizes are weighted to account for the fact that those from some studies are based on much larger participant samples than those from other studies.

To illustrate the basic elements of meta-analysis, we summarize the findings from a group of studies that compared the receptive vocabulary ability of young children who stutter (CWS) with that of children who do not stutter (CWNS) (Ntourou, Conture, & Lipsey, 2011). **Figure 15.1** shows the effect size for each study in a chart known as a *forest plot*.

In this forest plot, each row except the last represents the *effect size* on receptive vocabulary for an individual study. The last row shows the *mean effect size*. In this example, the effect size is *Hedges's g*, that is, an effect size that represents the difference between two means in standard deviation units. In each row the study authors are shown on the left, followed by the calculated effect size, the *p* value, and the sample size. The effect size for each study is then plotted with a circle whose location reflects the direction and the magnitude of the effect. In this example, negative effect sizes indicate higher receptive vocabulary skills for children who do not stutter (CWNS) compared with children who stutter (CWS), whereas positive effect sizes indicate greater skills for CWS. The size of the circle represents the weight assigned to the effect size when computing the mean effect size. Thus, in this example, studies with a relatively large sample size (e.g., Coulter, Anderson, & Conture, 2009) are weighted more heavily than studies with a small sample size (e.g., Murray & Reed, 1977).

As illustrated in the last row of the forest plot depicted in this figure, the estimate of the mean effect size was –0.52 and statistically significant ($p <.01$). This means that, on average, in this meta-analysis the CWS subjects scored about half a standard deviation below CWNS subjects on tests of receptive vocabulary.

### Meta-Analysis versus Narrative Review

Even though narrative reviews and meta-analyses share the common goal of summarizing, integrating, and interpreting the research evidence on a given topic, they are quite distinct entities (e.g., Borenstein, Hedges, Higgins, & Rothstein, 2009; Glass, McGaw, & Smith, 1981; Rosenthal & DiMatteo, 2001). Traditional narrative reviews are typically vague about the procedures used to search the literature and the criteria for identifying relevant studies. Systematic reviews and quantitative meta-analyses, by contrast, are expected to involve a systematic, rigorous, and comprehensive search of all

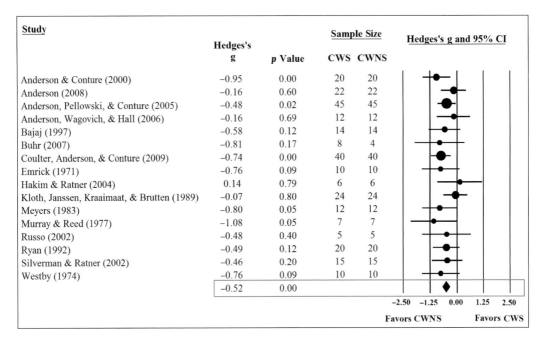

**Fig. 15.1** Effect sizes from individual studies and overall mean effect size for receptive vocabulary skills in young children who do (CWS) and do not (CWNS) stutter. CI, confidence interval. [Adapted from Ntourou, K., Conture, E. G., & Lipsey, M. W. (2011, Aug). Language abilities of children who stutter: a meta-analytical review. American Journal of Speech-Language Pathology, 20, 163–179.]

available research (published and unpublished) and to describe the search procedure in replicable detail. Furthermore, systematic reviews apply an explicit, predetermined set of rules for study inclusion and exclusion, for assessment of studies' methodological quality, and for assigning either a weight or a classification level to each study.

Also, narrative reviews often rely heavily on the statistical significance reported for each study to evaluate and compare studies, summarize findings, and ultimately reach conclusions (such as that the intervention reviewed was or was not effective). This often takes the form of "vote counting" where the reviewer counts how many results are statistically significant in one direction, how many are neutral (not statistically significant), and how many are statistically significant in the other direction (Cook et al, 1992) and generates conclusions about the literature based on the category with the most counts.

This way of appraising the cumulative results of research studies has been criticized (Hedges & Olkin, 1980). Statistical significance depends in part on the magnitude of the effect observed in a study, but is also heavily dependent on the size of the sample (Lipsey, 1990). That means that studies with small samples may find quite large effects that are not statistically significant, whereas, conversely, studies with very large samples may obtain statistical significance for small effects that have little practical significance. Much of the impetus behind the development of meta-analysis was the desire to find a more appropriate way to characterize the nature and magnitude of research findings.

The effect size statistics used in meta-analysis index the direction and magnitude of research findings without regard to sample size. It is only when aggregating those effect sizes that sample size comes into the picture to give more weight to effect sizes estimated from larger samples. Consider again the meta-analysis results presented in **Fig. 15.1**. The between-group differences were statistically significant in only five of the 16 studies, which could lead a reviewer using the vote counting procedure to the erroneous conclusion that there is no difference in the receptive vocabulary skills of young children who do and do not stutter. However, the direction of the effect favored children who do not stutter in 15 of the 16 studies and the magnitude of the mean effect showed a convincing and statistically significant difference in that direction. Meta-analytical techniques permitted aggregation of the results of all the studies, which in turn aggregated over their combined sample sizes. This procedure thus took full account of the direction and magnitude of the individual effect sizes and the total number of participants across all the studies, which finally led to a statistically significant mean effect size.

Another advantage of working with effect sizes in meta-analysis is that it facilitates examination of differences in study findings that are related to substantive methodological differences in the characteristics of the participant samples, settings, or interventions represented. Such *moderator analyses* are difficult to accomplish and elucidate from narrative reviews, and conclusions are likely to be erroneous if based on simple vote counting techniques. Meta-analysis thus has some distinctive advantages for explaining and reconciling inconsistencies in the research findings on a given topic.

For these and other reasons, narrative reviews generally lack the objectivity, rigor, transparency, and comprehensiveness of systematic reviews and thus often prove inadequate for reaching confident conclusions about the research findings at issue (for a more comprehensive discussion, see Borenstein et al, 2009).

## Criticisms of Meta-Analysis

Although meta-analysis has been accepted by many as a valuable tool for synthesizing research findings, it has not been without criticism (Bailar, 1997; Sharpe, 1997). Specifically, meta-analyses have been criticized for summarizing results from studies that vary, sometimes greatly, in their samples, methods, measures, and intervention variants (often referred to as the "apples and oranges" problem). This is recognized in meta-analysis as a real problem if the results of diverse studies are simply summarized by mean effect sizes. However, contemporary meta-analysis generally pays close attention to any heterogeneity in the findings of the studies examined and attempts to account for it in the statistical analysis. This can be done, for example, by coding relevant study characteristics into the meta-analytic database and including those variables in the analysis to investigate their relationships with the effect sizes derived from the different studies.

Another related criticism is often referred to as the "garbage in, garbage out" problem. According to this criticism, meta-analyses too often include studies that are not of the very highest methodological standards or that vary considerably in their methodological quality. Including methodologically flawed studies clearly can introduce biases into the results of a meta-analysis and consequently lead to misleading conclusions. However, there are no methodologically perfect studies and it is often not apparent which shortcomings will potentially or actually bias the results. Meta-analysts address this problem in several ways. The most straightforward way is to employ threshold criteria that exclude studies that fall below some explicit methodological standard. Setting that standard too high, however, can exclude studies that provide useful information and thus limit the scope and generalizability of the meta-analysis results.

A complementary approach to the hazards posed by methodologically flawed studies used by meta-analysts is to treat it as an empirical issue. Meta-analysts typically code key methodological characteristics of the studies included and then statistically explore the variation in methodological quality among the studies and its relationship to the study findings (Detsky et al, 1992). Studies with methodological characteristics that are clearly biasing can then be omitted from the final analysis or, if the distortions are not too great, statistically controlled in the analysis.

A third common concern about meta-analysis is one that has arisen largely from meta-analysts themselves. This is the problem of publication bias—the tendency for published studies to show stronger effects than unpublished studies (Song, Eastwood, Gilbody, Duley, & Sutton, 2000). This is presumed to stem from filters applied by authors, reviewers, and journal editors that are prejudiced against findings that are not statistically significant. Given that published studies are, obviously, more available than unpublished ones, any review—systematic, meta-analytic, or narrative—is thus likely to underrepresent studies that found small or null effects, and therefore may reach overly optimistic conclusions. In characteristic fashion, meta-analysts attempt to address this problem as systematically as possible. First, it is standard procedure to make concentrated efforts to identify and include unpublished studies along with the published ones and to attend to any differences in their findings. Also, techniques have been developed in meta-analysis to assess the potential for publication bias and estimate its influence on the mean effect sizes in any analysis (Duval & Tweedie, 2000; Rothstein, Sutton, & Borenstein, 2005).

## Basic Steps in Meta-Analysis

In view of the proliferation of meta-analyses conducted in our field, it may be useful to provide an overview of meta-analysis methods (**Fig. 15.2**) to enable readers to critically appraise published meta-analyses. For a more detailed review, interested readers are referred to Borenstein et al, 2009; Higgins & Green, 2011; Hunter & Schmidt, 2004; Lipsey & Wilson, 2001; Moher et al, 1999; Robey & Dalebout, 1998.

A good meta-analysis begins with well-defined research questions, represents the pertinent literature in as comprehensive and unbiased manner as possible, and uses appropriate methods to extract and analyze data from the source studies.

Like any other type of research, meta-analysis should start with clearly formulated research questions. This stage is critical because it establishes the scope of the meta-analysis by defining the population of interest, the empirical relationships to be examined, the choice of the appropriate effect size statistic, and so forth. Also, the nature of the questions yields a preliminary specification of the kinds of studies that will be relevant, which is then elaborated in the next step in the review process—specification of study inclusion and exclusion criteria. If the purpose of the meta-analysis is to assess the effectiveness of indirect stuttering treatment for young children who stutter, for instance, the meta-analyst would establish *a priori* explicit and detailed criteria about the nature of the studies to be included. These would identify acceptable *research designs* (e.g., randomized-controlled trials only, randomized-controlled trials and quasi-experimental designs, single subject studies), *outcome measures* (e.g., percent syllables stuttered, stuttering severity index, parental judgment), *types of treatment* (e.g., detailed criteria for considering a reported treatment as "indirect"), *participant populations* (e.g., age range of participants), and other factors (e.g., dates when the research was conducted, language of publication) (Meline, 2006).

As mentioned earlier, the validity of meta-analytic results can be compromised if the sample of studies included in the analysis is not representative of the population of studies actually conducted on the topic of interest (Hopewell, McDonald, Clarke, & Egger, 2003). Thus, the reviewer should attempt to identify and retrieve every eligible study, published or unpublished, by conducting an extensive and comprehensive literature search. This is typically done using several different approaches including key word searches in electronic databases, hand searching of journals and conference abstracts, contacting investigators in the field, and reviewing the reference lists of all relevant articles identified as well as those of any previous reviews and meta-analyses (Dennis & Abbott, 2006).

Once the sample of eligible studies is retrieved, an effect size estimate is calculated for each study and each outcome construct of interest. For example, if the purpose of the meta-analysis is to investigate changes in receptive and expressive language skills measured pre– and post–language intervention, the meta-analyst would calculate two effect sizes for each study: one for the expressive language construct and one for receptive language construct outcomes. Thus, the type of effect size statistic used is guided by the nature of the research questions (e.g., assessing group differences versus examining the covariation of two or more variables) and the type of the outcome measures (i.e., continuous versus categorical). For a detailed description of the different effect size statistics and the ways to compute them from the statistics available in the primary studies, see Ellis (2010, pp. 10–15) and Lipsey and Wilson (2001, pp. 34–72 and 172–207).

In addition, other information pertaining to study methods, measures used, participant samples, intervention characteristics, and the like is extracted by using a carefully designed coding scheme. This is an important step because even though computation of average effect sizes is a key element

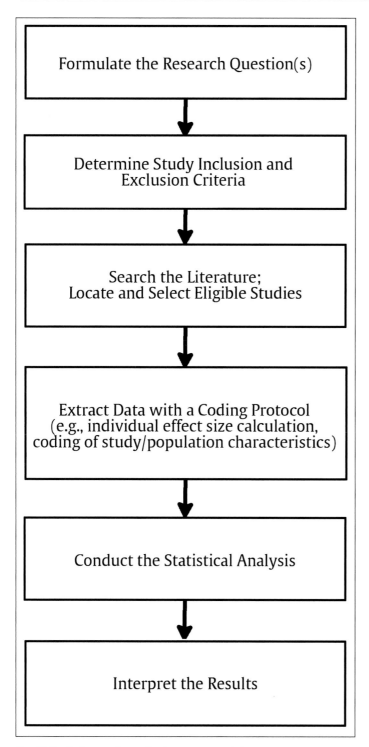

**Fig. 15.2** Basic steps in conducting a meta-analysis.

of meta-analysis, another important strength of this type of research synthesis is that it provides an opportunity to investigate the effect of moderating variables on the findings of the studies in the meta-analysis. As an example, consider the meta-analysis on the effects of Botox treatment in adductor spasmodic dysphonia (Boutsen, Cannito, Taylor, & Bender, 2002). Although, Boutsen et al reported that Botox treatment resulted in an overall moderate improvement, they also found that the degree of this improvement depended on such factors as measurement type. Specifically, effect sizes from physiological measures and patient self-ratings were higher than those from perceptual and acoustic measures.

After a set of statistically independent effect sizes from the primary studies is available (i.e., with each study contributing only one effect size from the same participant sample), the distribution of effect sizes is described in terms of *central tendency* and *variability*. The most commonly used estimate of central tendency is the weighted mean effect size, whereby each effect size is weighted by the inverse of its sampling variance. The sampling variance is based on the sample size used in the study, and weighting by its inverse gives greater weight to effect sizes from larger studies than those from smaller studies. Statistical *confidence intervals* may be placed around the mean effect size to indicate the precision of the estimate and a statistical significance test can be applied to determine if it is reliably greater than zero.

Another important step in the analysis is to determine whether the effect sizes obtained from the various studies estimate a common population effect size. This is done by examining the variation in the distribution of effect sizes with a statistical test for heterogeneity. For effect sizes to be heterogeneous, they must vary more than expected based on the sampling error stemming from the sample sizes of the contributing studies. Effect size heterogeneity must then be accounted for in the analysis and can be explored in relation to variation in study characteristics (moderator analyses).

Finally, the meta-analyst summarizes the key findings, provides an interpretation of the mean effect sizes in terms of their statistical and practical significance, identifies possible sources of heterogeneity, and evaluates whether there was enough evidence and statistical power to conclusively answer the original research questions.

## ◆ Evaluating and Interpreting Meta-Analysis Results

The interpretation of meta-analysis results, similar to other types of research, can sometimes be difficult and controversial. This section highlights several issues pertinent to the evaluation and interpretation of meta-analysis results to assist critical consumers of research to independently and objectively appraise findings and draw appropriate conclusions.

The credibility and validity of meta-analysis results depend heavily on the quality of the included primary studies. In cases where methodological quality does not constitute a study inclusion criterion, one would expect the primary studies to vary greatly, with some being of high quality (e.g., randomized-controlled trials) and others having weaknesses (e.g., observational studies, use of unreliable measures). In such cases, the consumer should assess whether the meta-analyst formally addressed this issue by conducting moderator analyses to explore whether the main findings vary as a function of methodological quality. However, this might not be feasible when the sample of included studies is small and thus the power to detect the effect of moderating variables on key results is insufficient, or when the majority of primary studies is of low quality. Nevertheless, readers need to be aware of the role of methodological quality in meta-analyses results, recognize possible limitations, and handle the interpretation of the findings accordingly.

Also, even though meta-analyses have greater statistical power to reject the null hypothesis and detect effects than do any of the individual studies included in the meta-analysis, nonsignificant findings should be interpreted with caution (Durlak & Lipsey, 1991; Kazdin & Bass, 1989). Results that fail to reach statistical significance might accurately describe the true state of affairs but may also be attributed to limited statistical power due to factors such as a small number of included studies, small sample size within the included studies, and a high degree of between-study variability.

Furthermore, mean effect sizes should not be interpreted solely on the basis of tests of statistical significance but also in terms of their meaning and practical significance. For example, consider for a moment a hypothetical statistically significant effect size of 0.35 standard deviation difference between preschool-age children receiving language therapy and those in the control group. What does this mean effect size really mean? Is it small or large? Were the effects of this type of therapy clinically significant?

Undoubtedly, these questions are fundamentally harder to address than those related to statistical significance. Thus, more often than not, researchers focus their discussion primarily on the *p* values and devote less attention to the real-world significance of their findings. However, it is essential that we confront the challenge of making informed judgments about the statistical results of meta-analyses.

One way to interpret mean effect sizes is to convert them into some other more intuitively comprehensible and readily understood metric. For example, in the aforementioned hypothetical example, knowing that the mean on the outcome variable for children in the treatment group was 0.35 standard deviation units greater than that for children in the control group may not mean much to the practicing clinician. A more effective way to communicate this finding might be to convert that effect size back into the original metric of one of the more familiar outcome measures. For example, if a well-known norm-referenced language test with a mean score of 100 and a standard deviation of 15 was used in several of the studies as the language outcome measure, we would know that, on average, the children who received therapy exhibited the equivalent of a 5.25 increase in their score on this measure (0.35 × 15) compared to their untreated peers. Even though this conversion was relatively easy, translating different effect sizes into less straightforward original metrics is feasible (see Lipsey & Wilson, 2001, pp. 148–151).

Another approach to interpret effect size results was proposed by Cohen (1988) and involves expressing effect sizes in terms of overlapping distributions of scores. Cohen proposed using a statistic called $U_3$ that describes the percentage of scores in the treatment group that is greater than the mean in the control group. For example, Ntourou and colleagues (2011) reported a mean effect size of −0.52 on receptive vocabulary skills for preschool-age children who stutter (CWS) compared with that of their fluent peers (CWNS). For this effect size, $U_3$ is approximately equal to 70, which means that 70% of the CWNS group exceeded the mean receptive vocabulary score of the CWS group versus only 50% of those in the CWS group (by definition for a symmetrical distribution).

Another common, but problematic, practice is to evaluate the magnitude of effect sizes in terms of the benchmarks introduced by Cohen (1988). Cohen reported that, across the range of effect sizes that appeared in social science studies, an effect size of about 0.20 or lower represented a relatively small effect, one of about 0.50 represented a moderate effect, and one about 0.80 or larger represented a large effect. However, interpreting effect sizes independently of their context and relying on Cohen's criteria is less than optimal and should serve only as a last resort (Thompson, 2002). Or, as Cohen (1988) himself suggested, "The terms 'small,' 'medium,' and 'large' are relative, not only to each other, but to the area of behavioral science or even more particularly to the specific content and research method being employed in any given investigation" (p. 25).

Some researchers argue that, rather than blindly applying Cohen's criteria to judge the magnitude of the obtained effect sizes, it is preferable to interpret effect sizes in the context of empirical benchmarks (e.g., learning trajectories in the absence of intervention) that are relevant to the area of study, the outcome measures, and the population studied (Hill, Bloom, Black, & Lipsey, 2008). However, due to the scarcity of such established empirical criteria in many areas of research, Cohen's general guidelines remain the default frame of reference for many meta-analyses.

Interpreting the practical significance of effect sizes in conjunction with their statistical significance is clearly neither simple nor straightforward. Thus, scholars and consumers of research should be continuously encouraged and supported to explore new strategies to assess and interpret the practical meaning of statistical results.

## Meta-Analysis and Single-Subject Research

Although meta-analysis has been used extensively to integrate and synthesize empirical findings from group-design studies, there is ongoing discussion concerning optimal statistical methods for synthesizing results from single-subject designs. Some of the distinctive characteristics of single-subject data (e.g., serial dependency of observations, trends in the data) render the statistical analysis of single-subject results and the calculation of effect-size metrics challenging and controversial (West & Hepworth, 1991). However, given the importance of single-subject methodology in evidence-based practice (Horner et al, 2005) and the large number of single-subject treatment research studies conducted in fields such as speech-language pathology (McReynolds & Thompson, 1986; Robey, Schultz, Crawford, & Sinner, 1999; Schlosser, 2003), ongoing efforts have focused on determining appropriate quantitative methods for calculating effect-size estimates and synthesizing results from single-subject design studies (for a brief review of different effect-sizes, see Beretvas & Chung, 2008). These methods include, but are not limited to, a variation on Cohen's (1988) *d* statistic as calculated by Busk and Serlin (1992), the *percentage of non-overlapping data* (PND) (Scruggs, Mastropieri, & Casto, 1987), the *nonoverlap of all pairs* (NAP) (Parker & Vannest, 2009), the *percentage of data points exceeding the median* (PEM) (Ma, 2006), as well as regression-based approaches (Center, Skiba, & Casey, 1986). Even though uncertainty still surrounds effect size estimation methods for single-subject research designs, it is hoped that methodological research on meta-analytical techniques for single-subject design studies will continue to evolve.

## ◆ Meta-Analysis in Speech-Language Pathology

The growing recognition of the importance of evidence-based practice (EBP) in the field of communication sciences and disorders (Dollaghan, 2004; Johnson, 2006) has sparked increased interest in meta-analysis methodology as an objective and unbiased approach to quantitatively synthesizing available scientific evidence for clinicians and stakeholders alike. In the area of treatment research, meta-analyses abound across a broad range of clinical populations and interventions, such as behavioral treatments for stuttering (Herder, Howard, Nye, & Vanryckeghem, 2006), augmentative and alternative communication interventions (Millar, Light, & Schlosser, 2006; Schlosser & Lee, 2000), and interventions for dysphagia (Carnaby-Mann & Crary, 2007), among others. Despite their undisputed value in clinical research and EBP, published meta-analyses should not be idly considered as the "gold standard" in the absence of critical appraisal of their quality, which, as discussed previously in this chapter, depends on several different factors. Thus, in evaluating the results of meta-analyses, clinicians should carefully assess whether there is sufficient high-quality evidence to support strong conclusions regarding the effectiveness of interventions.

Although, in the field of speech-language pathology, quantitative research synthesis methodology has been predominantly used in treatment research, a limited number of meta-analyses have aggregated and statistically synthesized findings from basic research studies. For example, quantitative reviews have investigated the abilities of clinical populations, such as sustained attention skills in children with language impairment (Ebert & Kohnert, 2011), general aspects of development (e.g., association between otitis media and language development; Casby, 2001), accuracy of diagnostic tests (Dollaghan & Horner, 2011), and so forth. In recent years, the number of basic research meta-analyses has been slowly increasing, and such research endeavors should be further encouraged and supported given that they could advance our field in different ways. For example, such meta-analytic reviews could explain inconsistencies and divergent findings in the literature, contribute to theory development by empirically examining relations not studied in the original studies, and highlight empirical findings that no longer require replication.

The appendix, below, lists references for several meta-analyses conducted in the field of speech-language pathology. The reader should note that this list, which was compiled by searching PsycINFO and four different clearinghouses for meta-analyses published in English (as of July 1, 2011), is not exhaustive. The searched clearinghouses and organizations that either produce or provide links to systematic reviews and meta-analyses were (1) the American Speech-Language-Hearing Association's Compendium of EBP Guidelines and Systematic Reviews (www.asha.org/members/ebp/compendium), (2) the Cochrane Collaboration (www.cochrane.org), (3) the Campbell Collaboration (www.campbellcollaboration.org), and (4) the National Center for the Dissemination of Disability Research (www.ncddr.org).

Finally, even though meta-analysis methodology has proven to be a valuable research tool for summarizing and statistically integrating existing empirical evidence, it also has the potential to shape future research in our field. For example, through the detailed literature search and coding of the different characteristics of the included studies (e.g., type of intervention, type of treatment setting, severity of disorder, types of measurement, etc.), knowledge gaps can be detected and areas where further research is needed can be identified. Furthermore, meta-analysis highlights and illustrates the importance of replication, which, as other authors have noted, is urgently needed in our field (Muma, 1993). And last, meta-analysis encourages improved and transparent publication practices by stressing the importance of including a full set of descriptive statistics in primary studies, both to provide full documentation and to allow their use for effect size calculation.

## ◆ Conclusion and Future Directions

"Scientists have known for centuries that a single study will not resolve a major issue. Indeed, a small sample study will not even resolve a minor issue. Thus, the foundation of science is the cumulation of knowledge from the results of many studies" (Hunter, Schmidt, & Jackson, 1982, p. 10). One of the issues that policy makers, reimbursement agencies, service providers, and consumers of our services often ponder is treatment effectiveness: "What works and for whom?" "How important or meaningful are the effects of an intervention?" "What is the strength of the evidence?" This chapter has illustrated the role that meta-analysis can play in providing answers to these questions and generating research-based recommendations for clinical practice. Also, quantitative synthesis of basic research can further our understanding of developmental processes (such as attentional skills, language skills) in typical and clinical populations, as well as facilitate theory refinement and development. Lastly, meta-analysis can guide further research by highlighting gaps in empirical knowledge, identifying areas in need of further investigation, and posing new research questions based on the synthesized evidence. However, despite its various merits and advantages, meta-analysis is not a panacea, and the quality and validity of meta-analysis results depend greatly on the quality and quantity of the primary research as well as the manner in which the meta-analysis is conducted. Thus, one of the objectives of this chapter was to present the basic methodological features of quantitative research synthesis and to identify common threats to the validity to help consumers of research to critically appraise the conclusions reached from meta-analyses and their application to clinical practice.

# ♦ Appendix: Examples of Meta-Analyses Conducted in Different Areas of Speech-Language Pathology

## Autism

Bellini, S., Peters, J. K., Benner, L., & Hopf, A. (2007). A meta-analysis of school-based social skills interventions for children with autism spectrum disorders. *Remedial and Special Education, 28,* 153–162

Campbell, J. M. (2003, Mar-Apr). Efficacy of behavioral interventions for reducing problem behavior in persons with autism: a quantitative synthesis of single-subject research. *Research in Developmental Disabilities, 24,* 120–138

Flippin, M., Reszka, S., & Watson, L. R. (2010, May). Effectiveness of the Picture Exchange Communication System (PECS) on communication and speech for children with autism spectrum disorders: a meta-analysis. *American Journal of Speech-Language Pathology, 19,* 178–195

Lee, S. H., Simpson, R. L., & Shogren, K. A. (2007). Effects and implications of self-management for students with autism: a meta-analysis. *Focus on Autism and Other Developmental Disabilities, 22,* 2–13

Ospina, M. B., Krebs Seida, J., Clark, B., Karkhaneh, M., Hartling, L., Tjosvold, L., et al. (2008). Behavioural and developmental interventions for autism spectrum disorder: a clinical systematic review. *PLoS ONE, 3,* e3755 10.1371/journal.pone.0003755

Spreckley, M., & Boyd, R. (2009, Mar). Efficacy of applied behavioral intervention in preschool children with autism for improving cognitive, language, and adaptive behavior: a systematic review and meta-analysis. *Journal of Pediatrics, 154,* 338–344

Zhang, J., & Wheeler, J. J. (2011). A meta-analysis of peer-mediated interventions for young children with autism spectrum disorders. *Education and Training in Autism and Developmental Disabilities, 46,* 62–77

## Neuroimaging

Brown, S., Laird, A. R., Pfordresher, P. Q., Thelen, S. M., Turkeltaub, P., & Liotti, M. (2009, Jun). The somatotopy of speech: phonation and articulation in the human motor cortex. *Brain and Cognition, 70,* 31–41

Ferstl, E. C., Neumann, J., Bogler, C., & von Cramon, D. Y. (2008, May). The extended language network: a meta-analysis of neuroimaging studies on text comprehension. *Human Brain Mapping, 29,* 581–593

## Developmental Speech-Language Disorders

Ebert, K. D., & Kohnert, K. (2011, Oct). Sustained attention in children with primary language impairment: a meta-analysis. *Journal of Speech, Language, and Hearing Research: JSLHR, 54,* 1372–1384

Graf Estes, K., Evans, J. L., & Else-Quest, N. M. (2007, Feb). Differences in the nonword repetition performance of children with and without specific language impairment: a meta-analysis. *Journal of Speech, Language, and Hearing Research: JSLHR, 50,* 177–195

Kan, P. F., & Windsor, J. (2010, Jun). Word learning in children with primary language impairment: a meta-analysis. *Journal of Speech, Language, and Hearing Research: JSLHR, 53,* 739–756

Law, J., Garrett, Z., & Nye, C. (2004, Aug). The efficacy of treatment for children with developmental speech and language delay/disorder: a meta-analysis. *Journal of Speech, Language, and Hearing Research: JSLHR, 47,* 924–943

Nye, C., Foster, S. H., & Seaman, D. (1987, Nov). Effectiveness of language intervention with the language/learning disabled. *Journal of Speech and Hearing Disorders, 52,* 348–357

Roberts, M. Y., & Kaiser, A. P. (2011, Aug). The effectiveness of parent-implemented language interventions: a meta-analysis. *American Journal of Speech-Language Pathology, 20,* 180–199

Scruggs, T. E., Mastropieri, M. A., Forness, S. R., & Kavale, K. A. (1988). Early language intervention: A quantitative synthesis of single-subject research. *Journal of Special Education, 22,* 259–283

Strong, G. K., Torgerson, C. J., Torgerson, D., & Hulme, C. (2011, Mar). A systematic meta-analytic review of evidence for the effectiveness of the "Fast ForWord" language intervention program. *Journal of Child Psychology and Psychiatry, and Allied Disciplines, 52,* 224–235

van Kleeck, A., Schwarz, A. L., Fey, M., Kaiser, A., Miller, J., & Weitzman, E. (2010, Feb). Should we use telegraphic or grammatical input in the early stages of language development with children who have language impairments? A meta-analysis of the research and expert opinion. *American Journal of Speech-Language Pathology, 19,* 3–21

Whitehouse, A. J. O. (2010, Aug). Is there a sex ratio difference in the familial aggregation of specific language impairment? A meta-analysis. *Journal of Speech, Language, and Hearing Research: JSLHR, 53,* 1015–1025

## Augmentative and Alternative Communication

Millar, D. C., Light, J. C., & Schlosser, R. W. (2006, Apr). The impact of augmentative and alternative communication intervention on the speech production of individuals with developmental disabilities: a research review. *Journal of Speech, Language, and Hearing Research: JSLHR, 49,* 248–264

Schlosser, R. W., & Lee, D. L. (2000). Promoting generalization and maintenance in augmentative and alternative communication: A meta-analysis of 20 years of effectiveness research. *Augmentative and Alternative Communication, 16,* 208–226

## Neurogenic Language Disorders

Faroqi-Shah, Y. (2007, Sep). Are regular and irregular verbs dissociated in non-fluent aphasia? A meta-analysis. *Brain Research Bulletin, 74*, 1–13

Greener, J., Enderby, P., & Whurr, R. (2001). Pharmacological treatment for aphasia following stroke. *Cochrane Database of Systematic Reviews*, (4, Issue 4). CD000424. 10.1002/14651858.CD000424

Henry, J. D., & Beatty, W. W. (2006). Verbal fluency deficits in multiple sclerosis. *Neuropsychologia, 44*, 1166–1174

Henry, J. D., & Crawford, J. R. (2004, Apr). A meta-analytic review of verbal fluency performance following focal cortical lesions. *Neuropsychology, 18*, 284–295

Henry, J. D., & Crawford, J. R. (2004, Jul). Verbal fluency deficits in Parkinson's disease: a meta-analysis. *Journal of the International Neuropsychological Society, 10*, 608–622

Henry, J. D., & Crawford, J. R. (2004, Oct). A meta-analytic review of verbal fluency performance in patients with traumatic brain injury. *Neuropsychology, 18*, 621–628

Henry, J. D., Crawford, J. R., & Phillips, L. H. (2004). Verbal fluency performance in dementia of the Alzheimer's type: a meta-analysis. *Neuropsychologia, 42*, 1212–1222

Henry, J. D., Crawford, J. R., & Phillips, L. H. (2005, Mar). A meta-analytic review of verbal fluency deficits in Huntington's disease. *Neuropsychology, 19*, 243–252

Laws, K. R., Adlington, R. L., Gale, T. M., Moreno-Martínez, F. J., & Sartori, G. (2007, Sep). A meta-analytic review of category naming in Alzheimer's disease. *Neuropsychologia, 45*, 2674–2682

Robey, R. R. (1998, Feb). A meta-analysis of clinical outcomes in the treatment of aphasia. *Journal of Speech, Language, and Hearing Research: JSLHR, 41*, 172–187

Stroke Unit Trialists' Collaboration (2007). Organised inpatient (stroke unit) care for stroke. *Cochrane Database of Systematic Reviews*, (Issue 4), CD000197. 10.1002/14651858.CD000197.pub2

Zakzanis, K. K. (1999, Oct). The neuropsychological signature of primary progressive aphasia. *Brain and Language, 70*, 70–85

## Learning Disabilities/Literacy

Burns, M. K., & Wagner, D. (2008). Determining an effective intervention within a brief experimental analysis for reading: A Meta-analytic review. *School Psychology Review, 37*, 126–136

Gersten, R., & Baker, S. (2001). Teaching expressive writing to students with learning disabilities: A Meta-analysis. *Elementary School Journal, 101*, 251–272

Herrmann, J. A., Matyas, T., & Pratt, C. (2006, Aug). Meta-analysis of the nonword reading deficit in specific reading disorder. *Dyslexia (Chichester, England), 12*, 195–221

Kim, A. H., Vaughn, S., Wanzek, J., & Wei, S. (2004, Mar-Apr). Graphic organizers and their effects on the reading comprehension of students with LD: A synthesis of research. *Journal of Learning Disabilities, 37*, 105–118

Mol, S. E., Bus, A. G., de Jong, M. T., & Smeets, D. J. H. (2008). Added value of dialogic parent-child book readings: A Meta-analysis. *Early Education and Development, 19*, 7–26

Sénéchal, M., & Young, L. (2006). The effect of family literacy interventions on children's acquisition of reading from kindergarten to grade 3: A Meta-analytic review. *Review of Educational Research, 78*, 880–907

Swanson, H. L. (1999, Nov-Dec). Reading research for students with LD: a meta-analysis of intervention outcomes. *Journal of Learning Disabilities, 32*, 504–532

Swanson, H. L. (2001). Research on interventions for adolescents with learning disabilities: A meta-analysis of outcomes related to higher-order processing. *Elementary School Journal, 101*, 331–348

Swanson, H. L., & Hoskyn, M. (1998). Experimental intervention research on students with learning disabilities: A meta-analysis of treatment outcomes. *Review of Educational Research, 68*, 277–321

## Language Development

Casby, M. W. (2001). Otitis media and language development: A meta-analysis. *American Journal of Speech-Language Pathology, 10*, 65–80

Dollaghan, C. A., & Horner, E. A. (2011, Aug). Bilingual language assessment: a meta-analysis of diagnostic accuracy. *Journal of Speech, Language, and Hearing Research: JSLHR, 54*, 1077–1088

Leaper, C., & Smith, T. E. (2004, Nov). A meta-analytic review of gender variations in children's language use: talkative-ness, affiliative speech, and assertive speech. *Developmental Psychology, 40*, 993–1027

Roberts, J. E., Rosenfeld, R. M., & Zeisel, S. A. (2004, Mar). Otitis media and speech and language: a meta-analysis of prospective studies. *Pediatrics, 113*(3 Pt 1), e238–e248

Scott, K. A., Roberts, J. A., & Glennen, S. (2011, Aug). How well do children who are internationally adopted acquire language? A meta-analysis. *Journal of Speech, Language, and Hearing Research: JSLHR, 54*, 1153–1169

## Stuttering

Andrews, G., Guitar, B., & Howie, P. (1980, Aug). Meta-analysis of the effects of stuttering treatment. *Journal of Speech and Hearing Disorders, 45*, 287–307

Brown, S., Ingham, R. J., Ingham, J. C., Laird, A. R., & Fox, P. T. (2005, May). Stuttered and fluent speech production: an ALE meta-analysis of functional neuroimaging studies. *Human Brain Mapping, 25*, 105–117

Herder, C., Howard, C., Nye, C., & Vanryckeghem, M. (2006). Effectiveness of behavioral stuttering treatment: A Systematic review and meta-analysis. *Contemporary Issues in Communication Science and Disorders, 33*, 61–73

Ntourou, K., Conture, E. G., & Lipsey, M. W. (2011, Aug). Language abilities of children who stutter: a meta-analytical review. *American Journal of Speech-Language Pathology, 20*, 163–179

## Feeding/Swallowing

Bath, P. M. W., Bath, F. J., & Smithard, D. G. (2000). Interventions for dysphagia in acute stroke. *Cochrane Database of Systematic Reviews*, (2, Issue 4), CD000323. 10.1002/14651858.CD000323

Bessell, A., Hooper, L., Shaw, W. C., Reilly, S., Reid, J., & Glenny, A. M. (2011). Feeding interventions for growth and development in infants with cleft lip, cleft palate or cleft lip and palate. *Cochrane Database of Systematic Reviews*, (2, Issue 2), CD003315. 10.1002/14651858.CD003315.pub3

Carnaby-Mann, G. D., & Crary, M. A. (2007, Jun). Examining the evidence on neuromuscular electrical stimulation for swallowing: a meta-analysis. *Archives of Otolaryngology–Head and Neck Surgery, 133*, 564–571

Pinelli, J., & Symington, A. J. (2005). Non-nutritive sucking for promoting physiologic stability and nutrition in preterm infants. *Cochrane Database of Systematic Reviews*, (Issue 4), CD001071. 10.1002/14651858.CD001071.pub2

## Voice

Boutsen, F., Cannito, M. P., Taylor, M., & Bender, B. (2002, Jun). Botox treatment in adductor spasmodic dysphonia: a meta-analysis. *Journal of Speech, Language, and Hearing Research: JSLHR, 45*, 469–481

Ruotsalainen, J., Sellman, J., Lehto, L., & Verbeek, J. (2008, May). Systematic review of the treatment of functional dysphonia and prevention of voice disorders. *Otolaryngology–Head and Neck Surgery, 138*, 557–565

Whurr, R., Nye, C., & Lorch, M. (1998). Meta-analysis of botulinum toxin treatment of spasmodic dysphonia: a review of 22 studies. *International Journal of Language and Communication Disorders, 33*(Suppl), 327–329

## Cognitive Rehabilitation

Clare, L., Woods, R. T., Moniz Cook, E. D., Orrell, M., & Spector, A. (2003). Cognitive rehabilitation and cognitive training for early-stage Alzheimer's disease and vascular dementia. *Cochrane Database of Systematic Reviews*, (4, Issue 4), CD003260. 10.1002/14651858.CD003260

Kennedy, M. R., Coelho, C., Turkstra, L., Ylvisaker, M., Moore Sohlberg, M., Yorkston, K., et al. (2008, Jun). Intervention for executive functions after traumatic brain injury: a systematic review, meta-analysis and clinical recommendations. *Neuropsychological Rehabilitation, 18*, 257–299

Martin, M., Clare, L., Altgassen, A. M., Cameron, M. H., & Zehnder, F. (2011). Cognition-based interventions for healthy older people and people with mild cognitive impairment. *Cochrane Database of Systematic Reviews*, (Issue 1), CD006220. 10.1002/14651858.CD006220.pub2

Park, N. W., & Ingles, J. L. (2001, Apr). Effectiveness of attention rehabilitation after an acquired brain injury: a meta-analysis. *Neuropsychology, 15*, 199–210

Sitzer, D. I., Twamley, E. W., & Jeste, D. V. (2006, Aug). Cognitive training in Alzheimer's disease: a meta-analysis of the literature. *Acta Psychiatrica Scandinavica, 114*, 75–90

Woods, B., Spector, A. E., Jones, C. A., Orrell, M., & Davies, S. P. (2005). Reminiscence therapy for dementia. *Cochrane Database of Systematic Reviews*, (2, Issue 2), CD001120. 10.1002/14651858.CD001120.pub2

## Other

Cook, C. R., Gresham, F. M., Kern, L., Barreras, R. B., Thornton, S., & Crews, S. D. (2008). Social skills training for secondary students with emotional and/or behavioral disorders: A Review and analysis of the meta-analytic literature. *Journal of Emotional and Behavioral Disorders, 16*, 131–144

Deane, K., Whurr, R., Playford, E. D., Ben-Shlomo, Y., & Clarke, C. E. (2001). Speech and language therapy versus placebo or no intervention for dysarthria in Parkinson's disease. *Cochrane Database of Systematic Reviews*, (Issue 2), CD002812. 10.1002/14651858.CD002812

Leaper, C., & Ayres, M. M. (2007, Nov). A meta-analytic review of gender variations in adults' language use: talkativeness, affiliative speech, and assertive speech. *Personality and Social Psychology Review, 11*, 328–363

Smith, J., Forster, A., House, A., Knapp, P., Wright, J. J., & Young, J. (2008). Information provision for stroke patients and their caregivers. *Cochrane Database of Systematic Reviews*, (2, Issue 2), CD001919. 10.1002/14651858.CD001919.pub2

# References

Bailar, J. C., III. (1997, Aug). The promise and problems of meta-analysis. *New England Journal of Medicine, 337*, 559–561

Beretvas, S. N., & Chung, H. (2008). A review of single-subject design meta-analyses: Methodological issues and practice. *Evidence-Based Communication Assessment and Intervention, 2*, 129–141

Borenstein, M., Hedges, L. V., Higgins, J. P. T., & Rothstein, H. R. (2009). *Introduction to meta-analysis*. Chichester, UK: Wiley

Boutsen, F., Cannito, M. P., Taylor, M., & Bender, B. (2002, Jun). Botox treatment in adductor spasmodic dysphonia: a meta-analysis. *Journal of Speech, Language, and Hearing Research: JSLHR, 45*, 469–481

Busk, P. L., & Serlin, R. (1992). Meta-analysis for single case research. In T. R. Kratochwill & J. R. Levin (Eds.), *Single-case research design and analysis: New directions for psychology and education*. Hillsdale, NJ: Lawrence Erlbaum Associates

Carnaby-Mann, G. D., & Crary, M. A. (2007, Jun). Examining the evidence on neuromuscular electrical stimulation for swallowing: a meta-analysis. *Archives of Otolaryngology–Head and Neck Surgery, 133*, 564–571

Casby, M. W. (2001). Otitis media and language development: A meta-analysis. *American Journal of Speech-Language Pathology, 10*, 65–80

Center, B. A., Skiba, R. J., & Casey, A. (1986). A methodology for the quantitative synthesis of intra-subject design research. *Journal of Special Education, 19*, 387–400

Cochrane Collaboration. (2011). *Glossary.* http://www.cochrane.org/glossary/5#letters

Cohen, J. (1988). *Statistical power analysis for the behavioral sciences* (2nd ed.). Hillsdale, NJ: Lawrence Erlbaum Associates

Cook, T. D., Cooper, H., Cordray, D. S., Hartmann, H., Light, R. J., Louis, T. A., et al. (1992). *Meta-analysis for explanation.* New York: Russell Sage Foundation

Coulter, C., Anderson, J. D., & Conture, E. G. (2009). Childhood stuttering and dissociation across linguistic domains: Replication and extension. *Journal of Fluency Disorders, 34*, 257–278

Dennis, J., & Abbott, J. (2006). Information retrieval. Where's your evidence? *Contemporary Issues in Communication Sciences and Disorders, 33*, 11–20

Detsky, A. S., Naylor, C. D. O., O'Rourke, K., McGeer, A. J. L., L'Abbé, K. A., et al. (1992, Mar). Incorporating variations in the quality of individual randomized trials into meta-analysis. *Journal of Clinical Epidemiology, 45*, 255–265

Dollaghan, C. A. (2004, Sep-Oct). Evidence-based practice in communication disorders: what do we know, and when do we know it? *Journal of Communication Disorders, 37*, 391–400

Dollaghan, C. A., & Horner, E. A. (2011, Aug). Bilingual language assessment: a meta-analysis of diagnostic accuracy. *Journal of Speech, Language, and Hearing Research: JSLHR, 54*, 1077–1088

Durlak, J. A., & Lipsey, M. W. (1991, Jun). A practitioner's guide to meta-analysis. *American Journal of Community Psychology, 19*, 291–332

Duval, S., & Tweedie, R. (2000, Jun). Trim and fill: A simple funnel-plot-based method of testing and adjusting for publication bias in meta-analysis. *Biometrics, 56*, 455–463

Ebert, K. D., & Kohnert, K. (2011, Oct). Sustained attention in children with primary language impairment: a meta-analysis. *Journal of Speech, Language, and Hearing Research: JSLHR, 54*, 1372–1384

Ellis, P. D. (2010). *The essential guide to effect sizes: An introduction to statistical power, meta-analysis and the interpretation of research results.* New York: Cambridge University Press

Glass, G. V. (1976). Primary, secondary, and meta-analysis of research. *Educational Researcher, 5*, 3–8

Glass, G. V., McGaw, B., & Smith, M. L. (1981). *Meta-analysis in social research.* Newbury Park, CA: Sage Publications

Hedges, L. V., & Olkin, I. (1980). Vote-counting methods in research synthesis. *Psychological Bulletin, 88*, 359–369

Herder, C., Howard, C., Nye, C., & Vanryckeghem, M. (2006). Effectiveness of behavioral stuttering treatment: A Systematic review and meta-analysis. *Contemporary Issues in Communication Science and Disorders, 33*, 61–73

Higgins, J. P. T., & Green, S. (Eds.). (2011). *Cochrane handbook for systematic reviews of interventions,* Version 5.1.0 (updated March 2011). The Cochrane Collaboration. www.cochrane-handbook.org

Hill, C. J., Bloom, H. S., Black, A. R., & Lipsey, M. W. (2008). Empirical benchmarks for interpreting effect sizes in research. *Child Development Perspectives, 2*, 172–177

Hopewell, S., McDonald, S., Clarke, M., & Egger, M. (2003). Grey literature in meta-analyses of randomized trials of health care interventions (Cochrane Methodology Review). In *The Cochrane Library, Issue 1.* Oxford, England: Update Software

Horner, R. H., Carr, E. G., Halle, J., McGee, G., Odom, S., & Wolery, M. (2005). The use of single-subject research to identify evidence-based practice in special education. *Exceptional Children, 71*, 165–179

Hunter, J. E., & Schmidt, F. L. (2004). *Methods of meta-analysis: Correcting error and bias in research findings* (2nd ed.). Thousand Oaks, CA: Sage

Hunter, J. E., Schmidt, F. L., & Jackson, G. B. (1982). *Meta-analysis: Cumulating research findings across studies.* Beverly Hills, CA: Sage

Johnson, C. J. (2006, Feb). Getting started in evidence-based practice for childhood speech-language disorders. *American Journal of Speech-Language Pathology, 15*, 20–35

Justice, L. M. (2008). Evidence-based practice in speech-language pathology: scaling up. *South African Journal of Communication Disorders, 55*, 7–12

Kazdin, A. E., & Bass, D. (1989, Feb). Power to detect differences between alternative treatments in comparative psychotherapy outcome research. *Journal of Consulting and Clinical Psychology, 57*, 138–147

Lipsey, M. W. (1990). *Design Sensitivity: Statistical Power for Experimental Research.* Newbury Park, CA: Sage Publications

Lipsey, M. W., & Wilson, D. B. (2001). *Practical meta-analysis.* Thousand Oaks, CA: Sage

Ma, H. H. (2006, Sep). An alternative method for quantitative synthesis of single-subject researches: percentage of data points exceeding the median. *Behavior Modification, 30*, 598–617

McReynolds, L. V., & Thompson, C. K. (1986, Aug). Flexibility of single-subject experimental designs. Part I: Review of the basics of single-subject designs. *Journal of Speech and Hearing Disorders, 51*, 194–203

Meline, T. (2006). Selecting studies for systematic review: Inclusion and exclusion criteria. *Contemporary Issues in Communication Science and Disorders, 33*, 21–27

Millar, D. C., Light, J. C., & Schlosser, R. W. (2006, Apr). The impact of augmentative and alternative communication intervention on the speech production of individuals with developmental disabilities: a research review. *Journal of Speech, Language, and Hearing Research: JSLHR, 49*, 248–264

Moher, D., Cook, D. J., Eastwood, S., Olkin, I., Rennie, D., & Stroup, D. (1999). Improving the quality of reporting of meta-analysis of randomised controlled trials: the QUORUM statement. *Lancet, 354*, 1896–1900

Muma, J. R. (1993, Oct). The need for replication. *Journal of Speech and Hearing Research, 36*, 927–930

Murray, H. L., & Reed, C. G. (1977). Language abilities of preschool stuttering children. *Journal of Fluency Disorders, 2*, 171–176

Ntourou, K., Conture, E. G., & Lipsey, M. W. (2011, Aug). Language abilities of children who stutter: a meta-analytical review. *American Journal of Speech-Language Pathology, 20*, 163–179

Parker, R. I., & Vannest, K. (2009, Dec). An improved effect size for single-case research: nonoverlap of all pairs. *Behavior Therapy, 40*, 357–367

Robey, R. R., & Dalebout, S. D. (1998, Dec). A tutorial on conducting meta-analyses of clinical outcome research. *Journal of Speech and Hearing Research, 41*, 1227–1241

Robey, R. R., Schultz, M. C., Crawford, A. B., & Sinner, C. A. (1999). Single-subject clinical-outcome research: designs, data, effect sizes, and analyses. *Aphasiology, 13*, 445–473

Rosenthal, R., & DiMatteo, M. R. (2001). Meta-analysis: recent developments in quantitative methods for literature reviews. *Annual Review of Psychology, 52*, 59–82

Rothstein, H. R., Sutton, A. J., & Borenstein, M. (2005). *Publication bias in meta-analysis: Prevention, assessment and adjustments*. West Sussex, England: John Wiley

Schlosser, R. W. (2003). *The efficacy of augmentative and alternative communication: Toward evidence-based practice*. New York: Academic Press

Schlosser, R. W., & Lee, D. L. (2000). Promoting generalization and maintenance in augmentative and alternative communication: A meta-analysis of 20 years of effectiveness research. *Augmentative and Alternative Communication, 16,* 208–226

Scruggs, T. E., Mastropieri, M. A., & Casto, G. (1987). The quantitative synthesis of single-subject research: Methodology and validation. *Remedial and Special Education, 8,* 24–33

Sharpe, D. (1997, Dec). Of apples and oranges, file drawers and garbage: why validity issues in meta-analysis will not go away. *Clinical Psychology Review, 17,* 881–901

Song, F., Eastwood, A. J., Gilbody, S., Duley, L., & Sutton, A. J. (2000). Publication and related biases. *Health Technology Assessment, 4,* 1–115

Thompson, B. (2002). "Statistical," "practical," and "clinical": How many kinds of significance do counselors need to consider? *Journal of Counseling and Development, 80,* 64–67

West, S. G., & Hepworth, J. T. (1991, Sep). Statistical issues in the study of temporal data: daily experiences. *Journal of Personality, 59,* 609–662

# V

# Graduate Education

# 16

# Outcomes Measurement in Graduate Clinical Education and Supervision

*Sue T. Hale and Lennette J. Ivy*

## ♦ Chapter Focus

This chapter addresses the means for fostering the development of competent and ethical professionals through clinical education and outcomes assessment. To assist students in developing desired clinical outcomes, there is a corresponding requirement that those who foster that development have an expected level of supervisory skill. This chapter emphasizes the roles of student learner and clinical educator in assessing the necessary skills and knowledge of each to achieve positive client outcomes.

## ♦ Introduction

University programs in speech-language pathology have wide-ranging objectives for graduate students. Training programs seek to develop competent and ethical professionals while fostering commitment to the science of the discipline, to lifelong professional learning, and to professional service and advocacy. To achieve these goals, training programs necessarily provide instruction in basic theory and science, in normal processes, in professional issues, and in disorders of communication and swallowing across the life span and for patients from diverse backgrounds. Instruction for speech-language pathology students occurs in the classroom, in laboratories, and in clinical settings. This chapter addresses the means for fostering the development of competent and ethical professionals through clinical education and outcomes assessment. Although the emphasis is on the skills and knowledge developed in clinical settings, learning outcomes from classrooms and laboratories that serve to enhance clinical skills are also addressed. The discussion focuses on the means by which clinical outcomes are developed, taught, and measured, regardless of the venue.

A discussion of clinical outcomes for graduate education in speech-language pathology must necessarily include a bidirectional emphasis. To assist students in developing desired clinical outcomes, there is a corresponding requirement that those who foster that development have an expected level of supervisory skill. Thus, the discussion of student clinical outcomes must be accompanied by a discussion of the necessary supervisory skills outcomes possessed by the clinical educators who contribute to student learning. It is this twofold topic that is the primary focus of the chapter.

Clinical outcomes for speech-language pathology trainees are further defined by several larger environments that influence what must be learned and when that learning must occur. Quality standards for graduate programs in the form of accreditation standards, particularly for professional accreditation, must be considered when developing learner outcomes. Requirements for state and national credentialing have a major influence on specifying learner outcomes. Quality indicators developed by entities that are internal to educational institutions must often be considered, particularly as these indicators relate to fiscal efficiencies and program effectiveness. These issues are addressed because they specifically impact clinical education outcomes. However, a fuller discussion of such topics occurs in other chapters of this text.

At the most fundamental level, learner outcomes may be influenced by factors largely out of the control of the department providing the training. Insufficient financial support from the institution, externally determined student enrollment figures, inability to recruit sufficient faculty, limited clinical education sites and opportunities, and factors in the larger regulatory environment that affect clinical practice may all serve to modify or impede achievement of desired clinical outcomes. For purposes of this discussion, the influence of these and other external factors are mentioned as needed but are not emphasized. The current discussion of the development, teaching, and measurement of clinical outcomes assumes that departments have the ability to determine appropriate outcomes within expected accreditation and certification standards and have sufficient human and financial resources and institutional support for program viability.

Finally, the term *clinical outcomes* is used here to refer to the skills and knowledge that students are expected to be able to utilize when formal clinical training within the graduate program has been completed. Other measures of knowledge are used throughout graduate training, including standardized and nonstandardized examinations. These sorts of examinations are typically based on input or process models rather than outcomes. Outcomes are *measurable* demonstrations of student knowledge or skills and, as such, differ significantly from the knowledge measured by *process* procedures. Until 2005, standards for achieving the Certificate of Clinical Competence (CCC) from the American Speech-Language-Hearing Association (ASHA) were highly process based. Pre-2005 standards required specific numbers of semester credit hours in certain topic areas as well as minimum numbers of clock hours in working with patients of specified ages and disorders. Until that time, most graduate programs were designed around those process standards. After 2005, the standards for the CCC in speech-language pathology included only a few process standards and rested largely on the achievement of skills and knowledge outcomes across the scope of practice in the profession. Currently, the construct of clinical training programs in speech-language pathology is heavily influenced by the skills and knowledge outcomes as specified by the requirements for the CCC.

# ◆ Development of Student Learning Outcomes in Speech-Language Pathology

Graduate training programs have some flexibility in determining the learning outcomes for the students they educate. However, the determination of such outcomes is also influenced by outside factors. Two sets of standards significantly impact the determination of desired student outcomes: (1) the standards for professional accreditation of programs as specified by the ASHA's Council on Academic Accreditation (CAA) in Audiology and Speech-Language Pathology, and (2) the standards for professional certification as determined by ASHA's Council for Clinical Certification (CFCC) in Audiology and Speech-Language Pathology. This chapter focuses on the standards for accreditation and certification as they apply to speech-language pathology.

It should be noted that graduate training programs were often engaged in outcomes measurement of graduates' skills and knowledge prior to the development of the outcomes-based standards for accreditation and certification. However, the influence of the CAA and CFCC standards can be credited with bringing consistency to the demonstration of a level of predictable competency across a wide range of specified knowledge and skills.

## Accreditation Standards

One of the reported purposes of the CAA standards (ASHA, 2011) is the promotion of excellence in preparing graduates to become speech-language pathologists (SLPs). These standards include requirements for a curriculum in which students acquire the necessary knowledge and skills across the entire scope of practice and from which they emerge prepared for individual professional practice (CAA, 2011). Some of the CAA standards are particularly relevant to this discussion. CAA-accredited departments are required to create a sequence of learning for students that is designed, organized, administered, and evaluated on an ongoing basis. Additionally, the students must undergo ongoing and systematic *formative* and *summative* assessments of performance (CAA, 2011). Specific requirements within the accreditation standards expressly target the development of student outcomes. The knowledge and skills outcomes in the accreditation standards parallel similar requirements within the certification standards, and those outcomes are addressed in the discussion of certification below.

## Certification Standards

National certification standards are developed by the CFCC of ASHA. Since 1952, SLPs have been able to achieve this nationally recognized credential, and the certification standards in place at a given time have strongly influenced state regulation of practitioners, notably since the 1970s when the first state licensure laws were developed. Certification standards are reevaluated every 8 to 10 years. The composition of the standards is dependent on a widely distributed Skills Validation Study, which determines what clinicians need to know and need to be able to do to enter professional practice. Results of this periodic study are compiled along with information from subject-matter experts participating in focus groups, and other information from the larger professional and regulatory community, and the information is used to determine current standards. At this writing, the most current standards for speech-language pathology certification are the 2005 standards including minor revisions made in 2009 (CFCC, 2005).

As mentioned previously, some of the standards for certification are process based (75 applicable semester credit hours overall, 36 of which must be at the graduate level; a total of 400 clinical clock hours, of which 325 must have been attained during enrollment in the graduate program). However, the 2005 standards were unique; they differed from all preceding requirements in that knowledge and skills outcomes were specified in detail and the numbers of semester credit hours and clock hour requirements were replaced with the requirement that skills/knowledge be assessed as outcomes.

Beyond prerequisite knowledge in the basic sciences, which may be obtained during undergraduate enrollment (biology, physical science, mathematics, and social science), and in order for graduates to be eligible for certification, students in graduate training programs are required to gain knowledge in principles of basic human communication and swallowing processes, ethical conduct, research and evidence-based practice, and contemporary professional issues and credentialing. The heart of the outcomes-based knowledge standards are standards III-C and III-D (CFCC, 2005). These standards are as follows:

- Standard III-C: The applicant must demonstrate knowledge of the nature of speech, language, hearing, and communication disorders and differences and swallowing disorders, including the etiologies, the characteristics, and the anatomical/physiological, acoustic, psychological, developmental, linguistic, and cultural correlates. Specific knowledge must be demonstrated in the following areas:

  —Articulation

  —Fluency

—Voice and resonance, including respiration and phonation

—Receptive and expressive language (phonology, morphology, syntax, semantics, and pragmatics) in speaking, listening, reading, writing, and manual modalities

—Hearing, including the impact on speech and language

—Swallowing (oral, pharyngeal, esophageal, and related functions, including oral function for feeding; orofacial myofunction)

—Cognitive aspects of communication (attention, memory, sequencing, problem solving, executive functioning)

—Social aspects of communication (including challenging behavior, ineffective social skills, lack of communication opportunities)

—Communication modalities (including oral, manual, augmentative, and alternative communication techniques and assistive technologies)

• Standard III-D: The applicant must possess knowledge of the principles and methods of prevention, assessment, and intervention for people with communication and swallowing disorders, including consideration of anatomical/physiological, psychological, developmental, and linguistic and cultural correlates of the disorders (CFCC, 2005).

When these standards were developed, graduate training programs accepted the requirement to develop a means of measuring these knowledge outcomes beyond the isolated use of process-based examinations. Such standards led to a closer relationship between the knowledge students learned in the classroom and the knowledge students demonstrated in the clinic. As a result of such measurements, students were asked to use higher order thinking to analyze, synthesize, and apply knowledge.

The standards that specify the required skills also include the requirement that students possess skills in oral and written communication sufficient to support professional practice. Other standards regarding skills outcomes address the number of total clock hours, requirements for sufficiency and credentialing of clinical supervisors, and the requirement that clinical learning take place with patients across the life span and with clients from diverse backgrounds who exhibit a wide variety of disorders (specifically those listed in standard III-C) (CFCC, 2005). Again, there are standards that specify the skills that must be attained and measured:

• Standard IV-G: The applicant for certification must complete a program of study that includes supervised clinical experiences sufficient in breadth and depth to achieve the following skills outcomes:

1. Evaluation

   a. Conduct screening and prevention procedures (including prevention activities).

   b. Collect case history information and integrate information from clients/patients, family, caregivers, teachers, relevant others, and other professionals.

   c. Select and administer appropriate evaluation procedures, such as behavioral observations, nonstandardized and standardized tests, and instrumental procedures.

   d. Adapt evaluation procedures to meet client/patient needs.

   e. Interpret, integrate, and synthesize all information to develop diagnoses and make appropriate recommendations for intervention.

   f. Complete administrative and reporting functions necessary to support evaluation.

   g. Refer clients/patients for appropriate services.

2. Intervention

   a. Develop setting-appropriate intervention plans with measurable and achievable goals that meet clients'/patients' needs. Collaborate with clients/patients and relevant others in the planning process.

   b. Implement intervention plans (involve clients/patients and relevant others in the intervention process).

   c. Select or develop and use appropriate materials and instrumentation for prevention and intervention.

   d. Measure and evaluate clients'/patients' performance and progress.

   e. Modify intervention plans, strategies, materials, or instrumentation as appropriate to meet the needs of clients/patients.

   f. Complete administrative and reporting functions necessary to support intervention.

   g. Identify and refer clients/patients for services as appropriate.

3. Interaction and personal qualities

   a. Communicate effectively, recognizing the needs, values, preferred mode of communication, and cultural/linguistic background of the client/patient, family, caregivers, and relevant others.

   b. Collaborate with other professionals in case management.

   c. Provide counseling regarding communication and swallowing disorders to clients/patients, family, caregivers, and relevant others.

   d. Adhere to the ASHA Code of Ethics and behave professionally (CFCC, 2005).

Graduate programs must assess students' performance on the delineated skills and verify that students have achieved them in order for students to qualify for the CCC. However, the skills are specified as final, if minimal, outcomes for entry into the profession. Each skill is actually a set of smaller skills that contribute to the whole. For example, skill item d under Evaluation requires adapting evaluation procedures to meet client needs. Although this standard necessarily requires using an evaluation instrument appropriate to the client's age and expected disorder, to demonstrate the ability to adapt to the client, the student learner might also need to use an appropriate amplification device during test administration to be certain that a client with a hearing disorder can benefit from the auditory presentation. Further modifications might require increasing the size of the visually displayed material for clients with visual challenges or taking short breaks from testing if the client exhibits poor attending skills. When to use an interpreter or different norms for testing clients whose primary language is not English would be subsumed under this skill. It is not enough for a graduate program to check skills acquisition off this master list but to carefully plan the classroom instruction, clinical experiences, and laboratory demonstrations that will in total ensure that a student has achieved the skills outcomes for entry into the profession. ASHA developed the Knowledge and Skills Acquisition (KASA) instrument (CFCC, 2009) as the summary recording form for the certification standards. Programs are free to use this instrument or one of their own design to document the acquisition of the requisite skills and knowledge for certification. An example of entries on the KASA from the clinical education program in speech-language pathology at Vanderbilt University is shown in **Table 16.1**. The exemplary skills are followed by information about where the knowledge that contributes to achievement of the skill was obtained by the student, including coursework, practicum experiences, and other types of learning.

Documentation of achievement of the skills and knowledge outcomes rests on appropriate and comprehensive program review. Course outlines include information about the skills and knowledge that will be achieved and measured during the course. Expectations for skills and knowledge achievement

**Table 16.1** Example of Knowledge and Skills Acquisition (KASA) Instrument Entries

| A | B | C | D | E |
|---|---|---|---|---|
| Standards | Knowledge/ Skill Met? (check) | Course No. and Title | Practicum Experiences No. and Title | Other (e.g., Laboratories, Research) (Include Description of Activity) |
| Receptive and expressive language (phonology, morphology, syntax semantics, and pragmatics) in speaking, listening, reading, writing, and manual modalities | | | | |
| • Etiologies | X | 305 Clin Princ & Proc; 306 Ch Lang Dis; 317 TBI; 331 Aphasia; 315 Intro Aut; 323 Assess/ Interv ASD; 313 Mgmt Com Dis Schools; 304 Ch Lang Acq | PLC; DD; AAC; PRAG; AUT; CI; AH; Pre-K; SA; CLIP; PBP; VA-; TVC-R; Metro-S; Cent-Peds | 305 Practical Laboratories; 306 Case Studies; 317 Practical Laboratories; 331 Practical Laboratories; 315 Obs/Lit Review; 323 Case Study; 313 Class Simulations; 304 Case Studies |
| • Characteristics | X | 305 Clin Princ & Proc; 306 Ch Lang Dis; 317 TBI; 331 Aphasia; 315 Intro Aut; 323 Assess/ Interv ASD; 313 Mgmt Com Dis Schools; 304 Ch Lang Acq | PLC; DD; AAC; PRAG; AUT; CI; AH; Pre-K; SA; CLIP; PBP; VA-; TVC-R; Metro-S; Cent-Peds | 305 Practical Laboratories; 306 Case Studies; 317 Practical Laboratories; 331 Practical Laboratories; 315 Obs/Lit Review; 323 Case Study; 313 Class Simulations; 304 Case Studies |
| Hearing, including the impact on speech and language | | | | |
| • Etiologies | X | 354 Coch Imp child; 217 Hrg Dis & Assess; 318 Hab/Rehab Hrg Imp; 313 Mgmt Com Dis Schools | AH; CI; HS-H; Metro-H | 354 Case Studies/ Practical Laboratories; 217 Practical Laboratories; 318 Practical Laboratories; 313 Class Simulations |
| • Characteristics | X | 354 Coch Imp child; 217 Hrg Dis & Assess; 318 Hab/Rehab Hrg Imp; 313 Mgmt Com Dis Schools | AH; CI; HS-H; Metro-H | 354 Case Studies/ Practical Laboratories; 217 Practical Laboratories; 318 Practical Laboratories; 313 Class Simulations |

from specific clinical placements are specified. Laboratory experiences, seminars, workshops, and independent study information may be included as sources of skills and knowledge development. In all instances, the outcomes of learning must be assessed, and if performance is unacceptable, sufficient planning and opportunity for remediation must be in place. In many instances, the achievement of the skills and knowledge outcomes are central to the graduation requirements for the student in speech-language pathology.

# ◆ The Stakeholders

Although the certification standards are helpful in designing the basic plan for student clinical education in graduate programs, the process of clinical education is far more complex than merely specifying required learner outcomes. To achieve those outcomes, clinical education includes three primary stakeholders at any given time, all of whom have significant roles in the learning process. These stakeholders are the student learner, the clinical educator, and the clients.

Throughout the training program for any individual, the student is the only constant in this paradigm. The student learns from several clinical educators with different skills and philosophies and in a variety of settings. Clinical assignments necessarily include numerous clients with wide-ranging disorders, some seen individually and others seen in groups. The student is required to participate in prevention activities, and to screen, assess, intervene, refer, collaborate, and communicate with many individuals. As the student negotiates the ever-changing milieu of clinical experience, it is hoped that what will be developed will not only be specific knowledge and skills but also, when necessary, the independent ability to access additional information. In one way or another since the first graduate programs were instituted, professors and clinical educators have stated that students need to "learn how to learn."

Those who engage in clinical education as supervisors are pivotal in the process as their students progress through wide-ranging clinical experiences, and supervisors must attend to their own skills and knowledge development to be effective as clinical educators. Additionally, client perspectives will further advise the learning process of students in the course of achieving appropriate clinical skills and knowledge outcomes. The technical report on clinical supervision (ASHA, 2008a) suggests that the goals of clinical supervision are that both supervisor and supervisee demonstrate professional growth that results in better client outcomes.

## Clinical Educators

Although ASHA (2008b) states the critical importance for clinical educators to obtain training in clinical supervision, the reality is that many clinical educators have not had such formal training. Apart from individuals employed in university settings in the role of clinical supervisors, many clinical educators are clinicians in real-world professional settings who provide training for students enrolled in practicum or externship placements. It is often the case that these clinicians, often masterful clinicians, have not had the benefit of instruction in the science of supervision. They employ strategies that they recall from their own clinical training, that they have gained from independent study of relevant literature, and that they have developed over the course of their experience to instruct students-in-training. For those clinical educators who have had the benefit of supervisory instruction, the instruction may have come from isolated seminars or workshops on supervision or a portion of an academic class, as few individuals have the benefit of participating in ongoing supervisory instruction except in the form of self-study. Fortunately, like classroom teaching historically, much of the requisite knowledge and skills for clinical education are learned with experience. However, in recent years more emphasis has been placed on defining and acquiring a specific set of skills and knowledge that lead to supervisory ability. This emphasis has been bolstered by the wealth of information available in textbooks, in Web resources, and through continuing education offerings. Additionally, for those individuals who wish to have interaction and information about supervision on an ongoing basis as an affiliate, ASHA's Special Interest Group 11, Administration and Supervision, is a valuable resource.

In addition to knowledge in clinical education, clinical supervisors must possess certain attributes to be successful in clinical teaching. Those individuals who cannot relinquish control in the clinical setting or who are too stressed by external factors in their job, such as employer demands for high productivity, may not be successful clinical educators. It can be assumed that clinicians who provide ethical and excellent clinical care and use evidence-based practice may become successful supervisors.

However, those individuals must be willing to become knowledgeable about the processes of supervision and of student learning as well as earnest in their interest to provide the time and attention the student requires to learn.

### Skills and Knowledge of Clinical Educators

Early pioneers in the area of clinical supervision for speech-language pathology (Anderson, 1970; Ward & Webster, 1965) described the role of clinical supervisors in terms of serving the welfare of the client while producing positive change in the knowledge and skill level of the student in training. Certainly, any discussion of clinical supervision owes a great debt to Anderson's contributions, and much of the current literature still incorporates her concepts and principles.

In 2008, ASHA's Ad Hoc Committee on Supervision in Speech-Language Pathology completed an impressive body of work that resulted in the publication of three documents. These documents included a technical report, a position statement, and a knowledge and skills document on the topic of clinical supervision in speech-language pathology (ASHA, 2008a–c). These three documents incorporated much of the historical thinking and current view of what clinical educators must know and what they must be able to do to effectively guide students.

In the position statement (ASHA, 2008b), supervision is identified as a specific practice area as well as being essential in student education. Building on the previous work of Anderson (1988), which suggests that supervision involves elements of professional development of both supervisor and supervisee, the ASHA technical report (2008a) expands the definition to suggest that professional growth is enhanced when both individuals engage in self-analysis and self-evaluation. Also central to this concept is that the most effective clinical teachers promote critical thinking or problem solving on the part of the supervisee (ASHA, 2008a).

The knowledge and skills document (ASHA, 2008c) provides a comprehensive list of necessary knowledge and skills for the supervisor in the broad areas of preparing for supervision, interpersonal communication, developing the supervisee's critical thinking and problem-solving skills, and developing the supervisee's clinical competence in assessment and intervention. Additional knowledge and skills include ability in conducting supervisory meetings; evaluating the clinical and professional growth of the supervisee; effectively addressing issues of diversity; developing and maintaining documentation; establishing knowledge and compliance with ethical, regulatory, and legal requirements; and becoming an effective clinical mentor (ASHA, 2008c). This document is available at http://www.asha.org/docs/html/KS2008-00294.html and has comprehensive information about the knowledge and skills outcomes for effective supervision.

Clinical supervisors are accountable not only for the students whose clinical work they guide and for client welfare, but also for their own supervisory skills. Assessing client progress and ensuring high-quality service delivery is central to the responsibility for any SLP providing clinical services. It is no less important when students participate in the clinical process. The assessment of supervisory effectiveness is often more difficult to determine, and few instruments exist to advise the process. The value of appraisal instruments completed by students is minimized by the students' lack of knowledge about what might contribute to effective supervision. Additionally, a perceived lack of anonymity for the respondent can make students reluctant to be completely forthright in the appraisal of supervision (ASHA, 2008a). For those reasons, continuing self-appraisal and professional development focusing on supervision are key to the acquisition and continual improvement of supervisory skills and knowledge.

Carozza (2011) elaborates some of the concepts from the ASHA document, suggesting that interpersonal communication, cultural and linguistic factors, personal resilience, and social power are critical contributors to supervisor effectiveness. She identifies interpersonal communication styles as an area in which increased knowledge can improve the supervisory process. Using self-assessment instruments or watching videos of interactions with the student clinician can provide insight into habitual conversational styles but also allow for modification of that style to enhance communicative effectiveness. She suggests that the ASHA (2008c) document accurately identified highly regarded interpersonal skills for supervisors, which included unconditional positive regard, earnestness, empathy, and concreteness.

Carozza (2011) further suggests that supervisors should make every effort to improve their cultural competence through a personal commitment and self-reflective tasks. She identifies the importance of personal resilience in creating a more accepting environment for the student clinician, and cites conflict resolution, stress management, and personal coping strategies as desirable characteristics of the mature clinical educator. Additionally, she emphasizes the importance of managing social/personal power in the clinical education. Power should relate to the clinical skills of the supervisor and not to the need to control another individual. The influence of power in the supervisory relationship is further underscored by ASHA (2008a) in suggesting that the power associated with grading a student's performance, validating clock hours, and completing performance evaluations requires awareness regarding the influence of such power. Awareness will allow the supervisor to avoid intimidating the student or reducing the student's willingness to participate in the supervisory partnership.

Although student appraisal instruments distributed and collected within a department often fail to provide highly useful information because of the power imbalance, student surveys that are not department-specific and that ensure anonymity of the respondent may provide useful information. Chabon (2006) surveyed students and inquired about specific instances of actions that supervisors exhibited that were particularly effective. The most frequently cited examples were related to good communication—that is, providing immediate, written, and concrete feedback and providing examples of what the student did right/wrong and suggestions for needed modifications. The second most frequently cited attribute was having the knowledge, skills, experience, and use of evidence to support procedures. Clearly, students value the input of supervisors who communicate effectively and are skilled in service provision.

If the ultimate goal for student development as a clinician is readiness for independent practice, then the supervisor must expect and allow for ever-increasing independence in the supervisory relationship. McCrea and Brasseur (2003), building on the work of Anderson and others, provide a comprehensive discussion of the supervisory continuum that ultimately leads to greater student independence. At the most basic level, the continuum has three stages: (1) *evaluation-feedback stage,* in which the supervisor takes the lead in determining the course of treatment and directing the student in achieving expected goals while providing frequent feedback regarding student performance; (2) *transitional stage,* in which the supervisee has obtained sufficient knowledge and skill such that aspects of joint problem solving can occur between the supervisor and supervisee; and (3) *self-supervision stage,* in which the supervisee has an ability to accurately assess personal performance and make corrections or alterations based on that assessment (McCrea & Brasseur, 2003). Clearly, the continuum is not a straight line for most students, and although a student might be at the self-supervision stage for a client with a particular disorder, the same student might be at the evaluation-feedback stage for a client with a more complex disorder or with more challenging behavioral or personal characteristics. An important skill for any clinical educator is to move students through the supervisory continuum, which involves recognizing readiness for increased responsibility and, more importantly, a willingness on the part of the supervisor to relinquish some aspects of control.

If the goal of clinical educators is to develop skilled clinicians, then Goldberg (1997) provides insight into the characteristics of master clinicians. He identifies the following important traits: *compassion,* intensely caring for the client's well-being and meeting that need with theoretically sound methods; *facilitation,* providing the necessary conditions for developing new behaviors; *timing,* knowing when to present and withhold information; *contingency thinking,* anticipating the client's response and providing the best response to it; and *consistency,* applying all of the other skills consistently. He suggests that the primary difference between student and master clinicians is the trait of *consistency.* Although the novice may display the first four skills in almost every session, these skills may be intermingled with errors in timing and judgment. Goldberg (1997) states, "The master clinician gets it right virtually all of the time" (p. 318). Based on the paramount importance of consistency, the job of the clinical educator is to help the student get it right as much as possible.

## Students

The master's degree in speech-language pathology is a practitioner degree, and students must gain not only theoretical knowledge regarding human communication and related disorders but also the skills and knowledge to enter professional practice. The view of speech-language pathology as a helping profession and the interest of the current generation of college students in engaging in such professions have led to large numbers of applicants to the 240 CAA-accredited speech-language pathology graduate programs (ASHA, 2011). The result is that only the most highly qualified students, based on individual university's admission criteria, gain entry into the clinical training programs. Due to the competitiveness of the applicant pool, training programs have every expectation that the admitted students will graduate from the program as skilled clinicians. These judgments are based on the applicants' strong undergraduate academic grade point averages, excellent scores on admission examinations, participation in service learning, and well-written statements of purpose, among other admission criteria.

Most students meet those high expectations, and graduate programs are justifiably proud of their graduates who become successful members of the profession. But it is also the case that each year some students are not successful in developing the required skills and knowledge, and they leave the graduate program before completion; other students graduate although members of the faculty consider them to have been only marginally successful in their endeavor to become SLPs. In these cases, usually, the problem is attributed not to poor academic performance but rather to the individual's inability to develop the clinical acumen required for entry into the profession. It may be assumed that most students who enter graduate programs have sufficient information about the profession to have the strong desire to engage in it. So, the question arises, Why do some academically gifted students with strong motivation to join the profession fail to achieve a sufficient level of clinical skills to become SLPs? Perhaps that question can best be answered by asking the opposite question: What clinical skills and knowledge do successful graduates achieve? Inherent to a discussion of student clinical outcomes is the underlying assumption that the graduate programs are doing everything that is needed to assist the student in being successful even when learning styles and rates of learning may differ significantly from one student to another.

### Skills and Knowledge of Students

Skills and knowledge outcomes for graduate students in speech-language pathology were discussed above, specifically in relation to the ASHA certification standards (CFCC, 2005). However, such outcomes are recognized as the end point for entry into the profession. Students require a program of academic instruction and many clinical experiences to get to that end point. Those who seek to instruct students must determine what progress is being made to reach the ultimate objectives and if that progress is sufficient or requires remediation along the way.

Just as the previously cited continuum of supervision requires the supervisor to relinquish control of a clinical situation to the student, the student has a corresponding requirement to acquire that same control. Novice clinicians require underlying theoretical information and well-articulated clinical instruction about specific clients. Although the student may not have the ability at the outset of training to effectively draw conclusions from case history or diagnostic information, that same student can benefit from being instructed in how the supervisor came to derive conclusions from such data. New clinicians may not be able to craft overarching objectives or discharge criteria for a patient, but they may be able to intuit how specific methods are relevant in achieving short-term objectives. To understand the process of moving students from these beginning levels and from highly dependent learners to independent practice, clinical educators must engage in evaluation and management of student supervisees. This process is not unlike the same kind of considered approach that must be used with clients.

In a study of clinical reasoning skills in speech-language pathology students, Hoben, Varley, and Cox (2007) determined that clinical reasoning challenges for speech-language pathology students were similar to those shown by students in medicine and other related fields. They found that most novice speech-language pathology students tended to rely on concrete observations or repeating reported data without making clinical judgments. The novice students had difficulty with conceptualizing an observed clinical problem, planning an evaluation strategy, organizing incoming information, assessing progress, and interpreting results. The authors concluded that, through direct instruction in clinical decision making, students benefitted from explicit teaching in diagnostic reasoning, particularly when the reasoning process was amplified with examples from previous theoretical teaching. This study suggests that many of the clinical outcomes required of graduate students in the areas of collecting and utilizing case history information, selecting and administering appropriate evaluation procedures, and drawing clinical judgments about intervention from evaluation information may be enhanced through strategic instruction. The use of simulated patients along with actual clinical experience can be useful for such learning.

The knowledge-based standards III-C and III-D for achieving the CCC (CFCC, 2005), which advise outcomes development for most graduate programs in speech-language pathology (shown above), delineate the areas in which knowledge must be gained and for which skills must be developed. These areas include articulation, fluency, voice and resonance, receptive and expressive language, hearing, swallowing, cognitive aspects of communication, social aspects of communication, and communication modalities (CFCC, 2005). When asked the intent of the standards in regard to knowledge and skills outcomes, members of the Council for Clinical Certification at the time of the development of the KASA summary instrument have been reported to have responded, and this is anecdotal, that students should have "knowledge in all, skill in all, and practicum in most" of the listed areas that have come to be called the *Big Nine*. Thus, graduate programs must show that academic and clinical instruction and the demonstration of knowledge and skills occurs across the listed disorder areas (CFCC, 2005). To achieve these student outcomes, training programs have necessarily placed skill requirements into academic classes. With direct instruction, and the opportunity to test and retest clinical knowledge in an applied situation (even in simulations), this direct instruction facilitates clinical reasoning when it occurs in the practicum setting.

As part of the supervisory process, clinical educators provide feedback on student performance. Although this is sometimes done verbally during or at the conclusion of the session, students often comment that they prefer written feedback that they can absorb and then use to guide future actions. Clinical supervisors expect the student to demonstrate growth in clinical skills across what is typically a semester (or academic quarter) of work with a given client. To facilitate understanding on the part of the student as to the expectations for growth that the supervisor intends, some form of goal setting for the student's performance is recommended at the outset of the assignment. The goals should be determined based on the student's level of knowledge, skill, and independence prior to the current placement as well as the supervisor's reasonable expectation for student growth and development based on the client, setting, and the supervisor's knowledge of the clinical dynamics that exist (good/poor family support, consistent/inconsistent attendance patterns, behavioral factors, etc.). It would not be expected that all clinical skills would show equal growth, as more complex skills may develop over a longer period of time. On the other hand, some skills may be expected to be demonstrated without instruction and at a mature level from the beginning. These might include professional behaviors such as consistent attendance and punctuality or basic requirements such as reviewing the patient chart prior to a clinical session. Skills requiring more complex sets of behavior will develop more slowly. Supervisors in graduate programs utilize a variety of means as well as formats for goal setting and for providing feedback to students in training. Most of the goal-setting forms have basic similarities.

The form for evaluating speech-language pathology students' performance used in the Vanderbilt University Department of Hearing and Speech Sciences is provided in **Table 16.2**. Developed by Rassi and Hancock (1999) with minor modifications in subsequent years, the form relates the student's level of ability in demonstrating a particular skill to the level of supervisory support that is necessary to achieve client progress. A system of this nature rests on principles of supervision outlined in the collaborative model and continuum of supervision of Anderson (1988). Levels of student independence are judged as absent, emerging, present, developed, or consistent. During an initial supervisory conference, the supervisor and student collaboratively determine the relevant goals to be targeted,

**Table 16.2** Form for Evaluating Speech-Language Pathology Students' Performance Used in the Vanderbilt University Department of Hearing and Speech Sciences

**Student Performance Review**

Department of Hearing and Speech Sciences
Vanderbilt University

Speech-Language Pathology Clinical Practicum

Student Name _____

School Term/Year _____

Supervisor Name _____ Site _____

Supervisor ASHA Certification Number _____

TO SUPERVISORS AND STUDENTS: The competency statements that compromise this document have been designed for purposes of practicum goal-setting and the monitoring and evaluating of students' clinical performance. Use the scale and descriptors shown on the dual-movement (supervisor and student) supervision continuum illustrated here.

Supervision Continuum with Rating Scale and Descriptors

Student:

| ABSENT | EMERGING | PRESENT | DEVELOPED | CONSISTENT |
|---|---|---|---|---|
| Competency/skill not evident | Competency/skill emerging | Competency/skill present but needs further development | Competency/skill developed but needs refinement and/or consistency | Competency/skill well developed and consistent |
|  |  |  |  |  |

Supervisor:

| MODELING/ INTERVENTION | FREQUENT INSTRUCTION | FREQUENT MONITORING | INFREQUENT MONITORING | GUIDANCE |
|---|---|---|---|---|
| Requires constant supervisory modeling/ intervention | Requires frequent supervisory instruction | Requires frequent supervisory monitoring | Requires infrequent supervisory monitoring | Requires guidance/ consultation only |

SUPERVISORS: Using the following key, circle the appropriate descriptor (starting on page 2) in the first column to indicate the student's initial goal for each competency and statement being reviewed. Then, indicate midterm status and final level of competency/skill development, respectively, by circling the appropriate descriptors in the second and third columns.

A = Absent
E = Emerging
P = Present
D = Developed
C = Consistent

**Table 16.2**   (*Continued*) Form for Evaluating Speech-Language Pathology Students' Performance Used in the Vanderbilt University Department of Hearing and Speech Sciences

| PLANNING | GOAL | MIDTERM | FINAL |
|---|---|---|---|
| 1. Reviews files from daily caseload to obtain pertinent information. | A E P D C | A E P D C | A E P D C |
| 2. Familiarizes self with available information regarding client and disorder prior to initial contact. | A E P D C | A E P D C | A E P D C |
| 3. Demonstrates an understanding of the client's communication problem and any related disorders or concerns. | A E P D C | A E P D C | A E P D C |
| 4. Familiarizes self with curriculum/therapy appropriate for clients. | A E P D C | A E P D C | A E P D C |
| 5. Familiarizes self with therapy techniques appropriate for individual(s) within group. | A E P D C | A E P D C | A E P D C |
| 6. Selects appropriate assessment tools. | A E P D C | A E P D C | A E P D C |
| 7. Plans logical sequence of assessment or activities within therapy session. | A E P D C | A E P D C | A E P D C |
| 8. Plans for each case separately, taking individual needs into consideration before choosing activity. | A E P D C | A E P D C | A E P D C |
| 9. Develops appropriate long-term goals for clients. | A E P D C | A E P D C | A E P D C |
| 10. Establishes appropriate short-term goals for clients. | A E P D C | A E P D C | A E P D C |
| 11. Plans appropriate daily activities to meet short-term goals. | A E P D C | A E P D C | A E P D C |
| 12. Develops instructional materials, as needed. | A E P D C | A E P D C | A E P D C |
| 13. Generates novel therapy tasks appropriate to goals. | A E P D C | A E P D C | A E P D C |
| 14. Demonstrates knowledge of normal development and expectations for age of client(s) (e.g., selects materials/ activities that are developmentally appropriate). | A E P D C | A E P D C | A E P D C |
| 15. Familiarizes/reviews materials prior to session. | A E P D C | A E P D C | A E P D C |

COMMENTS: _____

_____

_____

_____

_____

| IMPLEMENTATION | GOAL | MIDTERM | FINAL |
|---|---|---|---|
| 16. Outlines the purpose of the session and the sequence of events. | A E P D C | A E P D C | A E P D C |
| 17. Elicits relevant information in an organized manner and pursues pertinent points. | A E P D C | A E P D C | A E P D C |
| 18. Uses appropriate interview techniques. | A E P D C | A E P D C | A E P D C |
| 19. Records all pertinent information/data appropriately in an accurate and nondisruptive manner. | A E P D C | A E P D C | A E P D C |
| 20. Observes and records diagnostically significant behavior. | A E P D C | A E P D C | A E P D C |
| 21. Administers tests according to instructions. | A E P D C | A E P D C | A E P D C |
| 22. Modifies administration of formal tests for special cases. | A E P D C | A E P D C | A E P D C |
| 23. Identifies client's verbal and nonverbal cues (e.g., fatigue, on-off time). | A E P D C | A E P D C | A E P D C |
| 24. Uses appropriate verbal and nonverbal reinforces effectively. | A E P D C | A E P D C | A E P D C |
| 25. Uses behavior management techniques effectively. | A E P D C | A E P D C | A E P D C |
| 26. Uses allotted time efficiently. | A E P D C | A E P D C | A E P D C |

(*Continued on page 328*)

**Table 16.2** (*Continued*) Form for Evaluating Speech-Language Pathology Students' Performance Used in the Vanderbilt University Department of Hearing and Speech Sciences

| IMPLEMENTATION | GOAL | MIDTERM | FINAL |
|---|---|---|---|
| 27. When giving instructions, anticipates and reacts to individual needs of clients. | A E P D C | A E P D C | A E P D C |
| 28. Modifies planned activities and their order, when necessary, to obtain maximal relevant information. | A E P D C | A E P D C | A E P D C |
| 29. Instructs at level appropriate for individual client. | A E P D C | A E P D C | A E P D C |
| 30. Modifies level of instruction and/or activity by increasing or decreasing when appropriate. | A E P D C | A E P D C | A E P D C |
| 31. Provides opportunity for optimum participation by each client. | A E P D C | A E P D C | A E P D C |
| 32. Varies the level of structure imposed on client with appropriate (e.g., spontaneous versus clinician-directed). | A E P D C | A E P D C | A E P D C |
| 33. Utilizes suggestions given for modifying goals and/or techniques. | A E P D C | A E P D C | A E P D C |

COMMENTS: _____
_____
_____
_____
_____

| INTERPRETATION | GOAL | MIDTERM | FINAL |
|---|---|---|---|
| 34. Considers all pertinent information (e.g., test scores, background) prior to formulating recommendations or planning for therapy program. | A E P D C | A E P D C | A E P D C |
| 35. Formulates appropriate and realistic recommendations/ referrals. | A E P D C | A E P D C | A E P D C |
| 36. Evaluates and interprets client performance following a session. | A E P D C | A E P D C | A E P D C |
| 37. Evaluates own performance following a session. | A E P D C | A E P D C | A E P D C |
| 38. Recognizes client's goal attainment or client's need for goal adjustment. | A E P D C | A E P D C | A E P D C |

COMMENTS: _____
_____
_____
_____

| CASE MANAGEMENT | GOAL | MIDTERM | FINAL |
|---|---|---|---|
| 39. Demonstrates sensitivity to client and family members. | A E P D C | A E P D C | A E P D C |
| 40. Establishes appropriate relationship with family member and client(s). | A E P D C | A E P D C | A E P D C |
| 41. Communicates client's performance with family members as needed. | A E P D C | A E P D C | A E P D C |
| 42. Communicates client's performance with other professionals as needed. | A E P D C | A E P D C | A E P D C |

COMMENTS: _____
_____
_____
_____

**Table 16.2**  (*Continued*) Form for Evaluating Speech-Language Pathology Students' Performance Used in the Vanderbilt University Department of Hearing and Speech Sciences

| REPORT WRITING | GOAL | MIDTERM | FINAL |
|---|---|---|---|
| 43. Addresses all pertinent areas. | A E P D C | A E P D C | A E P D C |
| 44. Presents finding, programs, and recommendation clearly and concisely. | A E P D C | A E P D C | A E P D C |
| 45. Incorporates appropriate information into report content. | A E P D C | A E P D C | A E P D C |
| 46. Writes report in a professional manner (e.g., appropriate terminology, grammar). | A E P D C | A E P D C | A E P D C |
| 47. Makes recommended changes. | A E P D C | A E P D C | A E P D C |
| 48. Follows suggested format. | A E P D C | A E P D C | A E P D C |

COMMENTS: _____

_____

_____

_____

| SUPERVISORY CONFERENCES | GOAL | MIDTERM | FINAL |
|---|---|---|---|
| 49. Comes to supervisory conference prepared with questions, suggestions, and topics for discussion. | A E P D C | A E P D C | A E P D C |
| 50. Identifies and sets personal goals. | A E P D C | A E P D C | A E P D C |
| 51. Takes initiative to make suggestions regarding own clinical development. | A E P D C | A E P D C | A E P D C |
| 52. Other | A E P D C | A E P D C | A E P D C |
| 53. Other | A E P D C | A E P D C | A E P D C |

COMMENTS: _____

_____

_____

_____

TO SUPERVISORS AND STUDENTS: The competencies listed in this final section are expected to be attained, to their fullest extent, by all students in all stages of clinical practicum and in every setting. Thus, there are no degrees of expected competency development (hence, no specific goal-setting); these competencies are simply present or absent. The performance determinations in this section may or may not be a factor in grade calculation, at the discretion of the supervisor.

SUPERVISORS: In the checklist below, indicate whether a competency is present or absent. Add explanatory written comments at the end of this section.

| PROFESSIONALISM | MIDTERM | | FINAL | |
|---|---|---|---|---|
| | Absent | Present | Absent | Present |
| 54. Maintains professional appearance and conduct appropriate for job duties and work setting. | _____ | _____ | _____ | _____ |
| 55. Maintains professional relationship in all aspects of clinical practice. | _____ | _____ | _____ | _____ |
| 56. Is punctual for all appointments and, when necessary and appropriate, cancels/reschedules client sessions as well as supervisory conferences. | _____ | _____ | _____ | _____ |
| 57. Adheres to clinical policy regard absences. | _____ | _____ | _____ | _____ |
| 58. Maximizes learning opportunities provided by each clinical assignment. | _____ | _____ | _____ | _____ |

(*Continued on page 330*)

**Table 16.2** (*Continued*) Form for Evaluating Speech-Language Pathology Students' Performance Used in the Vanderbilt University Department of Hearing and Speech Sciences

| PROFESSIONALISM | MIDTERM | | FINAL | |
|---|---|---|---|---|
| | Absent | Present | Absent | Present |
| 59. Understands and adheres to ASHA Code of Ethics. | _____ | _____ | _____ | _____ |
| 60. Prepares physical environment prior to clinical session. | _____ | _____ | _____ | _____ |
| 61. Cleans up following clinical session. | _____ | _____ | _____ | _____ |
| 62. Completes lesson plans as requested. | _____ | _____ | _____ | _____ |
| 63. Turns in lesson plans on time. | _____ | _____ | _____ | _____ |
| 64. Provides written information as requested (e.g., feedback, test reviews, chart reviews). | _____ | _____ | _____ | _____ |
| 65. Maintains confidentiality. | _____ | _____ | _____ | _____ |
| 66. Reads or watches material recommended by supervisor within time guidelines. | _____ | _____ | _____ | _____ |
| 67. Brings appropriate forms/materials to supervisory and therapy/diagnostic sessions. | _____ | _____ | _____ | _____ |
| 68. Maintains own clinic records (e.g., feedback forms, hour sheets). | _____ | _____ | _____ | _____ |
| 69. Introduces self to patient/family appropriately. | _____ | _____ | _____ | _____ |
| 70. Follows departmental guidelines regarding file, material, and test checkout. | _____ | _____ | _____ | _____ |
| 71. Adheres to guidelines of professional conduct. | _____ | _____ | _____ | _____ |
| 72. Establishes and maintains own client work file. | | | | |

COMMENTS: _____

_____

_____

_____

_____

**GOAL ATTAINMENT/GRADE CALCULATION**

**STEP 1**
Total No. competency items scored _____

**STEP 2**
Add: No. of goals attained _____
No. of goals surpassed _____
Total No. of goals attained/surpassed

**STEP 3**
Divide Step 2 total by Step 1 total _____ Multiply result × 100 _____% **Basic Performance %**

**STEP 4** (optional—at supervisor's request)

BONUS PERFORMANCE % points may be added for **extraordinary** performances, as demonstrated in:
• Number of goals surpassed
• Number of CONSISTENT ratings obtained
• Amount of progress in key areas
• Excellence in quality of overall performance

Add: Basic Performance % _____%

Bonus Performance % _____%

_____% **Adjusted Performance %**

PENALTY PERFORMANCE % points may be subtracted for absent professionalism skills.

Subtract: Above Performance % _____%

Penalty Performance % _____%

_____% **Adjusted Performance %**

**Table 16.2**  (*Continued*) Form for Evaluating Speech-Language Pathology Students' Performance Used in the Vanderbilt University Department of Hearing and Speech Sciences

**STEP 5**

Using the table below, convert the final performance percentage (whether Basic or Adjusted) into a letter grade. Circle the FINAL GRADE IN THIS TABLE.

| If FINAL PERFORMANCE is | | | Then LETTER GRADE is | | |
|---|---|---|---|---|---|
| 90% or higher | A+ | or | A | or | A– |
| 80% to 89% | B+ | or | B | or | B– |
| 70% to 79% | C+ | or | C | or | C– |
| 60% to 69% | D+ | or | D | or | D– |
| Lower than 60% | F | | | | |

**Method of Grade Calculation (Check One)**

\_\_\_\_\_ Goal-attainment formula used.

\_\_\_\_\_ Other method or formula used, as described below.

\_\_\_\_\_ No method or formula used. Grade subjectively determined as explained here:

(NOTE: If any approach other than the goal-attainment formula is used, this must be discussed by the supervisor and student at the time of the initial goal-setting conference).

**VERIFICATION OF AGREEMENT AND COMMITMENT**

Goal-Setting Conference (Beginning-of-Term)

Our signatures below verify that we have set clinical and supervisory goals for the forthcoming term and that we are committed to working toward these goals. A goal-setting conference was held for this purpose.

| | | |
|---|---|---|
| Supervisor Signature | Student Signature | Date |

**Progress-Monitoring Conference (Midterm)**

Our signatures below verify that we have reviewed midterm goal status relative to beginning-of-term goals, noting progress in movement toward those goals, and making plans for the remainder of the term. A progress-monitoring conference was held for this purpose.

| | | |
|---|---|---|
| Supervisor Signature | Student Signature | Date |

**Evaluation Conference (End-of-Term)**

Our signatures below verify that we have reviewed end-of-term goal status relative to beginning-of-term goals and midterm goal status, noting final goal attainment and implications for the future. An evaluation conference was held for this purpose.

| | | |
|---|---|---|
| Supervisor Signature | Student Signature | Date |

OVERALL COMMENT/RECOMMENDATIONS (If additional space is needed, attach pages as necessary).

as not all goals apply to all clients, and not all goals applicable to a client need to be measured if the student has already successfully demonstrated achievement. The expected level of achievement for the targeted goals at the conclusion of the clinical assignment is also determined. Although feedback is provided about the student's performance on an ongoing basis, the goals are formally discussed at mid-term and at the conclusion of the semester. The student's success in achieving the targeted goals determines the practicum grade. Supervisors provide anecdotal commentary for each section of the feedback form as well. Such a form allows an objective measurement of the student's progress and allows future supervisors to assess what the student already knows and the level to which they can demonstrate that knowledge without supervisory support.

Some additions to the performance appraisal form may be used in specific settings when necessary. For example, in a voice center, students may be required to perform endoscopic procedures on each other or the supervisor, and such activities may be assessed separately. Using any form for clinical feedback is only as useful in the student's development of skills and knowledge as the skills of the supervisor in providing consistent and appropriate feedback. Students require readily accessible information about what is expected and how they are progressing in meeting those expectations. They also experience justifiable feelings of having been treated unfairly if they do not meet supervisor expectations during a final evaluation but have not received feedback prior to that time that performance was below that expectation.

In a survey of clinical educators regarding the most highly effective behaviors for student clinicians to develop, Chabon, Hale, Lee-Wilkerson, and Kellum (2008) found clinical supervisors to most highly value interpersonal skills, preparedness, and content knowledge in the students they supervised. In the same manner, the supervisors suggested that ineffective student behaviors included lack of preparation, poor judgment, and limited knowledge (Chabon, 2006). Although preparedness and content knowledge can be learned, interpersonal skills, while highly valued, may be challenging for some students to develop.

Throughout graduate education, students will engage in clinical experiences in which the supervisor is either present with them with the client or perhaps observing from another room or through video equipment. In being educated as a professional, a realistic goal is that the learner will have intrinsic motivation for what is being learned, and that the motivation is not dependent on the observation (or grade) afforded by the supervisor. Carozza (2011) describes the learning process for graduate students in speech-language pathology as the development of an adult learner in an authentic workplace. In that regard, she further states that adults are self-directed learners who bring varied past experiences to the clinical laboratory. She suggests that adults learn best when they possess a need to know and a task-centered point of reference (Carozza, 2011). With this in mind, clinical educators need to relinquish social power to students insofar as possible to best respond to the needs of the adult learner and to maintain high levels of motivation and engagement in the learning process.

A discussion of desirable student outcomes must address the importance of the development of skills for clinical writing. Historically, programs guided students in developing clinical reports that were cumbersome, multipage documents. It was argued that such reports gave students practice in writing all pertinent clinical observations and impressions. Although the value of such writing for case studies or problem-based learning cannot be ignored, real-world clinical practice requires efficiency in documentation. Today's graduate students must be able to develop skills for documentation specifically targeted for a variety of settings. Early intervention settings require individualized family service plans, whereas schools practice is guided by the individualized education plan. Health care settings may utilize SOAP (subjective data, objective data, assessment, and plan) notes, and each environment may have different requirements for the essential components of evaluation reports.

Many settings now utilize electronic reporting methods, often highly specific to the environment. Hospitals are increasingly using electronic health records (EHRs) as a result of public policy initiatives and the general movement toward greater use of informatics. Graduate training programs are charged with assisting students in learning appropriate and setting-specific clinical writing skills. An important component of clinical writing is the understanding that the clinical report is the essential documentation for a clinical contact. Clinical educators are often heard to comment, "If it is not documented, it did not happen." Students are required to learn that reports must be timely and accurate and must be filed in the appropriate format. This requirement is not just a part of good patient care but also an ethical responsibility. Documented clinical findings must be free of misrepresentation, particularly in regard to reimbursement for services. Student outcomes for documentation are an essential component of graduate education, and clinical educators must model timely documentation as well as assisting students in developing appropriate clinical writing skills and habits.

The ultimate assessment of clinical learning for students is workplace performance. If the essential knowledge and skills outcomes have been achieved and the student has also "learned how to learn," then employer assessments of new graduates should be positive. Asking employers about the performance of recent graduates who are nearing or at the end of their clinical fellowship can inform graduate programs about the quality of clinical education and the possible need for curricular modifications. A sample survey for such purpose is provided in **Fig. 16.1**.

A final helpful measure of graduates' clinical skills and knowledge may be gained by the use of a survey of those who have been employed in the profession for a relatively brief period of time, typically 1 to 3 years. During that period, students have a unique perspective on what they have been required to know and do and whether or not they had the requisite skills and knowledge. Savvy graduates will understand that education does not prepare them for every eventuality but that it is successful if they are knowledgeable about most clinical situations and have the problem-solving and critical thinking skills to access information that they do not have at other times. A self-assessment tool for graduates can be instrumental in program quality improvement. An academic department could use such a tool to collect information from graduates regarding the adequacy of their academic and clinical preparation once they have been in the workplace. These measures are in common use and may take the form of open-ended questions or surveys with questions specific to particular coursework or clinical assignments.

It is essential that students gain the necessary clinical skills and knowledge to become competent clinicians. Assessment instruments such as the student performance review, employer surveys, and graduate surveys can advise the process of measuring learning outcomes. However, there is no substitute for ongoing and consistent assessment of the learning process by engaged and caring mentors. Supervisors, faculty members, advisors, peers, and individual students reflecting on their own performance can all assist in determining if the student is making appropriate progress toward the goal of independent practice.

### Clients

The third stakeholder in the clinical learning paradigm is the client. At the most basic level supervisors who are effective clinical educators guide students in service provision that has a positive impact on the client's communication skills. Clinical outcomes from the client perspective should be equivalent to what would be expected if a student were not involved. Clinical expectations and methodology should be guided, as always, by evidence-based practice principles and governed by adherence to ethical standards. Clients have the right to know if they are being treated by a student, and should expect confidentiality and professionalism. Ethical principles regarding the responsibility to the profession and to the public should guide students and supervisors alike (Chabon, Hale, & Wark, 2008). Clients also have the right to expect that a fully credentialed professional is guiding their care and have confidence that their welfare is paramount.

## ◆ Conclusion and Future Directions

Positive outcomes from graduate clinical education in speech-language pathology rest on the highly varied skills and knowledge of clinical supervisors. Additionally, achieving these positive outcomes requires that student clinicians develop wide-ranging skills and knowledge across the course of the

Vanderbilt University - Department of Hearing and Speech Sciences
1215 21st Ave. S., Suite 8310
Nashville, TN 37232
Phone: 615-936-5000  Fax: 615-936-6914
www.vanderbiltbillwilkersoncenter.com

[ Submit by Email ]    [ Print Form ]

## *2011 Employer Survey of Program Alumni*

Please read the following statements. To answer the question, think about your overall impressions of your employee who graduated from our program.  Next to each statement there is a box; place a number from 1 to 5 corresponding to your level of agreement, from Strongly Disagree (1) to Strongly Agree (5), in the box.  If the statement is not applicable, place "N/A" in the box.

We encourage you to add comments at the end.
Thank you for completing this confidential questionnaire.

**This employee holds the following degree(s) from the Department of Hearing and Speech Sciences at Vanderbilt University** *(check all that apply)*

☐ Au.D.              ☐ M.S. - SLP              ☐ M.D.E.              ☐ Ph.D.

| **Strongly Disagree** | | | | **Strongly Agree** |
|---|---|---|---|---|
| 1 | 2 | 3 | 4 | 5 |

| |
|---|
| The clinician/teacher appropriately assesses and differentially diagnoses speech, language and other communication disorders. |
| The clinician/teacher consistently provides appropriate and effective treatment. |
| The clinician/teacher demonstrates critical thinking, appropriate independence, and problem-solving abilities to resolve clinical/instructional issues. |
| The clinician/teacher writes documentation that is technically accurate and complete. |
| The clinician/teacher interacts with colleagues in a professional and appropriate manner. |
| The clinician/teacher interacts professionally and appropriately with clients/students and families. |
| The clinician/teacher demonstrates genuine empathy and a caring attitude toward others. |
| The clinician/teacher abides by expected norms of ethical practice at all times. |
| The clinician's/teacher's overall performance meets all position requirements. |
| The clinician/teacher demonstrates on-going professional growth and development. |
| The clinician/teacher demonstrates the ability to work within interdisciplinary or multidisciplinary teams. |
| The clinician/teacher demonstrates leadership abilities. |

**Fig. 16.1**    An example of a survey of employers of recent graduates.

**Vanderbilt University - Department of Hearing and Speech Sciences**
1215 21st Ave. S., Suite 8310
Nashville, TN 37232
Phone: 615-936-5000  Fax: 615-936-6914
www.vanderbiltbillwilkersoncenter.com

[ Submit by Email ]    [ Print Form ]

Page 2

*If there are comments about this clinician/teacher you would like to share with us, please do so in the space below.*

### The following demographic information would be appreciated

| | |
|---|---|
| Your Title | |
| Name of employing institution/agency: | |
| Type of employment setting, disorders and ages served: | |

Mailing Address:

Email Address:

Telephone Number:

How many graduates from Vanderbilt's Department of Hearing and Speech Sciences are currently employed at your institution/agency?

In the past five years, approximately how many graduates from Vanderbilt's Department of Hearing and Speech Sciences have been employed at your institution/agency?

Overall, what is your satisfaction with the clinical preparation of our graduates in Audiology, Education of the Deaf, and Speech-Language Pathology?  Please feel free to comment, below:

Please submit this survey electronically by clicking on the "Submit by e-mail" button, or, if you prefer, please mail or fax to the attention of Penny Welch at the address on this form.

Thank you for completing this survey.*

*Survey adapted from MGH Graduate Program in Communication Sciences and Disorders' Employer Survey, with permission.

**Fig. 16.1**    (*Continued*)

graduate program. The venues for students to gain clinical skills and knowledge include classrooms, laboratories, and clinical settings, with clinical settings being the place where skills and knowledge are applied in real-life settings. Clinical educators foster student development during clinical placements, and to do that effectively, the educators must continually develop their own skills for supervision. Insight into what students must learn is provided in accreditation and credentialing standards. Assessing how students are learning can be done through student performance evaluations, employer surveys, and self-reports by the students.

Although clinical education has been positively influenced by technology in recent years, the basic paradigm has remained unchanged during the history of the profession. Supervisor, student, and client work simultaneously, and the desired outcome is that everyone emerges with improved skills and knowledge, although each stakeholder has a different focus for growth and development. Although it is unlikely that the clinical education paradigm will show significant changes in the immediate future other than technological influences, there are factors in the larger academic and regulatory arenas that will influence clinical education in the coming years.

University training programs in general and graduate programs in speech-language pathology and audiology specifically have felt the influence of budget exigencies, with those influences anticipated to continue. Demands for higher enrollments to meet budget targets, difficulty in recruiting academic and clinical faculty, program closings, expectations that university clinics generate departmental revenue, and a generally poor economy are sources of stress for training programs. Programs are being asked to do more with less, and clinical education is often a costly part of the training program. When university training clinics close or are scaled back, reliance on off-campus clinical sites increases. Speech-language personnel in those sites are experiencing their own challenges for high productivity and budget efficiencies. These factors sometimes lead to reluctance on the part of off-campus sites to take on the responsibility of providing clinical education to students.

Influences outside academia are having an effect on graduate training programs as well. Hale (2011) noted that state departments of education seem determined to lower credentialing standards to increase the work force addressing speech-language-hearing issues in the schools. Employers demand increased caseloads and use of support personnel to improve profitability. Regulatory bodies seem inconsistent on what is intended by phrases such as "qualified provider" and "line-of-sight" supervision. Graduate training programs are struggling to provide quality education to credential-worthy candidates in the face of these challenges.

As these obstacles are faced, it is important that the requirement for good outcomes, for the client, the supervisor, and the student clinician, is not compromised. Graduate training programs are charged with educating competent and ethical professionals who are prepared to serve a diverse client population with wide-ranging disorders. That charge will not change in the face of challenges. It will only become more important.

# References

American Speech-Language-Hearing Association (ASHA). (2008a). *Clinical supervision in speech language pathology* [technical report]. www.asha.org/policy

American Speech-Language-Hearing Association (ASHA). (2008b). *Clinical supervision in speech language pathology* [position statement]. www.asha.org/policy

American Speech-Language-Hearing Association (ASHA). (2008c). *Knowledge and skills needed by speech-language pathologists providing clinical supervision* [knowledge and skills]. www.asha.org/policy

American Speech-Language-Hearing Association (ASHA). (2011). CAA-accredited academic program statistics. http://www.asha.org/academic/accreditation/CAA_Program_Stats.htm

Anderson, J. L. (Ed.). (1970). *Proceedings of Conference on Supervision of Speech and Hearing Programs in the Schools.* Bloomington, IN: Indiana University

Anderson, J. L. (1988). *The supervisory process in speech-language pathology and audiology.* Austin, TX: Pro-Ed

Carozza, L. (2011). *Science of successful supervision and mentorship* (pp. 73–77). San Diego: Plural

Chabon, S. S. (2006). Platitudes on attitudes and the relevance of intelligence: The clinical education of graduate students. Annual Supervisor Conference, Vanderbilt University, October

Chabon, S. S., Hale, S. T., Lee-Wilkerson, D., & Kellum, G. D. (2008). Great expectations: A novel approach to quantifying student-clinician behavior. A presentation to the annual convention of the American Speech-Language-Hearing Association, Boston

Chabon, S. S., Hale, S. T., & Wark, D. W. (2008). Triangulated ethics: The patient-student supervisor relationship. *The ASHA Leader,* February 12

Council on Academic Accreditation in Audiology and Speech-Language Pathology (CAA). (2011). *Standards for accreditation of graduate education programs in audiology and speech language pathology programs.* www.asha.org/policy

Council for Clinical Certification in Audiology and Speech-Language Pathology (CFCC). (2005) *Membership and certification handbook of the American Speech-Language-Hearing Association.* www.asha.org/about/membership-certification/handbooks/slp/slp_standards.htm

Council for Clinical Certification in Audiology and Speech-Language Pathology (CFCC). (2009). Knowledge and skills summary form for certification in speech-language pathology. http://www.asha.org/uploadedFiles/certification/KASASummaryFormSLP.pdf

Goldberg, S. A. (1997). *Clinical skills for speech-language pathologists* (pp. 313–318). San Diego: Singular Publishing Group

Hale, S. T. (2011). Storm front approaching: The consequences of doing nothing. An invited plenary presentation to the Council of Academic Programs in Communication Sciences and Disorders, Tampa, FL

Hoben, K., Varley, R., & Cox, R. (2007, Mar). Clinical reasoning skills of speech and language therapy students. *International Journal of Language and Communication Disorders, 42*(Suppl 1), 123–135

McCrea, E. S., & Brasseur, J. A. (2003). *The supervisory process in speech-language pathology and audiology.* Boston: Allen & Bacon

Rassi, J. A., & Hancock, M. (1999). *Student performance review—speech-language pathology clinical practicum.* Nashville, TN: Department of Hearing and Speech Sciences, Vanderbilt University

Ward, L., & Webster, E. (1965). The training of clinical personnel: II. A concept of clinical preparation. *ASHA, 7,* 103–106

# 17

# Outcomes in Higher Education

*Michael L. Kimbarow, Celia R. Hooper, and Alex F. Johnson*

## ♦ Chapter Focus

This chapter provides a framework and cites resources to support the development and implementation of an outcomes assessment process for academic programs in communication sciences and disorders (CSD). It also reviews the external and internal imperatives that demand accountability in higher education enterprises to offer a context for CSD program assessment and make recommendations for integrating strategic planning at the department level with assessment of program and course outcomes.

## ♦ Introduction

State and private colleges and universities across the United States are suffering from economic woes. The cost of a college education is rising faster than many other sectors of our economy and the cost of attendance has almost tripled since 1980 (College Board Advocacy and Policy Center, 2010). The College Board reports that public universities are raising tuition even faster than expensive private schools. Lawmakers, parents, and students are beginning to ask whether the cost of higher education is justifiable. As legislators slash state budgets, they are slashing university budgets and laying off faculty and staff. Tuition increases tend to be the only sources of extra income found by administrators, leaving families to shoulder more and more college debt (Baum & Steele, 2010). But the families want to know if they are getting what they are paying for. Articles, blogs, and books in the popular press are addressing this issue; some recently published books on this subject are *Higher Education? How Colleges Are Wasting Our Money and Failing Our Kids and What We Can Do About It* (Hacker and Driefuss, 2011), *Academically Adrift: Limited Learning on College Campuses* (Arum & Roksa, 2011), and *Crisis on Campus: A Bold Plan for Reforming Our Colleges and Universities*, by Mark C. Taylor (2010). In addition, there is the Pew Research Center report, *Is College Worth It?* (Taylor et al, 2011), which found that 47% of the public believes "the main purpose of a college education is to teach work-related skills and knowledge," whereas 39% say the purpose of a college education is to "grow personally and intellectually." Whatever the mission, how do we know whether it is being accomplished? Is a college education a quality experience? Are faculties, tenured or untenured, delivering a quality education? Is the U.S. system of higher education falling from its number one ranking in the world? Does the Carnegie classification of colleges and universities matter in terms of quality? (McCormick & Zhao, 2005) Does it matter if a college is classified as "community engaged?" All of these questions and issues swirl as our society demands accountability in our higher education institutions, and campuses have responded with a push for better accountability. Terminology such as *outcomes, student learning outcomes, assessment,* and *outcomes assessment* have developed, and whole processes, professions, and organizations are now in place to attempt some form of accountability in higher education. Every college or university, or unit therein, faces this issue in formal processes, such as accreditation, and in informal processes, such as public scrutiny. In this chapter we explore ways to address the current climate and meet the challenges to higher education in CSD using outcome measures.

## ◆ Greater Accountability in Higher Education

### The Current Dialogue Regarding Outcomes

What do we mean by "accountability?" Some might define this in a higher education context as delivering the educational promises that the students and society expect at a reasonable cost. To do so, one must look at the promises made. These promises usually take the form of mission statements, and are achieved by a strategic plan. To know if the promise of the plan has been kept, a university measures something (assessment) and looks at the outcome of that measurement. For example, universities talk of "student learning outcomes." These are statements about what students will know and, through some action, be able to demonstrate when they have completed some course, project, activity or degree program. Universities, including faculty and administrators, struggle with two parts of accountability. First, they struggle to determine what outcome is desirable. Is it "to know," is it "to do," or is it a combination of the two? Are there differences in the outcomes of a history major and a speech-language pathology major? If we measure very broadly, the answer may be no, but is that meaningful? Second, they struggle with the best way to measure (assess) the desired outcome. These two struggles, not knowing what the desired outcome may be and not knowing the best way to measure it, has created a cottage industry of research, offices of assessment, assessment software programs, assessment organizations, and assessment mission statements. One of the authors' university Web site states: "The purpose of academic assessment is to give faculty a body of evidence on which to base decisions designed to improve teaching and learning. This body of evidence documents how well students are performing relative to faculty-defined student learning outcomes" (University of North Carolina Greensboro Office of Academic Assessment, 2008).

### How the Popular Press and Bestselling Books on Accountability Have Influenced Policy Makers

Many books and articles in recent years have attacked the status quo in higher education, but three of them can be highlighted here as representative of the important books that have been best sellers among the educated lay public. The authors of these books were interviewed in many educational journals and television programs, they were on the popular lecture circuit, and many spin-off articles were written in op-ed sections of newspapers and blogs all over America. The first book, *Higher Education?* by Hacker and Driefuss (2011), is dedicated to "our country's students, who deserve better." In this book, Hacker and Driefuss attack the world of the professoriate and review what an easy time of it the professoriate has, especially those who are "fireproof" with tenure. They attack the lack of teaching by many faculty, the failure to fire poor teachers, the cost of education, the extra (unneeded) amenities on most campuses (think fitness centers), and the arms race of athletics. The authors make several proposals that have started many campus conversations. They propose the abolishment of tenure, an end to reliance on loans, a demand for good teaching, an end to "vocational majors," an end to sabbaticals, an end to exploitation of adjuncts, and an increase in the role of university presidents as public servants. They recommended that universities cut ties with medical schools and research, including research centers and institutes, and instead have this role assumed by non-university institutions. They recommended that we examine what they call "techno-teaching" (such as distance learning), and that we spread the contributions of academic donors around to colleges that need it (such as Duke sharing with Appalachian State University). These authors, professors at Queens College and Columbia, lament the passing of an earlier time in academia when costs were more reasonable and higher education was valued for its own sake. Hacker and Driefuss reflect the current thinking of many on campus who have seen so much change.

In the second book, *Academically Adrift* by Arum and Roksa (2011), the authors examine student learning from the viewpoint of sociologists and express concern about what students are really learning in the climate of socializing and working long hours at an outside job. They comment on the many distractions of an institutional culture that puts undergraduate learning at or near the bottom of a priority list. Arum and Roksa take a very data-driven approach, using survey responses, student transcript data, and results from the standardized Collegiate Learning Assessment (CLA) administered during the first semester of college and at the end of four semesters. They found that there is very little student learning in areas of critical thinking, complex reasoning, and writing. In essence, they lay the groundwork for documentation that not enough learning is taking place in the first two years of undergraduate education. They offer ideas for educational reform, but propose that the real reform needs to be societal, including changes in K-12 education. They have a lively discussion in the book about helping students have a sense of purpose in college, about reorganizing student living and learning environments away from the current trend of individualization, and about improving the curriculum and instruction. Active learning, institutional transparency and accountability are themes in their recommendations for change. They propose a very structured system of externally mandated accountability, not unlike K-12 schools have. The CLA is recommended as a place to start in measurement, and the reader is encouraged to examine this instrument, used on many campuses in the U.S. (Driscoll, 2006). As a result of this book, and the higher education community discussions that followed, the CLA has been carefully scrutinized by many (Klein, Benjamin, Shavelson, & Bolus, 2007) and supported by the Council for Aid for Education (CAE, 2011; www.cae.org).

The third book is *Crisis on Campus* by Mark C. Taylor (2010). Taylor published an op-ed piece in the *New York Times* in 2009, "End the University as We Know It," in which he suggested we do away with tenure and academic departments (Taylor, 2009). The thousands of responses he received to that article prompted this book. Although the book is provocative and has been read by many, in and out of academia, it is not data-based. Nonetheless, his recommendation to abolish departments has provoked much discussion. Taylor states that the increase in specialization has not led to opportunity for intellectual exchange, and he argues that our colleges and universities are disconnected from a world that is defined by "webs, not walls." Instead of departments, he recommends divisions or "emerging zones" that would link the humanities, the social sciences, and the natural sciences. Many of our colleges and universities are moving in this direction as they realign within a division or merge one or more departments into a theme. Of course, the political (and alumni!) ramifications of that process are challenging, but Taylor would recommend these bold changes. Many universities are undergoing academic realignment, moving departments within the university to new schools, new colleges, and new configurations. Some examples in the past five years include Purdue University, Indiana University, Case Western Reserve University, University of North Carolina–Greensboro, Massachusetts Institute of Technology, University of Massachusetts–Amherst, University of Alabama, and Tennessee State University, to name a few. It is interesting to examine the realignment Web sites of these colleges to determine if more webs, not walls, are created.

## Stakeholders in Assessment

There are multiple layers of stakeholders in academic assessment. In addition to the obvious stakeholder, the student, there are stakeholders at every level in higher education and beyond. All experts in assessment suggest that stakeholders be involved as much as possible in the assessment process. Stakeholders can help evaluators understand that the right questions are being asked and that the process is valid. At the college/university level, a campus engages in effective outcomes assessment, as described by Banta (2002), that includes a *planning phase*, an *implementation phase*, and an *improvement* or *sustaining phase*. In these phases departments and programs utilize a variety of stakeholders, including faculty, administrators, students, employers, supervisors, and community advisory board members, not unlike an accreditation process. In the case of student learning, involving staff from all parts of the campus, such as student affairs professionals, technology professionals, and even business affairs professionals, can help everyone understand what a student might be learning. In an effective assessment process, involved stakeholders can determine if effective learning is taking place and if the intended outcomes of the program are occurring. The department or program reports to the next stakeholder, the unit or "school." In the case of CSD, that unit may be the arts and sciences school or a professional school (such as education or health professions). The unit characteristics can alter the stakeholders (those in health care versus education versus arts and sciences), but all units answer to the greater university stakeholders: administrators, boards of trustees, and legislators if it is a state university. Some external stakeholders, such as employers or alumni, can be involved in the process at all levels. Ultimately all universities answer to the public. How the process and outcome of assessment is explained to each level, beyond the department, can affect the perception of each level. Communication of the process and of the outcome of assessment is important in answering the question: "Is college making a difference in the life of the students in the nation and what is that difference?"

Some would argue that speech-language pathology and audiology, as part of a greater health professions group of disciplines, have an advantage when it comes to outcomes assessment and stakeholders. After all, our accreditation processes, described by Hale and Ivy in Chapter 16, have for many years required knowledge and skills assessment and planning, implementation, and improvement goals. The discipline has required student learning outcomes and program assessment in a very detailed way for quite some time. The stakeholders within the university and within the community (clinical supervisors, employers, medical advisory boards, etc.) have been involved in this process. Programs that are successful in assessment continue to use quality improvement within the program. But CSD faculty and other stakeholders would do well to engage within the greater university to make sure that the student learning goals and outcomes reach far beyond what we may focus on in our programs. General education outcomes are critical to the success of any pre-professional program, and the more that the faculty is involved in the scholarship of assessment at the most basic level, the stronger our communication sciences and disorders program will be and the more these outcomes become critical to the core mission of the university.

## ◆ Creating a Culture of Inquiry

A culture of inquiry, basic to successful assessment, begins campus-wide with a concern about general education of all students. As faculty and administrators, we are all accountable for the students on our campus, and if we fail to care about the basic education of students, we fail in this inquiry. For those faculty on a campus with traditional or distance education for four-year students, such basic outcomes as good writing, speaking, critical thinking, problem solving, information literacy, technology literacy, and mathematical literacy are very important to assess. Activities to help students attain these outcomes may include a residential college, service learning, international experiences, club and organization activities, honors programs, undergraduate research, and so on. There is a body of knowledge on *best practices* in these activities, and the more we are involved as CSD faculty, the more we will create a culture of inquiry on our campus and link our programs to the greater campus outcomes process. For those in professional schools and colleges, where undergraduates may not be present, or where there is a secondary admissions process to admit juniors and seniors, the link to the core mission of the university may not be as strong. But the need for a *culture of inquiry*, rather than a culture of discrete skill teaching, is equally important. All CSD programs, no matter where their academic home or format, depend on strong programs of institutional effectiveness, not just student learning and development outcomes.

Some faculty members think that such in-depth examination of coursework, activities within a curriculum, and standard syllabi, is a violation of "academic freedom" and that the outcomes assessment is a fad that will soon go away. In CSD, this is less common because evidence-based practice has been part of the culture for more than ten years (American Speech-Language-Hearing Association [ASHA], 2005). Although the original work in evidence-based practice focused on high-quality clinical care and research, it now includes the scholarship of assessment across the educational and practice spectrum (Banta, 2009). National work in designing effective assessment in educational outcomes is in line with the resources on academic assessment from ASHA (2011).

# ♦ The Institutional Perspective on Assessment and Outcomes

In this section we discuss the perspective of institutional leadership, with a focus on two specific questions:

1. What are the assessment and outcomes topics and issues of greatest interest to institutional leaders?

2. What are the tools that institutional leaders see as particularly useful in demonstrating the contribution of academic units?

Before discussing each of these topics, it is important to put these questions in context. There is extensive discussion of institutional assessment and academic outcomes in the literature. Leaders in the discipline of CSD who wish to have a general review of such information might consider one of the more general texts or reviews that have been published on the topic, such as Theall (2002), Palomba and Banta (2001), and Tierney (1999). These publications provide important review and background on the subject of assessment that is beyond the scope of this chapter. Rather than focus on the broad subject of assessment in higher education, in this discussion of outcomes in CSD we provide a perspective on the interdependent relationship among institutional leadership, the assessment process and outcomes, and the academic unit (usually, a department).

## Starting at the Top: What Do Institutional Leaders Care About?

Leaders of higher education institutions, both public and private, try to ensure that multiple institutional purposes are addressed simultaneously. The opportunity, and the challenge, of addressing divergent (sometimes competing) needs is complex; it calls for creativity, and often leaves various groups of stakeholders confused and occasionally feeling ignored. Institutions often develop a strategic plan (or map) as an expression of its values and a prioritization of attention and activities for a specified period of time. It is the institution's strategic planning documentation that provides a major clue as to the priorities of the board and academic administration. These priorities can be used to provide clarity and direction for various aspects of the academic community, including the department or program. Given the unlimited availability of "good ideas" for a program to consider, the strategic direction and plan of the institution provide a partial roadmap for decision making and prioritization.

Prior to developing or sharing a strategic plan, it is common for the leadership to ask stakeholders (staff, faculty, board, community, students) to contribute to the development of a collective pre-

**Table 17.1**   Common Themes Found in University Mission Statements

| Teaching | Scholarship | Service | Value/Edge |
|---|---|---|---|
| Excellence | Excellence | Excellence | Excellence |
| Technology | Research | Community | Student-centric |
| Cutting edge | Growing knowledge | Citizenship | Cost |
| Personalization | Innovation | Global | Distinctiveness |
| Innovation | Advances | Helping | Student services |
| Quality of faculty | Quality of researchers | Developing leaders | Location |
| Satisfaction of students | Contributions to knowledge | Professional leadership | Diversity |

ferred vision for the future and then to produce a mission statement for the institution. Although a strategic plan may take many forms, it usually consists of several key elements: a *mission* statement, a *vision* statement, and a summary of *core values* of the organization. Thus, the plan itself is really a set of operational directives and activities to reflect the superordinate ideas expressed in these background documents. Successful leaders in every level of an organization should understand and appreciate the purposes and values of the organization as well as the specific operational steps that have been developed.

The executive leadership of an institution is most concerned with demonstrating that the activities and resources of the institution are addressing the mission and values that have been expressed and agreed upon. Successful unit level administrators connect the work of their program or department to institutional missions and values in a manner that is completely transparent. Health professions programs, such as those in CSD, are particularly well positioned to address many of the typical "values" of most institutions. Attracting, retaining, and graduating great students, providing service to the community, and promoting scholarly faculty activity are typical activities.

However, in most universities the mission and values are expressed in a manner that calls for the distinguishing qualities of excellence, constant improvement, and advancement in performance. Similarly, strategic thinking requires a focus on the outcomes of the various activities and resources being expended. Measuring these distinguishing characteristics can be quite challenging.

Most CSD programs are administered within schools of health science or in the larger liberal arts and sciences domain. Only a few programs are identified as stand-alone schools of CSD, and even fewer are part of independent health sciences schools. Regardless of the larger "unit" that houses the program in CSD, it may be helpful to consider two categories of outcomes that a university board or president is most concerned about. **Fig. 17.1** summarizes these outcomes along several dimensions. All institutional leaders want to know that the programs are providing cost-effective, successful programs for students, and that the various units of the university or college are delivering value to the community—both geographically and to the professional environment. In addition, leaders are also concerned that those factors that differentiate their program from that of peer institutions, that align with regional and national goals, and that address the interests of various stakeholders are highly visible. It is these factors that distinguish the institution within the larger community.

**Table 17.1** lists common themes in university mission statements, which illustrate the types of outcomes that universities are striving to achieve across four dimensions: teaching, scholarship, service, and "value/edge" (or competitive edge). Under each of the categories several examples are listed around which specific objectives may be addressed. Note that none of these items is discipline-specific, but that many of them are applicable to most disciplines, including CSD.

In summary, academic leaders and governing boards are concerned with ensuring that the basic functions of the university (teaching, scholarship, service) are delivered effectively and efficiently and that the mission-specific goals that have been selected for emphasis are realized. It is these academic goals and features that are the central focus of assessment and outcomes measurement in higher education.

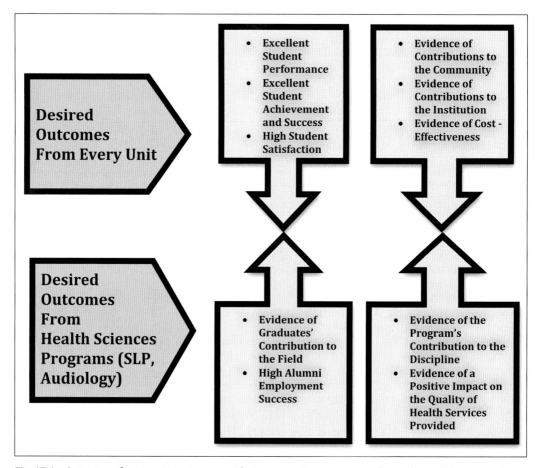

**Fig. 17.1** Outcomes of concern to institutions with Communication Sciences and Disorders (CSD) programs (and other health disciplines).

## What Are the "Tools" that Can Be Used to Measure Performance?

There are several features that serve as indicators and measures of performance in higher education programs. General categories of measures include general student achievement and outcomes measures; program review; disciplinary accreditation reports and measures; and faculty performance and productivity measures in teaching and scholarship. There is some overlap across these general measures, but each has a distinctive purpose.

### General Student Achievement and Outcomes

Assessing student achievement in the health professions, particularly at the graduate level, focuses on achieving competencies (skills and knowledge) that are specific to the discipline. In speech-language pathology and audiology, this content guidance is provided through two ASHA councils: the Council on Academic Accreditation (CAA) and the Council for Clinical Certification (CFCC). It is important to note that attainment of these competencies serves as the foundation for entering the professions.

Recently, leaders in medical and nursing education (Interprofessional Education Collaborative, 2011) have proposed that interprofessional competencies should be added to this portfolio. These competencies, along with the strong content knowledge and behaviors from the discipline, are presented as essential to the next generation of providers. In medicine and nursing, the discussion of these interprofessional competencies as the context for practice in the future has emerged as a major theme in health education circles. It is important that all health professions, including speech-language pathology and audiology, take note of this emergent trend and enter this important discussion. Appreciation for and implementation of instruction that includes development of interprofessional skills and knowledge will require new teaching strategies for faculty and alignment across disciplines for curricular and practicum opportunities.

Core disciplinary and interprofessional skills are assessed using a variety of techniques in the classroom and clinic. Several key outcomes measures are useful across all programs in the institution. These measures are quite familiar to program administrators, and include program retention and graduation rates, performance on high stakes (licensure, certification) examinations, job placement rates, and employer and alumni satisfaction measures.

Measures of student success in meeting the competencies of the discipline and in other outcomes measures are of critical concern to university leadership. Students come to every university professional program expecting a solid educational foundation that meets the entry-level competencies of their discipline, exposure to clinical situations that they are likely to encounter in the workplace, successful graduation, and employment. It is vital that, at the most basic level, every program documents that these basic expectations are met and continually reevaluated. When programs discover less than satisfactory performance in any of these outcomes measures, it is critical that they immediately document and implement improvement strategies. These measures are best viewed as the "vital signs" of the health of the educational program. Decreases or fluctuating performance suggests that immediate measures are in order.

### Program Reviews

Institutional program review is a widely used assessment approach in higher education and is particularly useful in assessing nonaccredited programs or, in the case of CSD, those aspects of the program that are not in the purview of the accrediting body (entry-level graduate education) such as undergraduate education, doctoral programs, research units, and clinical service delivery beyond student education. The typical model of institutional program review includes a self-study by the academic program, internal review by members of the larger university faculty and administration, and external review by one or more recognized experts in the discipline. The program review process results in a summary report that includes all of the information that has been collected and an assessment of program quality and efficiency.

Most university administrators consider the institutional program evaluation, along with regional accreditation of the institution, to be a key factor in assessing program quality and efficiency. Because of the use of independent outside experts and because the review can focus on specific questions and concerns of the administration (e.g., how does the program address the institutional goals as expressed in the strategic plan?), provosts and presidents rely heavily on the results of program review. Programs should heartily address the opportunity to use a program review as a time of serious reflection and planning. Additionally, the resources provided by the university at the time of review signal a serious commitment to the program. It also allows the chair and faculty within the program to highlight important information about the program and demonstrate a commitment to the institution's goals with particular clarity and focus.

### Faculty Performance Evaluations

Most universities have a standard approach to faculty evaluation in place that includes some aspects of self-assessment, peer review, review by an administrator, and assessment of teaching and research productivity. In some institutions this performance evaluation contributes to the annual merit raise or to promotion.

Assessment of teaching is usually completed through review of teaching portfolios, peer review of classroom or online instruction, and consideration of student course evaluations. Of these, student assessments of teaching are the most controversial. Multiple factors contribute to student assessments including complexity and demands of the course, personality of the instructor, and the student's inherent interest in the material. Regardless of this complexity and faculty concerns about student biases, these evaluations remain a primary measure of faculty teaching performance. Most can agree that the students' perspective is extremely important, as they are the key stakeholders and beneficiaries of the teaching, but administrators and faculty need to remember that multiple forms of assessment are critical, especially when there are concerns with an individual faculty member's teaching performance.

Research productivity standards vary considerably from institution to institution. Research-intensive institutions may view peer-reviewed publication productivity and research grants as the primary factor in evaluation of individual faculty members, whereas other institutions that are more focused on the teaching mission may view scholarly productivity in balance with teaching and other responsibilities. It is essential that faculty members understand the role and expectations of research productivity in their specific institution. In general, if research is a major part of the university mission, then all faculty members are expected to demonstrate productivity as evidenced by grants and peer-reviewed publications. A general guideline for department chairs and faculty members alike to consider: at every discussion of performance, address the faculty member's effectiveness in meeting institutional (not just departmental) expectations and the faculty member's progress toward promotion. Frank and clear discussion of this progress ensures fairness to both parties and allows for the faculty member to adjust effort or change course as needed.

How do university leaders view scholarly productivity and teaching? These factors are the heart of every university's contract with its stakeholders and are central to demonstration of this relationship. Measurement and reporting of these elements of academic productivity and performance are critical in the community's, the government's, and the accreditors' understanding of the contribution of an institution. Although there is significant variability in measures used to describe success in each of these areas, they should not be ignored. At the departmental level, in addition to using standard measures of teaching and productivity, measures of the impact in these areas should also be reported and brought to the attention of the administration.

## Disciplinary Accreditation

In professional disciplines, specialized accreditation is an essential and vital component of program operation. In most cases, and specifically in CSD, professional accreditation is a requirement for offering the degree and for students to be able to receive financial aid. Achievement of accreditation within the discipline, which requires a self-assessment and periodic site visits by peers from other institutions, provides an assessment from the perspective of the discipline as to the currency and quality of the curriculum, the academic and clinical faculty, the facilities, and the program leadership. Reports from accrediting bodies typically include a summary of the documentation provided, as well as commendations or concerns, and recommendations for improvement. These reports always include an accreditation decision; thus they constitute a "high stakes" review for the department and its leadership.

Because the stakes are high with regard to accreditation decisions, it is important to keep the nature of these assessments in perspective. Accreditation is necessary, but usually not sufficient as an indicator of program excellence in CSD or in other health fields. First, some aspects of the typical program—undergraduate education, interprofessional education, research, and scholarship—are not critical elements in accreditation. Second, by its nature, accreditation standards provide guidance as to the basic, minimal requirements for all academic programs in the discipline, not to the distinctiveness of the program. It is actually the attainment beyond these basic standards that differentiates programs and departments and distinguishes programs.

Although most academic units in the health professions are adept at demonstrating compliance with standards, the challenge of measuring performance beyond this most basic level is frequently not addressed in the real-world day-to-day life of higher education. The message to educational leaders in CSD programs is that although accreditation is essential, admirable, and demonstrates significant effort on the part of a program, it does not distinguish a program to the leadership of the institution. Certainly the president or the board would be extremely concerned when a particular program does not achieve accreditation from its disciplinary review body. However, accreditation is viewed primarily as an indicator that the program meets the *basic* requirements set by interprofessional peers.

## Reporting Outcomes Via Metrics

Producing evidence that demonstrates results and impact is incumbent upon both public and private academic institutions. Given the threat of reduced funding for higher education in the current governmental environment and the continuing increase of costs in private education, it is likely that meaningful metrics will be essential for all programs. Meaningful metrics are those measures that validate the strategic objectives of the institution, reinforce the key values expressed in mission and vision statements, demonstrate the program's essential value for students and the community, and provide strong evidence for the cost-effectiveness of the program.

Thus, institutional leadership typically views the assessment process as a system of providing metrics that allow for validation of programs, highlighting strengths and weaknesses, and identifying areas for investment or reduction. Programs that are most effective at attending carefully to measurement strategies that address these objectives are likely to be viewed as fulfilling the expectations of the leadership. Although there will be institutional variations in the reporting of metrics and outcomes, the need for the development of consistent periodic reports of academic program progress is increasingly expected. Using clearly understandable (and concise) data presentations and narrative report will get the attention of the leaders and be useful to them in their own work. It is important to note the critical importance of presenting data that show change in performance over time, variations against benchmark institutions or programs, and progress toward an institutional goal; these data will be highly valued by those who have to demonstrate institutional success to stakeholders. For example, a university with a goal of increasing scholarly productivity may be interested in showing metrics that demonstrate average new research grant dollars that are generated over time or the number of scholarly publications per faculty member plotted annually. Another institution attempting to demonstrate its commitment to the community might be interested in demonstrating increasing value, in terms of revenue generation, clinical teaching opportunity, or clinic visits, of the university's speech-language-hearing center from year to year. These simple examples illustrate the concept of linking the departmental activity to the institutional goals in a manner that may be useful to the administration.

## ◆ Department Level Assessment

### Strategic Planning

Strategic planning at the departmental level provides the framework and the foundation upon which a successful assessment program can be developed and implemented. Strategic planning is the formal consideration of an academic department's future direction. Generally a strategic plan will include a mission statement (a succinct summation of the reason a program exists) followed by a vision statement (a summation of the program's aspirations). The vision statement provides the inspiration, and the framework for the strategic plan. A sample of mission and vision statements obtained from selected CSD program Web sites can be found in Appendices A and B, below.

The effort to craft a strong strategic plan provides an opportunity for faculty members to reflect on the current state of their program and determine how they can leverage the present to construct a desired future. Strategic plans generally project out anywhere from 3 to 5 years. Anything less is too short a time frame to realistically achieve the plan's goals, and anything longer fails to acknowledge that the external and internal environment will likely be unrecognizable and unpredictable, making the plan outdated at best. A well-constructed strategic plan can support requests for additional resources for the program (e.g., new faculty lines, expanded space, or additional capital equipment), lead to new course or program development (e.g., online distance education), or expand degree options (e.g., adding a Ph.D. program).

There are a variety of approaches that can be used to develop a strategic plan. A generally accepted method for connecting a program's present state to its future path is though a SLOT/SWOT (strengths, limitations/weaknesses, opportunities, and threats) analysis. A SLOT analysis may be conducted on a macro-level for the program overall. The analysis requires programs to identify the external and internal variables that support or challenge achieving the strategic initiatives, as follows:

- *Strengths:* Internal characteristics of the program that give it an advantage over others and that can be effectively leveraged to achieve the strategic goals

- *Limitations*: Internal factors that place the department at a disadvantage and may inhibit change; these need to be identified and addressed to achieve the long-term desired outcomes

- *Opportunities:* An evaluation of the external environment to identify resources that may facilitate achievement of desired outcomes (e.g., the need for school speech-language pathologists)

- *Threats:* An evaluation of external elements in the environment that may hinder the program's achieving its desired strategic objectives (e.g., anticipated cuts in state funding for public universities)

The following program-reflective questions operationalize the SLOT analysis and may be useful to frame the initial discussion among department faculty:

- What works well in your program in terms of preparing your students for their profession?

- What things would you want to change in your program?

- What other programs/institutions are your competitors?

- How will your program distinguish itself from these competitors?

- What resources (faculty, staff, technologies, partnerships) do you have that will allow you to create/ maintain a distinctive program? What capacity do you have to offer the program?

- What resources might you need to create/maintain a distinctive program?

Conducting a SLOT analysis is essential because subsequent steps in the process of planning for achievement of the selected strategic objective may be derived from the SLOT. For example, a strategic initiative may target an effort to establish a specialty in augmentative and alternative communication (AAC) for the program. A SLOT analysis will identify the internal resources to achieve the objective (for example, faculty specializing in research and treatment of individuals using AAC devices), the internal limitations (small inventory of AAC devices), the external opportunities (program resides in a community with few available AAC resources), and external threats (growing private practice serving AAC needs of the community) that must be considered in planning the steps necessary to achieve the objective.

## Program Outcomes

A CAA-accredited program is required to collect data and make results available to the public on the following three macro-level program outcomes tracked continuously but reported only for the previous three academic years:

1. Number of students who completed the program within the expected time frame.

2. Number of students taking and passing the national Praxis Examination in Speech-Language Pathology.

3. Number of graduates employed in the profession within one year of graduation.

There are many methods for reporting the data; a sample table format is found in **Table 17.2**. Programs falling below national benchmarks are required to take corrective action to ensure that they come into compliance with national standards.

The CAA also requires that programs engage in systematic assessment of the quality currency and effectiveness of its degree program. A common method for doing so is through alumni surveys and employer surveys, which provide valuable information on how well prepared recent graduates were to start practice and how employers assess recent graduates' ability to fulfill their professional responsibilities.

## Student Learning Outcomes

The central focus of any academic enterprise must be the students and must hold paramount the identification of how well students can demonstrate knowledge and skills that are directly attributable to the program. This is how programs are able to demonstrate the cause/effect relationship

**Table 17.2**   Sample Reporting Matrix for Council on Academic Accreditation (CAA) Required Program Data Elements

| Academic Year | No. of Completed Program Within Expected Time Frame | No. of Completed Program Later Than Expected Time Frame | Number Not Completing | % Completing |
|---|---|---|---|---|
| 2010/2011 | 34 | 5 | 2 | 95% |
| 2009/2010 | 42 | 6 | 1 | 98% |
| 2010/2011 | 33 | 5 | 1 | 97% |
| **3-Yr. Avg.** | **36** | **5** | **1** | **97%** |

**PRAXIS Data (Institutional Data Reporting Method)**

| Period | No. of Students Taking the Praxis Exam | No. of Students Passed | Pass Rate |
|---|---|---|---|
| 2010/2011 | 35 | 32 | 0.91 |
| 2009/2010 | 25 | 24 | 0.96 |
| 2008/2009 | 32 | 29 | 0.90 |
| | | **3-Year Average** | **0.92** |

**Employment Data**

| | Employment Rate in Profession | |
|---|---|---|
| **Academic Year** | **Number of Graduates** | **Percent of Graduates** |
| 2010/2011 | 37 | 94% |
| 2009/2010 | 48 | 100% |
| 2008/2009 | 38 | 100% |
| | **3-Year Average** | **98%** |

between its goals for students finishing the program and the coursework and clinical practicum assignments that are designed to meet those goals.

A good place to start is for faculty to identify the attributes they expect their students to demonstrate upon graduation. In essence, this is the macro-level worldview on how the program curriculum relates to the achievement of knowledge, skills competencies, and dispositions necessary for clinical practice (see Appendix C, below, for examples of student attributes). Once those attributes are defined, program faculty are then in a position to develop an assessment program that will measure a student's progress toward achieving the program's desired outcomes—the student learning outcomes (SLOs). There is value in aligning the student attributes to the CAA and CFCC standards because those have been vetted by panels of experts and accepted by the CSD academic and professional community.

Once the curriculum level analysis is complete, a good next step is to identify where in the curriculum (i.e., the course level or the practicum level) a student is expected to have the opportunity to acquire knowledge, skills, and competencies. No single course can meet all the CAA/CFCC standards, but each course should be integral to meeting those standards; otherwise it may be difficult to justify and support allocating resources to teach it. A useful method for completing this analysis is to create a matrix in which each learning outcome is identified, and each outcome is attached to a course in the program. It is important to recognize that the same student-learning outcome may overlap among the various courses in the curriculum. For example, an outcome that defines the ability of a program graduate to treat individuals with a variety of communication disorders is likely to be addressed in some fashion across various courses that target specific communication disorders (e.g., voice disorders, aphasia, etc.). Curriculum matrices may be useful in identifying significant redundancies, misalignments, and gaps in the program that may lead to more efficient use of faculty and student time.

There is a common belief among faculty that student learning outcomes are already part of each course, and that when students achieve a passing grade they have met the learning outcomes specified in the course syllabus. However, there are several reasons why grades alone are not an adequate measure of student learning:

- Course content may vary among different faculty members teaching the same course.
- Course grading policies vary from instructor to instructor.
- Grades tell us nothing about what the student actually knows.
- Grades tell us nothing about the quality of the pedagogical process, and offer inadequate feedback necessary to make course or program improvements.

A good learning outcome is specific, well defined, achievable, bridges the gap between course and curriculum, and describes what the student will be able to do following completion of the program. But if the objectives are not grade based, then how does one know if a student has actually achieved them? One useful method is to tie the outcome to course assignments, which may include any of the activities required of the students as they complete a class such as exams or projects. **Table 17.3** shows an SLO tied to a signature assignment in an aphasia class.

## Rubrics

The next step in the process is to create a scoring rubric to assess student performance on the assignment. An effective rubric is used to assess student performance along task-specific performance criteria. A sample rubric tied to the final treatment project in an aphasia class is found in **Table 17.4**. The rubric defines the expected elements, which, if they appear in the project, would be accepted as evidence that the student has sufficiently demonstrated his/her understanding of the material across a continuum of mastery. An excellent compendium of rubric resources can be found at http://course1.winona.edu/shatfield/air/rubrics.htm.

**Table 17.3**  Sample Aphasia Course Objectives and Assignment Matrix Tied to Council for Clinical Certification (CFCC) Standards

Standard III-C: Students will be able to demonstrate knowledge of the nature of complex communication need by
1. explaining the neuropathology and secondary effects of hemorrhagic and ischemic stroke.
2. explaining the social/emotional effects of aphasia on the individual and his/her support systems.
3. providing a complete patient profile that completely and accurately describes an individual with fluent or nonfluent aphasia.

Standard III-D: Students will be able to demonstrate knowledge of the principles and methods of prevention, assessment, and intervention for children and adults with complex communication needs by
1. describing a treatment plan that includes three goals consistent with the deficits associated with fluent or nonfluent aphasia.
2. providing detailed instructions and descriptions of materials to be used in treatment.
3. developing a three-level cuing and prompting plan for each task.
4. developing alternative treatment goals designed to (a) simplify task treatment task demand and (b) increase the level of difficulty of the proposed task.

**Course Requirements Matrix**

| Student Learning Objective | Midterm | Assessment Project | Treatment Plan Project |
|---|---|---|---|
| III-C (1) | x | | |
| III-C (2) | x | | |
| III-C (3) | | | x |
| III-D (1) | | x | x |
| III-D (2) | | | x |
| III-D (3) | | | x |
| III-D (4) | | | x |

## Evaluation

An assessment system is only as good as its evaluation. The data collected must be analyzed. More importantly, assessment system should lead to change. The entire point of an assessment enterprise is for an academic program to engage in a continuous cycle of inquiry that leads to a continuous cycle of improvement of the program (Millett, Stickler, Payne, & Dwyer, 2007). In some respects this may be the most difficult step in the cycle for a department to embrace because with data analysis comes the possibility of discovering that the program is coming up short in meeting its goals. One way to minimize the fear factor is to frame the analysis and discussion of results as an opportunity to improve student outcomes rather than an exercise in identifying specific areas of weakness in a program. With this goal in mind, a program will fulfill the spirit of the assessment enterprise and will likely emerge stronger and well positioned to manage its own future.

## ◆ Conclusion and Future Directions

Academia is in the midst of a transformational shift in how the public perceives its role and mission in society. State universities have experienced unprecedented cuts in public funding, tuitions costs are increasing at an alarming rate, and consumers are demanding that their investment in higher education shows an acceptable return on investment. Assessment and accountability are the keys to survival for CSD programs. It is not enough to demonstrate that we are serving our communities by

**Table 17.4** Sample Rubric Tied to the Final Aphasia Treatment Project at San Jose State University

| Category | Mastery (15 Pts.) | Superior (10 Pts.) | Basic (6 Pts.) | Emerging (2 Pts.) | Unacceptable (1 Pt.) |
|---|---|---|---|---|---|
| Patient profile | Patient profile is clearly written and presents complete information on patient background, etiology, type of aphasia, language deficits, and other factors that may influence treatment outcome. | Patient profile is not presented in complete detail. There are two elements missing. | | There are at least two errors in the patient profile. | Patient description does not provide adequate information for a speech-language pathologist to fully understand client characteristics or variables that may influence outcome. |
| Diagnostic profile | Diagnostic test selected is appropriate for the patient description. Scores represent identified deficits and severity level. | Diagnostic test profile shows one inconsistency from patient description. | There are two errors in the test profile that are inconsistent with the patient description. | | Patient profile is inconsistent with patient description. Severity levels do not match the score profile. |
| Treatment goals CFCC Standard III-D, III-G | Treatment goals are appropriate to the aphasia type and severity indicated in the patient description and diagnostic profile. Goals are realistic and achievable in 1 semester. | One of the treatment goals is inconsistent with the patient profile and severity level. One treatment goal is unrealistic or not relevant to the client. | The description of the treatment program is incomplete and does not demonstrate a clear understanding of aphasia treatment principles. | | Three or more of the proposed goals are inconsistent or unachievable per the patient profile. |
| Treatment description CFCC Standard III-D | The treatment program is described in appropriate detail. Materials are clearly identified, instructions are included, and prompting and scoring procedures are presented with sufficient detail that anyone could conduct the session. | There is a key element missing from the description of the treatment activity. Prompting strategies are unclear or inconsistent with the treatment goal. | | There are two critical elements missing from the description of the treatment activity that would make it difficult for a new clinician to implement the program. | There are at least three critical elements missing in the description that would make it difficult for a new clinician to implement the program. |

**Table 17.4**   (*Continued*) Sample Rubric Tied to the Final Aphasia Treatment Project at San Jose State University

| Evidence | There are at least three acceptable sources of evidence provided to support the treatment approach. Use of published information is evident. If evidence is unavailable, a clear justification is provided. Minimal use of Internet sources. Sources are identified and cited properly. | There are two acceptable sources of evidence provided in support of the treatment program. There is one error in proper citation format. | There is one acceptable published literature source to support the proposed treatment plan. | There are no acceptable published sources to support the treatment approach. Two or more citation errors. |
|---|---|---|---|---|
| Writing 1 | Sentence structure is coherent and there are no grammatical errors. Paragraphs are well organized and contribute to a cohesive paper. Transition from one idea to the next is logical. No spelling or punctuation errors, no run-on sentences. No ambiguity in the use of pronouns. | There are two errors in spelling, grammar, paragraph structure, or sentence structure. Transition from one idea to the next is not clear. | There are three errors in any of the following: grammar, spelling, sentence structure, paragraph structure, pronoun referent. | There are four or more errors in grammar, word choice, tense, punctuation. |
| Writing 2 (10 pts. max.) | Paper is written consistent with APA style and all references are identifiable and formatted correctly. | | There is one error in APA format or reference list format. | |

graduating qualified professionals. We must demonstrate unequivocally that our graduates have the knowledge and skills necessary to go out and successfully perform their jobs.

As higher education funding shrinks, so will the financial resources that are allocated to programs. We believe there will be increased pressure for CSD programs to increase the number of students they admit. The days of being able to justify graduate programs designed for 15 to 20 students will soon be a distant memory for all. We can no longer hide behind the cloak of accreditation standards to counter-argue for fewer students and more faculty. Gone are the days when vacated faculty lines automatically return to the department. Approval to hire faculty will go to those departments that can demonstrate the greatest need through their assessment program. Resources will move to those programs that demonstrate efficiencies in program delivery, good records of program completion, alignment with institutional goals, and data that show they are successfully meeting the performance outcomes they set for the program.

Finally, we anticipate that there will be increasing pressure put on programs to consider entrepreneurial initiatives to generate increased revenue to fund operations. Look for a strong push to offer online, distance learning programs and to offer alternative pathways to degrees. The need for effective assessment programs generating hard data to drive campus resource allocation decisions is here and it will never go away.

## ♦ Appendix A: A Sample of Mission Statements Obtained from CSD Department Web Sites

The mission of the Communication Disorders Graduate Program is to educate students to become competent speech-language pathologists, audiologists, teachers, and/or researchers who are committed to scientific inquiry and lifelong learning, to add to the knowledge base of the discipline, to provide public service to enhance the lives and dignity of individuals with communication disorders, and to embrace diversity. (University of Cincinnati; http://homepages.uc.edu/csd/)

Our mission is to provide comprehensive programs of education and scholarship that will advance the understanding of human communication and related disorders; to build a foundation of knowledge and skills that encourages competent clinical practice for the professional lifetime; and to promote a culture of collaboration and respect for others. (University of Texas, Austin; http://csd.utexas.edu/about)

To provide an understanding of human communication disorders and their clinical management by emphasizing a scientific approach. Academic courses and clinical education experiences encourage a theoretical perspective and experimental orientation to develop an appreciation of current knowledge and future research needs. (University of Connecticut; http://www.cdis.uconn.edu/documents/MA _Brochure_Disorders_2011.pdf)

The Division of Communication Sciences and Disorders is dedicated to excellence in research and teaching undergraduate and graduate students who will be successful in future academic study and employment. (Ohio University; http://www.ohio.edu/chsp/rcs/csd/manage/upload/Graduate-Handbook .pdf)

The Mission of the Department of Communicative Disorders and Sciences is to provide high-quality academic and clinical preparation to students seeking careers working with individuals who have speech, language, and hearing disorders, and their families. Guided by principles of evidence-based practice and working in collaboration with other professionals, our graduates will adhere to the highest standards of ethical practice in serving the needs of our diverse community. (San Jose State University; http://www.sjsu.edu/cds/docs/Strategic_Plan_Dissemination.pdf)

# ◆ Appendix B: A Sample of Vision Statements Obtained from CSD Department Web Sites

Our vision is to be one of the best research and academics programs in Communication Sciences and Disorders in the United States. This vision is to be accomplished by achieving national and international recognition for its high-quality research, innovative graduate programs, outstanding undergraduate instruction, and model training approaches for educating superior researchers and practitioners. (University of Texas, Austin; http://csd.utexas.edu/graduate/speech-language-pathology-graduate-courses)

We believe that the Department of Communicative Disorders and Sciences is uniquely positioned to serve as the professional hub for speech-language pathologists and audiologists in the Silicon Valley. Utilizing CSD faculty expertise as well as department and University resources, the program will

a.  be a source for ongoing professional development;

b.  establish University/Community partnerships to serve individuals with communicative disorders across the life span;

c.  be a source of innovative models of professional preparation;

d.  contribute to the knowledge base of the disciplines; and

e.  align with campus models of environmental sustainability. (San Jose State University; http://www.sjsu.edu/cds/docs/Strategic_Plan_Dissemination.pdf)

The SFSU Communicative Disorders Program will meet the challenges of the present and future through dynamic response to the need for qualified professionals in Communication Sciences and Disorders. Through a commitment to addressing the needs of the workplace and professional excellence, SFSU CD faculty will provide mentorship for future professionals to gain experience with a wide range and diversity of individuals with communicative disorders; to understand their perspectives; and to integrate research with clinical practice in support of people with communication disorders across the life span. (San Francisco State University; http://www.sfsu.edu/~comdis/strategic.html#vision)

The Department of Communication Disorders and Sciences will be recognized as the clinical center and graduate education program of choice in the state of Illinois and among the very best in the United States. (Rush University; http://www.rushu.rush.edu/servlet/Satellite?c=content_block&cid=12087817 18576&pagename=Rush%2Fcontent_block%2FPrintContentBlockDetail)

# ◆ Appendix C: A List of Core Characteristics of CSD Graduate Students Upon Program Completion

1.  Graduates are knowledgeable about normal speech, language, and communication behaviors across the life span (including geriatrics). They are knowledgeable about the anatomy and physiology of the auditory and speech mechanisms and the neurological substrates of speech, language, and hearing.

2.  Graduates have a strong foundation in normal and bilingual speech, language, and communication development.

3.  Graduates utilize evidence-based assessment and treatment approaches by accessing, evaluating, and applying research within the framework of their own clinical experiences and their client's values.

4.  Graduates exhibit knowledge and skills in the identification and treatment of speech language disorders from a multicultural perspective. They know when to use interpreters in service delivery, can distinguish a disorder from a cultural difference, and know about formal and informal assessment tools that are valid for children and adults from a diversity of languages and cultures.

5. Graduates provide clinical services to individuals exhibiting a wide range of speech, language, and communication disabilities through the life span consistent with the professional scope of practice in speech-language pathology.

6. Graduates provide services in a variety of employment settings, including schools, hospitals, community agencies and clinics, and private practice.

7. Graduates make decisions regarding all aspects of the clinical process, including analysis of assessment data with resulting recommendations for designing and evaluating an effective treatment plan including family involvement and counseling.

8. Graduates are prepared to work with other professional disciplines to ensure effective treatment outcomes for persons served.

9. Graduates are committed to lifelong learning to maintain their currency and to use the best practices in the field. Graduates use a variety of learning opportunities throughout their careers, including workshop/seminar attendance, accessing literature for self-study, and Web-based learning.

10. Graduates utilize technology to support their clinical practice, including electronic documentation, augmentative/alternative communication systems, and educational presentations.

11. Graduates are prepared to provide professional services consistent with the American Speech-Language-Hearing Association and California State Codes of Professional Ethics.

12. Graduates are advocates on behalf of the persons they serve and their profession to ensure access, excellence, and equity in service delivery.

## ♦ Acknowledgments

The authors would like to acknowledge the work of Ashley Frazier, doctoral student at University of North Carolina at Greensboro, supported by the School of Health and Human Sciences and a university diversity scholarship.

## ♦ Resources

*Academe Magazine* special issue (online): Assessing Assessment: http://www.aaup.org/AAUP/pubsres/academe/2010/SO/.

Blog: Assess This!: http://assessory.blogspot.com/.

Bloomsburg University recommended assessment articles/books: http://orgs.bloomu.edu/tale/outcomesAssessment.html.

Higher Ed Resource Hub: extensive list of Publications and listservs: http://www.higher-ed.org/resources/Assessment.htm.

Journals with an assessment focus:
*Assessment and Evaluation in Higher Education*
*Assessment Update*
*Practical Assessment, Research, and Evaluation*
*Quality Approaches in Higher Education*
*Research and Practice in Assessment*

Learning Outcomes Assessment communities (listservs, organizations, etc): http://www.learningoutcomeassessment.org/LOAcommunities.htm.

Learning Outcomes Assessment organizations:
AAC&U: Association of American Colleges and Universities
AASCU: American Association of State Colleges and Universities

ACPA: American College Personnel Association

APLU: Association of Public and Land-Grant Universities

CAS: Council for the Advancement of Standards in Higher Education

CIC: Council of Independent Colleges

NAICU: National Association of Independent Colleges and Universities

NASPA: Student Affairs Administrators in Higher Education

List of award-winning university assessment programs: http://www.learningoutcomeassessment.org/Award-WinningCampuses.htm.

National Institute for Learning Outcomes Assessment (NIOLA):_http://www.learningoutcomeassessment.org/CollegesandAssociations.html.

NILOA has a model for how universities should be sharing information about student learning on institutional Web sites: http://www.learningoutcomeassessment.org/TransparencyFrameworkIntro.htm.

North Carolina State Office of University Planning and Analysis maintains an extensive list of assessment resources: http://www2.acs.ncsu.edu/UPA/assmt/resource.htm.

Office of Planning and Assessment (OPA): http://opa.uncg.edu/.

Portland State Institutional Assessment Council: http://iac.pdx.edu/content/accreditation. (Comprehensive site with links to plans, outcomes, activities supporting the robust assessment effort at Portland State.)

Sample of university assessment efforts: University of North Carolina Greensboro Office of Academic Assessment: http://assessment.uncg.edu/. (Web site has links to assessment materials, resources, and FAQs.)

University of Iowa, Iowa Outcomes Assessment: http://www.uiowa.edu/~outcomes/contact.htm. (This is a comprehensive assessment site that includes sections on "Tools," "Innovations," and links to assessment efforts by other top universities.)

University of Kentucky ASSESS: Assessment in Higher Education Listserv: http://lsv.uky.edu/scripts/wa.exe?A0=ASSESS.

University of Maryland, Provost's Commission on Learning Outcomes Assessment: https://www.irpa.umd.edu/Assessment/LearningOutcomes/. (Web site has links to resources, process, and UMD/departmental efforts.)

University of North Carolina at Chapel Hill, Office of Institutional Research and Assessment (OIRA): http://oira.unc.edu/. (Links to goals and university resources.)

University of Wisconsin: http://www.provost.wisc.edu/assessment/. (Web site has the following assessment links: presentations, plan, council, funds, manual, reports, and resources.)

# References

American Speech-Language-Hearing Association (ASHA). (2005). *Evidence-based practice in communication disorders.* www.asha.org/policy

American Speech-Language-Hearing Association (ASHA). (2011). *Assessment.* www.asha.org/academic/assessment.htm

Arum, R., & Roksa, J. (2011). *Academically adrift: Limited learning on college campuses.* Chicago: University of Chicago Press

Banta, T. (2002). *Building a scholarship of assessment.* San Francisco: Jossey-Bass

Banta, T. (2009). *Designing effective assessment: Principles and profiles of good practice.* San Francisco: Jossey-Bass

Baum, S., & Steele, P. (2010). *Who borrows most? Bachelor's degree recipients with high levels of student debt.* College Board Advocacy and Policy Center. http://advocacy.collegeboard.org/sites/default/files/Trends-Who-Borrows-Most-Brief.pdf

College Board Advocacy and Policy Center. (2010). *Trends in college pricing.* http://trends.collegeboard.org/downloads/College_Pricing_2010.pdf

Council for Aid to Education (CAE). (2011). *The Collegiate Learning Assessment.* www.collegiatelearningassessment.org

Driscoll, A. (2006). The benchmarking potential of the New Carnegie Classification: Community engagement. In B. Holland & J. Meeropol (Eds.), *A more perfect vision: The future of campus engagement.* Boston: Campus Compact

Hacker, A., & Driefuss, C. (2011). *Higher education? How colleges are wasting our money and failing our kids and what we can do about it.* New York: St. Martin's Press

Interprofessional Education Collaborative. (2011). *Core competencies for interpfrofessional collaborative practice.* http://www.aacp.org/resources/education/Documents/10-242 IPECFullReportfinal.pdf

Klein, S., Benjamin, R., Shavelson, R. J., & Bolus, R. (2007, Oct). The collegiate learning assessment: Facts and fantasies. *Evaluation Review, 31,* 415–439

McCormick, A., & Zhao, C.-M. (2005). Rethinking and Reframing the Carnegie Classification. *Change, 37,* 51–57

Millett, C. M., Stickler, L. M., Payne, D. G., & Dwyer, C. A. (2007). *A culture of evidence: Critical features of assessments for postsecondary student learning.* Princeton, NJ: Education Testing Service. http://www.ets.org/Media/Resources_For/Higher_Education/pdf/4418_COEII.pdf

Palomba, C. A., & Banta, T. W. (Eds.). (2001). *Assessing student competence in accredited disciplines: Pioneering approaches to assessment in higher education.* Sterling, VA: Stylus Publishing

Taylor, M. (2009). End the university as we know it. *New York Times,* April 27. http://www.nytimes.com/2009/04/27/opinion/27taylor.html.

Taylor, M. (2010). *Crisis on campus: A bold plan for reforming our colleges and universities.* New York: Alfred A. Knopf

Taylor, P., Parker, K., Fry, R., Cohn, D., Wang, W., Velasco, G., et al. (2011). *Is college worth it? College presidents, public assess value, quality, and mission of higher education.* Pew Research Center. http://pewsocialtrends.org/files/2011/05/higher-ed-report.pdf.

Theall, M. (2002). Evaluation and assessment: An institutional context. In R. M. Diamond (Ed.), *Field guide to academic leadership.* San Francisco: Jossey-Bass

Tierney, W. G. (1999). *Building the responsive campus: Creating high-performance colleges and universities.* Thousand Oaks, CA: Sage

University of North Carolina Greensboro Office of Academic Assessment. (2008). *Academic assessment FAQ.* http://assessment.uncg.edu/FAQ/

# Index

## A

AAC. *See* Augmentative and alternative communication
A-B-A-B withdrawal design, 285–286, 286*f*
Abresch, R. T., 50
ACA. *See* Patient Protection and Affordable Care Act
*Academically Adrift* (Arum and Roksa), 338, 340
Academy of Neurologic Communication Disorders and
    Sciences (ANCDS), 36, 39
    Practice Guidelines Project, 281
    systematic reviews from, 271, 272*t*
    treatment research and, 245, 258
Accelerated/Rapid-Cycle Change Approach, 231–232
Accountability in higher education, 339–341
    definition of, 339
    influences on policy makers, 339–340
    stakeholders in assessment of, 340–341
Accountable care, 142, 189
Accountable care organizations (ACOs), 86, 146, 149,
    172, 187, 192
Accreditation, 153–180
    definition of, 159
    disciplinary accreditation, 346–347
    evolution of, 166–172, 167*f*
    of hospitals, 159
    preventing medical errors and, 162–163, 168–169
    quality challenges in service delivery and, 172–175,
    174*f*
    in rehabilitation, 154–157
    standards, 317
    TJC and, 154, 159, 160–164, 161*t*, 162*t*
    transparency and, 153, 166–172
ACOs. *See* Accountable care organizations
Activities of daily living, 143
Activity
    activity limitations, 93, 109, 111*t*, 112
    types of, 93

Activity and participation
    definition of, 65
    ICF and, 48–49, 59, 64, 65, 93, 95, 253
    IRT in measuring, 48–49
Activity Measurement for Post-Acute Care (AM-PAC),
    49
Acute care hospitals, 75, 142. *See also* Hospitals
Adequate yearly progress (AYP), 117
Administration
    administrative concerns about CEA, 188–189
    administrator understanding and buy-in in,
    138–139
    district administrator's request for data, 134, 136
Administration Simplification Compliance Act, 31
Administrative outcomes, 9
Adverse events, 210, 211, 212
Advisory Commission on Consumer Protection and
    Quality in the Health Care Industry, 205
Agency for Health Care Policy and Research (AHCPR),
    16, 27, 210–211
Agency for Healthcare Research and Quality (AHRQ),
    212, 216. *See also* National Quality Measures
    Clearinghouse
Agency Patient-Related Characteristics Report, 76
AHCPR. *See* Agency for Health Care Policy and
    Research
AHRQ. *See* Agency for Healthcare Research and
    Quality
AIDET (acknowledge, introduce, duration, explanation,
    thank you), 233–234
AIMSWeb Assessment and Data Management for
    Response-to-Intervention, 126
Altman, D. G., 251
American Academy of Neurology, 18, 270
American Association for Accreditation of Ambulatory
    Surgery Facilities, Inc., 158–159

American Congress of Rehabilitation Medicine, 59, 172
*American Journal of Speech-Language Pathology*, 258–259, 261–262, 262*t*
American Occupational Therapy Association, 59
American Physical Therapy Association, 59
American Recovery and Reinvestment Act (ARRA, 2009), 40
American Society of Neurorehabilitation, 59
American Society of Physical Medicine and Rehabilitation, 59
American Speech-Language-Hearing Association (ASHA). *See also* National Outcomes Measurement System
  Ad Hoc Committee on Supervision in Speech-Language Pathology, 322
  CCC from, 155, 316, 325
  Compendium of EBP Guidelines and Systematic Reviews, 307
  Council on Academic Accreditation (CAA) and, 316–317, 344
  Council for Clinical Certification (CFCC) and, 316–319, 344
  EBP and, 36, 258, 265
  ICF and, 47, 59
  KASA and, 319, 320*t*, 325
  on MDS 3.0, 79
  during professional era, 167
  Quality Indicators for Integration of Clinical Practice and Research: Program Self Assessment, 259
  Scope of Practice for Speech-Language Pathology, 93
  on SLP caseloads, 224
  Special Interest Group 11, Administration and Supervision, 321
  Special Interest Group 11 Steering Committee, 241–242
  Task Force on Treatment Outcomes and Cost Effectiveness, 8
  on telepractice, 136
  treatment research and, 245
American Speech-Language-Hearing Foundation (ASHF), 8, 245, 258
Americans with Disabilities Act (1990), 48, 95
American Therapeutic Recreation Association, 59
AM-PAC. *See* Activity Measurement for Post-Acute Care
ANCDS. *See* Academy of Neurologic Communication Disorders and Sciences
Anderson, J. L., 322, 325
Anecdotal and qualitative data, 235–236
Angell, M. E., 253
APACHE (Acute Physiology, Age, and Chronic Health Evaluation), 7
Aphasia, 12, 63, 65
  case studies, 283–288, 288*f*, 291–294, 295*f*
  rubrics tied to treatment project for, 350, 352*t*–353*t*
  sample course objectives and assignment matrix, 351*t*
  SSEDs and, 280–281, 283–288, 288*f*, 291–294, 295*f*

Apples and oranges problem, 301
Applied behavioral analysis, 250
*Archives of Physical Medicine and Rehabilitation*, 49, 59
ARRA. *See* American Recovery and Reinvestment Act
Arum, R., 338, 340
ASHA. *See* American Speech-Language-Hearing Association
ASHA FACS. *See* Functional Assessment of Communication Skills for Adults
ASHA/N-CEP. *See* National Center on Evidence-Based Practice in Communication Disorders
ASHA Quality of Communication Life Scale, 94, 107
ASHF. *See* American Speech-Language-Hearing Foundation
Association of Rehabilitation Nurses, 59
Audbase, 234
Audit flag, 106
Augmentative and alternative communication (AAC), 163, 249, 348
AYP. *See* Adequate yearly progress

**B**
Bailey, R. L., 253
Bain, B., 63, 254, 276
Balanced Budget Act (1997), 74, 76, 78, 81, 145, 173
Ball, A., 294
Ballard, K. J., 248
Banta, T., 341, 342
*Baptist Health Care Journey to Excellence: Creating a Culture that Wows!* (Stubblefield), 220
Bar charts, 238
Barlow, D. H., 280
Barthel Index, 143
Baseline phase, 250, 283
Batavia, A. I., 12
Batcho, C. S., 48
Baylor, C. R., 44, 49, 259
Beaumont Health System of Michigan, 196, 197*f*, 197*t*, 198, 198*f*, 199*t*
Beaumont Outcome Software System© (BOSS), 8, 190–191
Beeson, P. M., 39, 293
Benchmarking, 189
  CEA in, 196, 197*f*, 197*t*, 198, 198*f*, 199*t*
Benefits Improvement and Protection Act (2000), 108, 204
Benesch, C., 177
Benninger, M. S., 15–16
Bernstein, J., 33
Berwick, D. M., 6
Best available evidence, 28, 271, 275
Big ideas in early reading, 126
Biklen, S., 256
Binger, C., 249
Bioinformatics, 29–30
Biological and physiological variables, 15
Blackboard, 30

Blackstone, Sarah, 163
Blenkarn, K., 249
Blosser, J., 129
Bode, R. K., 52
Body functions and structure, 47–48, 64–65, 93, 253
Bogdan, R., 256
Boone, B. J., 166, 168, 169, 170
BOSS. *See* Beaumont Outcome Software System©
Boston, B. O., 183–184
Bothe, A. K., 255, 257, 267
Boutsen, F., 304
Bowden, Mark, 29
Bradham, T., 52
Breeding, C., 294
Bright Outcomes, 50–51
Broca, Paul, 291
Brown, G. B., 199
Browner, W., 247
Bundling or bundled payments, 112–113, 172, 174
Burden of care, 142
Burden of Stroke Survival Scale, 94
Burton, E. C., 34
Busk, P. L., 306

**C**
CAA. *See* Council on Academic Accreditation
Camp, R. C., 230
Campbell, M., 271
Capacity qualifiers, 65
Capitation, 185
CAPS. *See* Consumers Advancing Patient Safety
*Cardiovascular Health Care Economics* (Weintraub), 184
CARE. *See* Continuity Assessment Record and Evaluation
CARF. *See* Commission on Accreditation of Rehabilitation Facilities
Carozza, L., 322–323, 332
Case-based approach, 38
Case-based reports, 39
Case-control studies, 19
Case managers, 147–148
Case-mix adjusted data, 92, 105, 108–109
Case-mix classification, 112–113
Case reports, 20, 291, 292
Case studies, aphasia, 283–288, 288f, 291–294, 295f
Cause-and-effect diagrams, 234, 236, 237f
CCC. *See* Certificate of Clinical Competence
CDC. *See* Centers for Disease Control and Prevention
CEA. *See* Cost-effectiveness analysis
Cebul, R. D., 169
Cella, D., 50, 52
Center for Medicare and Medicaid Innovation, 113
Center for Patient Safety (AHRQ), 212
Center for Rehabilitation Outcomes Research, 49
Centers for Disease Control and Prevention (CDC), 213, 215

Centers for Medicare and Medicaid Services (CMS, formerly HCFA), 74
    compliance rules for rehabilitation, 35
    CoPs and CfCs, 157–158, 158t
    deemed status and, 156, 158–159
    FCMs endorsed by, 100
    initiatives, 33, 166
    LTC payment system and, 145–147
    quality and, 207–209, 208f, 224
    validation surveys, 155–157, 159
CER. *See* Comparative effectiveness research
Certificate of Clinical Competence (CCC), 155, 316, 325
Certificate of Need, 154–155
Certification standards, 317–319
CETI. *See* Communicative Effectiveness Index
CFCC. *See* Council for Clinical Certification
CfCs. *See* Conditions for coverage
Chabon, S. S., 323, 332
Chalmers, Sir Iain, 298
Change, 224–225, 252–257
CHAP. *See* Community Health Accreditation Program
Charge efficiency, 190
Chartlinks, 35
Chart reviews, 214
Checklist for Appraising Patient/Practice Evidence, 274
Checklists, 213
Check sheets, 237, 238t
Chicago Patient Safety Workshop, 216
Child Health Outcomes Steering Committee, 85
Children's Health Insurance Program (CHIP), 85
Children's Health Insurance Program Reauthorization Act (CHIPRA, 2009), 85
Cirrin, F. M., 133, 136
Classical test theory, 43–44, 70
Classifications. *See also* International Classification of Functioning, Disability, and Health
    Nagi classifications, 13, 13f, 45
    of outcomes measurement methods, 16f, 17–20
    outcomes studies, 16t, 17–20
    WHO classifications, 11–13, 12f, 45–50, 46f
    Wilson and Cleary model, 14–15, 14f, 45, 49–50
Classroom-based service model, 136
Cleary, P. D. *See* Wilson and Cleary model
Clients, 333
    client-defined outcomes, 9
    client values and preferences, 246, 265, 268
Clinical anchor-based methods, 42
Clinical educators, 321–323
    skills and knowledge of, 322–323
Clinical efficacy, 184
Clinically derived outcomes, 9
Clinically important difference, 42
Clinical outcome data, 184–185
Clinical outcomes, as term, 316
Clinical quality measures, 33–34
Clinical writing, 332–333
Clinician expertise, 37, 265, 268

Clinician-scientist
    collaboration, 280–281, 290–294
    as term, 280
CMS. *See* Centers for Medicare and Medicaid Services
Cochrane Collaboration, 307
Code-Müller Protocols, 94
Codman, Ernest A., 4–5
Cohen, J., 305–306
Cohort studies, 19
Collaboration, 136–137, 149, 280–281, 290–294.
    *See also* Partnership outcomes
Collegiate Learning Assessment, 340
Commission on Accreditation of Rehabilitation
    Facilities (CARF), 8, 19, 154, 159, 164–166, 167
Committee on Quality of Health Care in America, 31,
    204
Committee to Design a Strategy for Quality Review
    and Assurance in Medicare, 203
Common Core Curriculum standards, 118, 119, 120,
    139
Communication Activities of Daily Living-2, 94
Communication disorders, 59–60, 93
Communication needs, 163
Communication sciences and disorders (CSD)
    higher education in, 338–357
    treatment research in, 245–246, 247, 257
Communication skills
    definition of effective communication, 215
    facilitated communication, 257
    low- and high-demand, 124
Communicative Effectiveness Index (CETI), 44, 94
Communicative participation, 49, 94–95
Communicative participation item bank, 44
Community Health Accreditation Program (CHAP),
    164
Comorbidities, 142–143, 172
Comparative effectiveness research (CER), 40
Compassion, 323
Comprehensive Integrated Inpatient Rehabilitation
    Program, 166
Computer-adapted testing (CT, CAT), 43
Computer-Assisted Interview, 51
Computerized Physician Order Entry, 32, 213
Computer Sciences Corporation (CSC), 82–83
Conditions for coverage (CfCs), 157–158
Conditions of participation (CoPs), 157–158, 158*t*
Consensus Development Process, 178
Consistency, 323
Consolidated Standards of Reporting Trial (CONSORT),
    270–271
Consumer-centric era (2000 and beyond), 40,
    170–172, 220
Consumer research, 6
Consumers Advancing Patient Safety (CAPS), 216
Consumer satisfaction, 257
Content collection, 30
Contextual factors, 93
Contingency thinking, 323

Continuity Assessment Record and Evaluation (CARE)
    tool, 42, 43, 109, 172–175
    postacute care and, 43, 147
    two converging tracks and, 173–175, 174*f*
Continuous performance improvement, 177–178
Continuous quality improvement, 225
Conversation, 235
CoPs. *See* Conditions of participation
Copy and Recall Treatment, 293
Core Competencies for Patient Safety Researchers,
    215
Core values, 343
Cost-benefit analysis
    definition of, 20, 186–187
    linking cost and benefit outcomes data, 192–195,
        193*t*, 194*t*, 195*t*
    reliance on, 92
Cost containment tactics, 168, 189–190
Cost data, 184
Cost-effectiveness analysis (CEA), 183–200
    in benchmarking, 196, 197*f*, 197*t*, 198, 198*f*, 199*t*
    caveats for, 199
    by clinician, 195–196, 196*t*
    conclusion and future directions for, 199–200
    definition of, 20, 187
    in speech-language pathology, 191–192
    uses of, 188–189
Cost-effectiveness questions, 249
Costello, J., 249
Cost per case, 185
Cost per procedure, 185
Cost *versus* charges, 185–186
Council for Aid for Education, 340
Council for Clinical Certification (CFCC), 316–319,
    325, 344
Council on Academic Accreditation (CAA), 316–317,
    344
    program outcomes, 348–349, 349*t*
Covenant Health, 171–172
Cox, R., 324–325
Cream, A., 248
*Crisis on Campus* (Taylor, M.), 338, 340
Critical Appraisal of Systematic Reviews and Meta-
    analyses, 274
Critical Appraisal of Treatment, 274
Critical paths, 21
*Crossing the Quality Chasm* (IOM), 31, 169, 180, 204
Crystal software, 35
CSC. *See* Computer Sciences Corporation
CSD. *See* Communication sciences and disorders
CSI (Computerized Severity Index), 7
CT, CAT. *See* Computer-adapted testing
Cultural coaching, 170, 220
Culture of inquiry, 341–342
Cummings, S., 247
Cumulative Index of Nursing and Allied Health
    Literature, 269
Current Procedural Terminology, 83

Customer satisfaction, 233–234
Customer value, 232

**D**
Dalvi, U., 60
Darwin, Sir Francis, 4
Data, 107. *See also specific data types*
    data-driven risk management, 31–32
    data mining, 30–31, 148
    exabyte, 25, 28, 29*f*
    security of, 29, 34
    structured and unstructured, 28–29
    validity and reliability of, 254–256
Data analysis, 101–102. *See also* Cost-benefit analysis;
        Cost-effectiveness analysis; Data collection and
        analysis; Outcomes data
    interpretation and, 255–257
    payment systems and, 105–106
Data-based research, 259
Data capture tools and support, 50–52. *See also* Data
        collection
    Web-based and phone survey tools for PROs, 50–51
    Web-based data capture and informatics support
        for translational research, 51–52
Data collection, 100–101
    mechanisms for, 189–190
    and monitoring, 234–235
Data collection and analysis
    for partnership outcomes, 127
    for program and system outcomes, 134, 135*t*
    for student outcomes, 124–126
Deemed status, 156, 158–160
Deficit Reduction Act (2005), 173, 175
DeJong, Gerben, 52, 172, 178–179
Deming, W. Edwards, 3, 5, 6, 11, 228
Deming wheel, 228
Department level assessment, 347–351
Department of Education, U.S., 130
Department of Health and Human Services (DHHS).
        *See* Health and Human Services
Dependent variables, 252–255, 282
de Riesthal, M., 39, 273, 294
Design standards, 290
Deutsch, A., 175, 179
DeVellis, R., 52
Developing Outpatient Therapy Payment Alternatives
        (DOPTA), 42, 82, 83, 92, 108–113
    activity limitation measures, 109, 111*t*, 112
    impairment measures, 109, 110*t*, 112
    participation restriction measures, 109, 112*t*
    uses for, 97
Devereaux, P. J., 37
Diagnosis-related groups (DRGs), 7, 145, 185
DIBELS. *See* Dynamic Indicators of Basic Early Literacy
        Skills
Dijkers, M., 48, 94, 96, 251
Direct and indirect costs, 185–186, 187
Disability, 12, 13

Disablement models, 45–50
Disease management risk stratification, 30–31
Disease-specific predictive models, 31
Disney Institute, 170
DMAIC (define, measure, analyze, improve, control),
        233
DNV Healthcare, 159, 163–164
Dollaghan, C., 37, 246, 274
Donabedian, Avedia, 5–6, 10
Donovan, N. J., 44
DOPTA. *See* Developing Outpatient Therapy Payment
        Alternatives
DRGs. *See* Diagnosis-related groups
Driefuss, C., 338, 339–340
Drug companies, marketing by, 171
Dynamic Indicators of Basic Early Literacy Skills
        (DIBELS), 126

**E**
Eadie, T. L., 49
EBM. *See* Evidence-based medicine
EBP. *See* Evidence-based practice
Economic era (1900–present), 166, 168–170
Education. *See* Graduate education and supervision;
        Higher education; Schools
Effectiveness, as term, 247
Effectiveness research, 27, 245–246. *See also* Treat-
        ment research
Effect sizes, 255
    meta-analysis and, 299–302, 300*f*, 304, 305
    in SSEDs, 39
Effect size statistic, 42
Efficacy
    clinical efficacy, 184
    of school service delivery, 132, 139
    as term, 247
Efficacy research, 8. *See also* Treatment research
    effectiveness research compared to, 245–246
    outcomes research *versus*, 15–16
    SSEDs in, 282
    as term, 9
    types of, 18, 27
EHRs. *See* Electronic health records
Einstein, Albert, 199
Eisenberg, John, 27
Electronic health records (EHRs)
    accessing, 34
    clinical quality measures with, 33–34
    CMS initiatives on, 33
    data privacy and, 34
    documentation audit report, 35, 35*f*
    electronic medical records (EMRs), 32–36, 332
    meaningful use and, 33–34, 175
    preventing medical errors and, 33
    speech-language pathology and, 34–36
Electronic Patient-Reported Outcomes, 51
Ellis, J. B., 254
Ellis, P. D., 302

Ellwood, Paul, 3, 4, 21
Empirical evidence, 268
Employees as new participants, 168–169
Employers
  advocacy during economic era, 169–170
  survey, 333, 334f–335f
End-results idea, 4–5
English/language arts standards, 118, 120
Environment factors, 64, 65–66, 93, 253
Epidemiological designs, 251
Episode of care
  definition of, 113
  definition of successful, 105
  fee-for-service compared to reimbursement for, 106
EuroQoL (EQ-5D), 50
Evaluation, 351
*Evidence-Based Communication Assessment and Intervention*, 37
Evidence-based medicine (EBM), 36
Evidence-based practice (EBP), 36–40, 265–277
  ASHA and, 36, 258, 265
  benefits of, 266
  challenges of, 266–268
  conclusion and future directions for, 276–277
  definition of, 27, 265, 271
  engaging in, 292
  evolving notions about, 37–39, 38f
  guidelines, 187–188
  how to make it work for you, 268–276
  interest in, 245, 306
  three critical components of, 246
*Evidence-Based Practice Brief*, 37
"Evidence-Based Practice in Communication Disorders" (ASHA), 258
Evidence-based systematic review, 133
Evidence standards, 290
Ewing, C., 249
Exclusionary criteria, 252
Experiential evidence, 268
Experimental control, 259, 270, 282
Experimental (or Class I) studies, 17, 18
Explanatory trials, 16
External evidence, 246

**F**
Facilitation, 323
Facility and staff licensure, 154–157
FACIT. *See* Functional Assessment of Chronic Illness Therapy
Faculty performance evaluations, 345–346
Fallon, K., 249
FCMs. *See* Functional Communication Measures
Federal Interagency Traumatic Brain Injury Research, 32
Federal programs, 73–87. *See also specific programs*
Fee-for-service
  as nonsustainable, 168

reimbursement for episode of care compared to, 106
  shift to VBP from, 146
Fey, M. E., 248
FIM. *See* Functional Impairment Measure; Functional Independence Measure
FIM-UDSmr™. *See* Functional Independence Measure–Uniform Data System for Medical Rehabilitation
Finan, D., 254
Financial outcomes, 9
Fineburg, H. V., 17, 22
Fishbone diagram, 236, 237f
Fisher, W. P., 34
5 Whys, 234, 236
Flow charts, 234
Focus on Therapeutic Outcomes, 51
FOCUS-PDCA model, 230
Forest plot, 299
Formative and summative assessments, 317
Fox, S., 33
Frattali, C. M., 36, 42, 45, 47–48, 59, 113
Freedom of Information Act, 7
FRGs. *See* Function-related groups
Friedman, Thomas, 52
Functional assessment, 176, 184
Functional Assessment of Chronic Illness Therapy (FACIT), 42, 50
Functional Assessment of Communication Skills for Adults (ASHA FACS), 8, 94
Functional communication, 123, 124–125
Functional Communication Measures (FCMs), 82, 98–104
  building, 99–100
  CMS endorsement of, 100
  data analysis and, 101–102
  data collection and, 100–101
  NOMS and, 82, 100, 101, 124–125
  NQF endorsement of, 100, 206, 206t
  sample, 99f
  speech-language pathology diagnosis and, 102f, 103–104, 103f, 104f
Functional Impairment Measure (FIM), 45
Functional Independence Measure (FIM™), 7–8, 79, 98, 173. *See also* WeeFIM
Functional Independence Measure–Uniform Data System for Medical Rehabilitation (FIM–UDSmr™), 190
Functional limitations, 13, 48
Functional Linguistic Communication Inventory, 94
Functional Outcome and Utilization System, 8
Functional outcomes
  definition of, 9
  ICF philosophy, 60–67
  in LTC, 141
Functional status, 15, 48
Functional Status Rating System, 143
Function-related groups (FRGs), 7

Functions, 144
Funding dictates form, 168

**G**

Ganz, Rick, 148
Gardner, G. M., 15
Garrett, K. L., 93
General health perceptions, 15
Gillam, R. B., 248
Gillam, S. L., 248
Ginsburg, P., 220
Glass, Gene V., 299
Glesne, C., 256
Goals, 225–227
Godfrey, A. B., 6
Goldberg, A. J., 169
Goldberg, S. A., 323
Golper, L., 93
Gonzalez-Rothi, L. J., 44
Google Scholar, 269
Goulding, W., 92
Government Accountability Office, 82
Grading of Recommendations Assessments, Develop-
     ment, and Evaluation (GRADE), 270
Graduate education and supervision, 315–336.
     *See also* Higher education
  accreditation standards, 317
  certification standards, 317–319
  characteristics of graduate students upon program
     completion, 355–356
  clients and, 333
  clinical educators and, 321–323
  conclusion and future directions for, 333, 336
  stakeholders in, 321–333
  student learning outcomes in speech-language
     pathology, 316–320
  students and, 324–325, 326*t*–331*t*
Grady, D., 247
Graphical tools, 236
Gray, J. A. M., 37
Grimby, G., 63–64
Grywalski, C., 15
Guba, E., 256
Guitar, B., 249
Guyatt, G. H., 37

**H**

Hacker, A., 338, 339–340
Hahn, E. A., 52
HAIs. *See* Healthcare-associated infections
Hale, S. T., 332, 336, 341
Hancock, H., 61
Hancock, M., 325
Handicap, 12
Handoffs and signouts, 213
Handwashing audits, 163
*Hardwiring Excellence* (Studer), 219, 225
Harris, Paul, 52

Harris Interactive survey, 209
Harvard Medical Practice Study, 210, 211
Hasham, Z., 249
Hayes, S. C., 280
Haynes, R. B., 37
Hays, R. D., 43
HCFA. *See* Health Care Financing Administration
Health
  continuum of measures of, 14–15
  definition of, 58
Health and Human Services (HHS), 7, 16. *See also*
     Agency for Healthcare Research and Quality;
     Centers for Medicare and Medicaid Services
  on ARRA, 40
  funding cuts in, 27
  quality "apps" development competition, 209–210
Health care, 91–114
  growth in costs of, 91, 169, 183, 223
  outcomes in, 10
  settings and levels of, 153–154
Healthcare-associated infections (HAIs), 213, 215
Healthcare Common Procedure Coding System, 83
Health care data, 32–36
Healthcare Effectiveness Data and Information Set
     (HEDIS), 75, 83–84
Health Care Financing Administration (HCFA), 7, 145,
     159. *See also* Centers for Medicare and Medicaid
     Services
Healthcare Flywheel™, 219
"Health Care Quality Transparency: If You Build It,
     Will Patients Come?" (Ginsburg and Kemper), 220
Health Equity Index, 171
Healthgrades, 218
Health insurance
  escalating cost of, 168
  pay out of pocket and reimbursement from, 159
  private insurers and P4P, 204–205
Health Outcomes Survey (HOS), 83–84
Health Plan Employer Data and Information Set
     (HEDIS), 210
Health plans, 159–160
Health-related quality of life (HRQoL), 49–50
Health service research, 247
Healthy People 2010, 95
Hedges, L., 255
HEDIS (Health Plan Employer Data and Information
     Set), 210
HEDIS (Healthcare Effectiveness Data and Information
     Set), 75, 83–84
Hegde, M., 247, 250
Heinemann, A. W., 49, 59
Hettenhausen, A., 70
HHC CAHPS. *See* Home Health Care Consumer
     Assessment of Healthcare Providers and Systems
HHS. *See* Health and Human Services
Higher education, 338–357
  accountability in, 339–341
  conclusion and future directions for, 351, 354

Higher education (*continued*)
  culture of inquiry in, 341–342
  department level assessment in, 347–351
  disciplinary accreditation in, 346–347
  institutional perspective on assessment and
    outcomes in, 342–347
  measures of performance in, 344–346
  mission statements in, 343, 343*t*, 354
  outcomes of concern in, 343, 344*f*
  reporting outcomes via metrics in, 347
  vision statements in, 343, 347, 355
*Higher Education?* (Hacker and Driefuss), 338, 339–340
Hilbert, M., 28
Histograms, 238, 239*f*
Hobden, E., 42–43
Hoben, K., 324–325
Holland, A. L., 18, 22
Holloway, R. G., 177
Home care, 161, 162*t*
Home health, 75–78
Home health agencies, 145
Home Health Agency services, 142
Home Health Care Consumer Assessment of Health-
    care Providers and Systems (HHC CAHPS), 76
Home Health Compare, 76
HOS. *See* Health Outcomes Survey
Hoshin Kanri methodology, 229, 229*f*
Hospital Compare, 166
Hospital Consumer Assessment of Healthcare
    Providers Survey, 217
Hospital Corporation of America, 230
Hospitals
  accreditation of, 159
  acute care hospitals, 75, 142
  adverse events after discharge from, 212
  discharge to LTC from, 142
  financial penalties for readmission to, 75, 142
  geographic area of, 145
  mortality rates of, 4, 7, 87
  payment systems and, 144–145, 147–148
  preventing readmission to, 212
  top compliance issues in, 161, 161*t*
  VBP and, 87
HRQoL, Health–related quality of life
Hubbard, Elbert, 227
Huber, W., 18
Hula, W., 44
Hulley, S., 247, 250
Human Genome Project, 32
Human Rights Campaign Foundation, 171

**I**

ICF. *See* International Classification of Functioning,
    Disability, and Health
ICF-CY. *See* International Classification of Functioning,
    Disability, and Health for Children and Youth
ICIDH. *See* International Classification of Impairments,
    Disabilities, and Handicaps

IEP. *See* Individualized education program
Iezzoni, L. I., 3
*If Disney Ran Your Hospital: 9½ Things You Would Do
    Differently* (Lee), 220
Impairment
  definitions of, 11, 13, 93
  measures, 12, 98, 109, 110*t*, 112
Implementation phase, 341
Implementation science, 246, 247
Improvement or sustaining phase, 341
Incident reports, 213–214
Inclusionary criteria, 252
Independent variables, 251–252, 282
Individualized education program (IEP), 119, 124
Individuals with Disabilities Education Act, 27, 119,
    123, 129–130
Infections, preventing, 163, 213, 215
Information elements, 30
Information literacy, 268
Ingersoll, B., 248
Inpatient rehabilitation facilities, 142, 145, 173
Inpatient Rehabilitation Facility-Patient Assessment
    Instrument (IRF-PAI), 79, 81*t*, 147
Institute for Healthcare Improvement, 209
Institute of Education Sciences, 246
Institute of Medicine (IOM)
  Committee on the Future of Disability in America,
    47
  *Crossing the Quality Chasm*, 31, 169, 180, 204
  definition of quality of care, 177, 224
  *To Err Is Human*, 31, 168, 202, 212
  Learning Health System Series, 113–114
Instrumental outcomes, 10
Integrated Healthcare Association, 204
Integrity, 252
Intermediate outcomes, 10
Internal clinical practice evidence, 246
International Classification for Patient Safety,
    215–216
International Classification of Functioning, Disability,
    and Health (ICF), 45, 46–50, 46*f*, 58–71, 92–97
  activity and participation and, 48–49, 59, 64, 65,
    93, 95, 253
  adopters of, 59
  ASHA and, 47, 59
  body functions and structures and, 47–48, 64–65,
    93, 253
  client-centered holistic goals of, 61–62
  communication disorders and, 59–60, 93
  conclusion and future directions for, 70–71
  contextual factors and, 93
  environment factors and, 64, 65–66, 93, 253
  functional outcomes philosophy of, 60–67
  integrating outcomes measurement across domains,
    96–97
  intervention and, 93–94
  measuring communicative participation with, 49
  measuring functional status and, 48

measuring QoL with, 49–50
outcomes and components of, 67–70
outcomes measurement and, 94–96
personal factors and, 64, 67, 93, 253
rehabilitation and, 62
severity qualifiers or rating scales with, 68–70
speech-language pathology and, 47
standardization and, 60
terminology and, 60
International Classification of Functioning, Disability, and Health for Children and Youth (ICF-CY), 58–59, 70
International Classification of Impairments, Disabilities, and Handicaps (ICIDH), 11–13, 12f, 45, 58
*International Journal of Speech-Language Pathology*, 59–60
International Organization for Standardization, 154, 170
International Society of Physical Medicine and Rehabilitation, 59
International Statistical Classification of Diseases and Related Programs, 58
Intervention, 93–94
    models for schools, 117–118
IOM. *See* Institute of Medicine
IRF-PAI. *See* Inpatient Rehabilitation Facility-Patient Assessment Instrument
IRT. *See* Item response theory
Ishikawa diagram, 236, 237f
Ishikawa Kaoru, 236
Item response theory (IRT), 43–44, 70
    in measuring activity and participation, 48–49
    PROMs and, 42
    Rasch analysis and, 43–44, 112
    in rehabilitation intervention research, 43–44
    in speech-language pathology, 44
Ivy, L., 341

**J**
Jacob, D. M., 33
Jacobson, B. H., 15
El-Jaroudi, R., 94
Jette, A. M., 48
Johnson, Wendell, 199
Joint Commission on Accreditation of Healthcare Organizations (JCAHO), 159. *See also* TJC
    Agenda for Change, 8
    on quality improvement, 19
    report on quality, 210
    on treatment efficiency, 17
Joint Commission Resources, 160
Joint Coordinating Committee on Evidence-Based Practice, 258
*Journal of Speech, Language, and Hearing Research*, 258–259, 261–262, 262t
Juran, Joseph, 229
Justice, L., 261

**K**
Kagan, A., 97
Kaiser Family Foundation survey, 209
*Kaizen* (improvement or change), 228
Kamhi, A. G., 37–38, 39
Kant, A., 60
KASA. *See* Knowledge and Skills Acquisition
Katz, L., 249
Kauffman, K., 134
Kearns, K., 39, 273, 284
Kellum, G. D., 332
Kelly, A., 177
Kemper, N. M., 220
Kendall, D. L., 44
Kendall, P., 17
Kent-Walsh, J., 249
King, D. L., 42
Knee osteoarthritis, outcome hierarchies for, 175, 176t
Knowledge and Skills Acquisition (KASA), 319, 320t, 325
Koul, R., 249
Krafcik, John, 232

**L**
Lalonde, K., 248
*Language, Speech and Hearing Services in the Schools*, 258–259, 261–262, 262t
LaPointe, L. L., 279
Lean method, 228, 229, 232, 239
Lean Six Sigma approach, 170
Leap Frog Group, 169
Least restrictive environment (LRE), 130
Lee, Fred, 220
Lee, J. S., 42–43
Lee-Wilkerson, D., 332
Length of stay (LOS), 142, 184
Lesbian, gay, bisexual, and transgendered (LGBT) population, 171
Level of Rehabilitation Scale III, 7
Levels of evidence, 270
Liberati, A., 251
Life Participation Approach to Aphasia Project Group, 93
Lincoln, N. B., 18
Lincoln, Y., 256
Lipsey, M. W., 16, 39, 251, 272, 302
Long-term care (LTC), 141–149
    conclusion and future directions for, 149
    functional outcomes in, 141
    future of outcomes in, 148–149
    hospitals discharge to, 142
    outcomes research on rehabilitation in, 143
    patterns of regulation and reimbursement in, 144–148
    review of outcomes usage in, 143–144
    setting of, 142–143
Long-term outcomes, 10
López, P., 28

LOS. *See* Length of stay
LOS efficiency, 190
Loxtercamp, David, 203
LRE. *See* Least restrictive environment
LTC. *See* Long-term care

**M**
Maag, A., 249
MacCourt, D. C., 33
Magasi, S., 49
Malcolm Baldridge National Quality Program, 154, 170
Managed care. *See also* Medicaid; Medicare Advantage (Part C)
    CEA and, 189
    during economic era, 168
    initiatives to define value, 147–148
    negotiating contracts for, 8
Managed care organizations, 147–148, 159
Management trials, 16
Manufacturing industry, 6, 177
Marshall, J., 36–37
Massof, R. W., 92
Mathematica Policy Research, Inc., 40
Matthews, D. R., 38–39
Mayo Clinic, 52
McCabe, P., 248
McCormack, J., 68
McDonald, J., 248
MCID. *See* Minimally clinically important difference
McReynolds, Leija, 8
MDS. *See* Minimum Data Set
Meaningful Use, 33–34, 175
Measure Applications Partnership, 87
Measurement development, 86–87
Medicaid, 84. *See also* Centers for Medicare and Medicaid Services
    legislation establishing, 73
    SNFs and, 142
    spending on, 223
    WeeFIM and, 125
Medical errors
    accreditation and preventing, 162–163, 168–169
    EHRs and preventing, 33
    trigger tools for, 214
    types of, 211, 212*t*
Medical evidence, 267
Medical Outcomes Study, 50
Medicare. *See also* Centers for Medicare and Medicaid Services; Physician Quality Reporting System
    assessment forms, 147
    Benefit Policy Manual, 106
    cost of, 73, 223
    legislation establishing, 73
    P4P and, 31, 147, 172, 204
*Medicare: A Strategy for Quality Assurance*, 203
Medicare, Medicaid, and SCHIP Extension Act (2007), 81

Medicare Advantage (Part C), 83–84
Medicare Improvements for Patients and Providers Act (2008), 75, 81, 205
Medicare Part A, 75–79
    acute care hospitals and, 75
    home health and, 75–78
    IRF-PAI and, 79, 81*t*
    SNFs and, 78–79, 142
Medicare Part B, 79
    PQRS and, 81, 82
    research projects, 82–83
    SNFs and, 142
    therapy caps, 81, 82, 105–106
Medicare Payment Advisory Commission (MedPAC), 74, 82, 84
Medicare Physician Fee Schedule, 78, 81
Medicare Prescription Drug, Improvement, and Modernization Act (2003), 204
Medicare Shared Savings Program, 86
Medication reconciliation, 209, 213
MediLinks, 234–235
MediServe, 35
MedisGroups, 7
Medline, 269
MedPAC. *See* Medicare Payment Advisory Commission
Mehta, S., 33
Meline, T., 134
Mendoza, D., 294
Merson, R., 36
MessageMate 40™, 294
Meta-analysis, 271–273, 272*t*, 298–310
    basic steps in, 302, 303*f*, 304
    conclusion and future directions for, 307
    criticisms of, 301–302
    definition of, 20, 251, 299
    effect sizes and, 299–302, 300*f*, 304, 305
    evaluating and interpreting results of, 304–306
    narrative review *versus*, 299–301
    single-subject research and, 306
    in speech-language pathology, 306–310
Metadata, 29–30, 34
Metz, D., 247
Michigan Keystone Intensive Care Unit Project, 215
Microsoft Excel, 234
MID. *See* Minimal important difference
Miller, B., 249
Minimal important difference (MID), 42–43, 44, 267
Minimally clinically important difference (MCID), 43
Minimally detectable difference, 42
Minimum Data Set (MDS), 78–79, 125, 145, 148
    MDS 3.0, 78–79, 80*t*
Mission statements, 343, 343*t*, 354
Modality-specific measures, 47–48
Moderator analyses, 301
Moher, D., 251
Montgomery, E. B., 276
Morales, L. S., 43
Mosteller, E., 20

*Muda* (waste or inefficiencies), 239–240
Mukundan, G., 60
Mullen, R., 79, 191, 249, 253–254
Multiple baseline designs, 286–290, 288*f*

**N**
N = 1 models, 39, 279–280
Nagi, Saad, 13
Nagi classifications, 13, 13*f*, 45
Nandurkar, A., 60
Narrative reviews, 271, 299–301
National Academies Roundtable on Evidence-Based
    Practice, 281
National Business Group on Health, 169
National CAHPS® Benchmarking Database, 217
National Center for Biotechnology Information, 269
National Center for Research Resources, 52
National Center for the Dissemination of Disability
    Research, 307
National Center for Treatment Effectiveness in
    Communication Disorders (NCTECD, N-CEP), 98
National Center on Evidence-Based Practice in Com-
    munication Disorders (ASHA/N-CEP), 36, 191, 281
National Committee for Quality Assurance (NCQA), 75,
    83, 159
National Forum on Quality Improvement in Health
    Care, 209
National Healthcare Quality Report, 210
National Institute of Disability and Rehabilitation
    Research (NIDRR), 48
National Institute on Deafness and Other Communi-
    cation Disorders, 258
National Institutes of Health (NIH), 51
    Division of Program Coordination, Planning, and
        Strategic Initiatives at, 260
    National Institute of Neurologic Disorders and
        Stroke, 32
    REDCap and, 51–52
National Integrated Accreditation for Healthcare
    Organizations, 163–164
National Outcomes Measurement System (NOMS), 8,
    48, 79, 92, 94, 97–104, 190, 191
    advantages of, 106, 144
    FCMs and, 82, 100, 101, 124–125
National Patient Safety Goals (NPSGs), 162–163,
    214–215
National Quality Forum (NQF), 49, 75
    aims and evaluation criteria of, 178–179, 205–206
    FCMs endorsed by, 100, 206, 206*t*
    measures endorsed by, 76, 82, 85, 176, 206
National Quality Measures Clearinghouse (NQMC),
    100, 206–207, 217
National Rehabilitation Hospital (NRH), 155–157,
    156*t*, 159, 169, 170, 220
National Strategy for Quality Improvement in Health
    Care (National Quality Strategy), 86
National Treatment Outcome Data Collection Project,
    191

NCQA. *See* National Committee for Quality Assurance
NCTECD, N-CEP. *See* National Center for Treatment
    Effectiveness in Communication Disorders
Nelson-Gray, R. O., 280
Neuro-Quality of Life (Neuro-QoL), 50, 51
New Freedom Initiative, 95
Newman, T., 247
NIDRR. *See* National Institute of Disability and
    Rehabilitation Research
Nightingale, Florence, 4, 5
NIH. *See* National Institutes of Health
No Child Left Behind, 27
NOMS. *See* National Outcomes Measurement System
Nonexperimental (or Class III) studies, 17, 20
Non-value-added items, 239–240
Northwestern University's Feinman School of
    Medicine, 50
Norton-Ford, J., 17
NPSGs. *See* National Patient Safety Goals
NQF. *See* National Quality Forum
NQMC. *See* National Quality Measures Clearinghouse
NRH. *See* National Rehabilitation Hospital
Ntourou, K., 39, 251, 272, 305
Number of procedures, 184–185
Nursing Home Compare, 79, 166

**O**
OASIS. *See* Outcome Assessment and Information
    Set
Obama, Barack, 32, 117, 192
OBQI. *See* Outcome-based quality improvement
OBQM. *See* Outcome-based quality management
Odds ratio, 255
OECD. *See* Organization for Economic Cooperation
    and Development
Oelschlaeger, M., 66
Olswang, L. B., 10, 18, 63, 245, 254, 276
Omnibus Survey, 183
Oral motor exercise, 94
Oregon Health and Science University, 52
Organizational behavioral management, 31
Organizational efficiencies, 223–242
    tools and resources for improving, 234–236
Organization for Economic Cooperation and Develop-
    ment (OECD), 153
Orlikoff, R., 247
OUTCOME (automated management system), 8
Outcome Assessment and Information Set (OASIS),
    76, 77*t*–78*t*, 78, 147, 173
Outcome-based quality improvement (OBQI), 76
Outcome-based quality management (OBQM), 76
Outcome measures, 177, 302
Outcomes. *See also specific outcome types*
    definition of, 5, 9–11, 60, 117, 316
    process compared to, 100, 316
    in schools, 117–118
    temporal order of, 10
    uses for, 141

Outcomes data, 20–21, 28–36
  differentiating, 184–185
  district administrator's request for data, 134, 136
  to improve programs and systems in schools,
    134–137, 135*t*
  information storage capacity and trend, 28–29, 29*f*
  linking cost and benefit, 192–195, 193*t*, 194*t*, 195*t*
  predictions about, 25
Outcomes management, 4, 5
  automated systems, 8
  definition of, 9, 21
Outcomes measurement, 3, 4
  advances in, 7–9
  classifications of, 16*f*, 17–20
  conclusion and future directions for, 52–53, 87,
    113–114
  historical perspective on, 4–9
  ICF and, 94–96
  integrating across ICF domains, 96–97
  issues and convergences in, 53*f*
  measures and methodologies for, 15–21
  multiple-attacks approach to, 20
  problems with, 9
  rehabilitation and, 7–8
  speech-language pathology and, 8–9
  systems, 190–191
  terminology for, 9–21
Outcomes research
  efficacy research *versus*, 15–16
  on rehabilitation in LTC, 143
  as term, 9, 247
Outcomes studies, 16*t*, 17–20
Outlier analysis, 186, 187
*Out of the Crisis* (Deming), 11
Overall quality of care satisfaction surveys, 41–42,
    41*f*
Overall quality of life, 15

**P**

P4P. *See* Pay-for-performance
Paired *t*-tests, 42
Palmer, R. H., 16
Palomba, C. A., 342
Pareto chart, 236–237, 238*f*
Pareto principle, 229–230, 236–237
Participant population, 302
Participation. *See also* Activity and participation
  definition of, 49, 93, 94
  measuring, 94–96
  as treatment end point, 45
Participation Objective-Participation Subjective Scale,
    107
Participation restrictions, 93
  measures, 109, 112*t*
  sources of, 95
Partnership outcomes, 122, 126–129
  data collection and analysis for, 127

  measuring efforts to collaborate, 127, 130*t*
  outcomes of collaborative speech-language
    intervention model, 127, 128*t*–129*t*
  teacher feedback survey and, 127, 129, 131*t*
Pathophysiologic rationale, 268
Patients
  care pathway for, 101
  clinical state and circumstances of, 37
  functions important to subacute, 144
  identifiers, rights and responsibilities for, 163
  patient complexity, 103–104, 104*f*
  patient factors correlated with amount of treat-
    ment, 102, 102*f*
Patient Assessment Instrument, 173
Patient-centric focus, 149
Patient Evaluation and Conference System, 7, 143
Patient-level payment limits, 112–113
Patient Protection and Affordable Care Act (PPACA,
    2010), 75, 86–87, 173, 175, 192
  passage of, 260
  patient safety and, 215
  patient satisfaction and, 216–217
  on quality, 210
Patient-reported outcome measures (PROMs), 42, 43,
    107
Patient-reported outcomes (PROs), 42–45, 50–51,
    107–108
Patient-Reported Outcomes Measurement Informa-
    tion System (PROMIS®), 51, 52
Patient safety, 210–216. *See also* Medical errors
  international focus on, 215–216
  key concepts of, 212–214
Patient Safety Indicators, 31
Patient satisfaction, 216–220
  with physicians, 217–218
  speech-language pathology and, 219
  surveys, 41–42, 41*f*, 217, 220
  typical measurements of, 218
  using data, 219
Pawson, R., 92
Pay-for-performance (P4P), 112–113
  Medicare and, 31, 147, 172, 204
  private insurers and, 204–205
  quality and, 178–180, 204
Payment systems. *See also* Bundling or bundled
    payments; Fee-for-service; Pay-for-performance;
    Value-based purchasing
  based on predictive modeling, 92, 148
  building payment mechanism, 105–106
  data analysis and, 105–106
  developing alternative, 112–113
  hospitals and, 144–145, 147–148
  LTC patterns of regulation and reimbursement,
    144–148
  pay out of pocket and reimbursement from
    insurance, 159
PBE. *See* Practice-based evidence

PDCA. *See* Plan, Do, Check, Act
PDSA. *See* Plan, Do, Study, Act
Pediatric Quality Measures Program (PQMP), 85
Percentage of data points exceeding the median, 306
Percentage of non-overlapping data, 306
Perception of difference, 69
Performance improvement, 177
Performance qualifiers, 65
Personal factors, 64, 67, 93, 253
Personal significance, 267
Peshkin, A., 256
Petersen, D. B., 248
Phillips, Sara, 164
Physician Quality Reporting Incentive (PQRI), 81, 146, 208
Physician Quality Reporting System (PQRS), 75, 81–82, 100
Physicians, patient satisfaction with, 217–218
Pimentel, J. T., 93
Plan, Do, Check, Act (PDCA), 228, 240
Plan, Do, Study, Act (PDSA), 6, 19, 228
Plan-Do-Study/Check-Act cycle, 177
Planning phase, 341
Poeck, K., 18
Pollard, R., 254
Porter, M. E., 175, 199
Post, M. W., 49
Postacute care
   bundling payments and, 113
   CARE tool and, 43, 147
   settings for, 145
Potentially Avoidable Event Report, 76
PPACA. *See* Patient Protection and Affordable Care Act
PPS. *See* Prospective Payment System
PQMP. *See* Pediatric Quality Measures Program
PQRI. *See* Physician Quality Reporting Incentive
PQRS. *See* Physician Quality Reporting System
Practice-based evidence (PBE), 27, 39–40
Practice guidelines, 28
Practitioner-reported outcome measures, 108
Predictive modeling, 30–31
   payment systems based on, 92, 148
President's Advisory Commission on Consumer Protection and Quality in the Health Care Industry, 169, 203–204
Procedural reliability or fidelity, 252
Process
   definition of, 5, 33, 177
   outcomes compared to, 100, 316
Professional era (1960–1980), 166, 167–168
Professional Services Board (PSB), 167
Program evaluation, 19
Program reviews, 345
Progress monitoring, 125–126
PROMIS®. *See* Patient-Reported Outcomes Measurement Information System
PROMs. *See* Patient-reported outcome measures

PROs. *See* Patient-reported outcomes
Prospective case reports, 292
Prospective Payment System (PPS), 78, 144–145, 168, 173, 185
Protected health information, 34
PSB. *See* Professional Services Board
PsycINFO, 306
Publication bias, 269, 301–302
Public policy, 86–87
Public reporting, 177, 205
Pull-out model for schools, 133
PULSES Profile (Physical condition, Upper limb function, Lower limb function, Sensory components, Excretory function, emotional or mental Status), 143

**Q**
QoL. *See* Quality of life
Qualitative data, 234, 235–236
Qualitative designs, 250–251
Qualitative research, 273
Quality, 203–210
   challenges in accreditation and service delivery, 172–175, 174*f*
   CMS and, 207–209, 208*f*, 224
   consumer use of data about, 209–210
   definition of, 27, 203, 205, 224
   initiatives for quality improvement, 203–204
   measuring improvement in, 210
   P4P and, 178–180, 204
   public reporting and, 177, 205
Quality/cost = value equation, 27
Quality data set, 175
Quality guidelines, 267
Quality improvement, 19, 177–178
   goals for, 225–227
   models and tools for, 228–240
Quality management, 223–242
   recommendations for, 241–242
   as term, 224
Quality measures
   clinical quality measures, 33–34
   implementation, 177–180
   for inpatient rehabilitation, 175–180
Quality of care
   assessment, 5–6
   definition of, 177, 224
Quality of Health Care in America project, 212
Quality of life (QoL), 15
   measuring, 49–50, 219
   SF-36, 42, 50, 107
   SF-36v2, 50
   as treatment end point, 45, 49–50
Quality of Life Index, 107
Quantitative research synthesis, 298
Quasi-experimental (or Class II) studies, 17, 18–20
Questionnaires, 236

**R**

Ramig, P. R., 254
Rand Health Corporation, 50, 79
Randomized-controlled trials (RCTs), 16, 18, 27, 205, 267–268
Rangasayee, R., 60
Rao, P., 40, 220
Rapid response teams, 209
Rasch analysis, 43–44, 112
Rassi, J. A., 325
Ratner, N. B., 187
RCTs. *See* Randomized-controlled trials
Reagan, Ronald, 173
Really important difference, 42
Rebitzer, J. B., 169
REDCap (Research Electronic Data Capture), 34, 51–52, 234–235
Regression analysis, 101–102
Rehabilitation
    accreditation in, 154–157
    CMS compliance rules for, 35
    ICF and, 62
    in LTC, outcomes research on, 143
    outcomes measurement and, 7–8
    quality measures for inpatient, 175–180
    rehabilitation intervention research, 43–44
Rehabilitation Institute of Chicago, 43, 49
Rehabilitation Institute of Chicago Functional Assessment Scale (RICFAS), 7, 79
Reinhardt, J. D., 63–64
Reise, S. P., 43
Renvall, K., 285
Replication, 250, 256
Report card, 192
Resar, R. K., 214
Research. *See also specific research types*
    asking good questions of, 268–269
    definition of, 15
    designs, 273, 302
    enhancing quality through, 27–28
    extracting useful information from, 273–276
    finding most helpful, 269–271
    integrating research for treatment planning, 276
    research evidence, 265, 268
Research Electronic Data Capture. *See* REDCap
Research Triangle Institute (RTI), 82, 108–113, 147
Resident Assessment Instrument–Minimum Data Set, 173
Resource Utilization Group, 78, 145
Response shift theory, 49
Response-to-intervention (RTI) strategies, 130
Restart model for schools, 117
Retrospective case reports, 292
Return on investment, 154, 184
Revenue and expenses as percent of gross domestic product, 26, 26f
Reversal designs, 284–286

RICFAS. *See* Rehabilitation Institute of Chicago Functional Assessment Scale
Richardson, J. D., 255, 257, 267
Richardson, W. S., 37
Riegelman, R. K., 44–45
Roadmap for Implementing Value Driven Healthcare in the Traditional Medicare Fee-for Service Program (CMS), 146
Roadmap for Quality Measurement in the Traditional Medicare Fee-for Service Program (CMS), 207–208
Robey, R. R., 39, 246, 248–251, 271, 291
Robin, D. A., 248
Roessner, J., 6
Rogers, M., 79
Roksa, J., 338, 340
Rolnick, Arthur, 184
Rolnick, M., 36
Rosenbek, J. C., 44, 279
Rosenberg, W. M. C., 37
Rounding technique, 233, 235
Royal College of Speech Therapists (UK), 36–37
RTI. *See* Research Triangle Institute; Response-to-intervention strategies
Rubrics, 350, 352t–353t

**S**

Sackett, D. L., 16, 37
Sampling bias, 269–270, 270f
Scale-up evaluations, 246, 247
Scatter plots, 237, 239f
Scenario review method, 134
Schiavetti, N., 247, 250
Schlosser, R. W., 37, 249
Schmitt, M. B., 261
Schools, 116–139
    administrator understanding and buy-in, 138–139
    benefits of outcomes assessment in school speech-language programs, 120–121
    conclusion and future directions for, 139
    curriculum, outcomes, and school-based SLPs, 118–119
    dropout rates for, 119–120
    intervention models for, 117–118
    outcomes data to improve programs and systems in, 134–137, 135t
    outcomes for students with disabilities, 119–120
    outcomes in, 117–118
    partnership outcomes, 122, 126–129
    program and system outcomes, 122, 129–134
    school closure model, 117
    school speech-language services outcomes, 122–134
    standardized assessment in, 119–120
    student outcomes, 122, 123–126
    training in, 137–138
School-based speech-language pathologists
    caseloads of, 224

curriculum, outcomes and, 118–119
   questions of, 116
   shifted roles and responsibilities of, 121
Schooling, T., 249, 254
School service delivery
   breaking with traditional, 136–137
   definition of, 132
   efficacy of, 132, 139
   five essential characteristics of good, 132
   options and variables for, 133–134, 135*t*
   telepractice, 136
Schultz, M. C., 291
Scientist practitioner, 280
SDCA. *See* Standardize, Do, Check, Act
Seattle Children's Hospital, 177–178
Semantic feature analysis, 94
Semantic knowledge, 30
*Seminars in Speech and Language*, 59–60
SeniorMetrix, 148
Serlin, R., 306
Service excellence, 219–220
Service-line management teams, 186
Severity
   definition of, 7
   severity measurement systems, 7
   severity qualifiers or rating scales, 68–70
   speech-language pathology diagnosis and, 103, 103*f*
Shared risk, 146, 149
Shelton, P., 218, 219
Shewhart, Walter, 228
Shewhart cycle, 228
Short-Term Alternatives for Therapy Services, 82–83
Short-term outcomes, 10
Sibelius, Kathleen, 32, 177
Sigafoos, J., 37
Simmons-Mackie, Nina, 48, 63, 97
Single-Case Experimental Design Scale, 273, 290
Single-subject experimental designs (SSEDs), 27,
      281–290
   aphasia and, 280–281, 283–288, 288*f*, 291–294,
      295*f*
   conclusion and future directions for, 294–295
   design considerations for, 282–283
   design options for, 283–290
   effect size in, 39
   in efficacy research, 282
   evaluating, 289–290, 289*f*
   experimental phases for, 283
   group designs compared to, 18, 273, 279–280, 282
Single-subject research, 39, 306
Six Sigma, 229, 232–233, 239
Skilled nursing facilities (SNFs), 78–79, 141, 142.
      *See also* Long-term care
Skills Validation Study, 317
SLOs. *See* Student learning outcomes
SLOT/SWOT (strengths, limitations/weaknesses,
      opportunities, and threats), 348
SLPs. *See* Speech-language pathologists

SMART goals (specific, measurable, attainable,
      realistic/relevant, timely), 227
Smith, K., 249
SNFs. *See* Skilled nursing facilities
SOAP (subjective data, objective data, assessment,
      and plan) notes, 332
Social comparison, 257
Social media, 170
Social outcomes, 9
Social Security Act, 158
Social validity, 257
Source Therapy Net™, 35
Spady, W. G., 117
Special education programs, 119, 121, 122, 132.
      *See also* Schools
SpeechBite™, 37
SpeechEasy, 254
Speech-language pathologists (SLPs), 42. *See also*
      Graduate education and supervision; School-
      based speech-language pathologists
Speech-language pathology
   amount of treatment, 101, 102*f*
   CEA in, 191–192
   challenges for, 267
   EHRs and, 34–36
   ICF and, 47
   IRT in, 44
   measures, 82
   meta-analysis in, 306–310
   outcomes measurement and, 8–9
   patient satisfaction and, 219
   SRs for, 36–37, 37*f*
   student learning outcomes in, 316–320
Speech-language pathology diagnosis
   FCMs and, 102*f*, 103–104, 103*f*, 104*f*
   patient complexity and, 103–104, 104*f*
   patient factors correlated with amount of treat-
      ment, 102, 102*f*
   severity and, 103, 103*f*
Spencer, T., 248
SRs. *See* Systematic reviews
SSEDs. *See* Single-subject experimental designs
Stamatis, D. H., 225
Standard error measurement, 42
Standardize, Do, Check, Act (SDCA), 228
Standardized assessment
   PROs and, 42–45, 107–108
   in schools, 119–120
Standardized mean difference, 255
Standardized regression coefficient, 255
Stiell, I. G., 42–43
Stiers, W., 94, 96
Stineman, M. G., 45, 98
Stoner, J. B., 253
Strategic planning, 342, 347–348
Strategy tip sheets, 127
Strength, 252
Structure, 5

Structure measures, 177
Stubblefield, Al, 220
Stucki, G., 63–64
Students, 324–325
    academic performance of, 123
    with disabilities, 119–120, 130
    skills and knowledge of, 324–325, 326t–331t
Student learning outcomes (SLOs), 349–350
    assessing student achievement and, 344–345
    definition of, 339
    in speech-language pathology, 316–320
Student outcomes, 122, 123–126
    data collection and analysis for, 124–126
    progress monitoring and, 125–126
Studer, Quint, 219, 225, 235
Studer Group, 170
*Studying a Study and Testing a Test* (Riegelman),
    44–45
Subjective evaluation, 257
Subjectively significant difference, 42
Survey Monkey, 50, 234
Surveys
    CMS validation survey, 155–157, 159
    employers, 333, 334f–335f
    Omnibus Survey, 183
    patient satisfaction, 41–42, 41f, 217, 220
    about quality, 209
    teacher feedback survey, 127, 129, 131t
    TJC survey, 160–161
    Web-based and phone survey tools for PROs,
        50–51
Swallowing Quality of Life Questionnaire (SWAL-QOL),
    94, 219
Symptom status, 15
Synthetic analysis, 20
Systematic reviews (SRs), 27–28, 251, 271–273
    from ANCDS, 271, 272t
    answerable and important question for, 274
    author of, 274
    definition of, 298
    items to include in, 274, 275t
    search strategies to locate studies for, 274–275
    for speech-language pathology, 36–37, 37f
    useful conclusions from, 275–276
System features, 268

**T**
Tate, R. L., 290
Tax Equity and Fiscal Responsibility Act (1982), 173
Tax Relief and Health Care Act (2006), 81, 146
Taylor, L. J., 169
Taylor, M., 338, 340
Taylor, S., 249
Teacher feedback survey, 127, 129, 131t
Teams, criteria for effective, 225
Technology assessment, 20
Teisberg, E. O., 199
Telepractice service delivery, 136

Ten-Step Benchmarking model, 230–231
Testing the test, 44–45
Tetzlaff, J., 251
Theall, M., 342
Thompson, J. P., 177
Threats, T. T., 93, 97
Tilley, N., 92
Time out, as part of Universal Protocol, 162
Timing, 323
Title I School Improvement Grant Program, 117
TJC (The Joint Commission, formerly JCAHO), 154,
    159, 160–164
    communication needs emphasis of, 163
    on goals, 226–227
    NPSGs and, 162–163, 214–215
    top compliance issues in home care, 161, 162t
    top compliance issues in hospitals, 161, 161t
*To Err Is Human* (IOM), 31, 168, 202, 212
Tonelli, M. R., 38, 268
"Top Standards Compliance Issues for the First Half of
    2010" (TJC), 161, 161t, 162t
Total quality control, 229
Tracer methodology, 161
Training, 137–138. *See also* Graduate education and
    supervision
Transformation model for schools, 118
Translational research, 27, 63, 247
    Web-based data capture and informatics support
        for, 51–52
Transparency, 180
    accreditation and, 153, 166–172
Treatment effectiveness
    definition of, 17, 246, 249
    treatment efficacy *versus*, 16–17
Treatment effects, 17
Treatment efficacy
    definition of, 246
    treatment effectiveness *versus*, 16–17
Treatment efficiency, 17
Treatment end point, 45, 49–50
Treatment phase, 250, 283
Treatment research, 245–262
    conclusion and future directions for, 259–261
    in CSD, 245–246, 247, 257
    definition of, 246
    designs for, 249–251
    five-phase model of, 248, 291
    impacts of, 257–259
    questions for, 247–249
    structure for, 246–247
Treatment studies, comparison of, 258–259, 261–262,
    262t
Triangulation, 256–257
Tsapas, A., 38–39
Turkstra, L., 276
Turnaround model for schools, 117
Tuttle, D., 177
Tweet, A. G., 230

**U**

UDSMR. *See* Uniform Data System for Medical Rehabilitation
Ultimate outcomes, 10
UnichartsTM, 35
Uniform Data System for Medical Rehabilitation (UDSMR), 7, 144, 190
Universal design instruction, 130
University of Buffalo Foundation Activities, 79
University programs, 10, 315. *See also* Graduate education and supervision; Higher education; *specific institutions*
User Test, 101

**V**

Value-added items, 239–240
Value analysis, 186–187
Value-based purchasing (VBP), 106–107, 173
 definition of, 74, 106
 fee-for-service shift to, 146
 hospitals and, 87
 implementation of, 217
 pilot test of, 178
Value equation, 27, 146
Value stream maps, 232, 234, 238–240, 240*f*
Vanderbilt University, 52, 234–235, 325
Varley, R., 324–325
VAS. *See* Visual analogue scale
VBP. *See* Value-based purchasing
Velozo, C. A., 44
Ventilator bundle, 209
Vision statements, 343, 347, 355
Visual analog scale (VAS), 42
Voice Handicap Index, 219
Voice Related Quality of Life, 219
Votruba, M. E., 169

**W**

Ware, J. E., 50
Warren, Reg, 148
Washington Quality of Life, 219

Web of Science, 269
Weed, J., 177–178
WeeFIM, 125
Weintraub, W. S., 184
Wells, G. A., 42–43
Wennberg, John, 6
Wernicke, Carl, 291
Wertz, R. T., 279
Western Aphasia Battery, 44
Westfall, J. M., 39–40
"What Is Value in Healthcare?" (Porter), 175
What matters, 41–42, 107
What Works Clearinghouse, 289
Whiteneck, G. G., 94, 96
Whiz bang effects, 257
WHO. *See* World Health Organization
Wilkerson, D. L., 187
Willmes, K., 18
Wilson, D. B., 302
Wilson, I. B., 14
Wilson and Cleary model, 14–15, 14*f*, 45, 49–50
Withdrawal designs, 284–286, 286*f*
Withdrawal phase, 250
Wolf, M. M., 257
World Health Organization (WHO). *See also* International Classification of Functioning, Disability, and Health
 classifications, 11–13, 12*f*, 45–50, 46*f*
 Disability Assessment Schedule, 59
 ICIDH, 11–13, 12*f*, 45, 58
 patient safety and, 215–216
 Quality of Life Assessment instrument, 107
 *World Report on Disability*, 70
*World Report on Disability* (WHO), 70
*Worm: The First Digital War* (Bowden), 29
Worrall, L., 68

**Y**

Yorkston, K. M., 49, 259
Young, L. M., 169
Young, M. E., 44